D1456702

# Core Pathology

## Fundamental Concepts and Principles

RB
111
.S48

# Core Pathology

## Fundamental Concepts and Principles

Chandler Smith, M.D.

241425

WITHDRAWN

THE LIBRARY
UNIVERSITY OF TENNESSEE
AT MARTIN

Medical Economics Company
Book Division
Oradell, New Jersey 07649

**Library of Congress Cataloging in Publication Data**

Smith, Chandler.
   Core Pathology.

   Includes bibliographical references and index.
   1. Pathology. I. Title. [DNLM: 1. Pathology.
QZ4 S643c]
RB111.S48      616.07      80-18504
ISBN 0-87489-239-2


Design by JoAnne Cassella

ISBN 0-87489-239-2

Medical Economics Company
Oradell, New Jersey 07649

Printed in the United States of America

Copyright © 1981 by Litton Industries, Inc.
Published by Medical Economics Company, a
**Litton** Litton division, at Oradell, N.J. 07649. All
rights reserved. None of the content of this publication may be reproduced, stored in a retrieval system,
or transmitted in any form or by any means (electron-
ic, mechanical, photocopying, recording, or otherwise)
without the prior written permission of the publisher.

To Dorothy, my grand companion, with love

Chandler

# Contents

# Foreword

The genesis of a true textbook is in the experience of its author. Knowledge and experience are cardinal values. These qualities can be transformed into a useful text if they are refined by the discipline, day after day, year after year, of teaching the subject. The obligation of knowing the material, and of knowing how to transmit it in the classroom, clears the mind of cobwebs. To know it, to teach it, to have evidence your students learned it, and to do it again next year and next year . . . that is the birth of a textbook.

Chandler Smith, M.D., has these qualities and this experience. He adds the other essential ingredients. He writes well, with a lean, spare clarity. His outstandingly clear illustrations perfectly augment his words. The student using this book will find a logical, sequential accrual of knowledge. This book is more than a primer and less than an all-out reference tome. It contains exactly what a medical student must know about pathology. It neither overkills nor underexposes.

In his teaching and in this textbook, Dr. Smith has followed his philosophy of instruction by stages. He has developed a concept of a "core" course with stepwise expansion of learning through graduated exposure and increasing clinical relevance and responsibility. The pathology curriculum of the University of Missouri—Kansas City School of Medicine has followed this same learning plan.

**E. Grey Dimond, M.D.**
Provost—Health Sciences
University of Missouri—Kansas City
Kansas City, Missouri

# Preface

*The knowledge a man can use is the only real knowledge, the only knowledge which has life and growth in it and converts itself into practical power. The rest . . . dries like raindrops off the stones.*

William Osler

A textbook is an informational resource used for the study of a subject. The book may have either of two purposes. One is to provide all the information that exists on the subject so that it becomes a comprehensive repository of information. The other purpose is to provide only the main aspects of the subject. In this case the book becomes relatively small and inexpensive. This text, though hardly diminutive in bulk, was written with the latter purpose in mind, for several reasons. First, pathology is too vast a subject to be covered in one volume or taught in a single course. This is especially true with the present tendency to curtail curricular time in the basic sciences. Nevertheless, all students of medicine need to understand a basic core of information shared by every specialty. Specialization then narrows and deepens the focus of study to the specific tissues and disease processes that are the focus of the individual specialty. Additional training and instruction are therefore important to such specialties as hematology, urology, and pediatrics, to name a few. Accordingly, pathology is best taught in two stages: an initial course that provides a core of knowledge for all students, and subsequent courses of detailed instruction that focus on particular anatomic systems or pathologic processes. This book is intended to be the basic text for the initial course.

There is, of course, no such thing as a clearly defined "core" of knowledge in pathology or any other subject. That notion is a disservice to the serious student with a lively intellectual curiosity. Furthermore,

what is too little information for one person is too much for another. The choice of what material to include and what to omit is therefore arbitrary, but nevertheless necessary for practical purposes.

At the University of Missouri—Kansas City School of Medicine, the core of information as presented in this text is sufficient for the initial course in pathology. A second course, mainly in clinical pathology, is given two years later, and weekly conferences demonstrating the gross and microscopic features of selected autopsy cases are held year round. The student is thus able to build a solid understanding of pathology around the central body of knowledge acquired in the initial course.

Most students expect to practice medicine, as opposed to devoting their careers to research or teaching. Therefore their interest lies not only in the pathologic changes of tissue reactions, but also in the ways in which those reactions are manifested clinically. For this reason the text provides accounts of the incidence, causes, and clinical manifestations of each pathologic process, as well as morphologic descriptions. Photographs further round out the descriptions of disease morphologies and enhance their relevance to clinical practice.

Pathology is not a subject to be learned entirely in one course for an entire career in medicine, but an ongoing engagement that begins with an initial course and continues with instruction suitable to the interests of the developing general physician and specialist. *Core Pathology* is designed to implement this concept of instruction.

# Acknowledgments

This book was written entirely by one author, and I am accordingly responsible for the entire text. Whatever credits accrue, however, must be shared with several others. Chief among these is my secretary, Marion Dotson, who typed every word of the manuscript more than once. Her indefatigable enthusiasm is much appreciated. The photographic department, under Fred Hissong, worked tirelessly to reproduce the photographs that embellish these pages. Thanks go also to his assistants, Bill Chisholm, Joe Martin, and Mark Scanlon, who were so capable and unfailingly cheerful about the task. The editorial and production staffs of Medical Economics Books spared no effort to produce a handsome text. Finally, to my wife, Dorothy, my heartfelt thanks for her persistent encouragement and willing allowance for the time spent on this project.

C.S.

# Publisher's notes

Chandler Smith, M.D., is Professor and Chairman of the Department of Pathology of the School of Medicine, University of Missouri at Kansas City, and the Truman Medical Center. He is a graduate of the University of Oregon School of Medicine and is certified by the American Board of Pathologic Anatomy and the American Board of Clinical Pathology.

Dr. Smith has twice received the Golden Apple award from George Washington University, is a member of Alpha Omega Alpha, and in 1978-1979 was named Outstanding Faculty Member by the student body of the University of Missouri—Kansas City School of Medicine. He is a member of several professional societies, including the American Medical Association, the American Association for the Advancement of Science, the American Association of Pathologists and Bacteriologists, the International Academy of Pathologists, the American Society for Experimental Pathology, and the Radiation Research Society.

Dr. Smith is the author of *Human Disease in Color* (Medical Economics Company, 1979) and has published more than 100 scientific papers.

Figures 13-21, 17-7, 21-3, and 22-12 were previously published in *Peery & Miller's Pathology: A Dynamic Introduction to Medicine and Surgery*, 3rd edition, 1978, and are reprinted here with permission of the publisher, Little, Brown and Company.

# Introduction

Given an understanding of anatomy and physiology, no course better prepares the student for the practice of medicine than pathology. It is pathology that relates anatomic structure to clinical manifestation. It is pathology that clarifies cause, explains mechanism, provides diagnosis, undergirds treatment, and estimates outlook. The physician cannot excel in the practice of medicine without a clear understanding of this special topic. It is thus pathology that lies at the center of medicine. Fortunately the topic is fascinating; it brings excitement to the understanding of disease. It is therefore to be given the most careful and thoughtful attention.

Pathology involves a special vocabulary whose words need to be understood and used with care. The word *disease*, for example, literally means "lacking in ease." It therefore encompasses any disturbance of the harmony between an individual and his/her environment. Disease is manifested by signs and symptoms. *Signs* are objective changes that can often be visualized and measured. Examples are swelling of the ankles, pigmentation of the skin, or a murmur of the heart. The degree of an objective change is expressed by such modifying words as *slight*, *marked*, or *pronounced*. *Symptoms*, on the other hand, are subjective. They consist of disturbances of comfort such as nausea, headache, or pain in the chest. The degree of a symptom, which is subjective, is therefore expressed by a modifier like *mild* or *severe*. Thus a headache is mild or severe but a heart murmur is slight or pronounced. A *syndrome* is a cluster of symptoms and signs that occur together and are characteristic of a particular disorder. *Pathognomonic* refers to a manifestation that is specific for a disease process. For example, a brown ring in the cornea close to the limbus is unique to Wilson's disease and is therefore pathognomonic of it. A *lesion* is a particular tissue alteration such as an ulcer of the stomach or carcinoma of the colon.

*Pathology* means the study of disease. The pathologist, however, limits his studies to the causes, mechanisms, morphology, and nature of those diseases that alter tissue structure. This excludes disorders of the mind, for which no abnormalities of tissue form are known. *Pathogenesis* is the mechanism by which a condition develops.

**Table I-1.**

## Estimated incidence of new cases of cancer in 1980

| Site | Number |
|------|--------|
| Lung | 117,000 |
| Colon-rectum | 114,000 |
| Breast | 108,900 |
| Prostate | 66,000 |
| Uterus | 54,000 |
| Bladder | 35,000 |
| Pancreas | 24,000 |
| Stomach | 23,000 |
| Leukemia | 22,200 |
| Ovary | 17,000 |

For example, erythroblastosis fetalis is the consequence of the transfer of antigens from the fetus across the placenta to the circulation of the mother. In response to this the mother produces antibodies that diffuse back across the placenta to the fetus, where they cause lysis of the fetal red cells. In this way hemolytic anemia becomes the mechanism, or pathogenesis, of the disease process.

*Etiology* is the study of cause. Staphylococci cause boils, chlamydiae cause urethritis, and viruses cause encephalitis. Atmospheric pressure changes cause nitrogen emboli, radiation burns tissue, and cold interferes with circulation. Although the topic is large, it is nevertheless proper to refer to the *cause* of a disease rather than to its etiology. The causes of all morphologic disease—i.e., disease in which tissue patterns are altered—may be classified in four main categories: biologic agents, such as bacteria, viruses, fungi, and parasites; physical agents, such as heat, cold, trauma, radi-

ation, and barometric changes; immunologic disorders; and congenital defects. Some conditions for which the cause remains unknown, such as malignant tumors, do not fall within any of these categories and, indeed, may bridge several of them. Entire chapters will be devoted to each of these etiologic categories.

*Incidence* refers to the frequency of an event in a population. For example, in the American population of 220 million, there are about 2 million deaths per year. The *mortality* rate, or incidence of death, is therefore about 890/100,000 per year. Almost half of these deaths are due to cardiovascular disorders, and approximately 20 per cent are due to malignant tumors.[1] Therefore, while immunization and antibiotics have controlled infectious disorders, heart disease, strokes, and cancer remain at the top of the list of the causes of death. The estimated incidence of malignant tumors in the American population for 1975 is given in Table I-1.[2]

*Morbidity* refers to the rate of disability from a disease process. For example, in one year Americans suffered 380 million acute illnesses, of which 200 million were respiratory infections, 55 million were nonrespiratory infections, 50 million were accidental injuries, and 20 million were disorders of the digestive system.[3] All these caused disability. To achieve an overall view, the morbidity of chronic diseases, estimated to affect 80 million Americans, must be added. These are especially important because chronic diseases such as arthritis, neurologic disorders, or mental disease often necessitate prolonged confinement. The infant mortality rate in the United States is about 15/1,000 live births, and the life expectancy is currently 69 years for males, 77 years for females.[1]

Hospital pathology has two main divisions: clinical and anatomic. *Clinical* pathology deals with the examination of body fluids, such as blood, urine, pleural fluid, ascitic fluid, joint fluid, and cerebrospinal

**Table I-2.**

## Normal weights of human organs

| Organ | Weight in gm |
|---|---|
| Heart | 250-400 |
| Lung | 300-400 |
| Liver | 1,200-1,600 |
| Pancreas | 60-120 |
| Spleen | 100-150 |
| Kidney | 140-160 |
| Adrenal | 5-7 |
| Thyroid | 25-40 |
| Prostate | 25 |
| Testis | 15 |
| Ovary | 10 |
| Brain | 1,200-1,400 |

fluid. These are processed in the service laboratories of biochemistry, hematology, urinalysis, serology, immunology, and microbiology. Thus in hospital practice the laboratories of clinical pathology provide diagnostic information as well as data that are used to monitor the progress of patients under treatment. *Anatomic* pathology deals with the examination of tissues, including autopsies, surgical specimens, and cytology smears. The *autopsy* includes a gross examination, in which the weights of organs and dimensions of lesions are registered along with a description of the shape, size, color, and consistency of the normal or abnormal structures. Normal organ weights are given in Table I-2; the student should become familiar with them. Surgical specimens are examined and reported in the same descriptive way. In addition, frozen sections are made when the surgeon needs to know the nature of a lesion during an operation. For this a small piece of tissue, or *biopsy* specimen, is frozen in a cryostat, cut on a microtome, and stained for histologic examination. Only a few minutes are required for this, so that such information as the presence or absence of malignant tumor tissue may be conveyed to the surgeon without any substantial delay in operative procedure.

Surgical specimens and autopsy tissues are also prepared for histologic examination. Representative blocks of formalin-fixed tissue are embedded in paraffin, cut on a microtome, and mounted on a glass slide. Since thin slices of tissue are virtually transparent, staining is necessary to make the tissue patterns visible. The standard stain is hematoxylin and eosin; hematoxylin imparts a blue color to nuclei, and eosin gives a red hue to cytoplasm. Special stains are used to identify various pigments or tissue components. Frequently used are the Masson stain for connective tissue (green) and muscle (yellow), the Prussian blue stain for iron (green), and the periodic acid-Schiff (PAS) stain for glycoproteins

and fungi (red). Also important are the phosphotungstic acid-hematoxylin (PTAH) stain for cross-striations in skeletal muscle (black), the mucicarmine stain for mucus (red), and the silver stain for reticulin (black). In addition, the acid-fast or Ziehl-Neelsen stain and the Gridley stain are used to identify tubercle bacilli and fungi.

Gross measurements are expressed in grams and centimeters or millimeters, but histologic examination involves magnification so that it is useful to understand the smaller units of the metric scale. A meter divided 1,000 times is a millimeter (mm), a millimeter divided 1,000 times is a micrometer or micron ($\mu$m), and a micron divided 1,000 times is a nanometer (nm). One nanometer is equal to 10 angstroms. Thus a millimeter is 1,000th of a meter, a micron is 1 millionth of a meter, and a nanometer is 1 billionth of a meter. The highest magnification of an optical microscope is about 1,200 times, and the highest resolving power is about 0.25 $\mu$m. The normal human red cell measures 7 $\mu$m in diameter, and most nuclei in human tissues measure 5 to 10 $\mu$m. Sections of tissue prepared for histologic examination measure 4 to 7 $\mu$m in thickness. The electron microscope carries magnification and resolution much further.

Educational pathology is also divided into two main divisions: general and systemic. *General* pathology includes those processes that occur anywhere in the body or affect it as a whole. Typical examples are inflammation, circulatory disturbances, and neoplasia. The first 10 chapters of this book deal with these general topics. *Systemic* pathology, on the other hand, deals with those alterations that are especially common in the various anatomic systems of the body. Chapters are thus devoted to the common pathologic processes that occur in the cardiovascular, respiratory, gastrointestinal, genitourinary, hemolymphatic, endocrine, musculoskeletal, and central nervous systems. Bringing all this information together through lectures, reading, and laboratory experiences constitutes a beginning education in pathology. It is in no sense, however, the full education; that is achieved by attendance at conferences, seminars, autopsy examinations, and constant reading. Education in pathology is a never-ending process.

## REFERENCES

1. U.S. Bureau of the Census: *Statistical Abstract of the United States: 1979* (100th ed). Washington, DC: US Government Printing Office, 1979

2. Singer RB, Levinson L: *Medical Risks*. Lexington, Mass: Heath, 1976

3. Linder FE: The health of the American people. *Sci Am* 214:21, 1966

# PART I
# General pathology

# 1

# DEGENERATION, NECROSIS, AND ACCUMULATIONS

## DEGENERATION

The structural unit for the consideration of disease is the cell. It is extremely complex and responsive to changes in its environment. The most common response, and the least important, is degeneration. There are three main kinds: cloudy swelling, steatosis, and hyalinization. The first two are reversible; the last is permanent.

All the molecular cell constituents, except protein, flow easily through the cell membrane. What the cell contains, therefore, is determined by the balance between ion transport, on the one hand, and diffusion from hydrostatic and osmotic forces, on the other. The sodium pump is located in the cell membrane and prevents sodium from accumulating within the cytoplasm. The slightest injury damages the pump, sodium enters the cell, and water follows. The cell swells, and the organ enlarges on this account to as much as one-third over its normal volume. This process is known as cloudy swelling or hydropic degeneration. Synonyms include albuminous or parenchymatous degeneration. As the mitochondria also take up water and enlarge, the cytoplasm becomes granular, as observed under the light microscope. The nucleus is unaffected. The process is most noticeable in liver, spleen, and kidneys. The functional reserve of these organs is so great, however, that no impairment is ordinarily detectable. Moreover, the causes are nonspecific and include such general disturbances as anemia, fever, infection, and

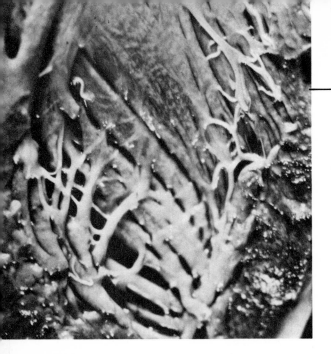

**Figure 1-1.** Fatty degeneration of endocardium of left ventricle

shock. The cellular damage is altogether reversible on elimination of the inciting cause. Cloudy swelling or hydropic degeneration is therefore a reversible cellular reaction that reflects morphologic injury but does not stand as a distinct clinicopathologic entity.

The second reaction indicating cellular damage is the accumulation of lipid within the cytoplasm, or steatosis. This term is preferable to "fatty metamorphosis," which is cumbersome, and to "fatty infiltration," which is imprecise. As nonspecific injury occurs, fine lipid droplets appear in the cytoplasm, or steatosis. This term is preferable to "fatty metamorphosis," that the nucleus is displaced to the side of the cell. This reaction occurs especially in hepatocytes in the pericentral region of the lobules, with later spread to the midzonal and periportal regions. Virtually all hepatocytes are eventually affected (see Figure 14-2). The process also occurs in the tubular cells of the kidney and in the endocardium of the heart, especially in the left ventricle. In the endocardium the surface becomes mottled so that it is said to resemble a thrush's breast (Figure 1-1). The reaction at all sites is reversible. In the liver,

however, the process may become so pronounced that the organ weighs up to 6,000 gm and presents a greasy cut surface that is pallid and tinged with yellow. While the process is still reversible, prolongation of the cause may be associated with the gradual development of cirrhosis or may result in unexpected death.[1]

Steatosis is associated with anemia, infection, diabetes, hepatotoxins such as phosphorus, intestinal disease, starvation, and nutritional impairment, especially from alcoholism. Alcohol plays a double role: It is associated with an inadequate diet and it also is a hepatotoxin.[2] Inadequate diet deprives the alcoholic of methionine, which is a precursor of choline. Choline is needed by hepatocytes for the synthesis of phospholipids. Without choline, phospholipid production is impaired, fat accumulates, and steatosis develops. The accumulating lipid evidently comes from extrahepatic sources, since a starved animal will not develop steatosis from the hepatic injury of phosphorus poisoning while a normal animal will.[3] Steatosis is therefore another reversible change, not ordinarily suppressive of measurable function, that arises from a variety of causes and denotes cellular degeneration rather than a discrete clinicopathologic entity.

The third degenerative change is hyalinization—the development of a structureless, acellular, pale pink appearance. Hyalinization takes place primarily in fibrous connective tissue. It is therefore seen in scars of the skin or in old infarcts of the heart. Cancers of the breast that stimulate much connective tissue often show extensive hyalinization. It is seen in the walls of blood vessels, as in the hyalinized plaques of aortic atherosclerosis, and in the walls of renal arterioles, especially in patients with hypertension (see Figure 15-9). The fibrosed glomeruli of chronic glomerulonephritis undergo hyalinization, as do the leaflets of the mitral valve in rheumatic disease. In the normal prostate and in the aging brain, spherules of hyalin form either as collections of degenerated cells or as deposits of inspissated secretions. At both these sites they are known as corpora amylacea because of a starchlike affinity for iodine. Nevertheless, all these deposits are proteinaceous and structureless, with loss of cellular detail. Figure 1-2 shows the appearance of a hyalinized scar of the myocardium. A most conspicuous formation of hyalin may occur over the capsule of the spleen, where it forms a thick layer resembling a sugar coat *(Zuckerguss)*. This phenomenon is mainly of unknown cause, although in some cases it is due to tuberculosis.[4] When the "sugar coating" affects the liver, spleen, and peritoneum, it is known as Concato's disease. When the pericardium is mainly affected, the condition is known as Pick's disease. Concato's disease is associated with intractable ascites; Pick's disease, with constrictive pericarditis. A photograph of the splenic involvement is shown in Figure 1-3.

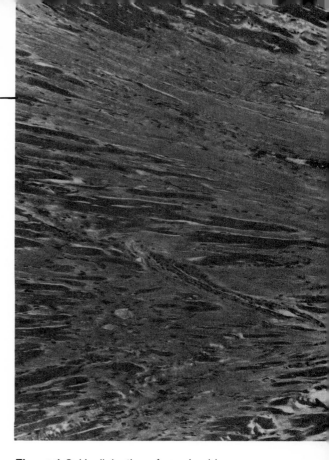

**Figure 1-2.** Hyalinization of scar in old infarct of myocardium

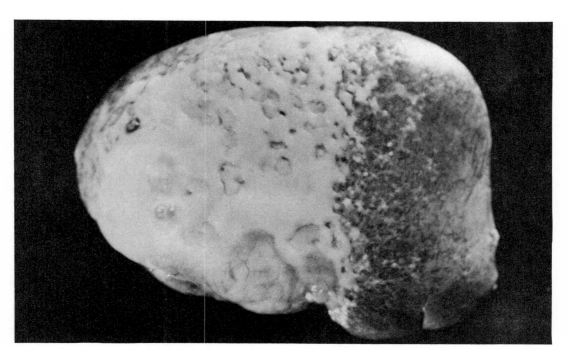

**Figure 1-3.** Hyalinization of splenic capsule

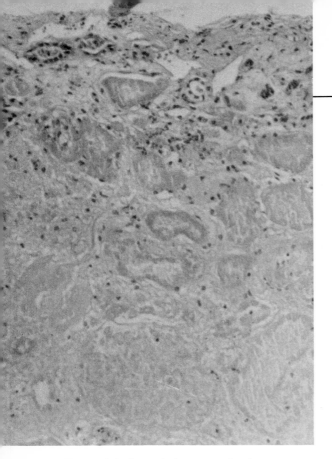

**Figure 1-4.** Coagulation necrosis of kidney

## NECROSIS

Necrosis is the term for tissue death. It occurs normally in the depletion phase of cell systems in constant renewal-depletion balance. These include many tissues, especially the intestinal mucosa, the seminiferous tubules of the testes, and the hematopoietic elements of the bone marrow. This process of normal cell loss is known as necrobiosis. When the whole body succumbs, for whatever reason, the term is somatic death. Different from both of these is the pathologic condition of focal tissue death. It is this to which the word necrosis ordinarily refers. It is, of course, irreversible. The usual cause is anoxia from arterial obstruction. Necrosis may also be due to bacterial or other exogenous toxins, to immunologic reactions, or to liberated enzymes. Depending on the cause, various different

morphologic types of necrosis are recognized: coagulative, caseous, fat, fibrinoid, and liquefactive.

When an arterial vessel is obstructed from any cause, the tissue served by that vessel becomes hypoxic or anoxic and tends to undergo necrosis. The sufficiency of the collateral vessels determines the outcome. When they are not adequate to maintain the viability of the tissue, it dies and undergoes coagulation so that the structural pattern of the tissue is not disrupted. Vascular obstruction therefore causes coagulation necrosis. The histologic lesion is shown in Figure 1-4, in which the tissue pattern is noticeably intact. Coagulation necrosis is common in the heart, spleen, kidney, and gut. It is also seen in the gumma of tertiary syphilis, although this lesion, because of the effectiveness of treatment, is now rare. The lesion, which is known as an infarct regardless of the type of necrosis, is discussed in detail in Chapter 3; the gross appearance of a renal infarct is described in Chapter 15.

Tissue infected with tubercle bacilli also dies but reveals a different kind of reaction. Instead of dying "in place," as with coagulation necrosis, it disintegrates so that all semblance of the tissue pattern is lost. Moreover, the focus discloses a dry, pale-gray cut surface having the consistency of cheese, and for this reason it is known as caseous necrosis. About the margins of the caseous reaction are epithelioid cells (large macrophages), a few lymphocytes, and occasional multinucleated giant cells. The last may be fused macrophages. The appearance is shown in Figure 1-5. Caseous necrosis is common where tubercles form, and it develops as they enlarge and coalesce. In this way cavities develop. Caseous necrosis is common in the lungs, liver, spleen, and lymph nodes.

Lipase is an enzyme that hydrolyzes triglycerides to fatty acids and glycerol. The enzyme is secreted by the glands of the pancreas and is found within fat cells as

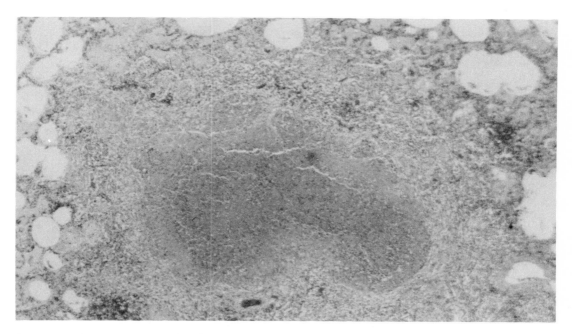

**Figure 1-5.** Caseous necrosis in tuberculosis of lung

well. When lipase is released into tissue, the glycerol is absorbed and the fatty acids combine with calcium to form a calcium soap. The process is known as saponification. At such sites a yellowish-gray, chalk-like deposit forms. Examined microscopically, the deposit consists of a focus of fat necrosis about which a variable but usually small number of leukocytes and macrophages accumulate. The appearance is unique (Figure 1-6). Eventually fibrous tissue replaces the necrotic site, or a cystlike space forms with fibrous margins that may undergo calcification. The process of fat necrosis with or without pseudocyst formation occurs in the breast, subcutaneous fat depots, mesentery, and peripancreatic adipose tissue. In the first two sites the cause is often trauma, although in some instances no cause is found. In mammary tissue the lesion is of little consequence, although it is important not to mistake it for a tumor. In the pancreas the reaction is usually subclinical, and the small "chalk deposits" found

at autopsy are of only incidental interest. In some patients, however, especially those with pancreatic disease, the lipase breaks into the substance of the pancreas so that autodigestion of that tissue and the retroperitoneal adipose tissue begins on a large scale. Proteolytic enzymes are also liberated, blood vessels are digested, and acute hemorrhagic necrosis of the pancreas and adjacent tissues results. The lipase and proteolytic enzymes also flow into the peritoneum, attacking the omentum and mesentery. At the root of this condition, which is a genuine abdominal emergency, is the process of fat necrosis. The clinical features are discussed in Chapter 14.

Fibrinoid necrosis, which is perhaps an immunologic reaction, is named for its resemblance to fibrin. The reaction occurs especially in vessel walls, and is seen most often in the arterioles of the kidney. The wall becomes thickened and separates into a fragmented eosinophilic mass that is smudgy and lacks cellular detail (Figure 1-7).

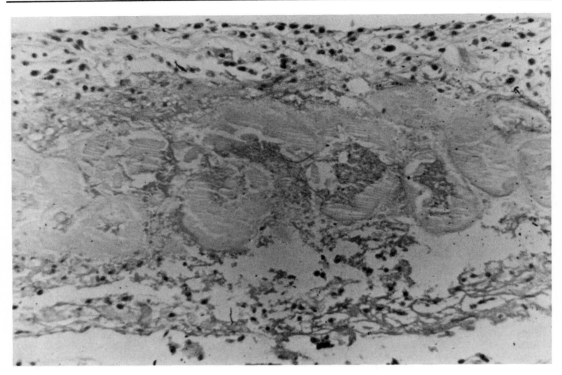

**Figure 1-6.** Fat necrosis of omentum

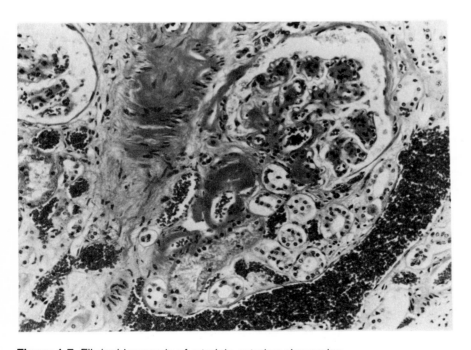

**Figure 1-7.** Fibrinoid necrosis of arteriole entering glomerulus

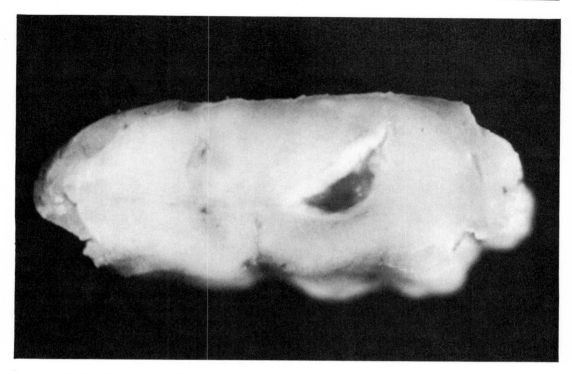

**Figure 1-8.** Liquefactive necrosis of spinal cord with cyst formation

The process tends to occur in the hyalinized arterioles of a patient with essential hypertension. The increased pressure may damage the wall, proteins may seep into it, or an immunologic reaction may initiate the process. Hemorrhage follows rupture of the wall, and the external surface reveals punctate discolorations known as flea-bitten kidney (see Chapter 15). With this necrotizing arteriolitis, the blood pressure rises abruptly to high levels and the patient suffers from both accelerated hypertension and renal failure.

The last type of necrosis is liquefactive. It occurs in tissue of the central nervous system, which is rich in proteolytic enzymes and poor in supporting stroma. As necrosis develops, the released enzymes dissolve the dead tissue so that a sterile fluid accumulates. This is then absorbed to leave a clean cyst. Cavitation of cerebral tissue is thus the result of the liquefactive process. The reaction in the spinal cord is shown in Figure 1-8.

Two other aspects of tissue death warrant description: gangrene and respirator brain death syndrome. Gangrene is necrosis complicated by infection with saprophytic bacteria. The organisms cause the dead tissue to decompose and putrefy. The tissue is wet, purple, soft, and foul-smelling. The reaction occurs in parts exposed to bacteria, such as the skin, mouth, bowel, lung, and cervix. Necrosis of a toe or foot from atherosclerotic disease in old age is not gangrene unless it has these properties. Usually the affected toe is dry, black, shriveled, and sharply demarcated from viable tissue, which is sustained by an adequate circulation. This is the reaction of ischemic necrosis rather than dry gangrene. Thus we should speak of gangrene and ischemic necrosis rather than of wet and dry types of gangrene.

Patients in congestive heart failure who are sustained on a respirator may develop whole-brain necrosis that proceeds to liquefaction of the cerebral tissue. In these instances the circulation is adequate for the viscera of the central body, such as the heart, kidneys, and liver, but inadequate for the peripheral structures, including the brain. The cerebral tissue dies, enzymes are released, and extensive liquefaction takes place. Clinically, neurologic disturbance progresses from paralysis to deepening coma. The electroencephalographic tracing goes flat. The condition is called respirator brain death syndrome.[5] Autopsy reveals a swollen brain that is soft and pale gray mottled with purplish red. The softening is so pronounced that the cerebral tissue may pour away from the skull on removal. The pathogenesis of this reaction is peripheral stasis complicated by cerebral vein thrombosis, especially of the dural sinuses. The pituitary frequently becomes necrotic as well. The arteries of the brain are uninvolved. Less often the reaction is seen in patients with congestive heart failure without the respirator, and in the brains of the newborn as well as those of the aged.

## ACCUMULATIONS

In the context of pathology, accumulation signifies a disease in which a normal or abnormal substance seeps into tissue spaces and causes pressure atrophy of the adjacent cells, or increasingly occupies the cells so that they gradually undergo deterioration. The main disorders of this kind are glycogen storage disease (see Chapter 11), lipid storage disease (see Chapter 22), amyloidosis, and calcification (see below). Many other conditions, each too infrequent to be assayed here, are congenital and are due mainly to heritable defects of lysosomes. In these disorders the normal digestive functions of the lysosomes are impaired so that undigested materials accumulate within

the cells and gradually injure them. The topic has been reviewed by Kolodny.[6]

**Amyloidosis**

Amyloidosis is an accumulation of proteinaceous material within tissue crevices and between cells that gradually causes pressure atrophy of the organs it affects. The accumulating material is structureless, pale pink, and translucent. It was discovered in the middle of the last century, when iodine was the main tissue stain; since a carbohydrate is attached to the protein, the material stains as if it were carbohydrate and therefore was named amyloid, meaning "starch." Nevertheless, it is mainly protein and is found on electron microscopy to consist of rigid, nonbranching, slender fibrils that are extremely small. Chemical analysis reveals that the building block of amyloid is the variable half of the light chain of the immunoglobulin molecule. These are produced in chronic infections by B lymphocytes and in plasma-cell tumors by plasmacytes. How the light chains of the

Table 1-1.

## Classification of amyloidosis*

Systemic amyloidosis
    With chronic infectious disease
    With plasma cell dyscrasia

Organ-limited amyloidosis
    Cardiovascular
    Respiratory
    Urinary

Focal amyloid deposits
    Islets of Langerhans in diabetes
    Thyroid gland in medullary carcinoma

*Omitted are cases of hereditary familial amyloidosis, which are systemic but extremely uncommon.

immunoglobulins are converted to the rigid fibrils of amyloid is not known. However, the disease usually occurs in association with chronic infections or with plasma-cell tumors, and the amyloid fibrils have been found to be present in macrophages. It is therefore possible to suppose that amyloidosis is a disorder of immunoglobulin synthesis and disposition. Under the stimulus of a strong antigenic load, as in chronic infection, or in the process of neoplastic transformation, as in multiple myeloma, light chains are produced in abundance by clones of B lymphocytes or plasma cells along with intact immunoglobulin molecules. It is then possible that the lysosomes of macrophages, which normally dispose of light chains by digestion, become saturated so that the process is impaired and the amyloid fibrils are formed. Although this notion is speculative, it has the virtue of giving a role in the process to those cells that are known to be affected.

There are three faults with this concept of pathogenesis. First, it does not explain deposits that are localized to a single organ and are unassociated with other disease. These are only a small proportion of the total, however, and are often subclinical as well. The second fault is that in many patients no evidence of plasma-cell neoplasia is found clinically. These were formerly regarded as examples of "primary" amyloidosis. Nevertheless, Glenner and Page stated that "most, if not all, cases of 'primary' amyloidosis result from deposition in tissues of a plasma cell product."[7] The third fault is that in many patients in whom the deposits are associated with a chronic infection, previously known as "secondary" disease, the amyloid fibrils are composed not of light chains, but of parts of a protein of unknown origin. The clinical and pathologic features of the two kinds of patients are nevertheless similar. Glenner and Page concluded that in both types of amyloidosis a similar, though not necessarily identical, immunologically related process occurs.

Overstimulation of immunoglobulin-producing cells and impaired disposal of their secretions may thus serve as a hypothetical pathogenic mechanism of the disorder.

The classification of amyloidosis may be based on the extent of the deposits rather than on the particular organs affected. This is shown in Table 1-1. In this scheme, a simplification of the scheme of Glenner and Page,[7] focal amyloid deposits are not regarded as examples of amyloidosis.

The two main forms of amyloidosis are systemic; together they accounted for 82 per cent of 236 cases reported by Kyle and Bayrd.[8] The proportion associated with infection varies in different series; the common disorders, however, are tuberculosis, osteomyelitis, rheumatoid arthritis, bronchiectasis, and leprosy. It also occurs in nearly half of paraplegics, perhaps from nonspecific infection.[9] Amyloidosis is seen in about 15 per cent of patients with multiple myeloma, and less often with heavy-chain disease or Waldenström's macroglobulinemia. In both systemic forms the same organs are affected, although predominance among them varies. In cases due to infection the cardiovascular system, lymph nodes, and gastrointestinal system, including the tongue, are affected early. In patients with myeloma early involvement is seen especially in the liver, spleen, kidneys, and adrenals. The Congo red stain is positive in all cases of amyloidosis, and under polarized light this stain gives a characteristic green birefringence.

The condition is rare under age 40, it affects men slightly more often than women, and the peak age is in the 60s. The onset is gradual, and the manifestations depend on the tissues affected as well as on the degree of involvement. The skin becomes indurated and bleeds easily, especially about the eyes. The tongue becomes large, the teeth indent it, and protrusion develops. Intestinal involvement causes diarrhea and malabsorption. The myocardial deposits, which are illustrated in Chapter

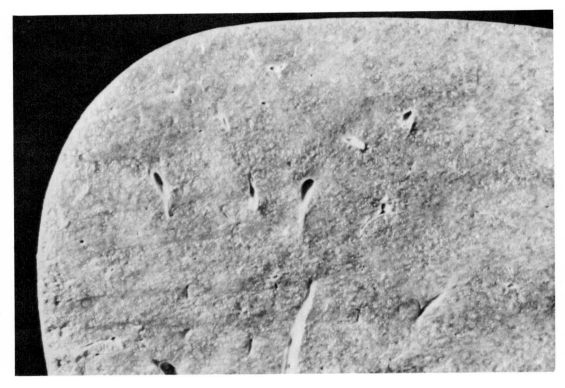

**Figure 1-9.** Cut surface of amyloid liver. The tissue is pale, waxy, and indurated.

11, produce conduction impairment, congestive failure, and low-voltage tracings on the electrocardiogram. The liver is large and palpable, although measurable hepatic dysfunction is slight. Cortical disturbance and even Addison's disease reflect involvement of the adrenals. The nephrotic syndrome (see Chapter 15) signifies renal deposition. Cardiac or renal disease eventually dominates the clinical events. Diagnosis of amyloidosis is established by biopsy of the gingivae, kidneys, or rectal mucosa. The full-blown clinical picture requires approximately one year to develop.

The effect of the intercellular deposition is to cause pressure atrophy of the parenchymal cells. As the tissue is gradually replaced with the translucent acellular deposit, the organs become large, waxy, pale, and indurated. The cut surface of an amyloid liver is shown in Figure 1-9. The material is also deposited in the walls of vessels, i.e., below the intima of capillaries and between the muscle cells of arteries. In the kidney the deposits are especially pronounced in the glomeruli (Figure 1-10). The spleen reveals a uniform indurated enlargement or a spotty deposit within the follicles, giving rise to the term sago spleen. In the intestine the vessels of the submucosa and the nerves of the wall are often involved. At no time is there inflammation about the sites of deposit; amyloid appears to be inert.

Treatment consists of removing the antigenic load when that is possible. Otherwise only supportive measures are available. Death from organ failure, usually of the heart or kidneys, takes place in about two years after the diagnosis is established.

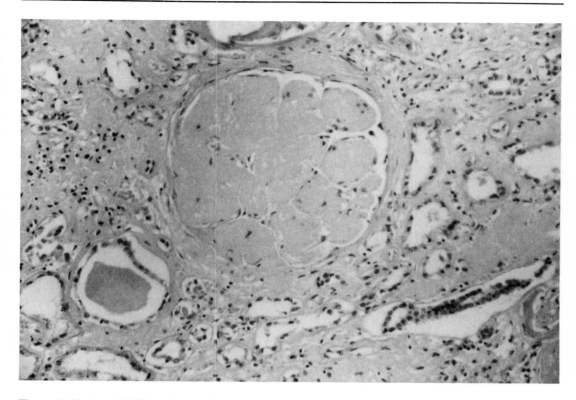

**Figure 1-10.** Amyloid filling glomerulus

## Calcification

Also falling loosely under the rubric of accumulations is the process of calcification. It occurs in two forms, dystrophic and metastatic. Dystrophic calcification refers to the accumulation of calcium in abnormal tissue. Examples include scars of the skin, old infarcts of the myocardium, atherosclerotic plaques of vessels, especially the aorta, and focal fat necrosis of the pancreas. The calcium is amorphous, intercellular, and dark purple when stained with hematoxylin and eosin. Dystrophic calcification is thus a consequence of focal tissue injury, in the nature of a deposition, that affects many tissue structures and is ordinarily not clinically evident.

Metastatic calcification, on the other hand, is the deposition of calcium in normal tissues, particularly the lungs, kidneys, and gastric mucosa. The reaction in the first two may be so pronounced as to become clinically evident, whereas the gastric mucosa usually shows only flecks of calcium as a histologic change. The pulmonary lesion is illustrated in Figure 20-13. The deposits in the kidneys may be so pronounced that the renal outlines become visible on abdominal X-ray. The process occurs when the blood calcium is high. This is caused by parathyroid adenoma or hyperplasia, widespread metastatic bone disease, excessive vitamin D intake, which increases intestinal absorption of calcium, and chronic renal disease. When renal function is suppressed, phosphorus is retained. Phosphorus and calcium have a reciprocal relationship so that, as the phosphorus rises, the serum calcium decreases. When the serum calcium is low, the parathyroids undergo hyperplasia, parathyroid hormone secretion is increased, and the calcium level tends to be restored. Thus renal disease, in a roundabout way, is a cause of demineralization of bone, hypercalcemia, and metastatic calcification.

The normal blood levels of calcium and phosphorus are 8.5 to 10.5 mg/dl and 2.5 to 4.5 mg/dl, respectively.[10] The product of the higher of these sets of numbers (10.5 × 4.5) is 47. When the product of the serum calcium and serum phosphorus values exceeds the number 75, metastatic calcification begins.[11] (The word metastatic is inappropriate in the context of a metabolic abnormality. It should be reserved for the process of malignant neoplasia. Nevertheless, the term in this context has the sanction of established usage and must be accepted as a word with two meanings.)

## REFERENCES

1. Graham RL: Sudden death and associated fatty liver. *Bull Johns Hopkins Hosp* 74:16, 1944

2. Lieber CS: Pathogenesis and early diagnosis of alcoholic liver injury. *N Engl J Med* 298:888, 1978

3. Farber E, Lombardi B, Castillo AE: The prevention by adenosine triphosphate of the fatty liver induced by ethionine. *Lab Invest* 12:873, 1963

4. Acheson RM: Tuberculous polyserositis. *Q J Med* 25:159, 1956

5. Towbin A: The respirator brain death syndrome. *Hum Pathol* 4:583, 1973

6. Kolodny EH: Lysosomal storage diseases. *N Engl J Med* 194:1217, 1976

7. Glenner GG, Page DL: Amyloid, amyloidosis, and amyloidogenesis. *Int Rev Exp Pathol* 15:1, 1976

8. Kyle RA, Bayrd ED: Amyloidosis: Review of 236 cases. *Medicine* 54:271, 1975

9. Epstein WV, Risk N: Amyloidosis—Medical staff conference, University of California, San Francisco. *West J Med* 130:354, 1979

10. Ravel R: *Clinical Laboratory Medicine*, 3rd ed, pp 500-501. Chicago: Year Book Medical Publishers, 1978

11. Smith JC, Stanton LW, Kramer NC, et al: Nodular pulmonary calcification in renal failure. Report of a case. *Am Rev Respir Dis* 100:723, 1969

# 2

# INFLAMMATION

Inflammation is the process by which the body removes, destroys, neutralizes, or in some other way obviates a toxic substance so that the form and function of the tissue may be restored as nearly as possible to normal. It is one of the most important and most frequent of all the general pathologic reactions. The causes of this process include living agents, physical effects, and immunologic disturbances. The process of inflammation is complex and dynamic; it has an onset, a course, and a resolution with or without various complications.

The clinical manifestations have long been known. They were outlined by Celsus, who recognized four main features, which he called *rubor, dolor, calor,* and *tumor*—in English, redness, pain, heat, and swelling. These clinical effects are due to five main tissue reactions that, in sequence, define the inflammatory process. These reactions are dilation of vessels, formation of edema, permeability of vessels, slowing of flow, and emigration of leukocytes. The vessels that dilate include arterioles, venules, and capillaries. The formation of edema is due to water that enters the extravascular compartment from the vessels. Permeability refers to the extravasation of protein molecules in addition to water. The decreased rate of flow in the vessels is a result of vascular permeability and increasing viscosity of the fluid remaining. The emigration of leukocytes is the response of ameboid cells to an increasing gradient of a leukotactic substance. It re-

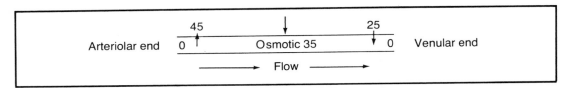

**Figure 2-1.** The factors that control fluid traffic in and out of a capillary under normal circumstances. Numbers indicate hydrostatic pressure in millimeters of mercury.

sults in the formation of the exudate. The understanding of inflammation requires a grasp of these five principal components of the process. It is to be understood that this compartmentalization is arbitrary and that the different reactions overlap.[1]

It may not be immediately apparent how such minute changes could be examined and monitored. Microscopic examination of living tissue is, of course, required. The techniques that have been developed include setting a microscope over the web of a frog's foot so that the capillaries, circulating cells, and interstitial tissues can be monitored before, during, and after a controlled injury. The same technique may be applied to the frog's tongue, pulled out and pinned to a transparent surface through which a subjacent light may provide illumination for the microscopic view. The extruded mesentery of the anesthetized rat can be examined similarly. In addition to these, a transparent membrane may be stretched across a hole punched in a rabbit's ear; as connective tissue grows in, capillaries can be observed and the events of inflammation followed. Because the device is permanent the observations may be repeated, and for this reason the ear chamber has been especially useful in following the more prolonged process of chronic granulomatous inflammation.

The capillary is the vessel that connects the arteriole to the venule. The most delicate of the blood-carrying vessels, it is composed of a single layer of flat endothelial cells with overlapping margins. The endothelial cells are enclosed within a basement membrane that is intact and reveals no evident seams.[2] Leukocytes within the capillary lumen are able to squirm between the overlapping margins of the endothelial cells and then, somehow, through the intact basement membrane to reach the extravascular tissue. A sphincter at the arteriolar end of the capillary controls the flow of blood through it. Under normal circumstances many capillaries are collapsed and represent potential vascular spaces rather than active ones. In general, fluid is given off from open capillaries. Some of this fluid is returned to the open vessels, some enters the collapsed capillaries, and some is returned to the circulation through the lymphatics.

The first component of the inflammatory reaction is hyperemia—the dilation and engorgement of vessels with blood. This begins in a slight way with constriction of small veins and dilation of venules, so that blood tends to accumulate in the latter. This reaction is transient, is accompanied by degranulation of mast cells, and is thought to be due to the release of histamine.[3] Somewhat later, the precapillary sphincters relax and the main development of hyperemia takes place. It is hyperemia that brings redness to the affected body part and raises the temperature.

The second component of the inflammatory process is edema formation. Normally water and electrolytes pass in and out of the capillaries with complete freedom. This traffic is controlled mainly by hydrostatic and osmotic factors, as revealed by Starling (Figure 2-1). The outward pushing force, or hydrostatic pressure, within the lumen gradually decreases as the blood moves from the arteriolar end to the venular end. The hydrostatic pressure at the arteriolar end, about 45 mm Hg, forces water and electrolytes out of the vessel and into the tissue. The proteins in the serum inside the vessel, however, exert an osmotic pressure of about 35 mm Hg, and this tends to pull the extravascular water back into the capillary. Thus the osmotic pressure is essentially constant while the hydrostatic pressure decreases as the venular end is approached. At the venular end the hydrostatic pressure is reduced to about 25 mm Hg. The transaction may now be understood: At the arteriolar end the hydrostatic pressure exceeds the osmotic pressure by 10 mm Hg and water is forced out of the vessel, while at the venular end the osmotic pressure exceeds the hydrostatic pressure by 10 mm Hg and the extravascular water is pulled back into the vessel. In this way the water inside the vessels bathes the extravascular tissues and returns to the intravascular compartment. What is left in the tissue from this imperfect transaction returns to the vessels through the lymphatic system.

In inflammation these values change. As the arteriole dilates, the pressure at that end rises to perhaps 50 mm Hg and decreases to only 35 mm Hg at the venular end. The transaction now is altogether different, because the net outward pressure at the arteriolar end is 15 mm Hg while the inward pull at the venular end is zero. On this account water accumulates in the tissue at the inflammatory site. This is the definition of edema. As a consequence of this accumulation of tissue fluid, lymphatic vessels open up and let some of the excess tissue fluid return to the circulation.

The third component of the inflammatory process is increased permeability of the vessel walls. Unlike water and electrolytes, which enter and leave the vessels with ease, proteins inside the vessels are not at liberty to make this crossing because the endothelium is normally not permeable to such large molecules. The largest molecule to pass through the normal vessel wall has a molecular weight of 40,000.[4] This is considerably smaller than most proteins. For instance, albumin, a relatively small protein, has a molecular weight of about 70,000. Thus the normal vessel wall discriminates among molecular sizes, a process called molecular sieving.

Increased permeability begins in the venule and spreads to the capillary.[5] As the lumen dilates, the spaces between the overlapping margins of the endothelial cells widen, and this, with the invisibly porous nature of the basement membrane, allows for escape of the larger molecules of protein into the extravascular space. As evidence of this, it is observed that in inflammation the protein content of lymph, which is normally about 2 gm/dl, rises to about twice that amount. The permeability may increase to such an extent that fibrin also passes into the tissue, where it reacts with thromboplastin and coagulates at the inflammatory site. Permeability, which relates to proteins, is thus altogether different from edema formation, which relates only to water and electrolytes in the inflammatory process.

The fourth component is slowing of the rate of flow through the capillaries and venules. While the hydrostatic pressure is increased and the lumens remain dilated, water and electrolytes continue to move from the vessels into the interstitial tissues. Some proteins also escape. As this persists, the large protein molecules and the cellular components of the blood become increasingly concentrated. Viscosity thereby increases, and the passage of blood through the lumens becomes more and more difficult. Increased permeability is generally accepted as the genesis of the reduced rate of flow.[5] The process may become so pronounced that the erythrocytes adhere to one another, stack up in columns, and display rouleaux formation. The flow of blood in some vessels may even come to a complete standstill, so that intravascular coagulation develops.

The fifth and last component of the inflammatory process is the emigration of leukocytes from the vessels into the tissues. Normally all of the cells in the vessel pass through the center of the lumen, the so-called axial stream, so that a zone of clear fluid is left at the perimeter overlying the endothelial cells. With inflammation, however, the rate of flow slows and the leukocytes move out of the central or axial stream to bump against the endothelial surfaces. The reason for this is unclear; it may be due to stickiness of the endothelium as a result of the decreased flow and relative hypoxia, or it may be due to a leukocyte-attracting substance (mediator) that diffuses from the inflammatory site into the vessel wall.[1] Whatever the explanation, leukocytes cover the endothelial surfaces of the venules first, and those of the capillaries later. The process is called pavementing or margination. After pavementing, the plastic leukocytes squirm through the gaps between the endothelial cell margins by their ameboid motion and the gaps immediately close after their passage into the tissues. The leukocytes then proceed to the site of injury, presumably because of an increasing gradient of leukocyte-attracting substance or substances collectively called leukotaxine.[3] The main observable components of inflammation are thus dilation of the vessels, formation of edema, development of permeability, slowing of the rate of flow, and emigration of leukocytes into the tissue. These components make up the beginning phase of the dynamic process.

It is one thing to observe these changes, and quite another to explain them. The central problem is to identify the chemical substances that mediate these reactions. It is evident that histamine plays a central role in the earliest phase of venular dilation. Mediation of the longer-lasting subsequent vascular changes is not so clear. Nevertheless, observation indicates that the mediating substances may be acquired, as with bacterial or other animate infections such as viruses and rickettsiae, or may come from normal tissue components, as occurs in burns or sterile traumatic injuries. The substances that may participate include histamine, serotonin, complement, the kinins, immunoglobulins, and, more recently, the prostaglandins.[6] Which of these substances, or what combination of them, mediates the inflammatory reaction is not yet understood. Nevertheless, the factors mediating vascular permeability seem to be independent and separate from those that mediate leukocytic emigration.[6] A possible mechanism is that Hageman factor (factor XII) is released from injured cells and combines with an inactive precursor substance in the blood (kallikreinogen), and the union causes kallikrein to form. Kallikrein then reacts with plasma globulins to form kinins, which are polypeptides composed of 9, 10, or 11 amino acids. Kinins are known to cause arteriolar dilation, increased vascular permeability, and margination or pavementing of the leukocytes in vessels.[3] In normal tissues kinins function as local hormones that control vessel caliber and perhaps permeability as well. Other factors that may be involved in the process include lymph node permeability factor, granulocytic substances, various components of complement, certain bacterial products, and permeability-increasing globulin.[3] It is accordingly evident that many substances may participate in the mediation of the inflammatory process, and it is a formidable undertaking to determine which and in what order they stimulate the five main components of the reaction.

The combined processes of edema, permeability of vessels, and emigration of leukocytes produce the exudate. The exudate consists of fluid, protein, and cells. It is defined by three qualities: a specific gravity over 1.015, a protein content over 3 gm/dl, and a large number of leukocytes. These properties serve to distinguish the exudate from a transudate, which is fluid that diffuses passively from vessels. A transudate has a specific gravity under 1.012, a protein content less than 3 gm/dl, and few if any leukocytes.

Five principal leukocytes are seen in exudates: neutrophils, eosinophils, lymphocytes, plasma cells, and monocytes. The neutrophilic segmented granulocytes appear first and accumulate in the largest numbers. Their function is to phagocytize bacteria, which are then destroyed by the liberation of lysosomal enzymes. Eosinophilic segmented granulocytes phagocytize antigen-antibody complexes, so that they tend to accumulate in conditions of allergy or parasitic infestation. The next cells to appear are the lymphocytes, which arrive at the locus, assimilate their antigen instructions, and begin to produce antibody. The first cells pass these instructions to their progeny, so that a clone of lymphocytes producing a specific antibody arises. Antibody is also produced later by plasma cells, which are derived from lymphocytes. The last of the exudative cells are the monocytes, which are called macrophages when in the blood and histiocytes when in tissue. The monocytes phagocytize such particulate material as bacteria, cell remnants, extravasated erythrocytes, foreign bodies, and hemosiderin particles. The cells of the exudate thus play a major role in the process of inflammation.

Although the cells are important, the protein and fluid components of the exudate have their functions too. The increased fluid serves to dilute the bacterial toxins or other noxious substances. Protein antibodies, such as opsonin, which coat bacteria and enhance phagocytosis, float to the site in the exudative fluid. The protein that escapes from vessels includes fibrin, which forms a coagulum that impedes bacterial spread. The exudative fluid leaves the tissue through the lymphatics and carries antigen to the lymph nodes, stimulating the immune response, i.e., the production of antibodies. Finally, the fluid of the exudate eases the movement of leukocytes to the locus of injury so that phagocytosis and debris removal can proceed. Although inflammation begins in complex ways, it is the exudate that is central to the process and reacts directly with the agent of injury at the inflammatory site.

Exudates have the common qualities described above, but they are defined according to their dominant component. For example, watery exudates are called serous, while fibrinous exudates are rich in this soluble protein that precipitates out of the serum. Viral infections often produce serous exudates, and the acute fibrinous exudates are commonly seen on serosal surfaces. Fibrin is a mesh of friable, elastic, pale yellow strands that forms a fuzzy mat on serosal surfaces and represents one of the first grossly evident features of acute exudative inflammation. Purulent exudates are characterized by accumulation of a thick, slightly viscid, turbid, pale yellow fluid, or pus. It is common in the peritoneum; combinations of fluid, leukocytes, and fibrin may produce thick puddles of pus that lie in the gullies and recesses of the peritoneal cavity. Such exudates often contain large numbers of bacteria. Hemorrhagic exudates are due to massive extravasation of red cells into such tissues as lung and gut; hemorrhagic pneumonia is a frequent reaction when this process occurs in the lung. Red cells enter the exudate passively by increased hydrostatic pressure, a process called diapedesis.

There are also combination exudates, e.g., fibrinopurulent or fibrinohemorrhagic, and exudates may progress through different stages, e.g., serous to fibrinous to suppurative. In addition, there are differences in distribution, e.g., focal or diffuse. Thus, in the peritoneum a ruptured appendix often produces a focal acute suppurative exudate, whereas a perforated gastric ulcer may produce an acute diffuse fibrino-purulent peritonitis. Acute fibrinous appendicitis is illustrated in Chapter 13.

Inflammation is a dynamic process. After it begins and the exudate forms, the process either resolves or goes on to some complication. The most common result is resolution. The hyperemia subsides, the sluggish flow quickens, the increased tissue fluid re-enters the capillaries or passes out through the lymphatics, the leukocytes degenerate, the fibrin is digested, and the macrophages carry away the debris. Finally, as the flow gradually resumes, the site of injury with its surrounding inflammation is restored to normal. A good minor example of resolution is the gradual disappearance of a pimple over several days. Resolution is not limited to such trivial events, however. A good major example is lobar pneumonia, in which an entire pulmonary lobe is the seat of massive inflammation with segmented granulocytes uniformly filling every alveolus. Still resolution takes place, the exudate clears, and the delicate alveolar walls are left intact. It is only in the event of complication that the process of resolution does not succeed.

The first complication is tissue breakdown. When the injurious agent persists, the inflammatory process continues and leukocytes emigrate to the site of injury without letup. As the exudate accumulates, pus forms, and tissue breakdown begins. Abscess or ulceration is the result. An abscess is a defect in solid tissue with an inflammatory margin. Abscesses are common in the lung, brain, kidney, and, less often, in the spleen, liver, and bone marrow (Figure 2-2). Subcutaneous tissue is also a frequent site, as illustrated singly by boils and, in multilocular form, by carbuncles. The abscess may continue to harbor the noxious agent, e.g., bacteria, parasite, or foreign body, which may eventually spread from the original locus to other parts of the body. Abscesses eventually heal. Because they heal by massive fibro-sis, a noticeable scar is ordinarily left.

An ulcer is altogether different; it is a defect of a surface with an inflammatory base. Externally ulcers are common over the lower legs because of impaired circulation, i.e., stasis ulcers; internally ulcers are frequent in the distal portion of the stomach and the first part of the duodenum. Ulcers tend to penetrate, and in the duodenum erosion into an artery with serious hemorrhage is common. In both the stomach and duodenum, penetration may carry the ulceration through the entire wall so that perforation follows and acute suppurative peritonitis forms. If the transmural penetration is slow, the peritoneal surface tends to bind to some adjacent structure so as to seal itself off against perforation. If the penetrating process continues, however, fistulae form so that inflammatory channels open up from one segment of gut to another (ileocolic), or from gut to urinary bladder (ileovesical), or from gut to skin (ileoabdominal). Such events are frequent in regional enteritis, which tends to cause penetrating ulcers and thus differs from chronic ulcerative colitis, which tends to remain a superficial inflammation. If these events do not take place, the ulcer gradually heals by the formation of dense fibrous connective tissue that leaves a scar and disfigures the surface. In the case of burns, for example, contraction deformities are frequent, and in the case of the gastric ulcer, pyloric stenosis may result from scar tissue of the healing process. The cut surface of a gastric ulcer with massive fibrosis of the base is shown in Figure 2-3.

The second complication is that the inflammation simply becomes chronic. The neutrophils leave and are replaced by lymphocytes. Plasma cells enter the region and macrophages follow. As the low-grade inflammation continues, granulation tissue gradually forms and, with maturation, a transition to mature fibrous connective tissue takes place. Eventually a scar develops and the structure becomes distorted. With

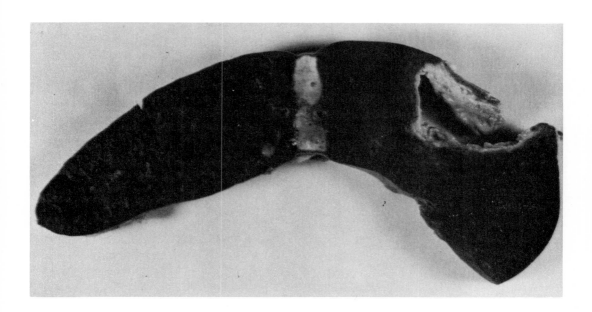

**Figure 2-2.** Abscess of spleen

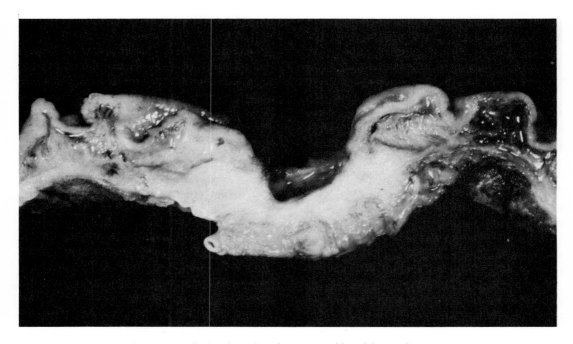

**Figure 2-3.** Section of gastric wall showing ulcer in center with subjacent layer of thick fibrous scar

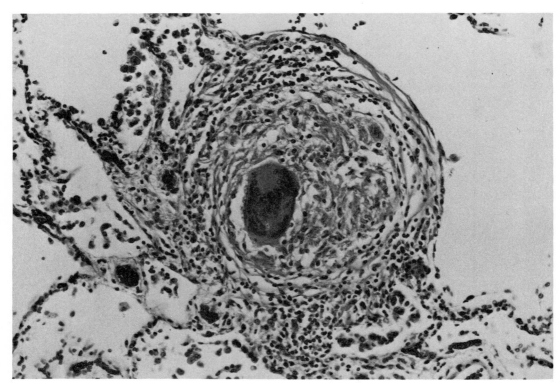

**Figure 2-4.** Hard tubercle with multinucleated giant cell, cluster of epithelioid cells, and peripheral rim of lymphocytes

distortion, function may become impaired. This is especially evident in chronic rheumatic heart disease, in which the thin, soft mitral leaflets become converted to thick, rigid, immovable ledges that obstruct the flow of blood. It is also characteristic of the bowel, which becomes thick, indurated, and stenosed in regional enteritis, and in the gallbladder, in which the wall is gradually converted to a firm, thick, pale gray casement after prolonged cholecystitis.

It is thus evident that exudative inflammation may be acute or chronic, and it may undergo resolution or progress to a complication such as abscess formation, ulceration, fistula formation, penetration of an artery with hemorrhage, penetration of a viscus with perforation, or the gradual formation of scar tissue that distorts the structure and may impair its function.

In contrast to exudative inflammation of any duration stands granulomatous inflammation, which is always chronic. The hallmark of chronic granulomatous inflammation is macrophages, which tend to form in clusters and give rise to multinucleated giant cells. The tubercle of pulmonary tuberculosis is the best example. The acid-fast organisms lodge in the pulmonary tissue of a sensitized host. At that site plump macrophages accumulate. Soon these merge, or nuclei undergo division within a nondividing cytoplasm, so that a multinucleated cell forms. At the periphery of this cluster of macrophages, now referred to as epithelioid cells, a collar of lymphocytes appears. This is the hard tubercle (Figure 2-4). As time passes, the center of the tubercle breaks down and the tissue becomes "emulsified" at this site—a process called

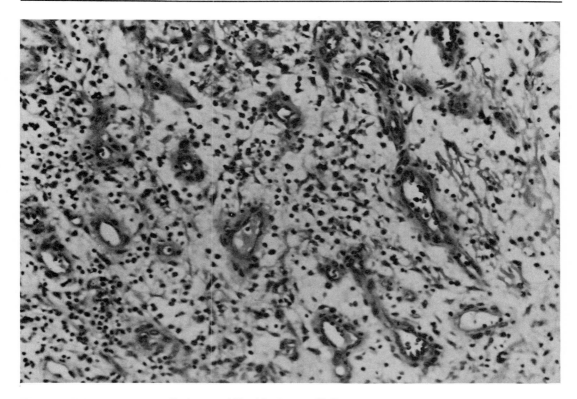

**Figure 2-5.** Leukocytes, capillaries, and fibroblasts constituting granulation tissue

caseation necrosis. At the periphery of the tubercle fibroblasts form, and from this point onward it is a contest between the virulence of the organisms, which tend to extend the necrosis, and the strength of the fibroblasts, which tend to seal off the process and limit its spread. The result is either a quiescent fibrous scar or expanding foci of necrosis that fuse and enlarge to produce cavity formation. Thus tuberculosis exemplifies the process of chronic granulomatous inflammation.

Although multinucleated giant cells identify chronic granulomatous inflammation, they are not always present. In typhoid fever, for example, the inflammatory reaction is almost entirely macrophagic, and clusters of such cells, especially in the liver, constitute the characteristic typhoid nodule. In almost all other examples, however,

multinucleated giant cells regularly form. In the gumma of tertiary syphilis they are almost always seen, and in fungal infections, such as coccidioidomycosis, multinucleated cells are common. In sarcoidosis they are again a hallmark of the disease, although the cause of this peculiar inflammation is not known.

The causative agent in chronic granulomatous inflammations does not have to be animate; multinucleated cells are a consistent feature of the inflammation that surrounds foreign bodies left in tissues. Silica particles, asbestos fibers, beryllium dust, talc granules, and suture remnants all evoke a chronic granulomatous inflammation, often with the foreign material embedded in the cytoplasm of the phagocytic giant cell. The consequence of this inflammation depends on the host-organism interaction; with subsidence, fibrosis forms in abundance, and with advancing activity, tissue destruction continues. Both processes occur in tuberculosis.

The resolution of inflammation implies healing. The process of healing depends somewhat on the nature of the wound. If the wound is clean, i.e., uncontaminated with bacteria or foreign material, and if the sides of the wound can be apposed, healing is prompt. This is called healing by first intention. If the wound is contaminated or the lesion gapes so that the sides cannot be apposed, the healing process is delayed. This is called healing by second intention.

A cut with a clean knife may heal by first intention. The sides of the incision are apposed and a blood clot seals the margins. Small numbers of neutrophilic leukocytes migrate to the wound margins in the first 24 hours. Epidermal cells proliferate and cover the surface defect. Along the sides of the wound granulation tissue forms, and endothelial sprouts develop by the third day (Figure 2-5). These extend into the blood clot and begin to bridge the sides of the defect. On the fourth and fifth days, fibroblasts emerge from mesenchymal cells in the region and produce reticulin fibers that transform into bridging collagen bundles within a week's time. By two weeks after injury the tensile strength of the tissue is nearly normal, and on the external surface the scar, which is pink and slightly raised, can be seen to be forming. Over subsequent days the scar gradually becomes flat, the pinkness disappears, and the wound is completely healed.

In contrast, healing by secondary intention is characteristic of wounds that are contaminated and have tissue destruction with nonapposable sides. Suppose that in an auto accident a chunk of flesh is torn away from the victim's buttock and particles of dirt are embedded in the wound. Bacteria are present in the tissue, of course, and the sides cannot be brought together because of the size of the defect.

Although debridement is carried out, inflammation is pronounced and a purulent exudate forms. Granulation tissue follows, and it forms abundantly because that is the only way to fill the defect. It is not until the defect is filled that the surface can be covered by epithelial cells, which grow in from the margins. The granulation tissue matures to a firm scar, which then contracts and may leave an inflexible deformity. Thus healing by second intention is prolonged and complicated by infection and scar tissue formation. Healing by first intention, then, is clean and prompt without deformity, and healing by second intention is dirty and delayed with deformity.

It should not be supposed from the foregoing discussion that the type of wound is the only factor that determines the promptness and quality of the healing process. Healing is impaired by several factors. Bacterial contamination is the first; staphylococci and streptococci are common, and their numbers and virulence have an effect on the reaction. An adequate blood supply is, of course, necessary. Low plasma proteins have a bearing on the rate of fibrous connective tissue formation, as does vitamin C, which is necessary to the process. All these factors determine the success or failure of the reaction by which inflammation subsides and wounds heal.

### REFERENCES

1. Spector WG, Willoughby DA: The inflammatory response. *Bacteriol Rev* 27:117, 1963
2. Wright GP, Symmers WC: *Systemic Pathology*, vol 1. New York: American Elsevier, 1966
3. Hersh EM, Bodey GP: Leukocytic mechanisms in inflammation. *Annu Rev Med* 21:105, 1970
4. Karnovsky MJ: The ultrastructural basis of capillary permeability studied with peroxidase as a tracer. *J Cell Biol* 35:213, 1967
5. Cotran RS, Remensnyder JP: The structural basis of increased vascular permeability after graded thermal injury—Light and electron microscopic studies. *Ann NY Acad Sci* 150:495, 1968
6. Ward P: The inflammatory mediators. *Ann NY Acad Sci* 221:290, 1974

# 3

# CIRCULATORY DISTURBANCES

Derangements of the circulation are among the most important and the most frequent of the general pathologic reactions. They include such conditions as edema, hyperemia, hemorrhage, thrombosis, embolism, infarction, and shock. Before proceeding, a review of normal circulation and the factors of fluid balance is appropriate.

About 70 per cent of the body weight consists of fluid. Body fluid is apportioned into three compartments: Approximately 72 per cent is intracellular, 21 per cent is interstitial, and 7 per cent is intravascular. The intracellular fluid is bounded by the cell membranes, and it is rich in potassium and protein. The intravascular fluid is bounded by the endothelial cells of the various vessels and is rich in sodium and protein. Between these two compartments is the interstitial fluid, which is protein-poor; it is in equilibrium with each of the other compartments and can move into the cells, in response to dehydration, or into the vascular compartment, in response to sudden fluid loss, as in hemorrhage. This is possible because the vascular endothelium and cell membranes are freely permeable to water and electrolytes, which compose the interstitial fluid, but are impermeable to the passage of protein. Because the circulatory system is closed, the fluid that leaks from the vessels or cells into the interstitial compartment drains out of the tissues through the lymphatics that converge to form the thoracic duct, which empties into the left subclavian vein.

The normal blood volume is about 5 liters; of this, approximately 3 liters are fluid and 2 liters are cells. The blood volume is dependent on certain organs, especially the lungs, skin, gut, and kidneys. Water is taken into the body by drinking and is released from the body by excretion. Excretion takes place from several sites. From the lungs 300 to 600 ml are lost daily as vapor in the breath. About the same amount emerges onto the skin and evaporates from it. About 100 ml are passed in the stool each day. The largest amount is excreted from the kidneys: normally 1,200 to 1,800 ml daily. These figures mean that the total fluid transaction of the body is approximately 2,500 ml/day.

While the kidneys excrete 1,200 to 1,800 ml of urine daily, they also produce about 182 liters of fluid each day by glomerular filtration. The difference between what is formed each day by glomerular filtration and what is excreted each day as urine is reabsorbed by the tubules. When dehydration develops, thirst follows and the hyperosmolarity of the blood stimulates the pituitary to produce antidiuretic hormone. Thirst encourages drinking, and antidiuretic hormone signals the renal tubules to reabsorb more water. Since the renal traffic in water is large, this mechanism is effective in counteracting dehydration. When hypervolemia arises, less tubular reabsorption occurs and more fluid is excreted in the urine. The kidney is therefore the main organ of fluid balance.

Fluid balance is also affected by the capillaries, which are the most delicate of the vessels of the circulatory system. The main factors are the osmotic and hydrostatic pressures. Hydrostatic pressure tends to push fluid out of the vessels into the interstitial compartment, while osmotic pressure tends to pull that fluid back into the vessels (see Figure 2-1). The two factors are normally in balance.

Even with these mechanisms, however, disturbances of blood volume occur. Blood volume is increased in heart failure, renal failure, and polycythemia. On the other hand, blood volume is decreased by conditions that cause fluid loss: internal and external hemorrhage, vomiting, diarrhea, excessive perspiration, and burns with plasma leakage over extensive surfaces.

## EDEMA

Edema is the presence of excessive fluid in the tissues. There are four main causes: high hydrostatic pressure, which forces fluid out of the vessels; low osmotic pressure, which fails to draw that fluid back into the vessels; endothelial injury, which increases the permeability of the capillaries; and lymph obstruction, which prevents normal return of interstitial fluid to the venous system.

Edema may be diffuse. Mechanisms include cirrhosis with insufficient production of serum protein, so that osmotic pressure is low in capillaries; renal disease with excretion of protein in the urine, giving the same effect; and failure to ingest sufficient protein, as in war, famine, or the African protein starvation disease kwashiorkor. In this connection it is useful to know that edema develops when the total serum protein falls to less than 4 gm/dl (normal, 6 to 8 gm/dl) or the serum albumin falls to less than 2.5 gm/dl (normal, 3 to 5 gm/dl). In congestive heart failure the hydrostatic pressure—i.e., the venous pressure at the level of the right atrium—rises from a normal value of 3 mm Hg to a value as high as 20 mm Hg. The edema of heart failure is usually dependent, being most pronounced over the ankles and lower legs when the patient is upright, and over the back and sacrum when the patient is supine. In contrast, the edema of renal disease affects the whole body and is also clinically evident over the face, especially around the eyes.

The organs grossly revealing increased tissue fluid are the brain and lungs. Both are increased in weight. In addition, the brain reveals flattening of the gyri, narrowing of the sulci, and grooving of the cerebellar tonsils as that structure is pushed downward into the rigid aperture of the foramen magnum. As the medulla is compressed, headache, seizures, coma, and death may follow. The pulmonary tissue becomes wet and, as fluid accumulates in the air sacs, gaseous diffusion is impaired. Dyspnea develops, rales may be heard, and effusion in pleural spaces may form. Hypostatic pneumonia is frequent if the edema persists.

Edema may also be localized. A thrombus obstructing a vein, blockage of lymph channels by metastatic carcinoma, a bandage too tight, a cast too constricting, a pregnancy compressing pelvic veins, or venous dilation that keeps valves from maintaining a unidirectional flow are all causes of localized edema. Accumulations of fluid in the peritoneum (ascites), the pleural spaces (hydrothorax), or the pericardium (pericardial effusion) tend to be transudates and, though not precisely edema, are nevertheless examples of excessive fluid between the tissues if not within them. There are also uncommon causes of localized edema, such as filariasis, which blocks the lymphatics (especially of the scrotum), Milroy's congenital obstruction of lymphatics, which usually affects the lower extremities, and the immune disturbances of capillary permeability that are seen with hives and angioneurotic edema.

## HYPEREMIA

Hyperemia is engorgement of vessels with blood. Since the word specifies blood, it is preferable to "congestion," which does not necessarily refer to blood. Hyperemia may be active, as in inflammation, exercise, and blushing, or passive, as in congestive heart failure or localized venous obstruction. When the left ventricle fails, the chamber empties incompletely and the unejected blood accumulates with each systolic

thrust. If an extra 1 ml of blood is left in the ventricle with each beat, and if the heart rate is 72 beats/minute, then 72 ml/minute, or over 4 liters/hour, of extra fluid must be accommodated within the circulation. Since this accumulation develops within the left ventricle, that chamber dilates, the mitral ring stretches, and a residue of blood begins to fill and dilate the left atrium. From there the pressure backs into the pulmonary veins and thence into the capillaries of the lungs. Hyperemia develops, the increased hydrostatic pressure forces fluid into the alveolar spaces, and dyspnea with frothy sputum arises along with the physical sign of rales. Diapedesis carries red cells from the hyperemic capillaries into the alveolar air sacs. Macrophages engulf the red cells, disassemble the hemoglobin into its constituents, and convert the heme into a brown granular pigment called hemosiderin. As dyspnea increases, the patient coughs, and the sputum looks rusty because of the pigmented macrophages it contains. Chronic passive hyperemia of the lungs with pulmonary edema thus characterizes left heart failure.

Without treatment the process continues on its backward course. The pressure is transmitted to the pulmonary conus, which causes a bulge in the X-ray silhouette of the heart, and to the right ventricle, which dilates and undergoes compensatory thickening. This is followed by stretching of the tricuspid ring, dilation of the right atrium, and transfer of increased pressure to the caval veins. That pressure is felt by the hepatic veins, which open into the inferior vena cava close by. In the liver, which now meets an obstruction to the passage of blood, the central veins of the lobules become dilated. As that pressure is transmitted to the pericentral sinusoids, dilation and pressure atrophy take place. In this way a mottling of dark brown (in the pericentral region) comes to alternate with pale pink (in the periportal region) so as to resemble the cut surface of a nutmeg (Figure

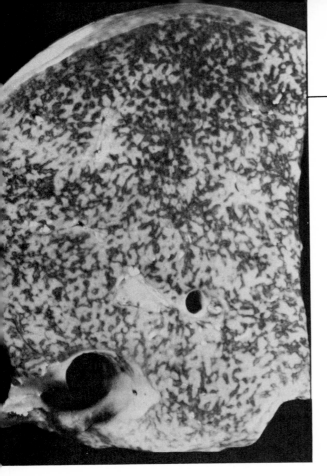

**Figure 3-1.** Chronic passive hyperemia of liver with "nutmeg" cut surface

3-1). "Nutmeg liver" is accordingly a gross characteristic of chronic passive hyperemia and most often results from right heart failure that occurs secondary to left heart failure. Eventually the intravascular pressure rises in the systemic and portal veins so that ascites, fibrosis of the spleen, dependent edema, and varicose ulcers of the legs develop. Heart failure is thus a long train of pressure consequences in a partially permeable vascular circuit.

## HEMORRHAGE

Hemorrhage is the flow of blood out of the vascular compartment. Since hemorrhages may be small or large, and internal, external, or on the skin surface, certain descriptive terms are useful. Petechiae are small punctate hemorrhages of the skin that measure only a few millimeters in diameter.

Purpura indicates a larger focus of bleeding measuring 1 to 2 cm. Ecchymoses are large, blotchy, irregular foci of hemorrhage into the skin. Solid masses of blood within the tissue are called hematomas, and collections of blood within the serous spaces are known as hemothorax, hemoperitoneum, or hemopericardium. The causes of hemorrhage include vascular disease, such as atherosclerosis, dissecting aneurysm of the aorta, and saccular aneurysms of the circle of Willis that tend to rupture. Trauma contributes, especially to external hemorrhage, as do diseases with a hemorrhagic tendency (hemorrhagic diatheses) such as hemophilia, Rocky Mountain spotted fever, and the leukemias.

An acute loss of only a moderate amount of blood is badly tolerated, whereas the gradual loss of even a large amount may not be disabling.[1] Small hemorrhages at critical sites, however, such as the brain or heart, may be devastating, whereas a large hemorrhage into a capacious site, such as the gut, is often clinically silent. Regardless of the site, the extravasated blood splits into heme and globin, the globin is reused, the iron is extracted from the heme, and the porphyrin residue is converted to bilirubin. For this reason the serum bilirubin may rise as large hemorrhagic lesions, such as pulmonary infarcts and sizable hematomas, undergo resolution. It is also the conversion of heme to the bilin pigments that accounts for the play of colors in the skin as a bruise undergoes resolution. A black eye is a good example.

Immediately after acute hemorrhage the hematocrit is normal, the blood volume is reduced, and whole blood given by transfusion is suitable treatment. Later, however, interstitial fluid shifts into the vascular compartment, the remaining red cell mass is diluted, and the hematocrit falls. At this stage the blood volume is normal and the patient needs packed red cells rather than whole blood, which overburdens the circulating volume.[1]

## THROMBOSIS

A thrombus is an intravascular mass of red cells, leukocytes, and platelets embedded in a fibrin mesh. Layers of fibrin and platelets alternate with layers of blood to form irregular bands of red and gray that are known as the lines of Zahn. Thrombi form only during life, so that the lines of Zahn help to distinguish the process from a blood clot that forms after death. In addition to this, the cut surfaces of a thrombus are dry, firm, reddish-gray, and lusterless. The margins are attached to the endothelial surface. In contrast, a postmortem clot is black, shiny, wet, and limpid, and the margins are unattached to the vessel wall.

Thrombi are occlusive or mural, bland or septic, and arterial, venous, or capillary. Most are occlusive, bland, and arterial. They form especially in the coronary, cerebral, splenic, renal, iliac, and femoral arteries. The abdominal portion of the aorta is also a frequent site. The causes are many, but endothelial injury and decreased blood flow are the most frequent.[2] The consequences of arterial thrombi depend on the site of the obstruction, abruptness of the process, need of the tissue for oxygen, and state of the collateral circulation. Serious consequences often occur in the heart and brain, where infarcts form. Ischemic necrosis of the lower extremities due to thrombi in the vessels of the leg is also common. Less likely to be life-threatening are infarcts of the spleen and kidneys.

Mural thrombi are frequent in the heart, especially in the left atrium or atrial appendage, in association with atrial fibrillation, and in the left ventricle, where they usually overlie a recent infarct of the myocardium. In atrial thrombi the flow slows, and in the ventricle the endothelial surface is injured by the underlying necrosis. Mural thrombi are often large and tend to undergo central degeneration, which transforms the center into a necrotic, thick, yellowish-gray semiliquid that is sterile and resembles pus. The process is accordingly known as puriform degeneration.

If the ischemic necrosis caused by the arterial thrombus is not lethal, the process of repair begins. Leukocytes accumulate about the margin, macrophages penetrate the thrombus, and phagocytosis of the cellular debris takes place. As the pigment is carried away, the color of the cut surface lightens. Capillary sprouts now penetrate from the periphery, and with time these extending tortuous vessels fuse to form irregular channels that course through the obstruction. Fibroblasts then emerge and a loose connective tissue supports the new capillary vessels. The new capillaries become more robust, the macrophages complete the task of debris removal, and the connective tissue matures and strengthens with the production of some collagen fibers. Thus the thrombus is repaired, the lumen is recanalized, and the circulation is partially restored.

Venous thrombi are also common, especially in the deep veins of the lower legs. They are attended clinically more by swelling, pain, and hyperemia than by ischemic necrosis. This is due to the lesser dependence of the tissue on oxygen in the veins, and to the more abundant collateral pathways for blood returning to the heart. The thrombi organize and repair in the same way as arterial lesions but have the additional characteristic of breaking loose and being carried by the vascular current as emboli. Emboli in the portal system, which are not frequent, pass to the liver. Emboli from the lower legs in the caval system, which are frequent, travel to the lungs. Thrombus formation in the veins of the leg is called phlebothrombosis when the process is bland and clinically silent, and thrombophlebitis when the process is septic and attended by pain, redness, and swelling. Phlebothrombosis has a higher tendency to embolus formation, whereas in thrombophlebitis thrombi tend to become fixed to the vessel wall by the process of

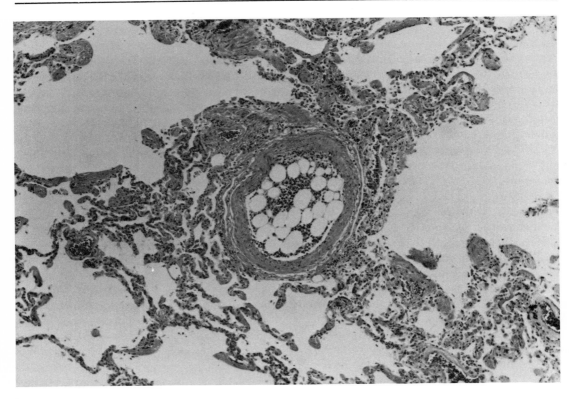

**Figure 3-2.** Bone marrow embolus in blood vessel of lung

organization. Pain on dorsiflexion of the foot indicates venous thrombi in the calf muscles and is known as Homans' sign.

Thrombi composed of fibrin and platelets also form in arterioles, capillaries, and venules. They are widespread and bland and affect especially the lungs, liver, kidneys, brain, and intestinal mucosa. The consequences are hemorrhage from endothelial injury, and ischemia from vascular blockage. The thrombi are so widespread that certain clotting factors are used up in their formation, i.e., platelets, fibrin, prothrombin, and factors V, VII, VIII, and X. The condition is thus regarded as a consumption coagulopathy and is called disseminated intravascular coagulation. The clinical consequences include shock, bleeding tendency, oliguria, pain in the back and abdomen, dyspnea, cyanosis, nausea and vomiting, convulsions, and coma. Heparin tends to

return the factors of the coagulation mechanism to normal.[3]

Although the precise cause of disseminated intravascular coagulation is not known, the process is initiated by a wide variety of conditions, including hemolysis, anoxia, endothelial injury, and the release into the circulation of bacterial endotoxin, tissue thromboplastin, proteolytic enzymes, and particulate or colloidal matter.[3] According to McKay, disseminated intravascular coagulation is the major pathogenic mechanism in microangiopathic hemolytic anemia and probably plays a role in the pathogenesis of acute renal failure from glomerulonephritis, certain cases of cirrhosis, certain vascular operations, hyaline membrane disease, fat embolism, malignant hypertension, the postpartum hemolytic uremic syndrome, and the rejection reaction to renal homografts.[3] The condition is thus extremely varied in its clinical manifestations, extremely diverse in the mechanisms of its causation, and remarkable in the number of conditions with which it is associated.

## EMBOLISM

An embolus is a structure that is swept in the vascular current to some site of obstructive lodgement. The structure is usually a thrombus, the vessel is usually a systemic vein, and the site of lodgement is usually the lung. Most frequently the systemic vein is one in the lower leg. Embolic structures other than thrombi include particles of bone, globules of adipose tissue, fragments of bone marrow, bubbles of nitrogen, cholesterol debris from aortic atheromas, foreign bodies such as bullets, amniotic fluid, and particles of talc from the injection of narcotics.[4] An embolus of bone marrow in pulmonary tissue is shown in Figure 3-2. The vessel of transport is not necessarily a vein; infected emboli break loose from mitral and aortic valves in bacterial endocarditis, and atheromatous ulcers of the aorta discharge cholesterol debris into the branches of that vessel. Nitrogen bubbles form in capillaries when ambient pressure suddenly decreases, and fat or bone marrow particles enter venules at fracture sites and are embolized to the lungs. Nor is the lung the only destination; large thrombi in the inferior vena cava pass through the right heart to land astride the bifurcation of the pulmonary artery and form the so-called saddle embolus. Sudden death results. Atheromatous emboli from the aorta are found in renal arteries as cholesterol clefts in organizing thrombi of those vessels. Abscesses form throughout the arterial system, especially in the brain and lungs, as septic emboli break away from infected heart valves, usually the mitral and aortic. Bacterial and fungal endocarditis occurs on the tricuspid leaflets, especially in alcoholic patients and narcotic addicts; it tends to seed the pulmonary tissue with disseminated abscesses.[5] Amniotic fluid, sucked into the venous sinuses of the uterus at the time of delivery, is later evidenced by squamae and lanugo hairs in the pulmonary vessels. Although the variety of embolic structures, vascular pathways, sites of lodgement, and pathologic consequences is wide, in clinical practice the process turns almost solely on thrombotic embolization, venous passage, and pulmonary lodgement. Thus pulmonary thromboembolism accounts for almost all of the clinical examples of the process. For an illustration, see Figure 12-6.

Pulmonary embolism tends to be followed by infarction only when passive hyperemia already exists in the vessels of the lung.[6] Initially there are edema and hyperemia. Fibrin then forms on the pleural surface, the alveolar walls undergo necrosis, and the infarct becomes hemorrhagic and dark bluish-red. Clinically the onset is characterized by fever, dyspnea, and leukocytosis. Cough, cyanosis, and chest pain may develop. The diagnosis is indicated by focal avascularity in a radioisotope scan of the lungs. Within two weeks fibroblastic repair is under way, and thereafter the infarct is gradually transformed into a pale gray fibrous scar that contracts and indents the pleural surface.

## INFARCTION

Infarcts are foci of coagulation necrosis due to sudden ischemia. The areas especially affected are the heart, lungs, brain, spleen, kidneys, and lower extremities. The ischemia is usually caused by arterial thrombosis or embolism, and the process is most frequent in vessels with pronounced atherosclerosis. Infarcts tend to form at the periphery of organs, assume a truncated cone shape with the base facing outward, become swollen early, and develop a peripheral margin of acute inflammation that is evidenced on external surfaces by the pres-

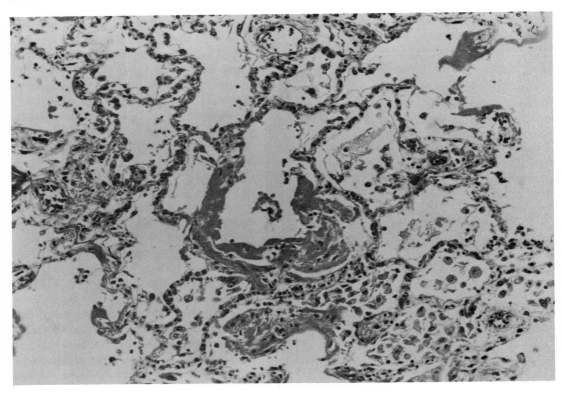

**Figure 3-3.** Macrophages, slight edema, and fibrin membranes lining alveolar walls, characteristic of adult respiratory distress syndrome (shock lung)

ence of fibrin. Microscopically there is a thin peripheral rim of recent hemorrhage and a central zone of nonstaining tissue in which the outlines of the structural pattern remain faintly discernible. Degeneration of the parenchymal cells follows. Thereafter the cellular debris and residual blood pigment diffuse out or are carried away by phagocytes, so that within several days the central region becomes decolorized, pale gray, and granular. A decolorized infarct of spleen is shown in Figure 1-3. In highly vascularized or loosely constructed tissues such as the lung or gut, infarcts are sodden with hemorrhage from the outset and tend to remain dark bluish-red. When the cause of ischemia is torsion of a pedicle, as occurs with the testis or a twisted loop of bowel, the veins are compressed while the arteries remain patent because of the higher intra-luminal pressure. The arteries thus continue to pump blood into a closed region from which it cannot escape. Large amounts of hemorrhagic fluid are impounded in such segments of bowel, and the tissue is regularly hemorrhagic and extremely dark red. Dehydration from this fluid loss and electrolyte imbalance often complicate the clinical state. Although emboli to the lungs are common, infarction is infrequent because of their dual blood supply, unless congestive heart failure has compromised the supply of oxygenated blood from the bronchial arteries. When pulmonary infarcts do form, they tend to be small and peripheral. Infarcts are also infrequent in the liver, where oxygen is likewise delivered through two separate vessels: the portal vein and the hepatic artery. In addition, the hepatic artery is seldom blocked by emboli because of its tortuous course as it proceeds from the celiac axis to the hilum of the liver.

Infarction is frequent in the brain and spinal cord, although in this instance enzymes dissolve the necrotic tissue so that liquefaction necrosis is characteristic and cavity formation is common. When bland emboli cause arterial obstruction, the necrosis tends to be sterile, but when septic emboli arise, as from the heart valves in bacterial endocarditis, the necrotic tissue becomes infected and abscess formation usually results.

The reaction of the infarct gradually subsides; the edema disappears and the pigment is carried away. Over several weeks, the repair process converts the necrotic zone into a fibrous scar that is shrunken, sharply demarcated, and pale gray.

## SHOCK

The heart pumps blood into a closed system of arteries against a pressure maintained by arteriolar constriction. Beyond the arterioles blood flows into the capacious capillary bed, which is controlled by vasomotor influences and in which only a few of the capillaries are open. The remainder are empty or collapsed. The veins are also under vasomotor influence and have a capacity, when dilated, that exceeds the total circulating blood volume.[7] Under normal conditions, therefore, the volume of the vascular bed is just matched to the volume of the circulating blood. Shock arises when the blood volume is inadequate to fill the vascular capacity. This occurs when the circulating blood is suddenly depleted or the vascular space is suddenly enlarged. The result is low cardiac output, insufficient perfusion pressure, and underoxygenation of tissue. Underoxygenation of tissue is the common denominator of all cases of shock.

Shock may be regarded as oligemic (hypovolemic), cardiogenic, or neurogenic. Oligemia may be due to hemorrhage, which depletes blood volume internally or externally, or to severe burns, which transude large amounts of plasma from the vascular compartment. An example of internal hemorrhage is rupture of an aortic aneurysm with massive hemorrhage into the peritoneal cavity. External hemorrhage results from such lesions as traumatic laceration of a femoral artery by a compound fracture of the leg, or incision of a carotid artery from self-inflicted or criminal stabbing. With burns, cardiac output drops, vascular permeability increases, and large volumes of fluid are lost from the burn surface as well as into the interstitial compartment.[8]

Cardiogenic shock is due to sudden pump failure, the most frequent cause of which is myocardial infarction. Less common causes include pulmonary embolus, rupture of a mitral leaflet or aortic cusp, rupture of a papillary muscle, or hemorrhage into the pericardial sac with cardiac tamponade. With these events flow slows, venous return decreases, and cardiac output falls so that there is no longer sufficient blood leaving the left ventricle to fill the arterial tree.

Neurogenic shock follows relaxation of arteriolar tonus so that arterial blood flows freely into the capacious capillary-venous bed. Although the mechanism of neurogenic shock is not altogether clear, it is observed with extreme pain, bacterial sepsis, and occasionally spinal anesthesia.[9] The sepsis is due to overwhelming infection, as in acute suppurative peritonitis with coliform organisms that produce endotoxins, and, less often, with gram-positive cocci that produce exotoxins, as in pneumococcal pneumonia with empyema.

The characteristic clinical features of shock include cool, moist skin, a tired, wan expression, and a thin, thready pulse. The blood pressure is usually low. Thirst is conspicuous. The skin is pale or ashen and wet with beads of cold perspiration. With pulmonary embolism, especially if massive, cyanosis may be seen. Respiration is often rapid and shallow. The sensorium is clouded, so that uninterest in immediate surroundings is evident. The psychologic alterations vary from obtundation to apathy, anxiety, restlessness, and fear. Acidosis develops as the metabolism shifts from aerobic to anaerobic and lactic acid is produced instead of carbon dioxide. The nephrons, suffering from low perfusion pressure and underoxygenation, reduce the rate of urine formation and oliguria develops. Thus the shock syndrome, though not uniform in all cases, is nevertheless conspicuous and complex. Moreover, the explanations proposed for the various aspects of the shock syndrome are complex and often speculative, involving hemodynamic alterations, vasomotor effects, and sympathetico-adrenal activity. To pursue these topics, the reader is referred to other published reviews.[7,9-12]

When death occurs, examination reveals wet, heavy, hyperemic lungs in which the vessels are dilated and the alveoli contain edema fluid and bands of fibrin that line the outer margins of the air sacs[13] (Figure 3-3). Fatty degeneration of myocardial fibers may be evident over the endocardium, although this is often slight. Vacuoles of lipid also accumulate in the hepatocytes, but the liver does not undergo marked enlargement. The intestinal mucosa is filled with dilated vessels gorged with blood, so that necrosis of the epithelium takes place and a large amount of hemorrhagic fluid may fill the lumen.[14] In the kidney tubular cells also display fatty degeneration; the glomeruli and vessels are not similarly affected. Necrosis may take place so that the lumens contain protein debris. With this, oliguria and renal failure develop. The kidney is grossly large, smooth, and pale, while microscopically the tubular degeneration is evident and the protein casts are conspicuous. The condition is variously called shock kidney, acute tubular necrosis, lower nephron nephrosis, and hemoglobinuric nephrosis.[15] If the patient survives, with the aid of hemodialysis or peritoneal lavage, the tubular cells regenerate and urine formation returns to normal in approximately 10 to 14 days. The lesions of shock are thus primarily circulatory and degenerative. With prompt restoration of the perfusion pressure and reoxygenation of the tissues, they are also temporary.

## REFERENCES

1. Linman JW: Physiologic and pathophysiologic effects of anemia. *N Engl J Med* 279:812, 1968

2. Deykin D: Thrombogenesis. *N Engl J Med* 276:622, 1967

3. McKay DG: Progress in disseminated intravascular coagulation. *Calif Med* 111:186, 279, 1969

4. Siegel H: Human pulmonary pathology associated with narcotic and other addictive drugs. *Hum Pathol* 3:55, 1972

5. Roberts WC, Dangel JD, Bulkley BH: Nonrheumatic valvular cardiac disease: A clinicopathologic survey of 27 different conditions causing valvular dysfunction. *Cardiovasc Clin* 5:334, 1973

6. Karsner HT: *Human Pathology*, 7th ed, p 110. Philadelphia: Lippincott, 1949

7. Simeone FA: Shock. In *Christopher's Textbook of Surgery* (Davis L, ed), 9th ed, pp 95-122. Philadelphia: Saunders, 1968

8. Moncrief JA: Burns. *N Engl J Med* 288:444, 1973

9. Shires GT, Carrico CJ, Canizaro PC: Shock. *Major Probl Clin Surg* 13:3, 1973

10. Thal AP, Brown EB Jr, Hermreck AS, et al: *Shock, A Physiologic Basis for Treatment*, pp 58-59. Chicago: Year Book Medical Publishers, 1971

11. Christy JH: Pathophysiology of gram-negative shock. *Am Heart J* 81:694, 1971

12. Zweigach BW, Fronek A: The interplay of central and peripheral factors in irreversible hemorrhagic shock. *Prog Cardiovasc Dis* 18:147, 1975

13. Blaisdell FW, Lim RC Jr, Stallone RJ: The mechanism of pulmonary damage following traumatic shock. *Surg Gynecol Obstet* 130:15, 1970

14. Drucker WR, David JH, Holden WD, et al: Hemorrhagic necrosis of the intestine. *Arch Surg* 89:42, 1964

15. Oliver J, MacDowell M, Tracy A: The pathogenesis of acute renal failure associated with traumatic and toxic injury, renal ischemia, nephrotoxic damage and the ischemuric episode. *J Clin Invest* 30:1307, 1951

# 4

# PHYSICAL AGENTS

All diseases that cause morphologic change are due to the effects of living agents, inherited defects, immunologic disturbances, or physical agents. These categories are inclusive except for the primary mental disturbances, i.e., psychoses, in which morphologic changes have not been identified. The physical agents that cause illnesses do so through mechanical, temperature, pressure, or radiation effects.

## MECHANICAL EFFECTS

Mechanical effects are usually due to trauma, and several words define these changes. An *abrasion* is a scrape, as when a child falls and the knees are denuded of skin. From this flat, superficial denudation serum and red cells appear if the lesion was caused during life; after death the surface remains dry—a point of forensic usefulness. A *laceration* is a tear of tissue, often liver or spleen, that tends to be ragged and frequently deep. In contrast, an *incision* is made by a sharp instrument, such as a knife, that produces a linear cut. A *bruise*, or contusion, is focal smashing of tissue in which small vessels break, blood diffuses into the injured tissue, and swelling develops. As the extravasated red cells break down and the porphyrin residues of the hemoglobin are converted to the various bilins, a play of colors develops so that the skin over the injured site gradually turns from red to blue to green to pale yellow to normal. These changes are discussed in detail in Chapter 8. A particularly severe bruise may cause hematoma formation. This solid mass of blood ordinarily is absorbed but may undergo cyst formation with or without calcification of the wall.

Mechanical injuries often cause *fractures*—disruptions of the continuity of bone. There are five principal types. A *simple* fracture is one in which the bone is separated into two discrete parts. In contrast, a *partial* fracture is one in which the cortex is broken on one side but only bent on the other. This is likened to the bending of a supple branch and is also known as a *greenstick* fracture. When the bone at the fracture site is shattered so that several separate fragments are present, the break is called a *comminuted* fracture. When any fracture ruptures the overlying skin, the break is called a *compound* fracture. A compound comminuted fracture, for example, is thus possible. Compound fractures are especially serious because of the probability of infection and the possibility of osteomyelitis. Finally, there are *pathologic* fractures, which tend to be spontaneous and are due to disease of the bone such as cyst formation (osteitis fibrosa cystica), primary tumors (chondroma), pronounced osteoporosis (multiple myeloma), and metastatic cancers. In elderly patients a pathologic fracture may be the first clinical evidence of metastatic disease.

Fractures heal by a process that tends to restore the bone to normal. Vessels are of course broken, and hemorrhage at the site of injury is the first reaction. Thereafter macrophages infiltrate the hematoma and the pigment is gradually carried away. Endothelial cells extend into the area, and capillary buds form. Fibroblasts infiltrate the fracture site, and granulation tissue begins to develop. Chondrocytes emerge, cartilage forms, and calcification begins. The assembly of cartilage, calcified connective tissue, and granulation tissue constitutes the callus. Its formation is promoted by growth hormone, testosterone, and para-

thyroid hormone. As the callus extends through the medullary cavity, across the bony cortex, and outside the fracture site, it is known as the internal, intermediate, and external callus, respectively. The external callus produces fusiform swelling about the site of the fracture. Calcified cartilage is gradually replaced by bone, compact cortex and cancellous medullary portions form, and the excess tissue of the external callus is progressively removed. After some remodeling, the new bone resembles the uninjured part and the site of the fracture becomes indiscernible. The process takes from six months to a year.

Complications of the healing process, of course, occur. The first is nonunion between fragments of bone. It may be due to infection, especially when the fracture is compound, to the interposition of soft tissue between the bone ends, or to impairment of blood supply as a result of nearby soft tissue injury. Excessive movement inside the cast may also cause soft scar tissue to form instead of new bone.

The second complication is injury to the soft tissues about the fracture site, due largely to laceration from the displacement of bone spicules. Examples include perforation of the urinary bladder with spillage of urine into the peritoneum or pelvic soft tissues, severance of an intercostal artery with hemothorax formation, and puncture of the pleura from a spicule of rib with pneumothorax and collapse of the lung. Severed nerves may cause paralysis, and severed arteries may result in ischemic necrosis of the affected part. Muscle atrophy may be the consequence of ischemic necrosis, and contracture may follow. In the muscles of the arm this is known as Volkmann's contracture. Hematomas may form, and the callus may ossify instead of gradually disappearing.

The last main complication of fractures is fat or bone marrow embolism. It is a complication of fractures of the long bones, especially those of the lower extremities, and occurs in 10 to 25 per cent of such fractures, often in young adults.[1] Clinically tachycardia, fever, dyspnea, and petechiae of the skin with central nervous system changes, including headache, irritability, and delirium, sometimes progressing to coma, begin within six hours to three days after the fracture. Thrombocytopenia, increased serum lipase, and mottling of the pulmonary X-ray, said to resemble a snowstorm, are characteristic. An open airway, the use of oxygen, and especially the administration of steroids relieve the pulmonary distress within a few hours. Whether the condition is due to the entrance of marrow particles into open vessels at the fracture site or to the emergence of fat globules in the plasma in association with shock is not resolved. Regardless of the mechanism, the principal lesions are minute hemorrhages throughout the brain and lungs in association with the embolic particles.

Joints are subject to mechanical injury. Displacement of apposite surfaces is known as luxation. When the displacement is partial, the condition is called subluxation. When the displacement is partial and temporary, the injury is known as a sprain. In all these injuries some soft tissues about the joint are affected, and this accounts for the swelling and hemorrhage that occur.

The spine is a column of joints, and the cervical portion is prone to a whiplash injury. In a car hit from behind, the driver's body is suddenly pushed forward, the head is moved less, and the sternocleidomastoid muscles vigorously contract to restore the normal alignment of the head with the body. In this snapping motion, subluxation of the cervical vertebrae may occur, the nucleus pulposus may herniate into the spinal canal (see Figure 21-10), and the cervical nerve roots may be squeezed in the process. The nerve root effect is called cervical radiculitis. Injuries of this kind are prevented by properly aligned headrests.

The brain is a soft tissue enclosed in a bony box. The brain is subject to move-ment within this rigid chamber, so that a blow to the head may cause a cerebral contusion at the point of impact. Bouncing inside the skull then causes a secondary contusion at the point opposite the site of the initial impact. The former is known as the coup; the latter, the contrecoup.

Hemorrhage within the skull but outside the brain occurs in the subarachnoid, subdural, and epidural spaces. Subarachnoid hemorrhage is the most common. The hemorrhage occurs within the arachnoid space so that it is contained by the surface of the brain beneath and by the intact pia mater on top. The blood thus spreads over the surface of the brain within this thin layer. Since the fluid in the arachnoid space circulates throughout the central nervous system, the cerebrospinal fluid is bloody at the outset and xanthochromic later as the pigment is degraded to a yellow bilin. The usual causes are trauma to the head with rupture of the delicate arachnoidal vessels. Less frequent is a primary intracerebral hemorrhage, often in a patient with pronounced hypertension, that extends through the brain substance to project into the subarachnoid space. Such strokes occur mainly in elderly persons. Least frequent are small saccular aneurysms of the circle of Willis, which rupture abruptly and bleed abundantly into the arachnoid space. These occur in adults and are characterized by extreme pain, sudden onset, and rapid progression of central nervous system signs.

The dura mater is firmly attached to the undersurface of the skull. Some vessels from the pia-arachnoid span the space from the pia to the dura, especially along the great venous sinuses of the dura. A traumatic laceration of the pia-arachnoid, or severance of the vessels bridging the space between the pia and dura, allows blood to flow into the subdural space. The fluid in this space also circulates throughout the brain coverings so that the spinal fluid is again discolored by blood. With an acute hemorrhage of this type the injury tends to be conspicuous, and the signs tend to be most pronounced at the outset and then gradually subside. Less frequently the trauma is slight and the clinical signs of cerebral injury are minimal and shortly disappear. The patient may even forget the event. Three to six weeks later, however, headache, confusion, and somnolence develop. The spinal fluid is xanthochromic, and arteriography may show an indented cortex or a shift of the hemispheres to one side. In this clinical pattern a chronic subdural hematoma arises. During the three- to six-week interval, fibroblasts and capillary buds have formed over the surface of the hematoma. The mass of hemoglobin exerts a high osmotic pressure so that fluid is drawn into the hematoma through its marginal neomembrane. As the mass swells, the brain is pushed aside and clinical signs escalate in severity with the passage of time. Unless the mass is evacuated, the displaced cerebrum may force the medulla into the foramen magnum, causing death from pressure on the vital centers.

Although the dura is tightly attached to the skull, fractures may create a shearing force that rips them apart. The middle meningeal artery runs in a groove on the undersurface of the temporal bone beneath the dura. When the injury separates the dura from the skull and the fracture severs the middle meningeal artery as well, a large hematoma may form in the space bounded by skull and dura. Since the hemorrhage is on the outer surface of the dura, it is known as an epidural hemorrhage. It is less serious than the other hemorrhages and is easily evacuated. It is important to realize that epidural hemorrhage produces no blood in the cerebrospinal fluid.

One of the consequences of trauma is shock. It is due to vascular collapse with decreased rate of flow and low perfusion pressure. The hypoxia occasioned by these changes has a pronounced effect on the kidneys, producing shock kidney or acute tubular necrosis, as described in Chapter 3.

Drowning also falls within the ambit of mechanical injury. The mechanism may be glottic spasm, in which case the body discloses only petechiae on the serosal surfaces, or it may be aspiration of large amounts of water, in which case the lungs are wet, airless, and extremely heavy. In the latter case water diffuses into the blood, hemodilution takes place, and the red cells swell and burst because of the hypotonic fluid. When this takes place in fresh water, the serum sodium and glucose are low because of dilution while the serum potassium is raised because of liberation from the lysed erythrocytes.[2]

## TEMPERATURE

Normally the gain and loss of body heat are in balance and the temperature is normal at 37.0°C or 98.6°F. Injury and death of cells take place when the temperature exceeds 42°C (107.6°F) or falls below 25°C (77°F).

The conditions caused by heat include heat cramp, heat stroke, and burns. Heat cramps are due to profuse perspiration with loss of sodium chloride. The individual may drink water to replace the lost fluid, which further dilutes electrolytes. Muscle cramping, nausea, and vomiting are the main effects. The condition is both prevented and treated by taking salt tablets.

Ninety per cent of heat loss occurs through the skin. When the ambient temperature is high, this process is impaired and the temperature-regulating mechanism may be overcome. As a consequence, unconsciousness develops. The condition is sometimes known as heat apoplexy. Although death seldom occurs, when it does the findings are limited to serosal petechiae, pulmonary edema, and hyperemia of the viscera.

Burn severity is classified by degree. A first-degree burn consists of hyperemia only; it subsides spontaneously and leaves no scar. A second-degree burn includes hyperemia and vesicle formation; it is also self-healing without residua. Third-degree burns extend through the full thickness of the skin, so that healing cannot take place by epithelialization from the epidermis or secondary skin appendages: hair follicles, sweat ducts, and sebaceous glands. Unless grafting is performed, therefore, scarring of the surface is unavoidable. Contraction of such scars disfigures the surface of the skin, often so severely that the function of the part is impaired.

Survival is threatened when a burn exceeds 20 per cent of the body surface. Extensive weeping of serum from the injured surface takes place. As serum protein is lost through this process, osmotic pressure falls, and the normal hydrostatic pressure pushes fluid out of the pulmonary capillaries into the alveoli. Pulmonary edema is the consequence. In addition, bacteria proliferate on the injured surface, and within 24 hours innumerable organisms occupy every square centimeter of injured surface. Gram-negative organisms predominate, especially *Pseudomonas aeruginosa*. The absorption of bacterial products from these organisms causes endotoxic shock.

Bacteria also penetrate into the subjacent tissue, to the extent of over 100,000 organisms/gm, and from this cellulitis with septic phlebitis develops.[3] Bacteremia then allows organisms to reach the pulmonary tissue, and pneumonia results. It is from these complications that burns of large areas threaten life.

Excessively low temperatures cause frostbite and freezing. Frostbite affects only the extremities, and the primary cause is impairment of the local circulation. Chilling causes constriction of arterioles, capillary flow stalls, and ice crystals form between cells. Because the water for the ice crystals comes from within the cells, the damage is due to dehydration, underoxygenation, and disruption of intracellular chemistry.[4] The affected parts swell, huge blisters form, and, unless the condition is relieved, ischemic necrosis takes place.

With whole-body freezing, metabolism is reduced, the flow of blood slows, and cerebral hypoxia develops. Carbon dioxide accumulates, drowsiness then develops, sleep follows, and ventricular fibrillation precedes death. There are no conspicuous pathologic changes.

## PRESSURE

Ambient pressure is the weight of an atmosphere 4.5 miles thick and amounts to 15 pounds/square inch (psi) at sea level. Disturbances are due to the degree of change and the rate at which it takes place. An increase is much better tolerated than a decrease; e.g., a pressure of 45 psi is rather well tolerated, while a decrease to 7 psi causes serious difficulty. If the change takes place gradually, however, physiologic adjustments can be made so that normal activity is possible. It is for this reason that Indians are able to live in the Andes at 15,000 feet above sea level. The adjustments that make this possible include an increase in the amount of hemoglobin per cell, an increase in the number of cells to 8 million/cu mm, and hypertension in the pulmonary circuit as a result of arteriolar constriction stimulated by hypoxia. These mechanisms provide a normal amount of oxygen even though the ambient supply is much reduced.

An abrupt decrease of pressure causes a serious illness called dysbarism. Understanding of this is improved by realizing that the human body consists of about 70 per cent fluid, so that a 70-kg adult contains about 49 kg of fluid. The atmospheric pressure drives gas into solution in this fluid just as carbon dioxide is dissolved in a carbonated soft drink. In the human, the gases consist of oxygen, carbon dioxide, and nitrogen. When the ambient pressure is suddenly reduced, gases emerge from solution just as bubbles appear when the cap is removed from a carbonated beverage. Emerging bubbles of oxygen and carbon

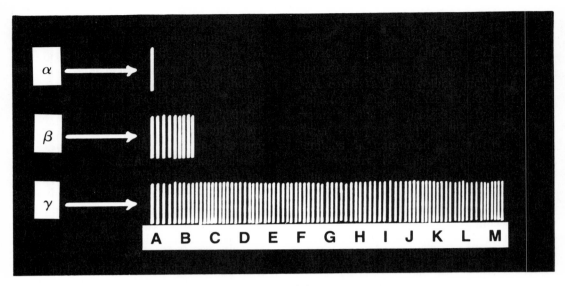

**Figure 4-1.** Relative penetrability of $\alpha$, $\beta$, and $\gamma$ rays of the same energy

dioxide are helped out of the human system through the lungs by the action of the enzyme carbonic anhydrase. Nitrogen, which makes up 80 per cent of inspired air, does not have such an assisting enzyme. Moreover, nitrogen is five times more soluble in fat than in water. The main disturbance is therefore due to nitrogen.

The bubbles of nitrogen sequester in the fatty tissues, which include myelin sheaths, bone marrow, adrenal cortex, pancreas, and subcutaneous fat depots. At these sites the bubbles cause vascular obstruction with focal necrosis, followed by hemorrhage and acute inflammation. In the belly such bubbles cause abdominal pain (the bends); in the ears, dizziness (staggers); in the lungs, an asthma-like dyspnea (chokes); and in the skin, producing vascular obstruction, pruritus (itch). These symptoms are characteristic of the deep-sea diver, acclimated to high pressure, who is brought to the surface too soon. Occasionally bubbles circulating in the retinal capillaries can be seen by funduscopic examination. Less frequently the skin is irregularly discolored by vascular obstruction (marbling), and,

rarely, half of the tongue is pallid from obstruction of one of the lingual arteries. Death may occur from nitrogen or marrow emboli. More often the patient survives with such complications as paralysis from spinal cord injury or arthritis from degeneration of articular surfaces. The condition is prevented by slow decompression in specially prepared chambers.[5]

## RADIATION

On the night of November 7, 1895, a 50-year-old professor of physics at the University of Würzburg stayed after work in his laboratory to observe the effect of a gas-evacuated tube in darkness. He was alone. The tube was turned on, and a sheet of barium platinocyanide lying on a bench six feet away began to glow in the dark. Barium platinocyanide emits light when exposed to radiation. That a sheet of paper covered on one side with this material happened to be lying that close to this experiment is one of the great serendipitous events of science. When Wilhelm Conrad Roentgen observed the glow, the thought first crossed the human mind that an invisible ray was passing from the tube to the bench. For want of a better term, Roentgen gave the name X-rays to the invisible phenomenon.

Over the ensuing 15 months Roentgen studied the rays, discovered their main properties, and recorded them in three scientific papers that secured for him a permanent place in the annals of science.

Within six months of Roentgen's revelation, Becquerel, in Paris, discovered the existence of radioisotopes. Thus, within six months, the fundamental discoveries for the science of radiology were made. Study then disclosed that the isotopes gave off $\alpha$, $\beta$, and $\gamma$ rays. Today these rays are encountered from cosmic sources, radioactivity in the earth's crust, contamination from radioactive waste disposal, and occupational sources involving nuclear reactors and uranium mining. Medical exposures from diagnostic and therapeutic procedures are also significant.

Radiation is interesting because of the small sizes and large numbers involved. Each cell is estimated to contain 100,000 billion (100 trillion, or $10^{14}$) atoms. If the nucleus of one atom were enlarged to the size of a BB shot and the BB were placed on the 50-yard line of a football field, the electrons circling about that nucleus would be down around the goal posts. Matter is therefore mostly space, and the particles that compose matter are extremely small.

Radiation consists mainly of $\alpha$ particles, $\beta$ particles, and $\gamma$ rays. The $\alpha$ particle is composed of two protons and two neutrons, so that it has a double positive charge and a large mass. For this reason, $\alpha$ particles ionize densely, lose their energy quickly, and fail to penetrate deeply. $\alpha$ particles will scarcely penetrate normal epidermis and therefore are not an external danger. Taken internally, however, they may be devastating because of the intense ionization. $\beta$ radiation consists of streams of electrons. Being light and having only a single charge,

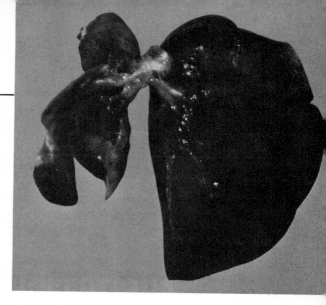

Figure 4-2. Postirradiation atrophy and fibrosis of rat lung

they penetrate deeply, ionize sparsely, and follow a zigzag course as they carom from one orbital electron of the target atoms to another. $\gamma$ rays are only perturbations of an electrical field; hence they have no mass and no charge. Reactions are caused only when they pass close to the nucleus or electrons of a target atom. Since these particles are so small in the structure of an atom and no interaction takes place unless the proton comes close to them, it is understandable that $\gamma$ radiation is extremely penetrating and only slightly ionizing in a comparative sense. At the site of impact the interaction is dependent on the energy of the ray: photoelectric, Compton recoil, or pair production. All these, however, cause ionizations, which are the basis for the radiation effect. The relative penetrability of the rays is illustrated in Figure 4-1.

Ionization chips electrons out of their perinuclear orbits so that a free electron is ejected and a free ion is formed. When this happens to an atom in a molecule in the nucleus of a cell, it is not clear whether the ionization by itself causes the disturbance (direct effect) or whether the ionization of water produces toxic radicals, such as hydrogen peroxide, that cause the injury (indirect effect). Direct hit and indirect effect are the two mechanisms by which the injury is eventually caused.

The biologic unit affected by radiation is the cell. It is composed of a cytoplasm with a large number of small molecules, and a nucleus with a small number of large molecules. The radiation strikes the cell in such a way that the ionizations are randomly distributed, i.e., as many in the cytoplasm as in the nucleus per unit of volume. In the cytoplasm duplicate molecules take the place of those that are injured so that the effect of injury is obscured. In the nucleus, however, no duplicate molecules are available, and an injury cannot be masked. The injury is revealed when the nuclear molecules undertake their complex process of mitotic division. Thus the nucleus is the most vulnerable portion of the cell, and injuries at that site are expressed by failure or impairment of mitotic division.

This biologic effect is illustrated by the experiment of Baldwin and Salthouse.[6] They found an insect in which cell division is synchronous and occurs only at the time of feeding. $\alpha$ radiation was applied to the breastplates of some of the insects. The controls were sham irradiated. Neither group was fed for several days; during this time the two groups were indistinguishable. On feeding, however, and the consequent stimulation of mitotic division, only the irradiated insects developed a focus of necrosis at the irradiated site. This experiment thus revealed that radiation impounds injury, the nucleus is most affected, and this effect is revealed by the mitotic process.

From the foregoing, radiation injury would be expected to be most pronounced in tissues that show the highest degree of mitotic activity. This is so; the specially affected tissues include the mucosa of the intestine, the spermatogonia of the testes, and the hematopoietic cells of the bone marrow. Whole-body irradiation, in suffi-cient dose, causes an intestinal syndrome characterized by denudation of the ileum and massive diarrhea, and a hematopoietic syndrome characterized by progressive leukopenia and anemia. One other cell is the most sensitive of all: the mature lymphocyte, which is a nondividing cell. The reason for the special sensitivity of this cell is not known.

Radiation in humans is given largely for the treatment of malignant disease. It is estimated that 50 per cent of patients with cancer will receive radiation therapy at some time during the course of their disease, and a large percentage of these patients will be treated with curative intent.[7] The rationale of this practice is that rapidly dividing cells are more susceptible to radiation injury than normal cells because there is less time for repair between cell divisions.[8] Although the practice is extremely useful, normal tissues are unavoidably affected. These often include bone marrow, gut, skin, and epithelium of the urinary bladder. The bone marrow depression, epilation, and gastrointestinal upsets all are ultimately due to failure of the proliferative compartments in cell systems that are normally in homeostatic balance with respect to cell renewal and cell depletion. The effects of such radiation on normal tissue have been reviewed by Bloomer and Hellman.[7] Late effects in normal tissues also develop after asymptomatic periods that last for months to years. They are characterized by the two pathologic processes of atrophy and fibrosis.[9] This is shown in Figure 4-2, in which experimental X-irradiation of the rat lung in a dose of 3,000 roentgens caused atrophy and fibrosis over a period of nine months. Carcinogenesis is also a late effect, but it occurs irregularly and after a latent period that is clinically silent and lasts for several years.

# REFERENCES

1. Herndon JH: The syndrome of fat embolism. *South Med J* 68:1577, 1976

2. Fatteh A: *Handbook of Forensic Pathology.* Philadelphia: Lippincott, 1973

3. Moncrief JA: Burns. *N Engl J Med* 288:444, 1973

4. Washburn B: Frostbite. *N Engl J Med* 266:974, 1962

5. Thorne IJ: Caisson disease. *JAMA* 117:585, 1941

6. Baldwin WF, Salthouse TN: Latent radiation damage and synchronous cell division in the epidermis of an insect. *Radiat Res* 10:387, 1959

7. Bloomer WD, Hellman S: Normal tissue responses to radiation therapy. *N Engl J Med* 293:80, 1975

8. Cohen BL: Impacts of the nuclear energy industry on human health and safety. *Am Scientist* 64:550, 1976

9. Smith JC: The pathogenesis of somatic radiation injury. *Am J Clin Pathol* 41:609, 1964

# 5

# INFECTIOUS DISEASE

All human disease has one of five major causes: inherited defects, physical agents, immunologic disorders, psychologic distress, and living agents. All but psychologic disorders cause structural changes in human tissues. An especially large segment of human disease is caused by living agents, which are, for the most part, infectious. Infectious diseases are due to six different types of organisms. These include bacteria, viruses, rickettsiae, chlamydiae, fungi, and parasites. Only the first four of these will be considered in this chapter.

## BACTERIA

Bacteria are microscopic prokaryotes—one-celled organisms without distinct nuclei—many of which are harmful to humans. They are classified according to their shapes and staining characteristics. The shapes are spherical (coccus), cylindrical (bacillus), and coiled (spirillum). The staining properties were discovered by Ehrlich, who applied aniline dyes, and by Gram, who found an unusual staining characteristic. Gram, a Danish physician working in Berlin, noticed in 1884 that an aniline dye could be fixed in some bacteria with a weak solution of iodine and would not be removed by subsequent immersion in alcohol. This was an empirical observation that bore no relationship to the pathogenicity of the organisms but provided a useful way of classifying them. The method is still in use and, as a consequence, we speak of gram-positive and gram-negative cocci and bacilli. No pathogenic gram-positive bacilli exist except for *Yersinia* (*Pasteurella*) and *Clostridium*, which cause diseases that are both exceptionally uncommon and clinically distinct. Table 5-1 lists the shape-stain classification of some of the main bacteria that affect humans. Omitted from this list are *Mycobacterium tuberculosis* and *Treponema pallidum,* both of which have special features, the former being acid-fast in its staining property, and the latter being coiled in its morphology.

All the coccal bacteria cause acute exudative inflammation and hence are known collectively as the pyogenic cocci. These organisms are of great importance because the infections they cause are both frequent and severe. The natures of the infections differ, however, and the sites of predilection are varied so that in these combinations certain characteristic diseases arise.

### Staphylococci

Staphylococci secrete toxins, among which are leukocidin, which destroys leukocytes, and enterotoxin, which causes the acute nausea and vomiting of staphylococcal food poisoning. The organisms also produce the enzyme coagulase, which causes plasma to clot in vitro and may cause thrombi to form in vivo. Thus staphylococcal diseases are characterized by infections that tend to remain localized and incite an acute suppurative inflammation with a pronounced tendency to abscess formation. Frequent sites of involvement include the skin, with boils and carbuncles; the lungs, with pulmonary abscesses; the kidneys, with acute suppurative pyelonephritis; the bones, with osteomyelitis; and the brain, with intracerebral abscess formation.

Different from these is staphylococcal food poisoning, which is not a tissue infection. It is due to the contamination and poor refrigeration of foods rich in carbohydrates, such as custards, into which the bacteria secrete enterotoxin. One to several hours after the ingestion of such food, severe nausea, vomiting, and diarrhea cause prostration and collapse. Recovery is spontaneous within a day's time. No lesions of the gut are found; the cause of the condition is discovered in the epidemiologic evidence that all those affected partook of the same meal, and by cultures of the food revealing staphylococci in large numbers.

### Streptococci

Streptococci are altogether different from staphylococci; they cause widely spreading infections that are characterized by cellulitis. This characteristic is due to the elaboration of fibrinolysin, hemolysins (streptolysins O and S), and hyaluronidase, which degrades mucopolysaccharides and enhances the spreading tendency. The streptococci are classified according to their ability to hemolyze blood: $\alpha$ designates partial

**Table 5-1.**

## Main bacterial pathogens

Gram-positive cocci
  Staphylococci
  Streptococci
  Pneumococci

Gram-negative cocci
  *Neisseria meningitidis*
  *Neisseria gonorrhoeae*

Gram-positive bacilli
  *Bacillus anthracis*
  *Clostridium*

Gram-negative bacilli
  Coliform bacteria
  *Salmonella*
  *Shigella*
  *Klebsiella*
  *Yersinia (Pasteurella)*
  *Haemophilus*
  *Corynebacterium*

hemolysis with a green border around the colony on the blood agar plate, β signifies a clear zone around the colony due to complete hemolysis, and γ registers no hemolysis. The α-hemolytic organisms, which comprise the *viridans* group of streptococci (virid means "vividly green"), cause low-grade infection especially of the heart valves, i.e., subacute bacterial endocarditis. The β-hemolytic organisms tend to be highly virulent, and the γ streptococci are scarcely virulent at all.

Another classification—that of Lancefield—is based on surface carbohydrates and divides the organisms into 12 groups designated by the letters A, B, C, D, E, F, G, H, K, L, M, and N. In this classification the most important organisms are found in group A, which are β-hemolytic. These include the causes of localized disease such as tonsillitis, the extending infections known as cellulitis, and the disseminated infections that spread to the whole body by the hematogenous route. In addition, the group A organisms are causative of the poststreptococcal immune disorders glomerulonephritis (strains 1, 4, and 12) and rheumatic fever. Both disorders are due to the consequences of a preceding infection rather than to the presence of the bacteria in the affected tissues.

Streptococci are ubiquitous and may affect any tissue. The most frequent sites of involvement, however, are the nasopharynx and recent wounds, either surgical or accidental. At both places the bacteria spread rapidly away from the site of the infection and the tissue becomes hyperemic, edematous, and warm. Leukocytes spread throughout the tissues but abscesses tend not to form. Fever, lassitude, sore throat, and pain on swallowing accompany the upper respiratory infections. Dehiscence of wounds may follow subsidence of the tissue edema at sites of surgical repair. The organisms respond to antibiotic therapy, and, unless hematogenous spread develops, the infections subside.

Two other distinct entities are due to streptococcal infection and both affect primarily the skin. The first is scarlet fever, which is due to strains of group A bacteria that produce a dermatophilic erythrotoxin. The condition is limited to children. Onset is heralded by acute nasopharyngitis accompanied by fever, chills, nausea, and vomiting. Within four to five days a bright red rash appears on the face, trunk, and extremities. Physical signs include acute hyperemia of the pharynx, "strawberry tongue," and a band of circumoral pallor. The rash stimulates skin growth, and scaliness follows its regression. The condition is controlled by antibiotics and subsidence is ordinarily uneventful, as the poststreptococcal immune disorders of glomerulonephritis or rheumatic fever rarely follow.

The second condition is erysipelas, which usually occurs after the age of 20, is ordinarily due to group A organisms, and consists of a cutaneous infection, especially of the face. It produces a wide, flat zone of raised, indurated, violaceous discoloration of irregular outline that is sharply demarcated from the adjacent soft, pliable skin of normal color. The inflammation penetrates no deeper than the subcutaneous tissue, and abscess formation is uncommon. The condition responds to antibiotic therapy and subsides without producing scarring or deformity.

## Pneumococci

Pneumococci are gram-positive streptococci (diplococci) with capsules containing specific carbohydrates that permit classification into more than 70 different strains. The organisms affect principally the respiratory tract, and the first three strains are most often involved. The capsules appear to protect the bacteria from phagocytes. The organisms enter the body through the respiratory tract. They are seen along with other organisms in bronchopneumonia, but cause nearly all cases of lobar pneumonia. Abscess formation may develop, and spread of the organisms through the pleura results in empyema. Other tissues less commonly affected include the paranasal sinuses, meninges, heart valves, and joint spaces.

## Meningococci

Meningococci (*Neisseria meningitidis*) are gram-negative and ferment glucose and maltose. The organisms cause a mild nasopharyngitis that is followed by spread to the meninges. The route and reason for this spread are not clear, although the meningitis may be preceded by a bacteremia, and extension through the cribriform plate of the ethmoid bone is possible. In the meninges an acute suppurative exudate forms, especially over the convexity of the cerebral hemispheres. The exudate is thick, opaque, and characteristically pale greenish-gray. The spinal fluid is cloudy and contains both neutrophilic granulocytes and bacteria. The patient experiences fever, headache, photophobia, stiff neck, and pain on movement of the eyes. Extension of the flexed leg is painful (Kernig's sign). The condition is responsive to treatment and healing is usually uneventful with dissolution of the exudate.

The meningococcemic phase may be associated with petechiae of the skin, which transform into minute pustules from which the organisms can be cultured. Occasionally the bacteremia also affects the adrenals, acute vasculitis develops, and hemorrhagic necrosis of both adrenals follows. This is accompanied clinically by a fulminant course ending in collapse and death attributable both to the overwhelming meningococcemia and to the bilateral hemorrhagic adrenal destruction. The combination of meningococcemia and hemorrhagic necrosis of the adrenals is known as the Waterhouse-Friderichsen syndrome and has an extremely high mortality.

## Gonococci

Gonococci (*Neisseria gonorrhoeae*) are also gram-negative and are distinguishable from meningococci by their ability to ferment only glucose. The organisms are suited to the mucosal surfaces of the genital structures of both sexes, where they cause urgency, burning on urination, and a purulent discharge that becomes a persistent thin leukorrhea. No immunity develops, so that repeated infections of the same surfaces are possible. The organisms shun squamous mucosa, sequester themselves in blind cul-de-sacs, and remain superficial in location. The entire male genital mucosa is affected, beginning with the urethra and extending through the epididymides; the testicular tissue is resistant. In women the infection begins in the urethra and in the vulvar glands of Skene and Bartholin. It skips the vagina and external cervix because of the squamous mucosa there. It also skips the endometrium, for unknown reasons. In addition to the vulvar structures, the infection spreads into the blind glands of the endocervix and the recesses of the uterine (fallopian) tubes, and onto the pelvic peritoneum. Eventually fibrosis develops, and this leads to tubal constriction, tubo-ovarian adhesions, tubo-ovarian abscesses, and pelvic peritonitis with fibrosis and fixation of the pelvic structures. Ectopic tubal pregnancy and sterility commonly result. In men urinary obstruction follows from fibrosis of the urethra with stenosis.

Two other conditions are caused by gonococci: epidemic vulvovaginitis of prepubertal girls, and ophthalmia neonatorum in either sex. Ophthalmia neonatorum is due to infection of the conjunctiva during passage through the birth canal. It was formerly a common cause of blindness but is now avoided by the instillation of penicillin or silver nitrate into the eyes of the newborn at the time of birth.

In the newborn girl the vaginal mucosa is thick in response to the mother's level of estrogen. At about three months after birth this subsides, and from this time until puberty the vaginal mucosa is thin and delicate from the lack of estrogenic stimulation. Vaginal infection with gonococci is possible during this period; the condition is related to careless sanitation and is not associated with sexual activity. It responds to antibiotics and is self-limited with the onset of puberty, which initiates the secretion of estrogen and thickening of the vaginal mucosa.

Only two main pathogens occupy the gram-positive bacillus classification: the anthrax and clostridial organisms. Anthrax is an extremely uncommon disease of humans that is contracted from an infected animal, begins as a skin pustule, and becomes an overwhelming infection that is often fatal. Clostridia cause the uncommon and serious diseases of tetanus, gas gangrene, and botulism. Because all these conditions are clinically conspicuous, gram-positive organisms observed in the laboratory from patients without overwhelming disease are ordinarily harmless nonpathogens.

## Clostridia

The tetanus organism is gram-positive and bacillary with a bulbous end that gives it the shape of a tennis racquet. The organism is widespread in nature and lives harmlessly in human and animal gut, and hence in the soil. It is introduced into tissue by contaminated injury and requires necrotic tissue and low oxygen tension to survive. The organisms remain at the contaminated site, cause focal acute inflammation, and produce a potent toxin that diffuses widely, affects motor nerve plates, and is associated with contractile spasms of voluntary muscles. The masseters are often affected first; hence the term lockjaw. Death results from respiratory difficulty. Autopsy examination reveals scant changes at the myoneural junctions although edema may be evident in the ganglion cells of the medulla and spinal cord. Since the disease is frequently fatal, it is important to cleanse wounds thoroughly, especially those contaminated with soil, and to give toxoid for the stimulation of immunity or antitoxin for the neutralization of toxin.

Gas gangrene, caused by the *C. perfringens*, *C. novyi*, and *C. septicum*, also begins by soil contamination of a deep wound in which necrotic fragments are present. The inflammation has three special properties: It spreads rapidly, causes extensive necrosis, and produces gas. The organisms are anaerobic and form an exotoxin as well as a wide range of proteolytic enzymes. The enzymes dissect tissue planes and allow the infection to spread rapidly. The toxin causes fever, and the bacteria produce gas. The infected part swells, the skin becomes tense and blanched, and crepitation may be felt. The skin may split from the pressure of the accumulated gas. The striated muscles turn soft and dark red and "dissolve" into wet, flabby structures that are widely necrotic. Eventually the bacteria become disseminated and gas bubbles form, especially in the liver. Prostration precedes death. Prevention requires careful debridement of wounds and opening of the tissue to provide exposure to oxygen so that bacterial proliferation is impaired. Antibiotics and antitoxin are also helpful.

Botulism is not an infection of tissue, but poisoning. The poison is produced by *C. botulinum*, which lives in the soil and contaminates imperfectly canned vegetables and poorly refrigerated meats, especially sausages. The organisms produce an exotoxin that accumulates in the food containers. No gas is produced, and the food appears normal. Shortly after ingestion paralysis of the face, neck, and muscles of respiration begins with or without headache, dizziness, nausea, and vomiting. The anatomic findings are slight and nonspecific. Antitoxin may be given, but the mortality is high. The toxin is inactivated by boiling for 10 minutes.

## Coliform bacteria

The coliform organisms are gram-negative bacilli that normally inhabit the intestinal tract. They consist of the various species of *Escherichia*, *Proteus*, *Enterobacter*, and *Pseudomonas*. Their tendency is to infect the urinary tract, causing pyelonephritis, cystitis, and urethritis. In addition, they are frequent contaminants of burns and postoperative wounds. As the organisms succumb to their environment, an endotoxin is released. Endotoxic shock thus often follows gram-negative bacteremia. With normal localization in the gut, these organisms are also common contaminants of the peritoneum when the intestine or related structures are opened or ruptured, as in acute appendicitis, bowel operations, or gallbladder disease. The coliform organisms tend to resist some antibiotics, so that they flourish when such agents inhibit the growth of staphylococci, streptococci, and other pyogens. The inflammation caused by the coliform organisms is acute, exudative, and in no way different from that produced by the common pyogenic bacteria.

### Typhoid fever

*Salmonella typhi* are flagellated, motile, gram-negative bacilli with somatic (O) and flagellar (S) antigens. The organisms cause typhoid fever by contaminating food, invading tissues, dying, and releasing the somatic antigen, which is a powerful endotoxin. The organisms affect only humans and are transmitted by carriers in whom the bacteria reside harmlessly in the gallbladder or biliary tract. In such persons the feces become infective and, through careless hygiene or vectors such as houseflies, the organisms contaminate food.

The ingested bacteria may be killed by gastric acid or may slip viably into the intestine. In the latter instance they invade the lymphoid tissue of Peyer's patches, where they evoke a pronounced hyperplasia of macrophages. As a result, the Peyer's patches become markedly thickened and sharply demarcated from the adjacent normal mucosa. Soon the macrophages rupture and the bacteria enter the portal vessels to be swept into the bloodstream. The organisms are then captured by the spleen, lymph nodes, and Kupffer cells of the liver, where typhoid nodules form. These are discrete clusters of plump macrophages that contain *Salmonella* organisms and erythrocytes. Indeed, the nodular accumulation of such macrophages with erythrophagocytosis is the anatomic hallmark of the disease. Neutrophilic granulocytes are conspicuously absent. The liver enlarges, and the spleen may undergo such rapid hyperplasia as to burst spontaneously. Degenerative changes, often with focal hemorrhage, take place in the renal tubules, striated muscle, and cardiac muscle. After hematogenous dissemination, the Peyer's patches also ulcerate, so that the bacteria are liberated into the fecal stream. If the bowel does not bleed or rupture and the spleen does not perforate, the toxemia may subside and the patient recover.

Clinically typhoid fever begins with fever, chills, abdominal pain, diarrhea, and prostration. Examination discloses bradycardia, leukopenia, and hyperemic foci of the skin, especially over the chest and abdomen, known as rose spots. Blood culture may become positive in the first two weeks of the disease. Later, stool culture may also become positive and agglutination of killed organisms by increasingly dilute samples of the patient's serum may be observed in the Widal test. Although recovery is frequent and ordinarily complete, a small number of patients continue to harbor the organisms and pass on the disease as typhoid carriers. Thus the condition is perpetuated.

Other species of *Salmonella* cause gastroenteritis and enteric fevers that are similar to but less severe than typhoid fever. The species include *S. enteritidis* (*paratyphi*), *S. schottmuelleri*, *S. hirschfeldii*, and *S. choleraesuis*.

### Bacillary dysentery

Bacillary dysentery is caused by various species of *Shigella*, including *S. dysenter-*

*iae, S. flexneri, S. boydii,* and *S. sonnei.* The condition differs from typhoid fever in three respects: The lesions affect chiefly the colon, the ulcers are superficial, and bacteremia does not occur so that the prospect of complication is slight. The organisms are transmitted by contaminated food and drink, the lesions begin in the colonic mucosa, and the ulcers are small and multiple with fibrin on the surface, neutrophils at the margins, and mononuclear cells at the base. The onset is heralded by fever, abdominal discomfort, and diarrhea. The illness is usually mild and sporadic, although it may become severe and epidemic. Diagnosis is made by stool culture and bacteriologic studies. Recovery is attended by only slight scarring of the mucosa. Chronic disease persists in some individuals, who thus serve as sources of infection.

### Klebsiella
Friedländer's bacillus, or *Klebsiella oxytoca (pneumoniae)*, is the one gram-negative bacillus especially prone to infect the pulmonary tissue of adults and cause pneumonia. Droplet infection of the airways is likely, the victims are often old, and emaciation from other disease is frequently seen. The organisms are aggressive and form a thick mucoid capsule. On this account the pneumonic process has two special features: The exudate is conspicuously slimy and mucoid, and abscess formation, usually multiple, is common. Otherwise the pneumonic process is not markedly different from that caused by the more common pyogenic bacteria.

### Plague and tularemia
Plague and tularemia are caused by two organisms formerly assigned to the genus *Pasteurella: Yersinia pestis* and *Francisella tularensis.* They are gram-negative, of uncertain morphology, and extremely virulent. Both infect chiefly animals and only occasionally are passed to humans. The most common plague reservoir is the rat, and the bacteria are occasionally transmitted to humans by rat fleas. The most common tularemic reservoir is the rabbit, and the organisms are transmitted to humans by the deerfly. Both bacteria affect lymph nodes, lung, and skin, and both cause extremely widespread acute suppurative inflammation with extensive necrosis. Neither condition is common, and both respond satisfactorily to antibiotics.

Other gram-negative bacilli are those of the genera *Haemophilus, Bordetella,* and *Corynebacterium.* All affect children, causing respiratory infection and meningitis *(H. influenzae),* whooping cough, or pertussis *(B. pertussis),* and diphtheria *(C. diphtheriae).* Whooping cough and diphtheria are now infrequent in the United States because of immunization programs.

### Chronic granulomatous disease
Although the foregoing organisms cause predominantly acute exudative inflammation, two additional organisms are the chief causes of chronic granulomatous inflammation. This is characterized by tissue infiltration with lymphocytes, macrophages, and multinucleated giant cells with or without necrosis. The two great granulomatous diseases are tuberculosis and syphilis. Both were formerly rampant, tuberculosis as the "great white plague" and syphilis as the widespread disease that mimicked so many others. With the advent of penicillin for syphilis, however, and of chemotherapy for tuberculosis, neither is currently seen in epidemic form in the United States. These diseases should not be dismissed, however, because both may reappear as drug-resistant organisms emerge or as inadequate treatment becomes evident.

**Tuberculosis.** Tuberculosis was unbelievably frequent in Europe and the United States during the 19th century. It reached epidemic proportions; approximately half the English population was affected. It struck at young and old, and at all levels of

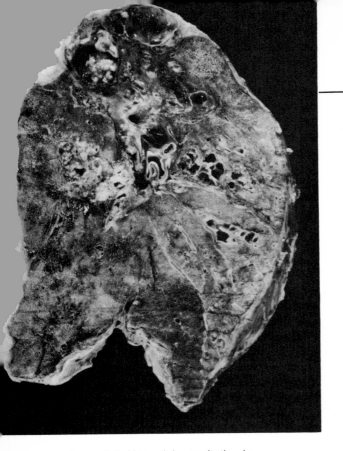

**Figure 5-1.** Upper lobe cavitation in pulmonary tuberculosis

al belief is in its non-communicability."[1] In the following year, Koch announced his discovery of the tubercle bacillus. It was one of the greatest victories medicine has ever achieved. Hope sprang forth. Isolation was given reason. Disinfection was ruthlessly enforced. Surgical techniques were soon perfected, and pneumothorax, followed later by pneumonectomy, was performed. In the 1930s streptomycin and *p*-aminosalicylic acid were found to have bacteriostatic properties against the organism and, within two more decades, isoniazid was found. At long last chemotherapy was effective, surgical treatment was sound, preventive measures were understood, and the greatest killer of the human race was subdued. Although endemic pockets remain, civilization had rid itself of a great malady.

Tuberculosis is a granulomatous disease, usually chronic, that affects many tissues but mainly the lungs, and is caused by *Mycobacterium tuberculosis*. The organism spreads from person to person by droplet infection. A small proportion of patients, perhaps 5 per cent, may contract the disease by ingestion of unpasteurized milk containing *M. bovis*. With the first infection, in which the organisms are usually inspired into the alveoli, a small focus of exudative inflammation arises, most often in the midportion of either lung closely subjacent to the pleura. From this site some of the organisms enter the pulmonary lymphatics to be carried to the hilar lymph nodes, where a second minute focus of exudative inflammation arises. No clinical illness ordinarily accompanies this trivial inflammatory process, which often takes place during childhood.

After some weeks the exudative inflammatory process becomes granulomatous. At each site, pulmonary and nodal, macrophages replace the neutrophilic granulocytes. The macrophages enlarge and form discrete clusters, and lymphocytes and fibroblasts are drawn to the periphery of each cluster, where they are loosely ar-

society. In 1844, in a workhouse in Kent, 78 of 78 boys and 91 of 94 girls were found to have the disease.[1] It was so frequent as to carry off nearly one-fourth the population of Europe, and so fatal as to deter many physicians from even attempting a cure. With the cause unknown, all manner of treatment was tried, from absolute immobility to vigorous exercise, from exotic foods to a starvation diet, and from the letting of blood to a change of air, a change of location, a change of temperature, a change of altitude, and even the change of a long sea voyage. But nothing worked; the disease progressed relentlessly. Despair prevailed. In 1881 a standard medical textbook dealt with the cause of tuberculosis, citing "hereditary disposition, unfavorable climate, sedentary indoor life, defective ventilation, deficiency of light, and depressing emotions." Moreover, it was added that "the doctrine of the contagiousness of the disease has its advocates, but general-

ranged. The large macrophages resemble epithelial cells and are termed epithelioid on that account. Moreover, some of the epithelioid cells fuse to form multinucleated giant cells of the Langhans type. The resulting structure is known as a tubercle, meaning nodule, and it is the hallmark of granulomatous disease.

The tubercle is "hard" so long as the center is viable; it is "soft" when the center becomes necrotic. A hard tubercle is shown in Figure 2-4. Either way, both sites, in the lung and hilar lymph nodes, regularly undergo healing, so that the inflammation process subsides and is replaced by fibrous connective tissue. Calcification follows. The combination of a focus of calcification measuring 0.5 to 1.0 cm in diameter in the lung, usually the subpleural midportion, and in a lymph node, usually in the hilar region, constitutes the Ghon complex, named after the Prague pathologist. It is the presence of this complex that testifies to a previous primary infection with the tubercle bacillus.

The significance of the primary infection is that this first exposure to the organism sensitizes the body to the tuberculoproteins of the bacterial wall. The bacterium produces neither endotoxin nor exotoxin, and the main disease process, which follows reinfection usually in adult life, is due entirely to this permanent, cell-mediated hypersensitivity. It is this hypersensitivity that changes the trivial exudative inflammation of the primary infection to the progressive, virulent, granulomatous inflammation of the secondary or adult infection. It is this hypersensitivity that causes the unique necrosis in which the debris of that reaction resembles cheese, in both appearance and consistency, and is hence called caseous. The microscopic feature of caseous necrosis is a finely granular, eosinophilic emulsification of the tissue at the center of the tubercle. It is the patient's hypersensitivity, ordinarily permanent, that provides a diagnostic skin test for the disease: Injection of sterile tuberculoprotein into the skin of a sensitized patient causes focal erythema and induration within 48 to 72 hours. The tuberculoprotein itself will not sensitize the patient; that requires the whole viable organism. Nor does the reaction reveal whether the patient has active disease; it only discloses that the patient has been exposed to the organism and has become sensitized. Moreover, the test does not absolutely exclude active disease since the result may be negative in overwhelming blood-borne tuberculosis as well as in some other conditions, including the lymphomas, measles, corticosteroid therapy, immunosuppressive treatment, and the characteristic anergy of Hodgkin's disease. Regardless of the clinical usefulness of the skin test, the central point is that the progressive and destructive disease of secondary or reinfection tuberculosis is due entirely to the sensitization of the host to the proteins of the bacterial wall.

The organism causing this devastating disease is a small, slender, slightly curved bacillus. It is acid-fast; i.e., it fails to decolorize in acid after having been immersed in heated stain. The reason for this is the high lipid content of the bacterial wall. These lipids may also account for two other properties of the organisms: They resist water-soluble drugs and they resist drying, which permits viability outside the body for long periods.

The main, secondary, or adult reaction may stem from the release of organisms from the connective tissue of old tubercles, in which they tend to remain viable (reactivation), or from external organisms that enter the lungs through droplet infection (reinfection). Reinfection is regarded as more common. Whichever the route, the reaction in the sensitized patient is now massive with abundant tubercle formation, early caseous necrosis, enlargement of the reactive sites, and fusion of the adjacent tubercles to form cavities and abscesses. This pronounced reaction has an additional remarkable feature: It tends to occur at the apices of both lungs. Although the reason for this particular localization is unclear, it is nevertheless true that apical reactions of the pulmonary tissue, especially with fibrosis, cavity formation, and focal calcification, are usually tuberculous. Tuberculosis flourishes in the apices of the lungs (Figure 5-1).

The course of the apical reaction is affected by the number of organisms, their virulence, and the sensitivity of the host. Other pulmonary diseases, such as silicosis, and general diseases or conditions, such as diabetes, malnutrition, senility, steroid therapy, and intercurrent disease, add their adverse effects. Depending on these factors, the apical pulmonary reaction has several possible outcomes. It may be overcome by the defenses of the host and subside so that the inflammatory site is gradually converted into a large, dense, fibrous scar, usually extending to the pleura with secure attachment to the overlying thoracic wall. Or, rather than subside, the apical tubercles may enlarge and coalesce to form sizable cavities filled with necrotic, bacteria-laden, caseous debris. A thick, reactive fibrous wall may form around these sites so that while the infection still smolders, it may nevertheless be contained. Failure of containment may allow a peripheral abscess to rupture into the pleural cavity and spill organisms into that chamber with the formation of a tuberculous empyema. The cavities are irregularly shaped, with shaggy walls, and display slender, thrombosed arteries that resist the erosion, remain intact, and pass across the open chambers. With progressive erosion and the passage of time, the necrotizing process may extend into a pulmonary artery with sudden hemorrhage that fills the lung, spills into the trachea, and issues from the mouth. Alternatively, the caseating process may extend into a bronchus, dumping necrotic debris and tubercle bacilli into an airway through which they are spread to other portions of the pulmonary tissue, including the opposite lung. Thus bronchial erosion and respiratory movement spread the infection widely in the pulmonary tissue. The acute reaction of massive, solid, tuberculous pneumonia may result.

The bacteria may ascend the trachea, infect the larynx, and cause extinction of the voice. Swallowing of the organisms infects the gut, causes ulceration of the bowel, and may be associated with hemorrhage. The apical cavities may also open into pulmonary veins, discharging bacteria into the systemic circulation, so that tubercles develop in a wide range of tissues, especially the liver, spleen, bone marrow, adrenals, kidneys, bone, meninges, and genital tract. Tissues seldom affected are thyroid, pancreas, myocardium, and striated muscle. The minute, pale gray tubercles, which are barely discernible to the unaided eye, resemble millet seeds, and the wide dissemination of these lesions is thus called miliary tuberculosis.

Last, the pulmonary process may persist without becoming clinically conspicuous while at the same time discharging small numbers of bacteria into the vascular stream. These organisms may flourish at a single susceptible site. Thus arises isolated organ tuberculosis, such as that of the spine, with gibbus formation, or of the adrenals, with Addison's disease. No tissue is invulnerable to the erosive reaction of the tubercle bacillus.

Just as the anatomic sites of tuberculosis vary, so do the clinical manifestations. Nevertheless, common among them are fever, weakness, night sweats, fatigability, anorexia, weight loss, and respiratory difficulties. The clinical appearance of the advanced case was described vividly by Thomas Beddoes in 1799:

> The emaciated figure strikes one with terror; the forehead covered with drops of sweat; the cheeks painted with a livid crimson, the eyes sunk; the little fat that raised them in their

orbits entirely wasted; the pulse quick and tremulous; the nails long, bending over the ends of the fingers; the palms of the hand dry and painfully hot to the touch; the breath offensive, quick and laborious, and the cough so incessant as to scarce allow the wretched sufferer time to tell his complaints.[1]

To this may be added the breathlessness, the abundance of sputum, the pain in the chest, and later the expectoration of blood. In the advanced stage, the clinical presentation is distinct.

With the availability of medical care and the effectiveness of therapeutic agents, few patients now come to such terminal disease untreated. With lesser manifestations, early diagnosis is important because therapy is most effective when the process is discovered at its outset. Diagnostic procedures include the skin test, pulmonary X-ray, and sputum examination with smear, culture, and guinea pig inoculation. The optic fundi may show tubercles in the retinae. Tubercles may be found in a needle biopsy of the liver or bone marrow, or in tissues curetted from the uterus. In one or another of these ways the diagnosis is established. Thus, in the course of 70 years, from 1882 to 1952, the cause of the disease was found, the principles of prophylaxis became evident, surgical therapy was perfected, and tuberculocidal drugs were discovered. The vast epidemic thus ended, and "the captain of all the men of death" finally yielded to the persistent attention of medical investigation. It is a remarkable chapter in the history of medical progress.

**Syphilis.** Syphilis appeared suddenly in Western Europe at the end of the 15th century and spread rapidly throughout the land. Although the source of the disease is obscure, it is widely presumed that it was brought to Spain by the sailors of Columbus on their return voyage. Syphilis spread through Spain, then Italy, and then all of Europe. This rapid propagation was enhanced by the nature of the disease, which is clinically silent for long periods but never leaves the body and remains infective for substantial intervals. It is a hideous disease that offends all. As quoted by Dennie:

If the primary lesion is not treated the disease may affect the entire body so that it is covered with eruptions that occur upon the head, face, arms and the legs. If the disease is allowed to progress, severe pains occur in the frontal region of the head, the shoulders, the arms, the tibia, around the breasts and the hips. This condition is followed by the appearance of hard tumors of the bones, which produce great pains at night and great apprehension in the daytime. These tumors are called gummata. They have a variety of form and characteristics. As the disease grows old it assumes many forms, such as corrosive and putrid ulcers, serpiginous eruptions (these are very common), chancre-like ulcers, gangrenous and virulent sores, cavernous lesions, fistulas, discharging sinuses from the bones, all very difficult to heal, but the pains are the most terrible of all of these conditions, as they may be arthritic in nature, affect the sciatic nerve, the feet and many other places.[2]

The revolting scenes included patients with great stinking ulcers that exposed the bone, noseless faces with powerful fetid breath, and broken-down gummas.[2] It was called the "serpentine disease" because of its loathsome nature.

The condition was widespread in Spain and Italy by 1498. In 1531 Hieronymous Fracastorius described the disease in a mythical poem in which a shepherd named Syphilis cursed the sun for its excessive heat and thereby offended the gods. As punishment for this he was felled by a morbid condition in which his face became an abomination even to himself, his body withered away, and his bones rotted. It is from the name of this "sinister shepherd" that the word syphilis comes. Fracastorius also recognized that the disease is sexually transmitted.

The condition was treated ineffectively and, without very good reason, with various preparations of mercury. Diagnosis and treatment remained at a standstill for the following four centuries, except for the useful addition of potassium iodide in 1835. All depended on finding the cause of the disease. In 1905 Schaudinn and Hoffmann were victorious; they identified the spirochete although they did not prove that the gimlet-like organism was in fact the cause of syphilis. That remained for Noguchi, who established the relationship with animal studies in 1913. In the interval Ehrlich had been experimenting with various organic preparations of arsenic. In 1909, after two years of work, and on his 606th attempt, success was achieved: A solution was found that would kill the organisms but not the animal. It was a preparation of arsphenamine trade-named Salvarsan (from *salvus* and *sanus,* meaning "healthy"), sometimes known as Ehrlich 606.

The central problems were now solved and treatment could be applied. The names of distinguished physicians were attached to characteristic features of the disease, e.g., John Hunter (Hunter's chancre), Jean Charcot (Charcot's knee), Sir Jonathan Hutchinson (Hutchinson's teeth), and John Clutton (Clutton's joints). The clinical stages were delineated, the pathologic changes were classified, serologic tests were devised, and, in 1943, Mahoney found penicillin to be an effective therapeutic agent that could avoid the toxic reactions of the arsenic compounds. Thus the violent "plague" that had ravaged Europe became understood and was finally controlled.

The organism causing syphilis is the spirochete *Treponema pallidum.* It is a slender, loosely coiled, slowly motile organism slightly longer than the diameter of an erythrocyte. It divides by fission, the replication time is about 30 hours, and the organism succumbs quickly outside the body.

There are six main clinicopathologic aspects of syphilis. These comprise the chancre, which is characteristic of the primary stage; mucous plaques and cutaneous eruptions, which occur during the secondary stage; and involvement of the cardiovascular and central nervous systems, which develops in the tertiary stage after a long latent period. The tertiary stage also includes isolated organ lesions. The sixth aspect is congenital syphilis, which is, of course, distinct from the others.

The temporal relationships of these stages involve the entire remaining lifetime of the patient. The initial lesion is usually on the external genitalia, where the spirochetes penetrate abraded skin or mucous membrane. The organisms become widespread throughout the body within a few hours.[3] The chancre develops at the point of entry three to four weeks after the exposure. It lasts for two to five weeks and then heals spontaneously. About six weeks later the secondary stage appears, and this consists of fever, widespread lymphadenopathy, and mucocutaneous eruptions. During this stage there may also be perineal plaques (condyloma latum) and "moth-eaten" alopecia. During this stage serologic tests for syphilis become positive. The secondary stage also subsides spontaneously, usually in two to six weeks, but occasionally recurs. It is followed by a long latent period lasting 10 to 20 years. At the end of the latent period about one-third of patients develop tertiary syphilis, which consists especially of cardiovascular disease or neurosyphilis. The other two-thirds remain asymptomatic and some spontaneously become seronegative. Without treatment, therefore, syphilis is a prolonged disease that is spread over most of the lifetime of the patient.

The two main pathologic reactions of syphilis are chronic interstitial inflammation and gumma formation. The interstitial inflammation is characterized by pronounced infiltration of tissue with lymphocytes and plasma cells, often with a conspicuous perivascular concentration. The inflammation tends to be focal and sharply delineated in the primary and secondary stages. Fibrosis, widespread perivascular inflammation, and associated tissue degeneration are the principle changes of tertiary disease. In addition, the gumma forms. It is a solid mass of firm, somewhat resilient, necrotic tissue that is sharply demarcated and measures 2 to 10 cm in diameter. The necrosis is coagulative, with discernible outlines of the normal tissue pattern. At the margins of the gumma there are lymphocytes, plasma cells, fibroblasts, and capillaries. In addition, a small number of multinucleated giant cells form. The lesion is thus distinct and differs from tuberculosis by the coagulative nature of the necrosis, the vascularization of the periphery, and the sparse number of multinucleated giant cells. In addition, gummas tend to be widely spaced, solitary lesions.

The chancre is a single, shallow, round superficial erosion that measures 1 to 2 cm in diameter and presents a clean, light red base from which clear serum transudes. The surface is ulcerated and the margins are not undermined. The transuding fluid contains spirochetes. The subjacent inflammation consists of plasma cells, lymphocytes, and histiocytes packed tightly into the dermis; the margins are sharply delineated. The chancre is thus firm and buttonlike, lying as a movable plaque in the otherwise soft skin. It is the hard or Hunterian chancre, and it differs from the soft, otherwise similar erosion of chancroid ("soft chancre").

In the secondary stage the skin eruption covers the entire body, including such unusual sites as the palms of the hands and the soles of the feet. The macular changes, often copper-colored, are slight except for scant infiltration with plasma cells and oc-

casional melanocytes. The flat papules, however, arise on the warm, moist surfaces of the body as condylomata lata, and these display pronounced acanthosis of the epidermis as well as dense infiltrations with lymphocytes and plasma cells. The surfaces of these wet plaques, which arise especially on the perineal skin, are covered with infectious spirochetes, as are the mucous "patches" of the buccal mucosa, which teem with organisms. The "shotty," painless enlargement of lymph nodes is due to nonspecific reticular hyperplasia.

The tertiary disease affects principally the cardiovascular system. The main lesion is aortitis that involves the portion above the diaphragm and may extend proximally to affect the ostia of the coronary arteries or the cusps of the aortic valve. The intima reveals an opaque, pearly white thickening that is longitudinally wrinkled. Microscopically the parallel fibers of the elastica show patchy destruction with fibrous replacement. In addition, the vasa vasorum extend deeply into the media and reveal perivascular "cuffing" with lymphocytes and plasma cells. The adventitia is occupied by small or "miliary" gummas, and sometimes is simply thick and fibrosed. The least effect of these changes is a slight dilation of the thoracic aorta.

The characteristic consequence is the formation of an aneurysm. These are regularly saccular and measure 5 to 25 cm in diameter with a large, discrete opening into the aorta (see Figure 11-37). About half occur in the ascending portion, one-third in the arch, and the remainder in the descending thoracic aorta.[4] The wall consists of thin layers of fibrous connective tissue infiltrated with lymphocytes and plasma cells. The lumen is often filled with laminated accretions of old and recent thrombi. Clinical manifestations are abundant as the large, bulky aneurysms press against adjacent mediastinal structures. Hoarseness and a brassy cough result from pressure on the recurrent laryngeal nerve as it loops underneath the aortic arch. Irritation of the superior cervical sympathetic ganglia causes dilation of the pupil, widening of the ocular slit, and eventually ptosis of the eyelid. Compression of the azygos vein is attended by a right hydrothorax, while compression of the superior vena cava causes edema and dusky cyanosis of the head and neck. The trachea may become compressed, leading to dyspnea, or attached to the aneurysm by fibrous adhesions, leading to a tracheal tug that is synchronous with the beating of the heart. Pressure may also affect the subclavian or innominate arteries so that the radial pulse is asymmetrical and may even disappear in one arm. The soft esophagus yields to the mass, and dysphagia results. On the posterior body wall the aneurysm abuts the spine; the vertebral centra give way and become atrophic while the intervertebral discs, for reasons not clear, resist the pressure and become projecting ridges between the atrophic vertebral bodies. On chest X-ray a mass distorts the outline of the mediastinum. As the aneurysm gradually enlarges, bone atrophies, the body wall yields, and a large, smooth, pulsating mass bulges below the skin. Eventually rupture occurs, especially into the pericardial sac, the pleural space, a large bronchus, or onto the anterior thoracic wall.

Whether or not an aneurysm forms, the pearly white intimal thickening and medial inflammation extend proximally and eventually reach into the sinuses of Valsalva, where the ostia of the coronary arteries lie. The ostia of these vessels gradually become stenosed and eventually may become totally occluded. In this event the myocardium is nourished by the thebesian vessels, which open through the endocardium into the ventricles.[4] This remarkable adjustment of the heart is possible because of the slow development of the stenosis. The ostial closures are frequently associated with angina but seldom cause infarction, and are often attended by sudden death.

Adjacent to the coronary ostia are the commissures of the aortic valve, and these structures are also caught up in the advancing syphilitic process. As the ascending aorta gradually dilates, a unique lesion arises: The upper surfaces and lateral portions of the aortic cusps are drawn toward the aortic wall, with which they fuse, so that the commissures are separated and a regurgitative channel is formed between them. It is of less consequence that the cusps themselves, while foreshortened at the lateral margins, also become thick, opaque, and fibrosed. The physiologic disturbance is aortic insufficiency so that the pulse pressure is wide, a bounding or water-hammer pulse is produced, and a "pistol-shot" sound is heard over the peripheral arteries of medium size. Even the smallest vessels may reflect this change; the retinae and nail beds may visibly blanch as the insufficiency allows the diastolic pressure to drop. Jet lesions of pale gray fibrosis form on the endocardium of the interventricular septum from the rushing backflow of the column of blood. The left ventricle, of course, undergoes dilation and hypertrophy, so that the heart may come to weigh in excess of 800 gm. Death occurs by congestive failure. The process does not affect any other valve. The principal cardiovascular consequences of tertiary syphilis are thus a chronic inflammation of the aortic media that weakens the wall, tends to aneurysm formation, and extends to involve secondarily the coronary ostia with angina pectoris, and the aortic valve with insufficiency and congestive failure.

The other anatomic structure especially affected by tertiary syphilis is the central nervous system. There are three main categories of involvement: meningovascular, paresis, and tabes dorsalis. Meningovascular syphilis is characterized by fibrosis of the pia-arachnoid, which becomes thick and pale gray, and by perivascular infiltration of the meninges that extends into the cerebral cortex. Thus lymphocytes and plasma cells "cuff" the meningeal vessels and extend into the Virchow-Robin spaces of the cortical tissue. In addition, medium-sized arteries show subintimal fibrosis with stenosis of the lumens. Thrombi form, and cerebral dysfunction is attributed to vascular closure.[5] Clinical manifestations include headache, irritability, loss of memory, dysfunction of cranial nerves, and occasionally delirium and convulsions.

Paresis is due to extension of the spirochetes into the cerebral tissue. Although gross changes are often inconspicuous, three lesions stand out in the advanced case. The frontoparietal lobes are atrophic, so that the brain is decreased in weight, and the gyri are narrow with widened sulci over the affected parts. The overlying meninges are thick and opaque, and on section the gray cortex is noticeably thin. Microscopically the cortical nerve layers are in disarray and various degrees of neuronal degeneration are observed. Lymphocytes and plasma cells are present around cortical vessels within the Virchow-Robin spaces. Clinically the patient with paresis displays obtundation, confusion, a change of personality, loss of memory, and inappropriate use of words as well as gestures. As the dementia progresses, outright psychosis develops.

Tabes dorsalis is a demyelinating process that affects the posterior columns of the lumbosacral portion of the spinal cord. Cross sections of the cord reveal shrinkage and contraction of the posterior columns. The overlying meninges are thickened and chronically inflamed. Microsections disclose demyelination, reactive gliosis, vascular thickening, and degeneration of axis cylinders. The process also extends into the dorsal nerve roots. Why the process affects principally the lumbosacral segment of the cord is not clear.

The functional disturbances are mainly proprioceptive, sensory, and autonomic. Autonomic disturbance produces loss of vesical tone, weakness of micturition, re-

tention of urine, and dilation of the bladder. The residual urine becomes infected, the infection ascends the urinary tract, and pyelonephritis results. The proprioceptive disturbance is characteristic: The patient becomes unsteady, walks with a wide gait, and learns to slap his feet against the pavement in order to stimulate a sensation of their position. Walking is especially difficult in the dark, and ataxia develops. The Romberg sign becomes positive: The patient cannot stand erect with eyes closed without wobbling. The ambulatory disturbances inspired the alternative term for the condition, locomotor ataxia.

Anesthesia of the skin develops, and as the sensation of pain is lost, trauma to the joints passes unnoticed and is repeated. As a result, large joints undergo degeneration, the articular surfaces split apart, and the joint spaces fill with particles of bone and fragments of cartilage. The joint becomes flail and the condition, which is especially frequent in the knee, is known as Charcot's joint. Trophic disturbances also affect the feet, on which painless perforating ulcers arise. The deep tendon reflexes are lost, as is the sense of vibration.

Also characteristic of tabes dorsalis are knife-like, intensely severe, shooting pains that "stab" at the extremities ("lightning pains") and, less frequently, at the abdomen ("abdominal crises"). The latter may be so severe as to cause nausea, vomiting, dehydration, and electrolyte imbalance.

Often associated with tabes dorsalis is some degree of optic atrophy. The incipient stage is evidenced by impairment of the periphery of the visual fields. The characteristic sign of neurosyphilis, however, is the Argyll Robertson pupil, in which the ciliary muscle is unresponsive to light but normally reactive to convergence. The visual disturbance is due to degeneration of the optic fibers, loss of neurons from the retinae, and inflammation of the meninges about the optic tract. It was formerly a common cause of blindness.

Finally, tertiary syphilis may be manifested by the formation of gummas. They most often arise in the liver, where the scarring is coarse and extreme so that a deeply scarred and creased "hepar lobatum" results. Less frequently gummas form in the bones, brain, testes, and skin.

Congenital syphilis is a different category of the disease process. It is transmitted to the fetus only after the fourth month of gestation. This means that treatment of the mother before that time will prevent infection of the fetus, that syphilis is not a cause of early abortion, and that malformation of structures formed before the fourth month cannot be attributed to the disease.[6] When placental transmission does take place, however, all the tissues of the placenta and fetus are subject to invasion by the spirochetes. The placenta becomes abnormally large and heavy, and the chorionic villi are coarse, thick, blunt, and fused. The abundant interstitial tissue is infiltrated with fibroblasts and scattered leukocytes.

The fetus may reveal the infection at birth, i.e., have early congenital syphilis, or may develop characteristic lesions later in childhood, i.e., display late congenital syphilis. The early lesions consist especially of shallow, red, weeping mucocutaneous erosions about the nose, mouth, and anus. The lesions teem with spirochetes and are highly infective. The skin tends to split, and the linear scars that result disfigure the complexion as rhagades (cracks) form. A desquamative rash may cover the entire body but is characteristic over the palms of the hands and soles of the feet. Shortly after birth, respiratory difficulty may be the cause of death. In this event the characteristic lesion is pneumonia alba, so-called because of the abundant interstitial fibrous connective tissue that obscures the pulmonary vessels and turns the lungs firm, heavy, and pallid. The process encroaches on the alveoli and the lining cells desquamate and fill the air sacs so that breathing and air exchange are impaired. Hepatic involvement is widespread: The sinusoids are disrupted, connective tissue replaces the lobules, and diffuse fibrosis results. Any part of the newborn, including the central nervous system, may be affected.

Late congenital syphilis becomes evident during childhood and adolescence. The widespread, silent, fibrosing reaction now becomes manifest in a variety of tissues, which show the effects of impaired development. The vomer fails to form, and a "saddle-nose" deformity results. The skull shows prominent bossing. The developmental process at the ends of the long bones is in disarray, so that slippage or dislocation of the epiphyses is common. Over the shafts of the long bones, the periosteum is inflamed, hemorrhage occurs, and organization of these processes causes thickening of the subperiosteal cortex. This is especially noticeable over the lower legs, which show anterior bowing. The condition is known as saber shins. Transient joint effusions, bilateral, painless, and especially of the knees, are known as Clutton's joints. In the eyes interstitial keratitis clouds the corneas and causes blindness. The incisor teeth may be pointed or notched, and the molars may show a nodular disfiguration of the biting surfaces, called mulberry molars. Eighth-nerve deafness and optic atrophy may develop. Punctate foci of atrophy discolor the retinal surfaces so that the characteristic "salt-and-pepper" fundi are observed. The combination of deafness, interstitial keratitis, and notched permanent incisors is known as Hutchinson's triad. Only cardiovascular involvement is infrequent in congenital syphilis. Although therapy may control the inflammatory process, the abnormalities of development are permanent. The importance of detecting syphilis during pregnancy is thus evident.

## VIRUSES

Viruses are infectious microorganisms of worldwide distribution that cause more human disease than any other class of living agents. The first human virus was identified in 1901 by Walter Reed in his investigation of the cause of yellow fever.[7] The technique that made discovery of viruses possible was the use of filters in which the apertures were too small to allow the passage of bacteria. Since these pioneering events, more than 300 viruses that infect humans have been found. These are segregated into eight major groups according to such factors as size, shape, lipid content, and nucleic acid composition. The major groups are shown in Table 5-2.

Viruses measure less than 200 nm in diameter and are hence below the resolving power of the light microscope. They consist of a core of nucleic acid and a shell of protein. The shell is called a capsid, and the combination of the shell and the nucleic acid is called a virion. The nucleic acid accounts for the heritable characteristics of the virus during multiplication, and the protein shell accounts for the stimulation of antibody on the part of the host. The nucleic acid may be RNA or DNA, but not both. Viruses live only within cells; on entry the capsid is shed and the nucleic acid aggregate attaches itself to the nucleus and saps energy from the host cell. The energy is used for multiplication of the separated virion parts, i.e., more nucleic acid and new capsid protein. On leaving the cell, the total virion is re-formed from its independent parts. In this process the host cell may recover or be injured beyond repair.

There are specific viruses for animals, plants, insects, and bacteria. Bacterial viruses are known as bacteriophages. Animal viruses have affinity for particular tissues, or target organs. There are accordingly dermatropic, pneumotropic, enterotropic, hepatotropic, and neurotropic viruses. The organisms enter the body through the mucous membranes of the respiratory and digestive tracts and, less frequently, may cross the placenta. After the initial infection the organisms spread throughout the body (viremia), localize in the target organ, proliferate in that tissue with adverse effects upon those cells, and are later released from the body as the host overcomes the infection. The pathologic changes in the host cells are primarily degenerative with edema, pyknosis, karyolysis, and rupture. Inflammation is lymphocytic and slight unless there is a secondary bacterial infection. The degenerative process may be slight or pronounced, and it may take place rapidly or over a long period of time. During the time of the infection, the host cell may disclose an inclusion body in either the cytoplasm or nucleus.

The host overcomes the infection by destroying the virions in the reticuloendothelial system, by developing antibodies against the virion, and by producing interferons. The protein of the capsid stimulates antibody formation, and the antibodies coat the virus, blocking its infectivity. Thus humoral immunity is stimulated by natural viral infection and by unnatural infection (vaccination), in which a nonvirulent form of the organism is introduced into the tis-

**Table 5-2.**

## Major groups of human viruses

| Virus | Disease |
|---|---|
| RNAviruses | |
| Picornavirus | Poliomyelitis |
| Reovirus | Possibly common cold |
| Arbovirus | Yellow fever |
| Myxovirus | Mumps, measles, rubella, influenza |
| | |
| DNAviruses | |
| Papovavirus | Verruca vulgaris (warts) |
| Adenovirus | Pharyngitis |
| Herpesvirus | Chickenpox, shingles, cold sores, genital herpes |
| Poxvirus | Smallpox |

sue. In some viral infections the immunity is transient, but in most it is permanent.

Virus-infected cells also produce soluble proteins that interfere with additional cell infection. These protein substances, called interferons, contribute to the recovery of the host by limiting the extent of the infection. The mechanism is not known, but it is not humoral immunity; interferons are not antibodies. Interferons are evoked by all major viruses, they are nonspecific in their antiviral effect, and they are useful in extremely small amounts. Moreover, interferons are nontoxic and only weakly antigenic, and exert their effects within 24 hours. The feature that limits their importance is species specificity, which means that they must be produced in human cells, or monkey kidney cells, to be therapeutically effective. It is nevertheless possible that interferons will have an expanding role in the treatment of viral infections as recombinant DNA research makes possible their large-scale production in bacteria.

The main viral diseases seen in the United States include smallpox, chickenpox, rubeola, rubella, mumps, and the simplex and zoster forms of herpes infections. Yellow fever is also of both historical and practical interest, the latter because of the burgeoning travel of Americans and others about the world. Hepatotropic viruses causing serum and infectious hepatitis will be considered in Chapter 14.

### Smallpox (variola)

Smallpox is a focal necrotizing reaction of skin and mucous membranes due to a DNA-containing poxvirus that produces a severe disease, especially in Asia (variola major), and a mild but otherwise similar disease (variola minor or alastrim). The virus is transmitted to the respiratory mucosa by dust or droplet infection. An incubation period follows, after which the onset is sudden with fever, headache, severe back pain, vomiting, and prostration. Within five days macules form on the face and extremities that progress to pustules, which are followed by scabs and crusts; these separate in three weeks to leave pockmarks from scarring of the dermis. Eosinophilic Guarnieri bodies form in the cytoplasm of infected epithelial cells. The lesions are all of the same age. The pocks may be discrete, confluent, or hemorrhagic, and the mortality worsens substantially with the last of these forms. In Asia the mortality from discrete variola major was formerly about 25 per cent, with death usually due to bronchopneumonia.[8] Alastrim is similar but less severe: Toxicity is slight, infection of the pocks is infrequent, and convalescence is rapid. The mortality is less than 1 per cent. Antibiotics are useful in aborting the pustular stage of both conditions. Immunity is strong and long-lasting. The viral particles survive in dust and remain infective for years.

Smallpox was a worldwide scourge in the 18th century. The mortality of the disease was 20 to 30 per cent, and in Russia every seventh child died of it; those who survived were grotesquely pocked. Late in that century a gentle country doctor, Edward Jenner, observed that milkmaids were immune to the disease. He also noticed that cowpox, or vaccinia (*vacca* means cow), occurred on the hands of these maids, who carried the infection from animal to animal. On both the udders of the cows and the hands of the maids, small pimples formed that progressed to vesicles, later scabbed, and finally left a punctate scar or pock. The systemic illness accompanying these skin changes was mild. Jenner conceived of protecting those vulnerable to smallpox by inoculating them with scrapings from the cowpox lesions. Although Jesty had done this earlier, no systematic evaluation of the procedure had been undertaken. The scheme was tried, and those inoculated became immune. The medical profession, however, scoffed at the idea. In 1796 Jenner's paper to the Royal Society was rejected. He persisted, gathering more evidence and pursuing his conviction. Finally the obstinate yielded as success became evident. Vaccination was widely undertaken and the disease was conquered. Although Jenner was lionized, he continued to practice medicine in the country, attending a charity patient two days before his death at the age of 74 in 1823. His fame had become great, and his statue replaced Nelson's for four years in Trafalgar Square. Later, his likeness in stone was removed to Kensington Gardens and Lord Nelson's statue was returned to the center of London. It has nevertheless been predicted that as the memory of history dims and events are placed in their proper perspective, Jenner will be revered while Nelson will recede into the shadows of obscurity; Jenner saved more lives than wars ever took.[9] On May 8, 1980, the World Health Organization announced the eradication of smallpox from the earth.

## Chickenpox (varicella)

Chickenpox is caused by a DNA herpesvirus that enters the respiratory tract, proliferates in the viscera, and localizes in the skin and occasionally the lungs. The onset is sudden, with a macular rash principally on the face and body that transforms into papules and then vesicles. The extremities are relatively spared. The rash comes on in crops, and pustules are infrequent. In these clinical ways the condition differs from smallpox. The dermal lesion consists of focal vacuolar degeneration of the epithelium with blister formation. In the epithelium lining the vesicles giant cells (Tzank cells) with large intranuclear inclusions may be seen. Rarely, disseminated lesions form in the viscera. Ordinarily the reaction subsides spontaneously, the condition is self-limited, and no scarring of the skin results. When chickenpox affects adults, however, a viral pneumonia with a mortality of 20 per cent may develop. Immunity is lasting and second attacks are rare. Maternal disease during pregnancy does not affect the fetus.[8]

## Measles (rubeola)

Measles is an exanthematous disease, chiefly of children, that is caused by an RNA myxovirus. The organism enters the respiratory tract by droplet infection, proliferates in the lymphoid structures of the body, and localizes in the skin. The clinical onset is abrupt, with catarrh, coryza, cough, and sore throat. In this pre-eruptive stage, the buccal mucosa reveals bright red foci of discoloration measuring 1 to 3 mm in diameter with minute white centers that are known as Koplik's spots. These are pathognomonic of the disease. The rash then appears, beginning behind the ears and on the forehead, and later spreading over the face, neck, trunk, and limbs. The rash is papular and discrete and consists of foci of epidermal necrosis and vacuolization with slight acute inflammation in the subjacent dermis. Multinucleated giant cells form in the lung and lymphoid tissues, including the appendix, and are known as Warthin-Finkeldey cells. The condition is self-limited and without residua unless a secondary bacterial infection develops or, less often, encephalitis or viral pneumonitis. The illness confers strong, lasting immunity. The clinical events may be aborted by giving $\gamma$-globulin containing neutralizing antibodies. Active and passive immunizations are practiced, the former with live attenuated organisms and the latter with formalin-killed organisms. There is no definite evidence that the embryo is harmed by maternal measles in early pregnancy.[8]

## German measles (rubella)

German measles is a highly infectious myxovirus disease of children over 1 year of age that is characterized by fever, catarrh, enlargement of cervical and axillary lymph nodes, and a macular rash that appears first on the face and then rapidly spreads over the body. Outbreaks among young adults are not uncommon. The condition is self-limited and recovery is complete. When the patient is a woman in her first trimester of pregnancy, however, the risk of fetal complications is high. The virus crosses the placenta and interferes with the cellular differentiation of certain organs. The characteristic triad includes congenital cataracts, deafness, and heart disease. Foremost are patent ductus arteriosus and interventricular septal defects. Maternal infection is also associated with abortion, stillbirth, low birth weight, and increased mortality during the first year of life. Protection against these complications is provided by injection of $\gamma$-globulin.

## Mumps
Mumps is an acute infectious disease caused by an RNA myxovirus that is contracted by droplet infection. It appears to spread from the mouth through Stensen's ducts to localize in the parotid glands. Children are most frequently affected. The parotids swell and become tender and painful because of edema and inflammation that is mostly interstitial and mononuclear. The condition subsides spontaneously without residua. The most frequent complication is an associated orchitis that causes necrosis of the seminiferous tubules and leaves the testis focally atrophic and hyalinized. Sterility is uncommon, however, as the condition is often localized to a part of the testis and is seldom bilateral. Secondary involvement of the pancreas, ovary, and meninges is uncommon.

## Herpes simplex (cold sore)
Infection with the herpes simplex virus causes vesicle formation on the skin and mucous membranes. The vesicles are popularly known as cold sores or fever blisters. They are due to a focal ballooning degeneration of the epidermis. The lining cells of the vesicles reveal intranuclear inclusion bodies and, in addition, multinucleated giant cells form because the virus interferes with the process of mitotic division. Hyperemia becomes pronounced in the tissue around the vesicles, and a small number of

inflammatory cells accumulate. Although the focal degenerative process is ordinarily localized to the skin and mucous membranes, wide visceral dissemination of the vesicles may occur. The process is self-limited and subsides without sequelae.

## Herpes zoster (shingles)
Herpes zoster refers to a painful eruption of the skin that is usually unilateral and is localized to one or more dermatomes corresponding to the associated dorsal root ganglia. In over half of cases the eruption occurs on the trunk, with the cervical and lumbar regions next in frequency. The cranial nerves may also be affected, and the ophthalmic branch of the trigeminal nerve is most often involved. The eruption consists of maculopapular plaques surrounded by zones of erythema that progress to vesicles which become pustular and then crusted. With trigeminal involvement, the lesion occurs over the upper third of the face on one side, extending frequently to the eye to cause a pronounced keratoconjunctivitis. The crusts fall away in one to three weeks, but resolution may be prolonged.

This infection is due to a virus different from that of herpes simplex, and evidence now suggests that herpes zoster is a localized recurrence of chickenpox in a person who has recovered from that disease and is partially immune to it.[7] The varicella-zoster organism is therefore referred to as the V-Z virus. The condition is not epidemic and occurs sporadically without seasonal or occupational incidence. Two-thirds of the patients are over 45, and the severity of the condition worsens with age. The illness usually subsides spontaneously, although the course may be long and the suffering, because of neural involvement, severe.

## Yellow fever
Yellow fever is an acute infectious disease caused by an arbovirus that is seen in the Caribbean and tropical Americas, from which it spread during the 17th and 18th

centuries to cause one of humanity's most devastating plagues. In the 19th century as many as 200,000 would succumb in a single epidemic as it spread through a large urban center. The mortality approached 10 per cent, the cause was unknown, and there were neither therapeutic methods nor preventive measures. In 1900 the Yellow Fever Commission was established, and Dr. Walter Reed was sent to Cuba to study the disease. He discovered that the causative organism circulates in the blood, that it is a filtrable agent, and that it is transmitted by the *Aëdes aegypti (argenteus)* mosquito. The disease was promptly controlled by antimosquito campaigns.

Subsequently it was found that yellow fever occurs in two forms. Urban yellow fever is transmitted from person to person by the mosquito, so that humans serve as both the reservoirs and the victims of the disease. In contrast, sylvan or jungle yellow fever occurs in monkeys and is transmitted among them by mosquitoes with only occasional, incidental transmission to humans. Endemic foci in jungle regions thus persist. Clinically the onset is abrupt, with fever, headache, nausea, vomiting, and muscle aches and pains. After a brief abatement the fever returns, jaundice appears, the heart rate slows, and bleeding from the gums, mouth, nose, and rectum develops. Leukopenia is characteristic, proteinuria and oliguria are frequent, and uremia follows. Finally the blood pressure falls, coma develops, and delirium precedes death. There is no specific treatment. The main lesions are in the liver and kidney. Extensive zonal hepatic necrosis is characteristic, with masses of acidophilic debris known as Councilman bodies forming in the hepatic lobules. The renal disease is tubular, secondary, and in the nature of nephrosis. For those who do not succumb, recovery may be prolonged but no sequelae are left. The disease has been preventable since Theiler showed in 1937 that a mutant form of the virus with low virulence nevertheless stimulates antibody formation that is strong and long-lasting.[7] Only those not vaccinated are vulnerable to the disease.

## CHLAMYDIAE

Chlamydiae are extremely small intracellular bacteria. They are the causes of trachoma, psittacosis-ornithosis, lymphogranuloma venereum, and urethritis. The organisms are morphologically similar and consist of gram-negative spherules measuring 300 to 1,000 nm in diameter. They live only within the cytoplasm of epithelial cells, where they produce a toxin and cause inflammation that progresses to necrosis. The chlamydiae differ from viruses in that they contain RNA and DNA, they divide by binary fission, and they display rigid walls in which muramic acid is found. The psittacosis-ornithosis organisms are transmitted from bird species to humans, while trachoma and lymphogranuloma organisms infect humans only. All are responsive to sulfonamide drugs or antibiotics.

### Trachoma

Trachoma is an infectious disease of the eyes that occurs principally in Africa and the Middle East, affects 400 million persons the world over, and causes fibrosis of the conjunctivae with gradual development of blindness. The organisms are spread by droplet infection, by dust, by scratching of the eyes, and by flies, which abound where sanitation is substandard. The palpebral and bulbar conjunctivae become inflamed, the process is chronic, reinfection is common, and the fibrous tissue that forms gradually dims the sight. The diagnosis is established by the finding of chlamydial organisms in cells scraped from the conjunctival surfaces. The condition is alleviated or cured by antibiotic therapy.

### Psittacosis-ornithosis

Two chlamydial diseases are transmitted from various species of birds to humans:

psittacosis from psittacine birds, especially parrots and parakeets, and ornithosis from other birds such as pigeons, ducks, turkeys, and chickens. Both cause febrile, flu-like respiratory distress that may progress to pneumonia. The organisms are found in the sputum and in the cytoplasm of the alveolar cells of the lungs. Psittacosis, or parrot fever, is seen in bird owners and pet shop attendants, while ornithosis is seen in poultry farmers and slaughterhouse workers. Without treatment, psittacosis has a mortality of 35 per cent; ornithosis is less severe and the mortality is less than 2 per cent.[8] Both conditions are effectively treated with antibiotics.

### Lymphogranuloma venereum

Lymphogranuloma venereum is a chlamydial disease transmitted by sexual intercourse. It develops in three clinical and pathologic stages. The primary stage consists of a herpetic lesion on the external genitalia of either sex. The organisms are then swept in the lymph current to the man's inguinal nodes, where soft, fluctuant, reddish-purple subcutaneous buboes form. The woman's different lymph drainage carries the organisms to the lymph nodes inside the pelvis so that subcutaneous buboes do not become evident. In the nodes of both sexes, however, minute abscesses form with characteristic palisading of marginal fibroblasts. It is the enlargement and fusion of the abscesses that give rise to the buboes. In the tertiary stage fibrosis becomes pronounced and lymph flow is blocked, resulting in elephantiasis of the external genitalia, especially in men, and pelvic fibrosis with rectal stricture in women. Diagnosis is aided by the Frei test, in which bubo material from a patient with the disease is heat-sterilized and injected into the forearm skin of a person suspected of having the disease. The development of a zone of erythema with central papulation at the injection site constitutes a positive test. Patients with lymphogranuloma venereum also have an elevation of serum globulins. The infection is responsive to sulfonamide treatment.

### RICKETTSIAE

Rickettsiae were discovered in the second decade of the 20th century by Ricketts in the United States and Prowazek in Austria. Both men died of the disease in the course of their investigations. Rickettsiae naturally infect humans and lice. The organisms are minute coccobacillary forms that are intermediate between bacteria and viruses. They resemble bacteria by containing RNA, DNA, and muramic acid, and they resemble viruses by being obligate intracellular parasites of small size. Their two own unique features include a selective preference for the endothelial cells of small blood vessels and a reliance on arthropods for transmission from person to person. There are four main rickettsial diseases, but one is not seen in the United States (scrub typhus) and another occurs in the United States only at a few endemic sites in cattle workers (Q fever). The main rickettsial diseases are typhus and Rocky Mountain spotted fever.

### Typhus

Typhus is carried by head and body lice living in unclean garments. Crowding and lack of sanitation are thus the conditions in which they thrive. These conditions have prevailed throughout history, as has the disease, especially in times of war when people are thrown together under adverse circumstances. Typhus is so easily spread that military campaigns have been aborted by the disease, and the course of history has been influenced by it. It is speculated that only malaria has been the cause of more human illness than typhus.

The louse *Pediculus humanus* bites the victim and defecates at the same time. The victim scratches the bite and pushes the rickettsiae into the wound. The organism, *R. prowazekii*, named after the original investigators, invades the endothelial cells of small vessels, proliferates there, and causes them to swell. The vessels become thrombosed and leukocytes accumulate in the perivascular tissue. Fluid leaks from the vessels, dehydration follows, and bronchopneumonia becomes a terminal event. These changes are widespread but have special predilection for the brain, heart, and skin.

The patient manifests high fever, severe headache, and a widespread macular rash. The condition subsides in about two weeks. During this time antibodies form and agglutinins in the blood cause a strain of *Proteus* (OX-19) to agglutinate. This is the unique Weil-Felix reaction, which is positive in 90 per cent of persons with typhus and therefore constitutes an important diagnostic test. Treatment consists of delousing the patient with soap, weak Lysol, and an insecticide and applying tetracyclines, which are effective against the organism. A vaccine of killed organisms is useful in aborting the illness.

Without treatment the organisms circulate in the blood during the febrile stage. During this time the louse, which takes four to six blood meals per day, ingests the organisms, which multiply in the intestinal cells and are deposited on the skin of the next person at the time of defecation. Thus the condition is spread. During the ensuing afebrile period, the lice scurry away from the patient, who then dies. The lice eventually succumb to the disease, but not before many more blood meals and spreading of the infection. Antilouse campaigns are the most effective prophylactic measures, although a vaccine exists.

The condition may recur in a mild form, when it is known as Brill-Zinsser disease. There is also a mild rickettsial disease caused by *R. mooseri* or *R. typhi*, which naturally infects rats and mice and is sporadically transmitted to man by the rat flea *Xenopsylla cheopis*. This is known as murine typhus.

## Rocky Mountain spotted fever

In the western United States rabbits and small rodents are the animals on which wood ticks live. The wood tick, *Dermacentor andersoni*, becomes infected with the organism *R. rickettsii*, which it harbors all its life. The tick infects the animals, and the animals infect more ticks. Occasionally the tick bites a human. Although Rocky Mountain spotted fever was first recognized in the western United States, the condition has now been seen nearly everywhere in the Western Hemisphere.

The onset is abrupt, with fever, chills, nausea, vomiting, and excruciating headache. Shortly after this a macular exanthem appears on the extremities, spreads onto the trunk, and becomes blotchy, dark purple, and hemorrhagic. There follow delirium, shock, dehydration, and renal failure. The cause of these events is spread of *R. rickettsii* to the endothelial cells of small vessels, where an acute angiitis develops. The organs most prominently affected include the brain, heart, skeletal muscles, lungs, and kidneys. In these tissues microinfarcts may form from the vascular occlusions. Diagnosis is aided by the Weil-Felix reaction, which is regularly positive, and by the nature of the exanthem, which is distinctive. The fever abates after two to three weeks. Either the patient recovers or shock, dehydration, uremia, and bronchopneumonia are the terminal events.

The overall mortality is about 20 per cent, although this rises to 50 per cent for patients over 40 years of age. In 1941 a vaccine was prepared by growing the organisms on the yolk sacs of eggs, and in 1948 broad-spectrum antibiotics were found to be effective against the organism.[7] As a consequence, treatment reduced the mortality to 5 per cent, and these developments mitigated the dread nature of the infectious disease. Prevention includes avoidance of tick-infested regions and immunization against the organism.

# REFERENCES

1. Dubos R, Dubos J: *The Great White Plague*. Boston: Little, Brown, 1952

2. Dennie CC: *A History of Syphilis*. Springfield, Il: Thomas, 1962

3. *Syphilis, a Synopsis*, Public Health Service Publication No. 1660. Washington, DC: U.S. Department of Health, Education, and Welfare, Bureau of Disease Prevention and Environmental Control, Jan 1968

4. Moritz AR: Syphilitic coronary arteritis. *Arch Pathol* 11:44, 1931

5. Moore RA: *A Textbook of Pathology*, 2nd ed. Philadelphia: Saunders, 1951

6. Dennie CC, Pakula SF: *Congenital Syphilis*. Philadelphia: Lea & Febiger, 1940

7. Horsfall FL, Tamm I: *Viral and Rickettsial Infections of Man*, 4th ed. Philadelphia: Lippincott, 1965

8. Rhodes AJ, Van Rohyen CE: *Textbook of Virology*, 5th ed. Baltimore: Williams & Wilkins, 1968

9. Riedman SR: *Shots Without Guns*. New York: Rand McNally, 1960

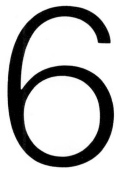

# IMMUNOLOGIC DISORDERS

In order to understand the immunologic disorders it is necessary to review the components of the immune system, study the mechanisms of immune injury, and apply them to the main categories of disease. These mechanisms are inadequate reactions (immunodeficiency disorders), excessive reactions (hypersensitivity diseases), and misdirected reactions (autoimmune diseases).

Immunologic reactions begin with the union of antigen and antibody. The antigen is harmful, the antibody is protective, and the purpose of the union is for the antibody to neutralize, immobilize, or destroy the antigen, which would otherwise be harmful to the host. An antigen is any substance that stimulates the formation of an antibody. Common antigens include bacteria, bacterial toxins, and protein-containing substances such as horse serum (tetanus antitoxin), animal dander, pollens, and molds. Some foods (shellfish) and certain drugs (penicillin) are also antigenic. The antigen may be attached to a carrier molecule, and on separation from this may lose its antigenicity. It is then a partial antigen, or hapten. Reattachment to a carrier molecule will restore its antigenicity. Different molecules may carry the same hapten.

Antibody is a protein produced by the reticuloendothelial system as a result of exposure to an antigen. The reaction may be specific, with the antibody reacting only with the antigen that stimulated its formation, or nonspecific, with the antibody re-

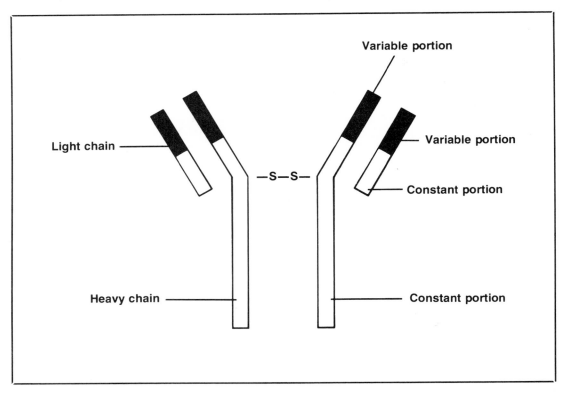

**Figure 6-1.** Structure of antibody. The light chain and the portion of the heavy chain with the variable segment from the tip to the disulfide bond are the fragments with the antigen-binding sites. They are accordingly known as the Fab portions of the compound.

acting with a variety of antigens. The non-specific reaction is attributable to the same hapten's being attached to different carrier molecules.

Antibodies are of two kinds: circulating (humoral) and fixed (cell-bound). Circulating antibodies consist of $\gamma$-globulins that are classified according to their chemical properties into five classes, designated by the letters G, A, M, D, and E. About 80 per cent of circulating immunoglobulin (Ig) is IgG, 20 per cent is IgA or IgM, and only small amounts of IgD and IgE are normally present. Each immunoglobulin consists of two light chains and two heavy chains, both consisting of polypeptides and connected by a disulfide (S—S) bond. Each chain has a constant sequence of amino acids that is characteristic of the class of immunoglobulin, and a variable sequence that provides it with antigenic specificity (Figure 6-1).

Humoral antibodies (immunoglobulins) are indirect products of B lymphocytes. These cells, which constitute 10 to 30 per cent of circulating lymphocytes, originate in the bone marrow, live only a few days, and on contact with an antigen change into plasmablasts. They then mature into plasma cells and secrete immunoglobulins. B lymphocytes are found in the follicles of the spleen, lymph nodes, and Peyer's patches of the ileum. They are morphologically identical with T lymphocytes and are distinguished from them by surface markers that allow for rosette formation with sheep erythrocytes.

Fixed antibody is cell-bound, evidently to T lymphocytes, which make up 70 to 80 per cent of lymphoid cells in the circulation. As T lymphocytes develop they pass through the thymus, which modifies their function and justifies the term thymus-dependent lymphocytes. Their life span is long (months to years), and they are found between the follicles in the spleen, lymph nodes, and Peyer's patches. They are also identifiable by special surface markers. On contact with antigens, some T lymphocytes secrete lymphokines while others become cytolytic (killer) cells. Lymphokines include activators of macrophages, which are then able to destroy bacteria and tumor cells; chemotaxins that attract neutrophilic leukocytes; a toxin that is lethal to tumor cells in vitro; and interferon, which protects host cells from further invasion by viruses. Thus macrophages, which circulate in the blood as monocytes and are widely distributed in lymphoid tissue as histiocytes, also participate in the immune reaction. Nevertheless, fixed antibodies are cell-bound and are not measurable in the serum.

In addition to the foregoing, the complement system participates in the immune reaction. Complement consists of 11 proteins linked together in a sequential cascade not unlike that of the blood coagulation factors. The system remains dormant until it is activated by the union of antigens with complement-fixing antibodies (IgG and IgM). Released from this activated cascade are histamine from mast cells, chemotaxins that attract neutrophils, and enzymes that lyse cell membranes, especially of bacteria, viruses, and parasites. The four main components of the immune system are thus B lymphocytes with circulating immunoglobulins, T lymphocytes with lymphokines, activated macrophages, and the complement system. These components interact to provide protection against harmful exogenous agents such as bacteria, toxins, viruses, and parasites.

There are three disturbances of this otherwise protective arrangement. The first is absence or a defect of one or more components of the system, which causes an immune deficiency disorder. The second is an excessive reaction of the system, which causes hypersensitivity diseases. The third is a misdirected reaction, which is the basis of autoimmune disorders.

## IMMUNODEFICIENCY

Immunodeficient states are rare, serious disorders that affect mainly infants and are inherited as autosomal or X-linked recessive traits. Bruton's disease is due to an X-linked trait in which B lymphocytes are deficient or absent. Thus there are neither plasma cells nor γ-globulins. The pathologic finding is absence of lymphoid follicles in spleen and lymph nodes. In Di George's syndrome the thymus fails to form so that T lymphocytes and cell-bound antibodies never develop. Immunoglobulins, however, are usually normal. In agammaglobulinemia both humoral and cell-bound antibodies are absent and the lymphoid tissue shows pronounced hypoplasia. The condition is inherited as an autosomal recessive trait. The Wiskott-Aldrich syndrome is similar, although it is X-linked and is characterized by eczema and thrombocytopenia; both humoral and cell-bound antibodies are deficient. In all these conditions ulcers and abscesses are common in early life, and death in childhood from overwhelming infection is frequent. Ataxia-telangiectasia also appears in childhood and is characterized by progressive ataxia, pulmonary infections, and dilation of small blood vessels over the face and neck. The fault is in a recessive autosomal gene that causes a combined deficiency of humoral and cell-bound antibodies. The brain discloses degenerative changes in the Purkinje and granular cells of the cerebellum. These disorders have been reviewed by Hayward.[1] Selective deficiencies of individual immunoglobulins, especially IgA, have also been reported.[2]

Leukocytes also reveal several immunodeficiencies. Among them is chronic granulomatous disease, in which neutrophils are able to ingest but not kill certain bacteria, notably staphylococci. This is evident by failure of the leukocytes to reduce nitro blue tetrazolium to a purple compound. The condition usually affects boys, is often X-linked, and is manifested by prolonged infections of lungs, liver, spleen, lymph nodes, and skin. Most victims fail to survive into adolescence.[3] The relationships of the primary immunodeficiencies are shown in Table 6-1.

Immunodeficient states are also acquired in certain diseases, including lymphoid leukemia, the lymphomas, plasma cell myeloma, and Hodgkin's disease. Immunosuppressive agents, including radiation, adrenocorticosteroids, and mitosis-inhibiting drugs such as cyclophosphamide, also cause deficient states. Malignant disease, especially the lymphomas, is more frequent in immunosuppressed patients.[4]

## HYPERSENSITIVITY

Excessive reactions of the immune system cause common clinical disorders. All occur in persons previously exposed to a particular antigen so that specific antibodies are already formed. It is the second encounter with the antigen that brings about the reaction. Four types occur.

In the first, previous exposure to an antigen has sensitized the patient by causing circulating antibodies to develop, especially IgE. These bind to basophils and mast cells. When the antigen is again encountered, it attaches to the antibody, which stimulates the basophils and mast cells to secrete histamine and a factor that is chemotactic for eosinophils. This accounts for the presence of eosinophils in such reactions, while the release of histamine increases vascular permeability and causes smooth muscle to contract. Complement does not participate. When the antigen is localized, as with inhalation, ingestion, or application to skin, such disorders as asthma, hay fever, food allergies, and hives result. When the antigen is not localized , as with the intravenous injection of antitoxin containing horse serum, the reaction is widespread with laryngeal edema, bronchospasm, and pulmonary edema. This is the reaction of anaphylaxis. It is immediate in onset, and it may be fatal within an hour. Steroids and theophylline are suitable agents for treatment.

The second reaction involves antibodies, especially IgG and IgM, that attach to antigens fixed on the surfaces of target cells. The union of antigen with antibody binds complement, and the complement activates enzymes that perforate the target cells and allow the contents to spill out. The target cells are usually erythrocytes, and for this reason the reaction is seen most often in hemolytic anemias, mismatched transfusions, and erythroblastosis fetalis. In transfusions the antigens of the mismatched cells interact with the natural antibodies of the host and the reaction is initiated. In erythroblastosis the same ar-

Table 6-1.

# Primary immune disorders

Humoral antibody deficiency

Bruton's disease

Cell-bound antibody deficiency

Di George's syndrome

Combined antibody deficiency

Agammaglobulinemia

Wiskott-Aldrich syndrome

Ataxia-telangiectasia

Macrophage deficiency

Chronic granulomatous disease

rangement prevails: Fetal erythrocytes leak into the maternal circulation, where antibody formation is stimulated. The maternal antibodies cross the placental barrier; as they reach the fetus, hemolysis ensues and erythroblastosis results. It is a triumph of modern medicine that the condition can be prevented by giving the mother specific antibodies against the fetal red cells. The erythrocytes are thus rendered nonimmunogenic and the condition is prevented. This second reaction, involving cell-bound antigens, is referred to as cytotoxic hypersensitivity.

The third reaction depends on the formation of immune complexes consisting of antigen, antibody, and complement bound together. These form when a previously sensitized person encounters antigen for the second time; IgG or IgM binds to the antigen, complement is fixed, and the immune complexes thus formed attach to the basement membranes of blood vessels. At these sites the chemotactic factors of complement cause acute inflammation, and the lysosomal enzymes of the leukocytes cause tissue destruction. If the antigen is deposited locally, as by subcutaneous injection, hemorrhage and edema develop at that site in 30 minutes to an hour. This response, which involves the small blood vessels of the skin, is known as the Arthus phenomenon. If the antigen is given intravenously, as with the injection of an antitoxin containing horse serum, the reaction will also be prompt if the patient was previously sensitized. If not, the immune complexes form gradually and the reaction is delayed, developing a week or 10 days after the injection. In both, however, the complexes are deposited widely in small vessels or focally in joints, lymph nodes, and the glomerular filters of the kidneys. They are visible as lumpy deposits at these sites when examined by immunofluorescence microscopy. The clinical manifestations are acute serum sickness if the deposits are distributed widely, and arthritis or glo-merulonephritis if their deposition is localized. Serum sickness is characterized clinically by fever, lymphadenopathy, and urticaria. It is to be understood that only complement-fixing antibodies, IgG and IgM, cause the reaction, which is also known as immune complex hypersensitivity. Poststreptococcal glomerulonephritis and possibly viral hepatitis are also disorders in which immune complexes have been found to play important roles.[5]

The last reaction is delayed and cell-mediated. When a patient is exposed to a particular antigen, surface receptors specific for that antigen arise on a clone of T lymphocytes. On second encounter the T cells lock onto the antigen, and this union causes the T cell to destroy the antigen by injection of a toxic substance into it. In addition, the T lymphocytes secrete lymphokines that are both chemotactic and macrophage-activating. The activated macrophages become "killer" cells. As a result of these changes, inflammation develops, and this has the purpose of protecting the host against antigens from bacteria, viruses, fungi, protozoa, and parasites. The reaction is especially apparent with the intradermal injection of tuberculoprotein into a sensitized person; redness and swelling begin in 12 hours, become pronounced at 48 to 72 hours, and then subside. The histologic feature is perivascular cuffing of lymphocytes and macrophages, which becomes pronounced. However, at this focus of cellular activity only a small proportion of the lymphocytes are activated; somehow the T cells recruit "normal" lymphocytes and plasma cells in large numbers. The important aspect of this reaction is the absence of circulating antibodies; all the antibodies to the antigen in question are attached to the T lymphocytes.

Rejection of transplanted organs is also a hypersensitivity reaction. The donor tissue contains histocompatibility antigens, which are especially strong on lymphocytes and platelets. To these the T lymphocytes of the host develop cell-bound antibodies that react against the human lymphocyte antigens. The T lymphocytes cause cytolysis of the donor cells and secrete lymphokines as well. The lymphokines stimulate acute inflammation and macrophage aggressiveness against the donor cells. The reaction is cell-mediated, type IV, and it is the same in all transplanted organs. In the kidney it is characterized by lymphocytic infiltration and focal tubular necrosis that begin within days to weeks and respond to immunosuppression. Later on, rejection vasculitis may develop with acute inflammation, subintimal proliferation of fibroblasts in arteries, and patchy necrosis of the cortex. This inflammatory process is slowed by immunosuppressive agents, so that intimal fibrosis of cortical arteries and atrophy of renal parenchyma are the dominant changes in chronic rejection.[6] The process develops over a four- to six-month post-transplantation interval and is attended clinically by steadily decreasing renal function. The features of the four types of hypersensitivity reactions are summarized in Table 6-2.

## AUTOIMMUNITY

Reactions in the immune system may be either deficient or excessive but they may also be misdirected. Misdirection lies at the root of the autoimmune disorders. Normally most lymphocytes are compatible with host tissues because cells that might bear antigens against the self have been suppressed. Various kinds of defects, however, allow host lymphocytes to become intolerant of the body's own tissues. For example, a hapten may disassociate from one carrier molecule, attach to another, and then be recognized by the immune system as foreign. Or genetic factors that regulate the immune system may allow self-antigens to become overly reactive. It is also possible that viruses can activate the immune system by altering the genome of the cell. Thus hapten associations, genetic alterations, and viral effects may modify the ability of host cells to recognize their own

**Table 6-2.**

## Hypersensitivity reactions

| Term | Antibody | Clinical |
|---|---|---|
| Type I, anaphylactic | IgE | Anaphylaxis <br> Asthma <br> Hay fever <br> Hives |
| Type II, cytotoxic | IgG, IgM | Hemolytic anemia <br> Mismatched transfusions <br> Erythroblastosis fetalis |
| Type III, immune complex | IgG, IgM | Serum sickness <br> Glomerulonephritis <br> Arthritis |
| Type IV, cell-mediated | T lymphocyte | Tuberculin reaction <br> Transplantation rejection |

tissues. Whatever the mechanism, the classical diseases attributed to autoimmunity are disseminated lupus erythematosus, scleroderma, dermatomyositis, and polyarteritis nodosa. Hashimoto's thyroiditis and rheumatoid arthritis, which are described in Chapters 20 and 21, respectively, are also important members of the autoimmune disease group. Several other conditions are suspected of being autoimmune and are listed in Table 6-3.

## Disseminated lupus erythematosus

Lupus erythematosus is a multisystem disease, affecting mainly young women, who develop fever, joint pain, renal disease, pleuritic pain, and sensitivity to sunlight. The manifestations of the renal disease are hypertension, hematuria, and proteinuria. The photosensitivity causes hyperemia and blisters of the skin, especially over the face in a "butterfly" distribution involving the bridge of the nose and both malar eminences. Mental dysfunction develops and convulsions occur. The disturbance is

Table 6-3.

## Probable autoimmune diseases

Systemic lupus erythematosus

Idiopathic thrombocytopenic purpura

Rheumatoid arthritis

Dermatomyositis

Polyarteritis nodosa

Scleroderma

Graves's disease

Pernicious anemia

Primary biliary cirrhosis

Hashimoto's thyroiditis

Temporal arteritis

Chronic ulcerative colitis

chronic, with remissions, exacerbations, and gradual progression.

Autopsy examination reveals widespread vasculitis with fibrinoid necrosis and infiltration with segmented granulocytes and mononuclear cells. These reactions are most frequent over serosal surfaces, including joint spaces, and they are otherwise seen in the kidneys, heart, brain, lungs, and skin. At all these sites immunofluorescence microscopy discloses lumpy deposits of immune complexes. These are pronounced on the basement membranes of glomeruli and in peritubular tissue as well, giving rise to immune complex nephritis.[7] The basement membrane thickening of glomeruli gives rise to the so-called wire loop lesion that is characteristic of lupus. Fibrin accumulates over pericardial and pleural surfaces; it is sterile and eventually either dissolves or progresses to dense fibrous adhesions. The heart also discloses minute nodules of vasculitis and fibrinoid necrosis that appear at unusual locations such as ventricular endocardium or the undersurface of the mitral leaflets. These constitute Libman-Sacks endocarditis. The spleen is large and follicular hyperplasia is pronounced. In the pulmonary tissue, fibrosing alveolitis progresses to widespread interstitial fibrosis. Vasculitis of the brain causes thrombosis of small arteries with microinfarcts of cortical tissue. Immune complex deposits are present in these inflamed vessels, as well as on the choroid plexus.[8] The skin reveals hyperemia, vesicle formation, subepidermal vasculitis, and a layer of immune complexes along the dermal-epidermal junction. Thus, although the lesions are widespread throughout many systems of the body, the unifying aspect is the regular presence of acute vasculitis, fibrinoid necrosis, and infiltration with inflammatory cells. In addition, the immune complex deposits signify the autoimmune nature of the process.

The cause of disseminated lupus is unknown. However, a wide range of anti-

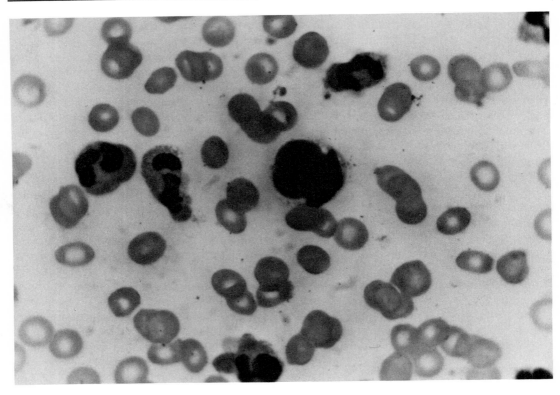

**Figure 6-2.** The "LE cell"; swollen nucleus being phagocytized by a segmented granulocyte

bodies to many nuclear and cytoplasmic constituents of cells are present in the serum. It is therefore supposed that the disease is due to a failure of the immune system to preserve self-tolerance. Why this failure should develop is not clear, although genetic factors, viral infections, or hormonal disturbances may activate the process. The important serum immunoglobulin is antinuclear antibody, without which the diagnosis is in doubt. This antibody also causes the lupus erythematosus (LE) cell to form. Nuclei of leukocytes in blood are normally protected by their cytoplasmic envelopes. When venous blood is withdrawn, however, some of the envelopes are injured and the nuclei are then exposed to the circulating antibody. As a result the nuclei swell, become homogeneous, and are phagocytized by leukocytes. The LE cell is

thus a swollen nuclear mass within a phagocytizing leukocyte (Figure 6-2).

A similar reaction occurs in tissue, so that a homogeneous nuclear remnant constitutes the hematoxylin body; this is most often found in biopsies of renal tissue and is pathognomonic of the disease. Other laboratory findings include increased serum globulins, decreased serum complement, leukopenia, and occasionally hemolytic anemia. False-positive tests for syphilis also occur. The disease has an unpredictable course and often lasts for many years. During this time corticosteroids and immunosuppressive drugs are helpful. When death occurs, renal failure and intercurrent infection are common causes.

Discoid lupus reveals the "butterfly" rash over the face but lacks the systemic aspects of the disseminated disease. Cer-

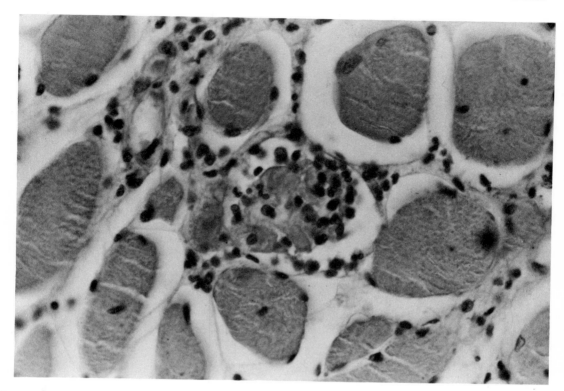

**Figure 6-3.** Focal degeneration and chronic inflammation of skeletal muscle in dermatomyositis

tain drugs, including hydralazine and procainamide, also induce antinuclear antibodies and a syndrome that mimics disseminated lupus. The condition subsides on withdrawal of the drug.

## Scleroderma

This condition, also known as progressive systemic sclerosis, arises between the ages of 30 and 50 years, in women four times more often than in men. The presenting signs are arthritis of the fingers, Raynaud's phenomenon,* and atrophy of the skin of the distal parts. The skin of the fingers becomes thin and shiny, the process advances proximally, and eventually the skin of the face becomes tight, drawn, and shiny. The atrophy and fibrosis also affect

*Vasoconstriction in fingers and toes associated with cold or emotional distress.

internal structures, especially the kidneys, lungs, skeletal muscles, and esophagus. The renal lesion is vascular, consisting of proliferation of intimal cells in medium-sized arteries; this is associated with hypertension, often "malignant," and renal failure.[9] The pulmonary tissue discloses extensive interstitial fibrosis that progresses to "honeycomb lung" (see Figure 12-14). Skeletal muscle is replaced with connective tissue, and sterile inflammation develops in joints. A characteristic feature of scleroderma is dysphagia associated with atrophy of the muscle fibers of the esophagus and replacement with connective tissue so that the esophagus becomes stiff and stenosed. The cause of scleroderma is unknown. The course of the disease is slowly progressive, and death is often attributable to renal failure or pulmonary insufficiency.

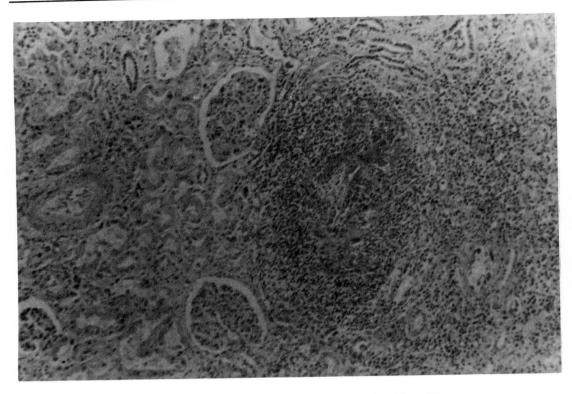

**Figure 6-4.** Fibrinoid necrosis and transmural inflammation of artery in kidney. The changes are characteristic of polyarteritis nodosa.

## Dermatomyositis

Dermatomyositis is a rare disease of skin and skeletal muscle that affects women slightly more often than men and begins in the 40- to 60-year age range. The onset is manifested by muscle weakness and skin rash. The former affects the proximal muscles of the extremities first, then spreads to the trunk, and may involve the diaphragm. On this account the patient may be confined to a wheelchair or bed. The rash, which is violaceous and desquamative, occurs over the face, simulating lupus erythematosus, and also over the neck and upper torso. Associated aspects include fever, weight loss, and lassitude. Although the skin changes are not diagnostic, biopsy of muscle reveals degeneration, chronic inflammation, and fibrosis (Figure 6-3). Diagnosis is indicated by the typical muscle changes, the viola-

ceous rash, a characteristic low-voltage electromyographic tracing, and elevation of serum aldolase and creatine phosphokinase. In addition, the excretion of creatine in the urine is increased. A peculiar aspect is the high frequency of associated malignant disease; viz. eight of 45 cases in the account of Bohan and colleagues, arising in breast, colon, stomach, uterus, prostate, and urinary bladder.[10] The identical condition also exists without skin involvement and is called polymyositis. The course is long and indefinite, although the response to corticosteroids, which may have to be continued for years, causes the serum enzymes to return to normal and muscle strength to improve. Immunosuppression, especially with methotrexate, is also useful. There is scant threat to life except in the case of malignant tumor with metastases. Although their cause is unknown, antibodies in the serum that react with purified myoglobin have been reported.[11] The reason why autoantibodies to skeletal muscle develop is also not clear.

## Polyarteritis nodosa

Acute inflammation of vessels occurs in a wide spectrum of disorders, some of which are described in Chapter 11. Not reported there, and chief among these disorders, is polyarteritis nodosa. This condition is unique in that the vascular lesions are widely scattered throughout many anatomic systems. Moreover, the lesions are segmental with a predilection for bifurcations and the formation of aneurysms that measure as much as 1 cm in diameter. These are revealed by angiography and are pathognomonic. The process affects small and medium-sized arteries, which show smudgy fibrinoid necrosis and transmural infiltration of the wall with neutrophilic and eosinophilic granulocytes (Figure 6-4). Thrombi may form, and microinfarcts occasionally develop. The inflammation subsides so that a canalized lumen or a fibrous cord is left. At any one time, different arteries show various stages of acute inflammation and repair.

The organs often affected are the kidneys, heart, intestine, testes, urinary bladder, prostate, and brain. The patients are young to middle-aged adults, more often male than female, who experience fever, weight loss, malaise, and evidence of multisystem involvement: hypertension, hematuria, abdominal cramps, melena, peripheral neuritis, and muscle pain. In addition, eosinophilia and a history of allergic disease are frequent. It is generally accepted that polyarteritis is an immune disorder due to deposition of immune complexes on vessel walls, and in many cases the complexes consist of hepatitis B antigen-antibody unions.[12, 13] These do not differ from other antigen antibody unions except that the hepatitis B antigenemia persists and the liver enzymes are elevated in the serum. The course of polyarteritis may be fulminant or intermittent. Death from progressive disease is often due to renal failure or intestinal hemorrhage. Corticosteroids and cytotoxic drugs (cyclophosphamide) materially improve the outlook, especially when given early in the course of the disease.[12]

## REFERENCES

1. Hayward A: Immunodeficiency. In *Immunology in Medical Practice* (Taylor G, ed), p 33. Philadelphia: Saunders, 1975

2. Hang R, Ammann AJ: Selective absence of IgA. Autoimmune phenomena and autoimmune disease. *Am J Pathol* 69:491, 1972

3. Elgepors B, Olling S, Peterson H: Chronic granulomatous disease in three siblings. *Scand J Infect Dis* 10:79, 1978

4. Penn I: Second malignant neoplasms associated with immunosuppressive medications. *Cancer* 37:1024, 1976

5. McCluskey RT, Hall CL, Colvin RB: Immune complex mediated diseases. *Hum Pathol* 9:71, 1978

6. Rowlands DT Jr, Hill GS, Zmijewski CM: The pathology of renal homograft rejection. *Am J Pathol* 85:774, 1976

7. McCluskey RT, Colvin RB: Immunologic aspects of renal tubular and other interstitial diseases. *Annu Rev Med* 29:191, 1978

8. Johnson RT, Richardson EP: The neurologic manifestations of systemic lupus erythematosus. A clinical-pathological study of 24 cases and review of the literature. *Medicine* 47:337, 1968

9. Oliver JA, Cannon PJ: The kidney in scleroderma. *Nephron* 18:141, 1977

10. Bohan A, Peter JB, Bowman RL, et al: A computer-assisted analysis of 153 patients with polymyositis and dermatomyositis. *Medicine* 56:255, 1977

11. Nishikai M, Homma M: Antimyoglobin antibody in polymyositis. *Lancet* 2:1205, 1972

12. Fauci AS, Haynes BF, Katz P: The spectrum of vasculitis. Clinical, pathologic, immunologic, and therapeutic considerations. *Ann Intern Med* 89:660, 1978

13. Michalak T: Immune complexes of hepatitis B surface antigen in the pathogenesis of periarteritis nodosa. *Am J Pathol* 90:619, 1978

# 7

# GENETIC AND CHROMOSOMAL DISORDERS

The four main causes of morphologic disease are living agents, physical effects, immunologic disturbances, and inherited defects. Although the last of these may seem to be the least frequent, major congenital malformations, most of which are inherited, are grossly evident in approximately 2 to 4 per cent of live births. Moreover, this figure rises to 4 to 6 per cent by the end of the first year of life because of developments not evident at birth.[1] Minor anomalies are more frequent. Most of them are negligible, of course, but the frequency of abnormal genes in the population is obviously considerable.

In order to understand the mechanisms of inherited disease, certain definitions are helpful. *Proband* refers to the first family member with the abnormality. *Sibs*, or siblings, are brothers and sisters. $P_1$ refers to the parent generation, and $F_1$ to the first-generation offspring. *Alleles* are the genes at the same locus on each of a pair of chromosomes. The individual is *homozygous* when the alleles are identical, and *heterozygous* when they are different. A *dominant* gene is clinically evident even when its allele is missing. A *recessive* gene is evident clinically only when its allelic partner is identical with it, i.e., when the patient is homozygous. *Autosomes* are the nonsex chromosomes, of which there are 22 pairs in humans. The 23rd pair consists of the sex chromosomes, the X being derived from the mother or father, and the Y from the father only. Every somatic cell of the human body normally carries 46 chromosomes, which are divided into 22 pairs of autosomes and one pair of sex chromosomes. *Phenotype* is the clinical expression of a genetic composition, while *genotype* refers to the gene structure regardless of the clinical appearance. Finally, *consanguineous* means that the parties are related. Because related individuals are more likely to carry the same recessive genetic defect, consanguineous marriages are more likely to produce genetic defects in the offspring than are marriages between unrelated people. *Congenital* means "born with," so that congenital disease is not necessarily an inherited defect but may be the result of an environmental stress that causes a fault in development, e.g., phocomelia after the use of thalidomide.

The sex of an individual is determined by the X and Y chromosomes. Mothers produce only X chromosomes while fathers produce X and Y chromosomes. After meiotic division of the germinal cells, each ovum contains only one X chromosome while each sperm carries one X or one Y chromosome. An X chromosome in a sperm that fertilizes an ovum produces a female with two X chromosomes. A Y chromosome in a sperm that unites with an ovum produces a male with an XY set of chromosomes. Maleness is thus determined by the Y chromosome alone.

The characteristics of a person are determined by the genes he/she inherits from his/her father and mother. Each chromosome has many genes, and each gene has a specific locus on the chromosome. Certain patterns of inheritance indicate whether a particular gene is carried on an autosome or on a sex chromosome, and whether it is a dominant or recessive character. An autosomal dominant gene, for example, gives a pattern of inheritance with three characteristics: It affects both sexes, it is present in all generations (parent and child), and the unaffected offspring neither have the gene nor transmit it to their offspring. An example of a dominant gene carried on an autosome is the disease of congenital spherocytic anemia.[2] An autosomal recessive gene is indicated by a somewhat different pattern: It affects both sexes equally, it appears in some offspring but not in the parents, and it is more likely to appear in the children of a consanguineous marriage than in those born to parents who are unrelated. An example of a recessive gene carried on an autosome is that of cystic fibrosis, which occurs once in every 2,000 live births and is carried silently in one of every 20 adults.[3]

The sex chromosomes consist of an X from the mother and an X or Y from the father. No significant disease is carried on the Y chromosome so far as known.[4] No important disease is carried on the X chromosome as a dominant gene.* Therefore all significant diseases carried on the sex chromosomes are located on the X member as a recessive character. Such conditions are said to be sex-linked. This means nothing more than that they are carried on the X chromosome, whether it is derived from the mother or the father. X-linked diseases are almost always passed from mothers to sons because the gene is recessive and has to be present on both X chromosomes to be clinically evident in a female; thus both parents must have it. X-linked disease is never passed from a father to his son because the father contributes only the Y sex chromosome to his male offspring. Examples of conditions carried on the X chromosome, or sex-linked diseases, are hemophilia and color blindness.

Although the patterns of inheritance follow inviolable rules, there are nevertheless difficulties in recognizing these patterns. The reasons for this are that clinical severity may vary from slight to extreme, onset of the condition may vary from birth to old age, the incidence of the condition may

*The exception is glucose 6-phosphate dehydrogenase deficiency.

vary in the two sexes, and the genotype may be only partially expressed by the phenotype. The terms used for these variations, given in the same order, are variable expressivity, variable onset, variable sex limitation, and variable penetrance.

Variable expression of the phenotype is a matter of special interest. Whereas the male sex chromosomes are X and Y, the female sex chromosomes are X and X. Thus, in the female, one X comes from the father and one from the mother. Both are active in all cells of the developing embryo until the 12th to 16th day after conception. At that time one of the X chromosomes in each cell becomes permanently inactive. All the progeny of these early cells thereafter retain the same inactive chromosome as a vestigial body. It is this mechanism, described by Lyon, that prevents the female from having twice the complement of enzymes from X chromosomes as the male.[5] Regardless of sex, therefore, the somatic cells of all normal persons carry only one active X chromosome.

Whether the father-derived X chromosome or the mother-derived X chromosome undergoes inactivation on the 12th to 16th day is a random matter. The probability is that the distribution is about equal. Therefore women are *mosaics* with respect to the X chromosome because the active member of the pair is sometimes maternal and sometimes paternal in origin. If a hereditary trait is carried on the maternal X chromosome, and if that chromosome becomes inactive by random chance during embryologic development, the progeny of that cell will also no longer carry that trait. The degree with which the trait is expressed, i.e., is evident clinically, will therefore depend on the proportion of cells carrying the trait that became inactive. Since the possible range extends from none of the cells to all, the degree of expression of the phenotype is extremely broad. Thus the proportion of X chromosomes carrying the mutant gene that escape inactivation determines the

phenotype of the individual. It is this explanation that is given for the variable expression of the phenotype as it relates to the characteristics that are carried on the sex chromosomes.

The inactive X chromosome is carried in female cells as a vestigial body, and it is easily seen in two locations. One is the circulating neutrophilic segmented granulocytes, in which a minute nuclear projection, called a "drumstick," represents the inactive X chromosome. The drumstick is present in about 5 per cent of neutrophils in females. The other is the squamous cells from the buccal mucosa, 20 to 50 per cent of which reveal a minute pyknotic mass on the inside of the nuclear membrane. It is known as the Barr body.[6]

Fundamental to an understanding of heritable diseases is the realization that most are caused by defective genes transmitted on the autosomes of the parents. In these instances there is no observable effect in the chromosome; the alteration is at the molecular level and is too fine to be seen even with the electron microscope. The second, much less common mechanism is an accident of gametogenesis that causes a chromosomal alteration that can be seen in the karyotype of the abnormal cells.

The causes of gene abnormalities include radiation, viral infection, and chemical agents. In addition, some mutations appear to arise spontaneously. Regardless of the cause, abnormalities derived from these faults may be structural and for the most part evident at birth, or functional with gradual development that becomes evident some time later. Structural faults, functional diseases, and chromosomal disorders due to errors of gametogenesis are summarized in Table 7-1.

## STRUCTURAL GENETIC DISORDERS

### Achondroplasia

Achondroplasia is a form of dwarfism in which the trunk is normal, the limbs are short, and the face presents a characteristic appearance. The limb defect is due especially to shortening of the humerus and femur. Lumbar lordosis is pronounced, the legs are usually bowed, and the gait is waddling. The face has a recessed nose, hypoplastic maxilla, and relatively protuberant mandible. Defective chondrocranial development often leads to hydrocephalus. The cause of this dwarfism is not known.[7] It is a dominant autosomal trait, and 80 per cent of the cases are due to new mutations. Fathers of individuals with sporadic achondroplasia tend to be somewhat older than those with normal offspring. The condition does not flourish because of difficulty in finding mates and, for females, in completing childbirth. Marriages between achondroplastic individuals produce homozygotes that are often stillborn. Achondroplastic dwarfs are hardy, and survivorship is approximately normal.

### Osteogenesis imperfecta

This condition is due to an autosomal dominant genetic defect that prescribes a generalized disorder of connective tissue. It is uncommon but not rare. It affects the sexes equally and may be evident at birth or develop during childhood or adulthood. The principal clinical features are the triad of brittle bones, deafness, and blue sclerae. The bony change is a deficiency in the formation of the bone matrix. This causes fractures, which occur easily and repetitively. They are nearly painless and heal normally. The legs become short from bowing and fracturing. Kyphoscoliosis is common. The forehead is prominent and domed while the temporal regions bulge outward so that the ears point outward. The face is triangular and the distance between the eyes is increased (hypertelorism). Radiographic examination reveals pronounced osteoporosis with corresponding radiolucence. The most constant of the major features is blue discoloration of the sclerae, which is due to the choroid showing through the thin scleral layer. Deafness is also a major feature and is attributed to sclerosis of the petrous portion of the temporal bone. The skin is thin and the tendons

Table 7-1.

## Hereditary mechanisms with disease examples

I. Defective gene transmitted from parent

A. Structural
1. Achondroplasia
2. Osteogenesis imperfecta
3. Arachnodactyly
4. Polycystic kidneys
5. Clidocranial dysostosis
6. Cleft lip/palate
7. Clubfoot
8. Spina bifida
9. Hypospadias

B. Functional
1. Glycogen storage disease
2. Galactosemia
3. Phenylketonuria
4. Gaucher's disease
5. Neimann-Pick disease
6. Ochronosis
7. Porphyria
8. Gout
9. Sickle cell anemia

II. Defective chromosome transmitted from parent

A. Autosome
1. Down's syndrome
2. Trisomy E syndrome

B. Sex chromosome (X)
1. Klinefelter's syndrome
2. Turner's syndrome

and ligaments are lax. The fundamental defect appears to be a failure of collagen to mature.[7] There is a wide range of severity of the condition; some patients die at birth and others live to old age. There are no pathognomonic changes in the blood, the calcium and phosphorus values are not remarkable, and intelligence is normal.

### Marfan's syndrome

Marfan's syndrome is a hereditary fault of connective tissue metabolism that affects the skeletal, ocular, and aortic tissues. It was described by Marfan in 1896, and renamed arachnodactyly in 1902.[7] The patients are tall and slim with loose joints and slender, elongated hands and feet. The fingers are so long that with the fist clenched over the thumb the latter still projects from the ulnar side. The ocular fault is due to looseness of the suspensory ligaments of the eye so that bilateral dislocation of the lenses is characteristic. The aorta reveals a defect of the media closely resembling cystic medial necrosis. The consequence of this is dilation of the ascending portion, which stretches the aortic cusps and causes insufficiency of the valve at a young age. In addition, dissecting aneurysms of the aorta are common, and it is this lesion, with or without congestive failure from aortic insufficiency, that usually terminates life. Absence of calcification of the ascending aorta helps distinguish this condition from syphilitic aortitis. Although life may run its normal course, death in the fourth decade is more common. The basic fault is not certain but may be a metabolic defect that causes an abnormality of elastic or collagenous tissue. The condition affects the sexes equally and is transmitted as a dominant autosomal character.

## FUNCTIONAL GENETIC DISORDERS

In 1941 Beadle and Tatum announced their one-gene/one-enzyme hypothesis:[8] Each gene directs the production of one enzyme, and that enzyme catalyzes a specific reaction. This relationship may be conceived of as the reaction of substrate A catalyzed by a specific enzyme to form normal product B. A defect in the gene causes an abnormality of the enzyme, which interferes with the reaction. The consequence is either too much A, which produces an accumulation disease, too little B, which produces a deficiency disease, or a new product, which produces a synthetic disease (Figure 7-1).

### Glycogen storage disease

Glycogen storage diseases are due to genetic faults of carbohydrate metabolism. The common fault is a deficiency of the enzyme that converts glycogen to glucose, which causes the condition known as von Gierke's disease. The enzymatic fault results in accumulation of glycogen in the liver and kidneys. The principal clinical effect is hypoglycemia with convulsions. The illness becomes evident soon after birth, and causes death in childhood. It is transmitted as an autosomal recessive trait. Less common but similar defects of glycogen metab-

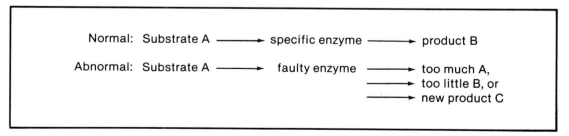

**Figure 7-1.** The genesis of accumulation, deficiency, and synthetic diseases

olism include Pompe's disease and McArdle's disease, in which other enzymes are deficient and other organs, such as the heart and skeletal muscles, are the sites of glycogen accumulation.[9] The various forms of glycogen storage disease are referred to by Roman numerals I through VII.

## Galactosemia

An additional fault of carbohydrate metabolism is galactosemia, which is also inherited as an autosomal recessive trait. Lactose is normally hydrolyzed to galactose and glucose, but the galactose cannot subsequently be converted to glucose because of a deficiency of the transferase enzyme necessary for this reaction. As a result, galactose accumulates in the blood, spills into the urine, and causes nausea and vomiting as well as failure to thrive. There are also lenticular cataracts and mental retardation. These clinical manifestations begin soon after birth. Organ changes include hepatic steatosis, which may progress to portal cirrhosis, and gliosis with nerve cell loss in the cerebellum and medulla. Occasionally there is also a striking hyperplasia of the islets of Langerhans.[10] Withdrawing milk from the diet is effective treatment.

## Phenylketonuria

Phenylketonuria is a rare hereditary disease, transmitted as a recessive autosomal trait, that is due to a deficiency of phenylalanine hydroxylase, which normally converts phenylalanine to tyrosine. The result of this deficiency is too little tyrosine and too much phenylalanine. The tyrosine deficiency is not harmful, although on this account patients are fair, blue-eyed, and blond. However, accumulation of phenylalanine in the blood and urinary excretion of its metabolite, phenylpyruvic acid, cause demyelination of the brain and spongy lesions of the white matter. The outstanding clinical characteristic is gradual, irreversible mental retardation. The EEG tracing is usually abnormal.

The serum level of phenylalanine rises above 25 mg/dl. The urine turns green on addition of a 10 per cent solution of ferric chloride, and this may be used as a screening test. Both abnormalities may be detected by the third week of life, and clinical manifestations begin soon thereafter. Detection is important because the progress of the disease may be halted by excluding phenylalanine from the diet. Heterozygotes are not clinically evident, and homozygotes occur only once in approximately 20,000 live births.[11]

## Gaucher's disease

Leukocytes and erythrocytes contain glycolipids. When these cells are disposed of in normal fashion, glycolipids are released. The catabolism of glycolipids includes the formation of glucosylceramides. When the enzyme that normally cleaves glucose from this compound is deficient, glucosylceramide accumulates and is phagocytized by macrophages. In this way Gaucher's disease begins. The macrophages accumulate in the spleen, liver, bone marrow, and lymph nodes. The spleen is the focus of the disease; it is affected early and becomes markedly enlarged. As the normal elements of the bone marrow are crowded out, anemia, leukopenia, and thrombocytopenia arise. A bleeding tendency from the low platelet level is common. The bone marrow effects include destruction of trabeculae, elevation of serum acid phosphatase, infarct formation, and pathologic fractures. Biopsy of the liver or bone marrow reveals the characteristic Gaucher cells. These are macrophages with abundant cytoplasm containing finely fibrillar material that resembles wrinkled tissue paper and differs from the foamy cytoplasm of other lipid storage diseases. The Gaucher cells are so large that they obstruct pulmonary capillaries and also cause chest pain, cough, and recurrent pneumonitis.

The condition is familial but of uncertain inheritance. It begins at any time of life and is slowly progressive. Bone pain is the most disabling feature. There is no specific treatment. Less common forms occur in children and are rapidly progressive, involve galactosylceramides, and also affect the central nervous system.[12]

### Niemann-Pick disease

In 1914 Niemann, a Berlin pediatrician, described a patient who he thought had Gaucher's disease but whom Pick later showed to have a new disease. The disorder, subsequently given the names of both men, is due to excess sphingomyelin, a phospholipid present in all cells. Catabolic degradation requires an enzyme that is deficient because of a genetic defect transmitted as an autosomal recessive trait.

The excess sphingomyelin accumulates in macrophages of the reticuloendothelial system, the lungs, and the central nervous system. The macrophages are distended with lipid globules that give a foamy appearance to the cytoplasm. Clinically the neonatal period is normal, after which hepatosplenomegaly develops in association with psychomotor disturbances so that the child rapidly regresses to a vegetative state. In the brain there are foci of gliosis, loss of cells, and accumulation of macrophages of irregular distribution. Loss of neurons from the macula may produce a cherry-red spot on the optic fundi. Diagnosis is suggested by hepatosplenomegaly in a child with a neurologic disorder, and confirmed by biopsy of liver or bone marrow. There is no specific treatment. Other forms of the disease are chronic and less frequent. No way is yet available to identify carriers of the trait.[13]

### Gout

Primary gout is an inherited fault of purine metabolism that is characterized by hyperuricemia, recurrent arthritis, and deposits of urates in connective tissues. The pattern of inheritance is complex and unclear. The metabolic fault is presumably enzymatic and results in the overproduction or underexcretion of uric acid. Maximum solubility of uric acid is approached by the upper normal serum level, which varies from 6.5 to 8.4 mg/dl, depending on the method. At levels only 1 mg/dl higher, supersaturation occurs and precipitation of urate crystals in synovial fluid may begin. The crystals are slender rods 10 $\mu$m long and are found free in the synovial fluid or within the cytoplasm of segmented granulocytes. The joints of the lower extremities are most often affected, especially that of the great toe. The inflammation is exudative, abrupt in onset, and excruciatingly painful. Fever and leukocytosis attend the process, which subsides spontaneously in a few days. The disease tends to begin in middle age, affects principally men, and recurs over long periods. After several years deposits of urates called tophi form in tendon sheaths, periarticular structures, and subcutaneous tissues. At these sites the inflammation is granulomatous with multinucleated giant cells, which distinguish the deposits from the nodules of rheumatic disease. Urate crystals also precipitate in the renal pyramids, where they block the collecting ducts and lead to pyelonephritis. Excretion into the renal pelvis causes stone formation in about 15 per cent of cases. The diagnosis is suggested by a high serum uric acid, a history of exquisitely painful arthritis of the great toe, and occurrence of the condition in members of the family. The diagnosis is established by demonstration of sodium urate crystals in synovial fluid or subcutaneous tophi. Oral colchicine gives dramatic relief in 24 to 48 hours. Prolonged therapy is effective with allopurinol, which inhibits an enzyme necessary for the synthesis of uric acid, or with probenecid, which blocks tubular reabsorption and increases the excretion of uric acid.

Secondary gout is clinically similar and is due to the increased turnover of nucleic acid associated with such conditions as polycythemia, leukemia, multiple myeloma, and sickle cell anemia. As would be expected, it begins earlier, affects women more often, and is not seen in other family members.[14]

Porphyria and ochronosis-alkaptonuria are also metabolic accumulation diseases and are described in Chapter 8. Instead of causing accumulation diseases, however, inherited metabolic errors may cause too little of a normal product to form so that a deficiency state arises. Examples of such conditions include albinism, adrenogenital syndrome, and cretinism.

## Albinism

Albinism is the clinical manifestation of a rare metabolic fault of melanin production. It may be restricted to the eyes or may affect the skin as well. Ocular albinism is passed as an X-linked recessive trait, while oculocutaneous albinism is carried as an autosomal recessive gene. The faulty gene dictates a deficiency of tyrosinase, which is needed to convert tyrosine to dopa (3,4-dihydroxyphenylalanine) and thence to melanin. The enzyme may be only partially absent (tyrosinase-positive) or totally absent (tyrosinase-negative). Some pigmentation is present in tyrosinase-positive patients, but in tyrosinase-negative oculocutaneous albinism the skin and hair are strikingly white, the irides are gray to light blue, and the optic fundi show a red reflectance to light. Visual acuity is impaired, nystagmus is common, and photophobia is pronounced. In addition, there is strong sensitivity to sunlight, and exposure frequently causes skin cancer. Tyrosinase-negative oculocutaneous albinism has an incidence of about one in 35,000 adults.[15]

## Adrenogenital syndrome

The steroidal hormones of the adrenal cortex are synthesized from cholesterol through several complex reactions. Each is controlled by an enzyme which, when faulty, prescribes a deficiency of a normal product or the accumulation of an intermediate product. Either may be harmful. When the enzymatic defect of this syndrome, which is a recessive autosomal trait, results in a deficiency, feedback inhibition from the adrenal is lost and excessive stimulation by the pituitary from adrenocorticotrophin (ACTH) secretion follows. When an intermediate product accumulates, diversion of metabolic pathways may lead to excessive production of androgens. The most frequent clinical consequence is virilization, which is evident in females at birth and in males at 2 to 3 years of age. Clitoral hyperplasia, rugate labioscrotal folds, and a penile urethra are seen in girls and may lead to an error in sex assignment. In the male, premature development of the penis, rapid growth, deepening of the voice, and excessive muscular development characterize the condition. Hyperplasia of the zona reticularis of the adrenal cortex is the main morphologic finding in addition to those already mentioned. Diagnosis is aided by examination of the buccal smear for Barr bodies, and of the urine, which usually discloses increased secretion of 17-ketosteroids. Treatment by the administration of cortisol usually corrects the abnormal pattern of steroid secretion.[16]

## Cretinism

The synthesis, storage, secretion, and utilization of thyroid hormone form a complex process that takes place in many steps, each controlled by a specific enzyme system. Genetic faults that interfere with these enzymes lead to hypofunction of the thyroid through several different pathways, which may be evident at birth or develop shortly thereafter. The clinical effects include thick, coarse skin, scant body hair, low metabolic rate, retarded growth, and impaired mental and sexual development. The thyroid is small and may be hypoplastic with few glands, much connective tissue, and little colloid. Low thyroid function values indicate the diagnosis. Therapy with desiccated thyroid may be helpful, but much depends on the stage of the condition at the time treatment is begun.

### Sickle cell anemia

There exist conditions in which a gene defect prescribes a faulty enzyme that leads to a new substance. An example of this is sickle cell anemia, which is inherited as a recessive autosomal trait. When the patient is homozygous the consequence of this fault is the production of hemoglobin in which valine replaces glutamic acid in the globin protein. This minute change in a structure composed of 574 amino acids causes rigid tactoids to form when the cells are under low oxygen pressure. Because of this the cells cannot slip through the capillary constrictions, and the subsequent vessel obstructions produce the clinical and pathologic events described more fully in Chapter 19.

It is concluded that genetic effects may be structural and obvious at birth, or functional and obscure at birth with gradual development later. Moreover, the function-

al effects may be diseases of accumulation, deficiency, or new product formation. It is a large chapter in medicine, and the examples cited give no more than a glimpse of this enormous and fascinating field.

## CHROMOSOMAL DISORDERS

While the foregoing cites examples of gene defects that are too small to be seen, there are also chromosomal abnormalities, which are relatively large and conspicuous. These arise at the time of gametogenesis and are often due to nondisjunction at the time of meiotic division. In order to prepare for an understanding of this mechanism it is helpful to review the chromosomal activity of normal somatic cells undergoing mitotic division and of normal germinal cells undergoing meiotic division.

In Figure 7-2 a single pair of chromosomes is shown. Although this is necessary for simplification, it is to be understood that 23 pairs of chromosomes are involved in each cell in the actual process. All, however, behave as indicated by the single pair in the diagram. In somatic cells each chromosome replicates and divides so that the daughter cells are exact copies of the parent cell and are diploid in chromosomal number. The straight chromosome is of paternal origin; the wavy one of maternal origin. The division produces exact copies of the parent cell. A fault in this process is clinically obscure, and an abnormal cell presumably succumbs and is disposed of in the reticuloendothelial system.

Meiosis takes place in germinal cells, i.e., sperm and ova. The parent cell is diploid while the daughter cells are haploid. This is achieved by two reduction divisions, indicated by A and B in Figure 7-3. When fertilization takes place the complementary chromosome is added to the gamete, a zygote is formed, and the diploid number is restored. Errors of gametogenesis are obscure if the cell succumbs. If it survives, however, every cell of the individual who

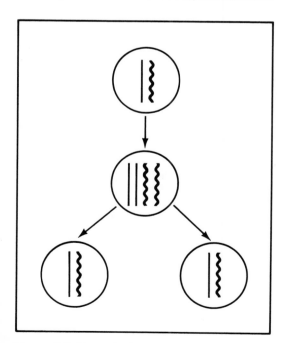

**Figure 7-2.** Normal mitosis

develops from that fertilization will be abnormal. Thus gametogenesis is critical to the normality of the developing embryo and of the individual who emerges from it. Errors of the gametogenic process are attributable to viruses, chemicals, radiation, and, in Down's syndrome, to advanced maternal age.

The kinds of faults seen in gametogenesis are simple loss, in which a portion of a chromosome wanders away in the cell and disappears; deletion, in which a chromosomal fragment breaks off and fails to reattach; translocation, in which a wandering fragment reattaches to the wrong chromosome; and nondisjunction, in which the chromosome does not divide properly. Many of the main faults of gametogenesis are due to nondisjunction (Figure 7-4). In the first re-

duction division (A) the chromosomes fail to disjoin, and as a result both come to occupy one daughter cell while the other daughter cell gets neither chromosome. After the second reduction division, therefore, two cells have one too many chromosomes and two cells have one too few. Thus nondisjunction at the first reduction division leaves all cells abnormal.

Nondisjunction may also take place at the second reduction division (B, Figure 7-4). In this event half the progeny are normal and half are abnormal; i.e., one daughter cell has an extra chromosome and the other has none of that pair.

The importance of nondisjunction may be seen from the effect of fertilization of the four gametocytes (Figure 7-5). Suppose each of these cells represents an ovum

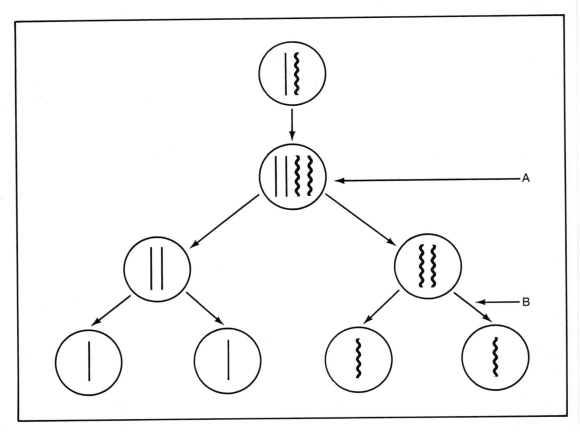

**Figure 7-3.** Normal meiosis

ready to be fertilized, and the chromosome shown therein is autosome 21. A sperm comes along with a normal complement of chromosomes. The first two ova produce normal zygotes (A). The third ovum, however, has one too many of autosome 21 so that when fertilization takes place, a trisomy 21 fertilization forms (B). This is the genesis of Down's syndrome. When a normal sperm encounters the ovum on the right, 45 chromosomes result.

It may also be supposed that the chromosomes of the gametocytes of Figure 7-5 are X chromosomes rather than autosomes. In this event the sperm fertilizes the first two ova shown in Figure 7-5. If the sperm carries the X chromosome, a female is conceived or, if a Y chromosome, a male. If the sperm carries an X chromosome and fertil-izes the third ovum, however, a triple-X female is conceived and will have two Barr bodies in her buccal cells. If the sperm carries a Y chromosome and fertilizes the same cell, an XXY genotype is formed, and this is the genesis of Klinefelter's syndrome. Finally, an X-carrying sperm that fertilizes the last ovum on the right creates an X0 genotype, which is the basis of Turner's syndrome. A Y0 conceptus does not survive.

## Down's syndrome

In 1959 Lejeune and colleagues discovered that patients with Down's syndrome have 47 chromosomes.[17] The extra chromosome is autosome 21, and nondisjunction was later found to be the cause of most of the examples of this condition. Infants with

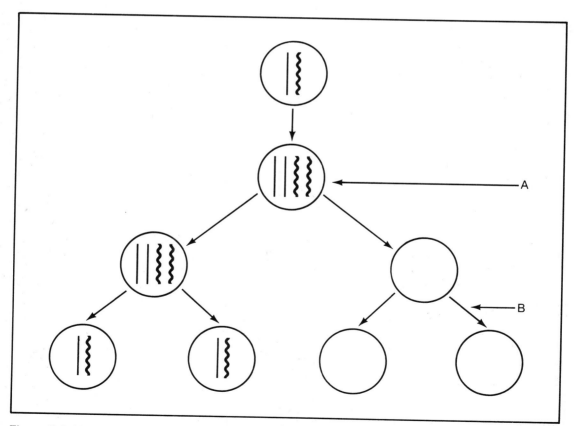

**Figure 7-4.** Meiosis with nondisjunction at first reduction division

Down's syndrome show prominent epicanthic folds, giving them a so-called mongoloid appearance, and they tend to have hypotonic muscles, an easy disposition, a flat facial profile, a protruding tongue, and a single palmar crease that is horizontal. In addition, mental deficiency is characteristic, and retarded development becomes evident later. Only a small fraction of 1 per cent of children of young mothers are afflicted, but the incidence rises to 2 per cent among children born to mothers over 45 years of age.[4] The age of the father has considerably less bearing on the frequency of the condition.

Trisomy of other autosomes also causes malformations of the newborn that tend to be more pronounced and less frequent than Down's syndrome.

## Klinefelter's syndrome

In 1942 Klinefelter and colleagues described males with Barr bodies in their buccal cells who were sterile and developed gynecomastia. Examination of such a patient reveals normal external genitalia except for small testes, in which the seminiferous tubules are hyalinized. There are also lack of libido, scant body hair, and increased secretion of pituitary gonadotrophin in the urine. Approximately half of these individuals are also mentally retarded. The genotype is XXY, and meiotic nondisjunction is presumed to be the main cause of this abnormality.[18]

## Turner's syndrome

A second type of sex chromosome disorder is Turner's syndrome, which was described

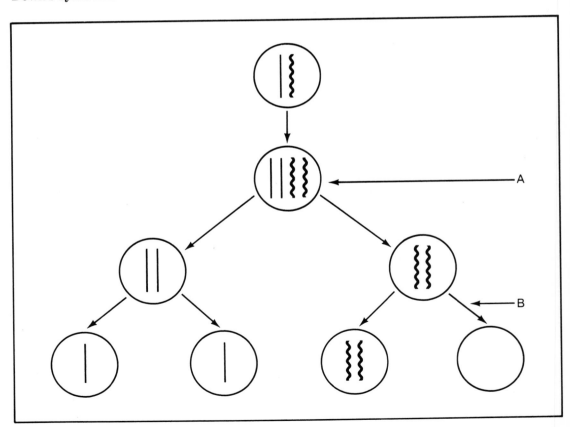

**Figure 7-5.** Nondisjunction at the second reduction division

in 1938. It occurs in girls; they are short, display webbed necks, and fail to develop secondary sex characteristics. They accordingly have scant pubic hair and slight breast development, and are sterile. The ova are composed of stroma without follicles. The patients do not menstruate. Diagnosis is made by the absence of Barr bodies in buccal cells and by the karyotype, which reveals only 45 chromosomes with an X0 genotype. The condition occurs approximately once in every 3,000 female births.[18]

The other sex chromosome disorders are less frequent and consist of XXX females and XYY males. Triple-X females are sexually normal but often display mental retardation, which is their outstanding characteristic. XYY males tend to be tall, thin, and aggressive. This behavior has been associated with a tendency toward violent crime, although environmental factors also incline individuals in this direction, and studies are still lacking in sufficient evidence to establish such a conclusion.[19]

## REFERENCES

1. Riccardi VM: *The Genetic Approach to Human Disease*, p 4. New York: Oxford University Press, 1977

2. Beutler E: Genetic disorders of red cells. *JAMA* 233:1184, 1975

3. Di Sant'Agnese PA, Talamo RC: Pathogenesis and patho-physiology of cystic fibrosis of the pancreas. *N Engl J Med* 277:1287, 1344, 1399, 1967

4. Stern C: *Principles of Human Genetics*, 3rd ed. San Francisco: Freeman, 1973

5. Lyon MF: Gene action in the X-chromosome of the mouse. *Nature* 190:372, 1961

6. Barr ML, Bertram EG: A morphological distinction between neurones of the male and female, and the behavior of the nucleolar satellite during accelerated nucleo-protein synthesis. *Nature* 163:676, 1949

7. McKusick VA: Heritable disorders of connective tissue. St. Louis: Mosby, 1972

8. Beadle GW, Tatum EL: Genetic control of biochemical reactions in neurospora. *Proc Nat Acad Sci USA* 27:499, 1941

9. Hsia DY: The diagnosis and management of the glycogen storage diseases. *Am J Clin Pathol* 50:44, 1968

10. Smetana HF, Olen E: Hereditary galactose disease. *Am J Clin Pathol* 38:3, 1962

11. Blaskovics ME, Nelson TL: Phenylketonuria and its variations. A review of recent developments. *Calif Med* 115:42, 1971

12. Fredrickson DS, Sloan HR: Glucosyl ceramide lipidoses: Gaucher's disease. In *The Metabolic Basis of Inherited Disease* (Stanbury JB, Wyngaarden JB, Fredrickson DS, eds), 3rd ed, pp 730-759. New York: McGraw-Hill, 1972

13. Fredrickson DS, Sloan HR: Sphingomyelin lipidoses: Niemann-Pick disease. In *The Metabolic Basis of Inherited Disease* (Stanbury JB, Wyngaarden JB, Fredrickson DS, eds), 3rd ed, pp 783-807. New York: McGraw-Hill, 1972

14. Rodnan GP, McEwen C, Wallace SL, eds: *Primer on Rheumatic Diseases*, 7th ed. *JAMA* 224:662, 1973

15. Fitzpatrick TB, Quevedo WD Jr: Albinism. In *The Metabolic Basis of Inherited Disease* (Stanbury JB, Wyngaarden JB, Fredrickson DS, eds), 3rd ed, pp 326-337. New York: McGraw-Hill, 1972

16. Bongiovanni AM: Disorders of adrenal steroid biogenesis (the adrenogenital syndrome associated with congenital adrenal hyperplasia). In *The Metabolic Basis of Inherited Disease* (Stanbury JB, Wyngaarden JB, Fredrickson DS, eds), 3rd ed, pp 857-885. New York: McGraw-Hill, 1972

17. Lejeune J, Gautier M, Turpin R: Les chromosomes humains en culture de tissus. *R Hebd Sem Acad Sci Paris* 248:602, 1959

18. Hsia DY: *Human Developmental Genetics*. Chicago: Year Book Medical Publishers, 1968

19. Court-Brown WM: The development of knowledge about males with an XYY sex chromosome complement. *J Med Genet* 5:341, 1969

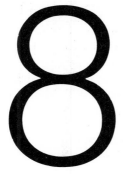

# PIGMENTARY DISORDERS

The pigmentations of the body are customarily regarded as either exogenous or endogenous. Exogenous pigments are largely inhaled and induce various lesions of pulmonary tissue. These are collectively known as the pneumoconioses and include such substances as carbon (anthracosis), silica (silicosis), iron dust (siderosis), cotton fibers (byssinosis), and asbestos fibers (asbestosis). These conditions are discussed in Chapter 12.

The normal endogenous pigments include hemoglobin, melanin, and lipofuscin. The last is a finely granular, dark brown pigment associated with old age or wasting disease, where it is found especially in the hepatocytes and at the poles of the nuclei of the myocardial fibers. These atrophic organs are distinctly brown and give rise to the term brown atrophy. The pigment is not associated with any conspicuous clinical illness, is not precisely identified, and does not take the stain for melanin or iron.

## HEMOGLOBIN

Most endogenous pigmentation is due to heme, the precursor of hemoglobin. Hemoglobin is constantly being renewed and depleted, and this cycle is the setting in which these pigmentary disorders may be understood. Hemoglobin is synthesized mainly in the bone marrow, functions in the circulating red cells for about four months, and then is degraded and disposed of in the reticuloendothelial system. Abnormalities arise in each of these phases of the hemoglobin cycle (Figure 8-1).

The porphyrias are inherited faults of hemoglobin synthesis whereas jaundice is an impairment of hemoglobin degradation. Hemosiderosis is not a disorder of clinical significance and is included here only for completeness. Hemochromatosis is an iron storage disease rather than a fault of degradation but is nevertheless due to a pigment related to hemoglobin. Of these conditions, jaundice is by far the most frequent. The anemias and polycythemia are the principal diseases of hemoglobin but are not primarily pigmentary disorders. They are considered in Chapter 19. The main disorders associated with hemoglobin pigment thus consist of the porphyrias, jaundice, and hemochromatosis.

Hemoglobin consists of three components: heme, iron, and globin. Synthesis begins with the production of heme; iron and globin are added later. Heme is produced mainly in the liver and bone marrow. The hepatic tissue produces heme-containing enzymes such as cytochromes, catalase, and peroxidase. The bone marrow synthesizes hemoglobin. In both liver and bone marrow the sequence begins with the union of glycine from the protein pool with succinate from the carbohydrate pool to form adipic acid (Figure 8-2). Specific enzymes catalyze each reaction.

Porphobilinogen is a monopyrrole. Four monopyrroles join to make a tetrapyrrole, and iron locks into the central bonding of the tetrapyrrole to form heme. The four pyrroles are the porphyrin component of the heme molecule. With the attachment of globin, the complete hemoglobin molecule is formed. About 8 gm of hemoglobin are formed daily.

**Porphyria**

Porphyria is a clinical disturbance caused by a fault in the production of heme in either the liver or bone marrow. It may be acquired, as with poisoning by a porphyrogenic agent (hexachlorobenzene) that gets into food, but it is usually due to hereditary defects in the enzymes that control the production of heme. This occurs separately in liver and bone marrow so that it is natural to classify the porphyrias as either hepatic or erythropoietic. The classification is shown in Table 8-1.

By far the most common of these disorders is acute intermittent porphyria. It begins in young adulthood, affects women and men in the ratio 3:2, and is characterized by severe abdominal colic, hypertension, bizarre behavior suggestive of hysteria or psychosis, and a central and peripheral neuropathy that may progress from paresthesia to paralysis and later to coma. The attacks last for days to months and are accompanied by tachycardia, fever, and occasionally leukocytosis. Vomiting occurs and causes dehydration with electrolyte imbalance; constipation is suggestive of intestinal obstruction. Laparotomy is often performed, although it is futile. Scars attest to

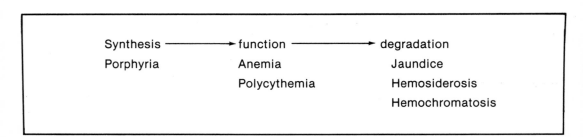

**Figure 8-1.** Disorders associated with the hemoglobin cycle

previous incorrect diagnoses of a surgical abdomen. The attacks can also be brought on by barbiturates, narcotics, and steroids, including oral contraceptives. Another difficulty thus arises: Hysteria is diagnosed, sedatives are ordered to calm the patient, and the condition is worsened. The skin is not sensitive to sunlight.

The cause is a dominant autosomal gene of variable expressivity that prescribes an excess of the enzyme determining the rate of heme synthesis in the liver.[1] The excess enzyme, aminolevulinic acid synthetase, causes overproduction of aminolevulinic acid and porphobilinogen. The latter accumulates in the blood and is excreted in the urine. How an excess of these substances causes the clinical disturbance is not known. Diagnosis depends on identifying porphobilinogen in the urine; porphobilinogen turns red on addition of Ehrlich's aldehyde reagent, and the pigment is not extractable with chloroform, which distinguishes it from urobilinogen. The excess synthetase activity is inhibited by heme, so that injection of this material may have therapeutic value.[2] Occasionally death occurs from respiratory failure during an attack; porphobilinogen is seen in hepatic cells and demyelination occurs in nerves. Changes are otherwise slight.

The other hepatic porphyrias are less common but clinically similar, except for photosensitivity of skin. This is due to the intense fluorescence of porphyrins; by absorbing and re-emitting energy they damage the epidermis.

The erythropoietic porphyrias are rare autosomal recessive disorders in which anemia is frequent. In the congenital form, uroporphyrin is diverted to a stereoisomer (uroporphyrin I) that is incapable of progressing to the formation of heme. Beginning in infancy the pigment spills into the urine, discoloring it burgundy red, stains the teeth red, and makes the skin extremely sensitive to sunlight.[3] As a result sores, blisters, and ulcers develop on exposed surfaces and necrosis occurs on distal parts such as the fingers, nose, and ears. The condition is extremely disfiguring. Fewer than 100 cases have been reported.[1]

## Jaundice

The most important disorder of hemoglobin degradation is jaundice. When hemoglobin is degraded, iron is extracted, globin is detached, and both are reused. The porphyrin residue is then broken down to a linear tetrapyrrole, which is the basic structure of bilirubin. These changes take place in the reticuloendothelial system. As the bilirubin enters the circulation from these sites, it is attached to albumin and in this form is carried to the liver. The bilirubin-albumin complex is not soluble in water. In the liver the albumin is separated, the bilirubin is conjugated with glucuronide, and the conjugated pigment is transferred from the hepatocyte to the bile canaliculi. The conju-

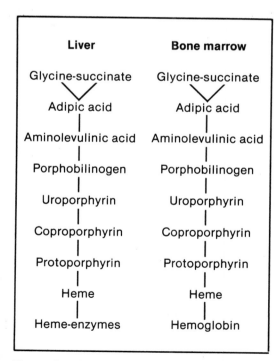

**Figure 8-2.** Sequence of steps in the production of heme in the liver and bone marrow

gated bilirubin is soluble in water. The water-soluble pigment now passes out of the liver in the biliary channels to be concentrated in the gallbladder, and then passes into the duodenum through the common bile duct. In the small intestine bacteria convert the bilirubin to urobilinogen, a colorless compound. Some of the urobilinogen is absorbed through the mucosa and returns to the liver in the portal circulation, where it is reconverted to bilirubin and re-excreted into the duodenum as bile. A very small part of this urobilinogen gets through the liver into the general circulation, where it is carried to the kidneys and, being water-soluble, is excreted in the urine. This is normally an extremely small amount, 0 to 4 mg/24 hours. The bulk of the urobilinogen in the intestine is reduced by bacteria to a brown pigment (bilin), which gives the normal color to the stool.

If 8 gm of hemoglobin are formed daily, 8 gm of hemoglobin are broken down each day. The porphyrin component constitutes 3.5 per cent of the hemoglobin molecule. Thus 0.28 gm or 280 mg of porphyrin pigment are disposed of each day. Since very little of this is eliminated through the urine, the normal porphyrin residue (bilin) in the stool is 100 to 250 mg/day. Stools of normal color thus indicate in a general way that the liver is functioning, that the bile ducts are patent, and that the rate of hemoglobin breakdown is neither excessive nor insufficient.

Jaundice, or icterus, is caused by the diffusion of the tetrapyrrole pigment from heme (bilirubin) into the tissues. It is clinically evident as yellow discoloration of the skin and sclerae. The normal serum bilirubin is under 1.5 mg/dl; jaundice is detectable clinically when the serum bilirubin reaches 3 to 5 mg/dl. Jaundice is often attended by a serum level of 6 to 15 mg/dl, although it may occasionally rise to more than 40 mg/dl.

In clinical terms jaundice may be thought of as due to excessive breakdown of heme pigment before it has reached the liver (prehepatic jaundice), to liver disease (hepatic jaundice), or to obstruction of bile ducts after the pigment has left the liver (posthepatic jaundice). The significance of this classification is that prehepatic jaundice and hepatic jaundice are generally medical problems but posthepatic jaundice often requires surgical treatment. Prehepatic jaundice is most often due to the hemolytic anemias, in which large amounts of heme are disassembled in short periods of time, as with erythroblastosis or the hemolytic crises of sickle cell anemia. Other causes include resolution of a hemorrhagic infarct, especially of the lungs, the absorption of heme from intraperitoneal hemorrhage, as with ruptured tubal pregnancy, and such uncommon conditions as mismatched transfusions, the hemolytic toxin of a snakebite, or the effect of a disseminated infection with hemolytic streptococci. Hepatic or hepatocellular jaundice is, of course, due to liver disease, and the most frequent causes include viral hepatitis, cirrhosis, and drug toxicity. Posthepatic jaundice is usually due to bile duct obstruction. The most common causes of bile duct obstruction include cholelithiasis, scarring of the common duct from adjacent inflammation, e.g., duodenal ulcer, and carcinoma of the head of the pancreas.

Table 8-1.

# Classification of porphyria

Hepatic
    Acute intermittent porphyria
    Porphyria cutanea tarda
    Hereditary coproporphyria

Erythropoietic
    Congenital erythropoietic porphyria
    Erythropoietic protoporphyria

These three types of jaundice may often be distinguished in the laboratory. The key test was provided by van den Bergh, who discovered that a certain diazo compound* produces a color when combined with bilirubin. When the bilirubin is still attached to albumin (prehepatic), the color development is slow (30 minutes), but if the bilirubin has passed through the liver and is no longer attached to albumin, so that it is water-soluble, the color development is rapid (1 minute). The importance of the test is that it tends to distinguish prehepatic from posthepatic bilirubin. Bilirubin in prehepatic jaundice is spoken of as delayed-reacting, indirect, or unconjugated, and bilirubin in posthepatic jaundice is termed prompt, direct-reacting, or conjugated. For consistency of expression, this book will speak of unconjugated and conjugated serum bilirubin.

With prehepatic jaundice, the liver is overloaded with bilirubin and cannot process the pigment fast enough to keep up with the rate of its formation. The excess pigment that accumulates in the blood is still attached to albumin and is unconjugated. The flow of bilirubin through the liver is unimpeded, however, so that the stool contains an excess of urobilinogen and is therefore unusually dark. The unconjugated bilirubin is not water-soluble, so that it cannot be excreted into the urine, although urobilinogen, which is colorless, is present in increased amount. An icteric person with normally colored urine is sometimes said to have acholuric jaundice.

With posthepatic jaundice the pigment has passed through the liver and thus is water-soluble and conjugated. The pigment therefore passes into the urine, which becomes dark. Passage into the gut is blocked so that the stool becomes pale yellowish gray because of the lack of pigment and the absence of digestion of fat, which requires

bile. Urobilinogen in the stool and urine also decreases. Persistent absence of urobilinogen from the urine is the most reliable sign of total biliary obstruction.

Although the pre- and posthepatic types of jaundice are sharply different, hepatic jaundice tends to be less distinct. The serum bilirubin is part conjugated and part unconjugated (biphasic), and the other values tend to fluctuate because of the varying proportions of these pigments that accumulate. Some bilirubin as well as some urobilinogen is thus found in the urine, and the stool is paler than normal but not altogether devoid of pigment (bilin) or urobilinogen.

It is to be understood that jaundice is not a disease; it is the consequence of a pathologic process. Symptoms are infrequent, and itching of the skin, which may be severe, is due more to the associated retention of bile salts than to the accumulation of bile pigment. Bilirubin is toxic to the renal tubules, however, and bile nephrosis with renal failure may develop, especially when shock and jaundice coexist. In the newborn, and especially the premature infant, the enzyme that conjugates bilirubin in the liver (glucuronyltransferase) may not be fully developed. When this is coupled with a hemolytic crisis, as occurs in erythroblastosis fetalis, the unconjugated bilirubin, which is lipophilic, seeps into the brain, discolors the basal ganglia, and often causes serious neurologic disease. The condition is known as kernicterus.

### Iron storage disease
When hemoglobin is broken down, most of the iron is used for the production of new hemoglobin. Some, however, is stored as a reserve. There are two storage forms of iron: ferritin and hemosiderin. Ferritin is a protein-ferric hydroxide complex, and hemosiderin may be a denatured form of ferritin.[4] Ferritin is widely distributed in the body whereas hemosiderin is found principally in the reticuloendothelial tissues, where it may be recognized in macrophages

*Commonly referred to as Ehrlich's diazo reagent (p-dimethylaminobenzaldehyde).

as coarse, yellowish-brown granules that show a positive stain for iron, i.e., the Prussian blue reaction. Stored iron is subject to wide variations in health and disease. Hemosiderosis and hemochromatosis are iron storage diseases.

Hemosiderosis is the deposition of hemosiderin in tissues. It occurs mainly in the macrophages of the reticuloendothelial organs, does not cause tissue damage even when the overload is pronounced, and has no specific clinical meaning.[4] Hemosiderosis is thus a pathologic reaction of little clinical significance. Local forms take place at the margins of hematomas or hemorrhagic infarcts, where macrophages degrade the extravasated red cells and convert the heme pigment to hemosiderin. Macrophages laden with hemosiderin are also abundant in pulmonary alveoli in patients with congestive heart failure; diapedesis and increased hydrostatic pressure carry erythrocytes into the alveoli, where phagocytosis and red cell breakdown take place. It is the abundance of these cells, with their yellowish-brown granules, that produces the "rusty" sputum of patients with congestive heart failure. Excessive breakdown of red cells also occurs in the hemolytic anemias, and in these instances the reticuloendothelial tissues become laden with hemosiderin. Multiple transfusions also result in an excess of heme that contains iron and has to be processed in the reticuloendothelial system before it is available to the other body tissues. So long as the deposition is principally in the macrophages of the reticuloendothelial system, clinical signs do not arise and the reaction is regarded as an innocuous transfusional hemosiderosis.

Hemochromatosis is a disease of iron overload in which intestinal absorption is excessive, conversion to hemosiderin follows, and storage takes place mainly in the epithelial cells of various organs rather than in the macrophages of the reticuloendothelial tissues. Although the mechanism of the process is uncertain, the intestinal derangement is functional and no lesions of the mucosa are described. The process may affect the liver, spleen, lymph nodes, pancreas, heart, and endocrine organs. The liver is large and develops micronodular cirrhosis with abundant hemosiderin pigmentation so that the external surface is nodular and the cut surface is chocolate brown. Portal hypertension tends not to develop, ascites is rare, and primary carcinoma is frequent in long-standing cases. Hemosiderin granules are present in the hepatocytes, bile duct epithelium, Kupffer cells, and scar tissue of the cirrhotic process. In addition to brown pigmentation, the pancreas reveals interstitial fibrosis, although this is slight in other organs except for the liver. Hemosiderin granules are present in the islets as well as the exocrine cells. Diabetes mellitus develops and the skin turns dark from melanin pigmentation. For these reasons the condition has been known as bronze diabetes. In a small proportion of cases cardiac arrhythmias and congestive failure develop; the latter is often refractory to treatment.[5] Testicular atrophy, loss of libido, and gynecomastia may also occur.

The patients are often alcoholic, the condition occurs almost exclusively in men, and the frequency of increased iron absorption in close relatives suggests an inherited defect of uncertain transmission.[6] Male dominance may be due to the inability of men to eliminate iron whereas women are protected by the repeated blood loss of menstruation. Onset is extremely gradual; over a period of 20 to 40 years the total body iron store, which is normally about 5 gm, rises to a total of 15 to 50 gm. The plasma iron is normally 120 to 140 mg/dl, but it rises to 250 mg/dl in hemochromatosis. Diagnosis is aided by a high plasma iron level, a liver biopsy showing parenchymal iron storage, and excessive excretion of iron in the urine after injection with a chelating agent.[7] Phlebotomy mobilizes and eliminates iron stores and improves the outlook for the patient.

## MELANIN

The second normal endogenous pigment is melanin, after the Greek *melas*, meaning "black." It is a dark brown, finely granular pigment found in the cytoplasm of melanocytes. Melanocytes are located in the skin, iris, retina, and meninges. The cells are derivatives of melanophores, which originate in the neuroectoderm of the fetus. The function of melanin is to protect skin and eyes against actinic rays. The pigment is formed by the enzyme tyrosinase, which converts the amino acid tyrosine to dopa (3, 4-dihydroxyphenylalanine). Dopa is then polymerized and attached to a protein to form melanin.[8]

Melanocytes lie in the deepest layer of the epidermis. They produce melanosomes, which are organelles that mature to melanin. Dendritic processes extending from melanocytes convey melanin granules to adjacent squamous cells, into which they are "injected." This process is stimulated by exposure to sunlight and accounts for tanning of the skin. As the epidermal cells exfoliate from the skin surface, the pigment is lost and the tan fades.

Skin pigmentation may be increased or decreased. Increased pigmentation may be focal or diffuse. Freckles are foci of pigmentation due to clusters of melanocytes that have an increased rate of melanin production. They are not related to skin cancer. Moles, or nevi, are also foci of pigmentation due to clusters of melanocytes that may be found in the dermis, in the epidermis, or between the two as junctional lesions. They are sharply circumscribed, show no mitotic figures, and are ordinarily of only cosmetic significance. The malignant tumor of the melanocyte system is the melanocarcinoma, or melanoma. It may arise from nevi, and occurs predominantly on the skin but may originate in the retina

or meninges. Melanocarcinomas and pigmented nevi both take the stain for melanin, but only the former display central mitotic activity and marginal inflammation. The tumors show wide degrees of malignancy, tend to be unpredictable in their spread, and often produce deeply pigmented metastases. The occasional unpigmented melanocarcinoma is presumed to originate from undifferentiated melanoblasts that are not sufficiently mature to produce pigment.

Diffuse melanin hyperpigmentation of skin is a particular feature of Addison's disease. Normally melanin production is stimulated by adrenocorticotrophin (ACTH) and melanin-stimulating hormone from the pituitary, and the secretion of ACTH is regulated by adrenocortical steroids. In the absence of adrenal function, the production of ACTH is uncontrolled and diffuse pigmentation results. Diffuse melanin pigmentation of skin also occurs in hemochromatosis. In hemochromatosis the plasma iron-binding capacity is saturated and diabetes mellitus may be present; in Addison's disease the plasma 17-ketosteroid level is low and does not respond to ACTH.

The most pronounced example of decreased melanin pigmentation is albinism, in which a hereditary trait prevents the synthesis of tyrosinase (see Chapter 7). Without this enzyme, melanin cannot be produced. Albinos are accordingly white-haired, their skin is pink, and their irides are nearly transparent. They suffer from visual disturbance and vulnerability to sunlight, causing an increased incidence of skin cancer.[8] In patients with phenylketonuria, a metabolic block impairs the conversion of phenylalanine to tyrosine so that fair skin, blond hair, and hypopigmentation are also common in this disorder.[8]

## WILSON'S DISEASE

Also under pigmentary disorders is the rare condition of copper accumulation. It was described in 1912 by Wilson, who noted cirrhosis and signs of a neurologic disorder.[9] Kayser and Fleischer independently described the yellowish-green rings that discolor the periphery of the cornea, and subsequently Hall pointed out the inherited nature of the illness as an autosomal recessive trait.[10] He suggested the term "hepatolenticular degeneration," linking the liver with the lenticular nuclei of the brain. More recently it was found that ceruloplasmin, the protein that carries copper in the serum, is absent or deficient. Copper normally bound to this protein is thus free to be deposited in tissues, especially the liver, brain, and cornea.

Wilson's disease begins gradually, mainly in children and young adults, and is manifested by hepatic disorder, neurologic disease, and pigmentation of the eyes. The first may appear as chronic active hepatitis that progresses to cirrhosis. The neural signs include drooling, dysarthria, tremor, and rigidity. The order of onset of these manifestations is variable, although the hepatic disease generally precedes the neurologic signs and corneal pigmentation. The last, known as Kayser-Fleischer rings, is virtually pathognomonic of the disease. Without treatment the course is variable. Most patients suffer progressive neurologic deterioration and die from intercurrent infection within five years of the onset. Chelating agents such as penicillamine, however, increase the urinary excretion of copper and, along with a diet low in copper, can prolong life and diminish the manifestations of the disorder.

When death occurs, autopsy examination reveals a small, cirrhotic liver that varies from micronodular to postnecrotic. Secondary splenic enlargement and portal hypertension may develop. The copper content of each dry-weight gram of hepatic tissue rises from an upper normal value of 50 $\mu$g to between 1 and 3 mg.[11] In the brain, astrocytosis is widespread, cavities form in the lenticular nuclei, and special stains re-

veal pericapillary deposition of copper. In the eyes the copper pigmentation is found in Descemet's membrane of the cornea adjacent to the limbus.

## OCHRONOSIS

The last of the pigmentary diseases is due to a melanin-like substance whose chemical structure is not precisely known. The disease, called ochronosis, is rare and is due to hereditary lack of the enzyme homogentisic acid oxidase, which is an intermediate in the metabolism of tyrosine. Homogentisic acid accumulates behind this metabolic block because it has no alternative pathway of degradation. These relationships are shown in Figure 8-3.

The accumulated acid is transformed into a pigment that resembles melanin, and this, for some unknown reason, binds to cartilage and connective tissue. The carti-

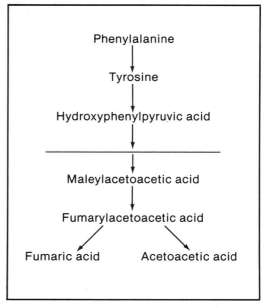

**Figure 8-3.** Intermediate steps in the metabolism of tyrosine. The horizontal line indicates the point at which the process is blocked by the absence of homogentisic acid oxidase.

lage turns dark blue to black, becomes friable, and causes degenerative arthritis, especially of large joints. The condition tends to be progressive and may become completely disabling. The dark blue discoloration is evident clinically in the nose, ears, and sclerae, where cartilage or connective tissue is exposed or lies close beneath the skin surface. Tendons and heart valves also take up the pigment. Sweat may be blue-black, and the urine, which is laden with homogentisic acid, turns dark on standing. Diagnosis depends on finding homogentisic acid in the urine; a screening test for this is available.[12] The morbid changes include black discoloration of cartilage, tendons, and heart valves as well as degenerative arthritis and accelerated atherosclerosis.[13]

From a historical perspective, the black urine was noticed before homogentisic acid was identified. This acid in the urine is a strong reducing agent, so that the urine is avid for oxygen. The term alkaptonuria, derived from the Greek *hapto* ("to seize"), was created because of this affinity. Later the morphologic changes were described. Although the cartilage is discolored blue-black, the tissue microsections, as observed by Virchow in 1866, reveal an ochre or pale yellow color.[14] Virchow therefore named the condition ochronosis. The connection between alkaptonuria and ochronosis was not realized until almost 40 years later. Alkaptonuria was thus found to be only a sign of ochronosis rather than a disease separate from it.

Ochronosis is carried by a recessive gene on an autosome. Although the clinical course is long, black-stained diapers may indicate the diagnosis shortly after birth. Staining of cartilage does not become evident until near the age of 20, and arthritis sets in between 20 and 40 years. The condition is nevertheless consistent with a long life, as noted by McKusick, who cited the description by Garrod taken from a report published in 1649:[14]

> The patient was a boy who passed black urine . . . and who, at the age of fourteen years, was submitted to a drastic course of treatment which had for its aim the subduing of the fiery heat of his viscera which was supposed to bring about the condition in question by charring and blackening his bile. Among the measures prescribed were bleedings, purgation, baths, a cold and watery diet, and drugs galore. None of these had any obvious effect, and eventually the patient, who tired of the futile and superfluous therapy, resolved to let things take their natural course. None of the predicted evils ensued, he married, begat a large family, and lived a long and healthy life, always passing urine black as ink.

Although ochronosis is rare, it is not unimportant. It was the study of alkaptonuria that led Garrod to his pioneering investigations of inborn errors of metabolism. In doing this, Garrod brought medical attention to a whole new concept of human disease.

## REFERENCES

1. Stanbury JB, Wyngaarden JB, Fredrickson DS, eds: *The Metabolic Basis of Inherited Disease*, 4th ed. New York: McGraw-Hill, 1978

2. Dhar GJ, Bossenmaier BA, Petryka ZJ, et al: Effects of hematin on hepatic porphyria. *Ann Intern Med* 83:20, 1975

3. Illis L: On porphyria and the etiology of werewolves. *Proc R Soc Med* 57:23, 1964

4. Williams WJ, Beutler E, Erxlev AJ, et al: *Hematology*. New York: McGraw-Hill, 1972

5. Buja LM, Roberts WC: Iron in the heart. Etiology and clinical significance. *Am J Med* 51:209, 1971

6. Balcerzak SP, Westerman MP, Les RE, et al: Idiopathic hemochromatosis. *Am J Med* 40:857, 1966

7. Harker HA, Funk DD, Finch CA: Evaluation of iron storage by chelates. *Am J Med* 45:105, 1968

8. Fitzpatrick TB, Seiti M, McDugan AD: Melanin pigmentation. *N Engl J Med* 265:328, 374, 430, 1961

9. Wilson SAK: Progressive lenticular degeneration: A familial nervous disease associated with cirrhosis of the liver. *Brain* 34:295, 1912

10. Goldstein NP, Owen CA Jr: Symposium on copper metabolism and Wilson's disease. *Mayo Clin Proc* 49:363, 1974

11. Sternlieb I: Diagnosis of Wilson's disease. *Gastroenterology* 74:787, 1978

12. Kang ES, Gerald PS: Alkaptonuria: Rapid semiquantitative determination of homogentisic acid in urine. *J Pediatr* 76:939, 1970

13. Cooper JA, Moran TJ: Studies on ochronosis. *Arch Pathol* 64:46, 1957

14. McKusick VA: *Heritable Disorders of Connective Tissue*, 4th ed. St. Louis: Mosby, 1972

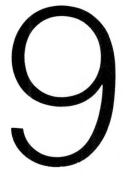

# NUTRITIONAL DISORDERS

Food consists of nutrients that are needed in small and large amounts. The small needs are the vitamins, minerals, and trace elements. The large needs are the proteins, fats, and carbohydrates. The nutrients of large need are quantified in terms of energy units or calories. Fats and carbohydrates provide calories for the physical and metabolic needs of the body, while proteins provide amino acids for the replenishment of tissues lost through the normal process of necrobiosis. Micronutrients facilitate the utilization of calories and proteins. Sound nutrition requires all of these components, each in its appropriate amount. The disturbances of nutrition may be classified as those of too little and those of too much of these components.

## CALORIES

Sunlight initiates all biologic processes by photosynthesis, which takes place in green plants and converts carbon dioxide and water to carbohydrates. The carbohydrates contain chemical energy, which is stored in the body when the plants are eaten. Eventually the metabolic processes of the body utilize this energy. Energy may be measured in the laboratory as the amount of heat given off from the combustion of the carbohydrate with oxygen. Combustion takes place quickly in the laboratory but occurs in the body at a slower rate.

The calorie is the amount of heat needed to raise the temperature of 1 gm of water

1°C, e.g., from 14.5° to 15.5°C. Measurement reveals that each gram of combusted carbohydrate gives off several thousand calories. Since this necessitates unwieldy numbers, a larger energy unit is used. It is the kilocalorie—the amount of heat required to raise 1,000 gm (1 kg) of water 1°C. This larger unit is abbreviated Cal.

It should be understood that while the energy of foods may be expressed as heat in Calories, the same energy may also be expressed as mechanical work in joules. The reason is that energy can be converted from one unit to another. For example, the unit of work energy is the erg, which is the amount necessary to move the mass of 1 gm a distance of 1 cm. The joule is 10 million ergs. One Calorie is equal to 4,180 joules. Thus the energy of food can be expressed in terms of work units just as well as in terms of heat units. It is only because of convention and the practical needs of uniformity that the Calorie is used.

The fuels of the body are proteins, fats, and carbohydrates. On combustion with oxygen they yield 4, 9, and 4 Cal/gm, respectively. This energy is utilized for the metabolic needs and physical activities of the body. Since these needs vary, the total body requirement for energy depends on several factors, including age, sex, work habits, metabolic rate, pregnancy, lactation, and the presence or absence of disease. For these reasons, energy requirements vary among individuals depending on personal circumstances. Nevertheless, the total requirements for the average normal adult is between 1,500 and 3,500 Cal/day. With vigorous work, as in hard manual labor, the total requirement may rise to as much as 6,000 Cal/day.

The American diet is composed of about 50 per cent carbohydrate, 40 per cent protein, and 10 per cent fat. The carbohydrate is the chief source of energy in most diets; it is metabolized to carbon dioxide and water. The second largest source of energy is fat, which is present in food mainly as tri-glycerides. Animal fats are firm at room temperature and their carbon atoms are saturated with hydrogen. Most vegetable fats are liquid at room temperature and their carbon atoms are connected by double bonds without hydrogen saturation. This difference has a bearing on blood cholesterol, and hence atherosclerosis, and is discussed in Chapter 11. About 5 per cent of dietary fat is passed in the feces, while the intermediary products of diacetic acid and its derivative, hydroxybutyric acid, are passed in the urine. The urinary amounts are extremely small. When carbohydrate metabolism is reduced, however, fat is utilized for energy and the amounts of these acids increase in the blood and urine. This is the genesis of ketoacidosis, which is a complication of diabetes mellitus.

Protein in the diet is used to replace the tissue lost in the normal processes of necrobiosis, e.g., desquamation of skin, sloughing of old cells from the intestine, and degradation of effete erythrocytes in the spleen and bone marrow. The amount of dietary protein needed per day for these purposes by the average adult, with a margin to spare, is about 1 gm/kg of body weight.[1] The ingested protein is composed of about 20 amino acids, of which eight cannot be synthesized by the body and hence are regarded as essential. The essential amino acids are valine, methionine, threonine, leucine, isoleucine, phenylalanine, tryptophan, and lysine. Two additional amino acids, arginine and histidine, are needed in the diet during infancy. The ingested protein is broken down into its amino acids, which are absorbed and recombined to form the tissues of the individual.

In the synthesis of body protein, different amounts of specific amino acids are needed. A protein that contains a sufficiency of all of the needed amino acids is a "good protein." One that is deficient in one or more essential amino acids is a "poor protein." A protein that contains a sufficiency of all but one of the essential amino acids can be utilized only to the extent of the insufficient amino acid. Such a protein is therefore "poor," and the insufficient member is known as the limiting amino acid. Milk and egg white contain nearly the right proportion of amino acids for the body's needs. Other proteins may be compared with these nearly ideal mixtures: The smaller the difference, the higher the quality of the protein. From such comparisons comes the concept of the biologic value of a protein: The more nearly similar to an ideal mixture, the higher the biologic value. Most of the proteins in the American diet have biologic values that range between 40 and 80 per cent.[1] The end product of protein digestion is urea, which is excreted in the urine. Comparing the nitrogen of the protein eaten with the nitrogen of the urea excreted reveals whether the individual is gaining or losing protein from his tissues. He is accordingly said to be in positive or negative nitrogen balance.

The body minerals, which contribute importantly to the serum electrolytes, include calcium, chloride, magnesium, phosphorus, potassium, sodium, and sulfur. The trace elements, which are needed in extremely small amounts, include copper, fluorine, iodine, manganese, molybdenum, selenium, and zinc. Altogether over 40 different elements and molecules are needed for the nutrition of the body.

Good nutrition is a balance between too much and too little. Too much leads to obesity and shortening of life. Too little leads to the specific avitaminoses and the general conditions of starvation. Obesity is prevalent in the prosperous nations of the world, while starvation is common in those nations that are impoverished.

## UNDERNUTRITION

There are three main causes of undernutrition: decreased food supply, increased metabolic needs, and failure of assimilation. Decreased supply of food affects those who cannot afford protein, those who live in countries where protein is scarce, and those who follow food fads or prefer alcohol to a nutritious diet. Metabolic needs are increased in mothers during pregnancy and lactation, in the young during adolescence, and in workers at hard physical labor. They are also high in hyperthyroidism and in disease states in which protein is lost, such as large burns or glomerular disease, or in which tissue turnover is rapid, as in leukemia, febrile states, and polycythemia. When food is abundant and metabolic processes are normal, undernutrition may still be due to disease states that retard assimilation of the ingested nutrients. Examples include mucosal impairment, as in nontropical sprue and Whipple's disease; diffuse inflammation, as in regional enteritis; bypassing of the absorptive surface, as in ileojejunal fistula; and deficiency of the digestive juices, as in biliary stricture or pancreatic disease, especially cystic fibrosis. The causes of undernutrition are therefore largely covered by the mechanisms of insufficient supply, increased needs, or defective utilization.

The general diseases of undernutrition include prenatal, postnatal, and adult starvation. Of the fetal organs, the first to achieve complete growth is the brain. The growth phase begins before birth, extends into early postnatal life, and is complete at about 18 months after birth. During this growth spurt, maternal malnutrition may retard cerebral development. This has been demonstrated in pregnant animals in which maternal deprivation of nutrients curtails brain growth to such a degree that the damage is irreparable.[2] Pronounced maternal undernutrition also causes the human brain to be diminished in weight.[3] Whether the diminished brain weight of the newborn also causes mental retardation in later life is a complex question that is still unanswered. Although it has yet to be established in humans, the possibility is of grave concern because millions of children,

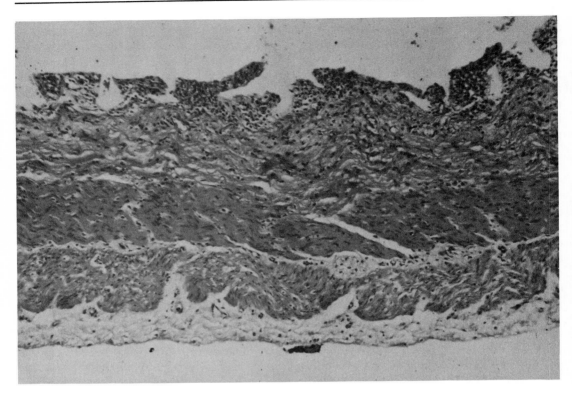

**Figure 9-1.** Atrophy of the ileal mucosa in kwashiorkor

especially in the impoverished countries, are enduring the consequences of prenatal and postnatal starvation.

Undernutrition may also begin in infancy. The reason is famine or impoverishment, and the result is infantile starvation, called marasmus. The body shrinks, the fat depots disappear, and brown atrophy affects the heart and liver. The intestinal mucosa becomes smooth and flat while the skin becomes thin and fragile. As the serum proteins diminish, subcutaneous edema forms. The temperature drops, the heart rate slows, and the psychologic disturbance of restlessness alternates with apathy. Inactivity supervenes, infection develops, and diarrhea follows, with death preceded by cardiovascular collapse.

Whereas marasmus is due to insufficient calories, kwashiorkor is due to insufficient protein with an adequate supply of calories.

The result is not a baby thin and wasted as in marasmus, but a baby with apparently abundant flesh who is nevertheless severely malnourished. Kwashiorkor vaguely means "deposed one," and it refers to the fate of the newborn who has been thriving on the "good protein" of breast milk but who is deposed at perhaps 1 year of age in favor of a younger sibling. The deposed baby thereafter subsists on protein of low biologic value. In Africa this consists of matoke (plantain banana) and cassava root. Malnutrition gradually sets in, and the clinical manifestations become evident at 2 to 3 years of age. They include anorexia, diarrhea, retardation of growth, and apathy alternating with irritability. The color of the hair changes, often to red, and the skin reveals keratosis, desquamation, and irregular pigmentation. Subcutaneous edema forms. The serum albumin is low, and autopsy examination reveals pronounced steatosis of the liver. Atrophy of the ileal mucosa is shown in Figure 9-1. Without proper treatment the mortality is seldom less than 30 per cent and may be much higher.[4] Although kwashiorkor has been more or less recently delineated as a clinicopathologic entity, it nevertheless affects millions of children throughout the world and is one of the most widespread of the scourges of modern mankind.

Starvation in the adult is usually due to famine. In the 19th century approximately 1 million deaths from starvation took place in Ireland when blight destroyed the potato crops repeatedly.[4] In the modern day, and for the first time in history, such terrors can be prevented. Nevertheless, three famines have occurred since 1950: in India from floods and drought, in the Middle East from locusts and earthquake, and in Africa from drought and civil war.[4] It was reported that 3.5 million persons starved to death in 1968; this amounts to nearly 10,000 human beings each day.[5] Nor can complacency prevail; the National Academy of Sciences has predicted grave agricultural disturbances in the event of nuclear war, a development that cannot be altogether dismissed.[6] Whatever the reason, adult starvation causes pathologic changes like those of marasmus with the addition of amenorrhea in women and testicular atrophy and loss of libido in men.

The specific diseases of undernutrition are due largely to the absence of vitamins. In the second decade of the 20th century it was found that animals given a diet of pure protein, fat, and carbohydrate did not thrive, and this evoked the idea that supplemental substances of a vital nature were needed. In 1913, a Polish chemist named Funk found an amine that was helpful in the treatment of experimental beriberi. Knowing about vital supplements and presuming that these would be amines, he coined the word *vitamine*, from which the last letter was later dropped. The first vita-

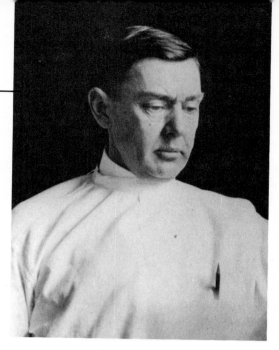

**Figure 9-2.** Elmer McCollum, discoverer of the first vitamin (courtesy National Library of Medicine)

min to be identified was retinol, or vitamin A, which was discovered by Elmer McCollum in 1913 (Figure 9-2). Since then 12 additional vitamins have been found, the last being cyanocobalamin in 1948. Cyanocobalamin, along with folic acid, is reviewed in Chapter 19. Riboflavin ($B_2$) deficiency causes cheilosis but is usually seen in conjunction with other avitaminoses. Vitamin K deficiency is due to liver or intestinal disease rather than to dietary failure. Four vitamins—tocopherol (E), pyridoxine ($B_6$), pantothenic acid, and biotin—have been revealed experimentally but are not associated with dietary deficiency in humans. This leaves five vitamins, shown in Table 9-1, that are associated with classical deficiency diseases.

Vitamins are essential nutrients that have three common properties: They cannot be synthesized by the body, they are needed in extremely small amounts, and they function as reusable catalysts in metabolic reactions. Vitamins are pure proteins or proteins that have attached prosthetic groups; many are components of enzyme systems. The 13 vitamins may be divided into those that are water-soluble and those that are fat-soluble. Fat-soluble vitamins are absorbed after bile salts have emulsified them to fine droplets and pancreatic lipase has hydrolyzed the droplets to fatty acids and glycerol. Deficiencies of fat-soluble vitamins thus tend to be associated with diseases that interfere with these digestive steps, such as biliary obstruction, pancreatic fibrosis, and nontropical sprue. After absorption the fat-soluble vitamins are stored in the liver so that excretion is slow and overdosage is possible. The fat-soluble vitamins are A, D, and K. Overdosage of vitamin A causes pruritus, bone pain, alopecia, and neurologic disturbance.[7] Excess vitamin D occasions metastatic calcification, especially in the lungs, kidneys, and gastric mucosa.[8]

The water-soluble vitamins are easily absorbed and excreted. They are therefore associated with inadequate diets more than with internal disease, and they are not subject to overdosage because of their ready elimination. These vitamins include C and the B complex: thiamine, riboflavin, nicotinic acid, folic acid, and cyanocobalamin.

Lack of vitamins causes five classical deficiency diseases—xerophthalmia, rickets, beriberi, scurvy, and pellagra—as well as the coagulation disorder due to vitamin K deficiency. In addition, lack of folic acid and cyanocobalamin leads to progressive macrocytic anemia (see Chapter 19).

## Xerophthalmia

Vitamin A, or retinol, is necessary for the replenishment of visual purple (rhodopsin), a photosensitive pigment that is bleached from the retina by light. Without replenishment, the rod cells are not stimulated and poor sight in dim light results. Night blindness, or nyctalopia, is thus the first sign of vitamin A deficiency. Retinol is also needed for the orderly renewal and depletion of epithelial cells. In its absence superficial cells accumulate and deep cells undergo squamous metaplasia. As a result, the skin becomes rough and scaly because of follicular keratitis. In glands, especially the lacrimal, salivary, bronchial, and pancreatic, squamous metaplasia develops so that secretions dry up. The same process occurs on other mucosal surfaces, particularly the renal pelves, ureters, and urinary bladder, which become rough and may provide the nidus for stone formation. In the eyes, dryness from lacrimal gland failure and thickening from retention of corneal cells lead to blindness and eventually to infection that may destroy the eyes. This process occurs in thousands of children in the impoverished nations of the world every year.[1] In the mucous glands of the respiratory tract, squamous metaplasia and cellular retention lead to bronchial obstruction, infection, and various degrees of inflammation, including pneumonia, bronchiectasis, and abscess

Table 9-1.

# Vitamins essential for human nutrition

| Name | Designation | Disease | Source |
| --- | --- | --- | --- |
| Retinol | A | Xerophthalmia | Liver, dairy products |
| Calciferol | D | Rickets | Liver, sunlight |
| Ascorbic acid | C | Scurvy | Citrus fruits |
| Thiamine | $B_1$ | Beriberi | Yeast, whole grains |
| Niacin | | Pellagra | Yeast, whole grains |

formation. It is thus the visual and respiratory tracts that are especially affected.

## Rickets

Vitamin D, or calciferol, is found in fish oils, especially cod liver oil, and is formed in the skin by the action of sunlight on the epithelial oils. The vitamin controls the absorption of calcium from the gut, affects the level of phosphorus in the blood, and induces the mineralization of osteoid in the formation of bone. Deficiency thus causes low blood calcium and phosphorus as well as poor mineralization of epiphysial cartilage. The consequences of these changes are rickets in children and osteomalacia in adults. Rickets occurs in the first two years of life and is characterized by soft bones that bend, as well as accumulations of cartilage that bulge at the sites of osteogenesis. The cartilage accumulations cause prominent bossing of the frontal bones, nodules along the costochondral junctions (rachitic rosary), distortion of the thorax (pigeon breast), and indentation of the lower ribs along the line of diaphragmatic attachment (Harrison's groove). These clinical findings, along with deformities such as bowing of the lower legs, are the hallmarks of rickets. The condition is unknown in the tropics because of the abundance of sunlight and the conversion of skin oils to calciferol. After adulthood the bones have formed, so that defects of shape no longer occur and demineralization takes place instead. Osteomalacia is manifested by spontaneous fractures and radiolucency of cortical and medullary bone.

## Beriberi

Beriberi is characterized by atrophy of muscles, paralysis of nerves, and sometimes congestive heart failure. It is mainly a disease of the Orient, where milled rice is abundant, inexpensive, and a natural staple of the diet. When the Dutch occupied the East Indies, this malady overcame their soldiers in large numbers. At that time bacteria had just been recognized as a cause of disease, and for this reason a team of Dutch scientists was dispatched to the East Indies to search for a bacterial cause of beriberi. After two years without success, Eijkman made the thoughtful and critical observation that chickens fed table scraps of milled rice developed droop neck, a sickness resembling beriberi, while chickens eating unmilled or whole-grain rice were not so affected. This led eventually to the realization that the husks of whole rice contain an ingredient that prevents the disease. It was not until 1936, however, that Williams identified thiamine as the vital ingredient of the whole-grain husks.

Thiamine is needed for carbohydrate metabolism. Without it, nerves degenerate and muscles atrophy. The first nerves to be affected are those at the periphery of the body. The characteristic clinical signs are wrist drop, foot drop, and tenderness and atrophy of the leg muscles. The condition often occurs in infants suckled by undernourished mothers, who may describe numbness of their feet during the increased metabolic needs of pregnancy. The name beriberi is taken from the paralysis and muscle weakness; it means "I cannot." The nerves reveal demyelination, fragmentation of axis cylinders, and foci of Wallerian degeneration. The illness with these neuromuscular defects is known as dry beriberi.

Independently of the foregoing, congestive heart failure may also develop. The central feature is lowering of peripheral resistance, which causes the blood pressure to rise, the circulation to accelerate, and the heart to work harder and become dilated and markedly hypertrophic. Sodium and water are retained, anasarca develops, and the condition is known as wet beriberi. It is a prime example of high-output failure. There are three diagnostic keys: The venous pressure is raised, the circulation time is reduced, and the congestive failure responds dramatically to thiamine but not to digitalis.

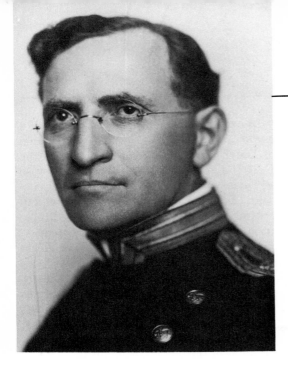

**Figure 9-3.** Joseph Goldberger, the conqueror of pellagra (courtesy National Library of Medicine)

Beriberi is seldom seen in the United States except in alcoholics who are undernourished and rely on white bread made of milled grain for calories. In such a person, oculomotor weakness with confusion leading to coma constitutes Wernicke's syndrome. A mild degree of this confusion, often seen as the syndrome subsides, is called Korsakoff's psychosis. The practice of fortifying white bread with a supplement of thiamine guards against these conditions. In whatever form, beriberi responds quickly to oral or intravenous thiamine.

## Scurvy

Lack of vitamin C causes scurvy, which is characterized by bleeding of the gums, loosening of the teeth, and painful, swollen joints. The condition was rampant in the Middle Ages and accounted for the deaths of more Crusaders than did the Saracen's blade. It became especially prominent in sailors at sea; in 1497, 100 of 160 men with Vasco da Gama on his long voyage around the Cape of Good Hope died of scurvy. In 1752 Lind found that fresh fruits prevented the disease, and shortly before 1800 lemon juice was dispensed daily to British sailors,

who became known as "limeys" on that account. It was not until 1928 that ascorbic acid was identified as the vital ingredient of the lemon juice.

Ascorbic acid is needed for the production of intercellular ground substance. Without it, fibroblasts, osteoblasts, and odontoblasts fail to produce collagen, osteoid, and dentin. As a result, capillaries rupture and connective tissue loosens. The gums become spongy and swollen, hemorrhage takes place, and necrosis may develop. The teeth become loose and may fall out. Fever arises. Scars break down and wounds fail to heal. The skin develops follicular keratitis that becomes hemorrhagic. Hemorrhage also arises under the periosteum, especially of the legs. Bone formation is impaired, osteoid is lacking, and epiphyses slip so that weight bearing is curtailed. With these disturbances also come weakness, fatigue, and aching of the bones, joints, and muscles.

Although scurvy is no longer common, it is occasionally seen in infants 6 to 12 months old who have lived on processed milk without fruits or vegetables. The diagnosis is based on a nutritional history, the appearance of the gums, and a positive capillary permeability test. Response to ascorbic acid by mouth is dramatic: The weakness and bleeding subside in 24 hours, the pain and fever abate in 48 hours, and the gums, skin, and hemorrhages heal in 10 to 12 days.

## Pellagra

Pellagra is a chronic disease characterized by scaly thickening of the skin, a red tongue, sore mouth, nausea and indigestion, and later by weakness, diarrhea, and mental disturbance. It was prominent in Europe from 1700 to 1900, especially in Italy and Spain, and it became epidemic in the southern United States in the early 20th century. It was a disease of the poor, widely regarded as infectious and communicable. Thousands died of pellagra each year in the United States alone.[9] This vast disease was conquered by one man, Joseph Goldberger (Figure 9-3). He was a Public Health Service physician sent to the South in 1914 to investigate the condition. In asylums and prisons he noted that inmates suffered the illness while members of the staff escaped. His observations then disclosed that the diets of these groups were different: The staffs enjoyed milk, butter, eggs, and meat while the inmates were given grits, corn mush, molasses, and sowbelly. Providing the inmates with the diet of their custodians cured the disease. It thus became evident that some factor in the protein-rich foods would both cure and prevent pellagra. The factor turned out to be niacin, but it was not chemically identified until 1937. Niacin is now added to carbohydrate foods and this, together with the improved American diet, has all but eradicated the disease.

Niacin stands for nicotinic acid and nicotinamide, which are needed by all living cells for glycolysis, tissue respiration, and fat synthesis.[10] Without niacin, skin that is exposed to sunlight becomes thick, dry, scaly, brittle, and cracked. In fact, the word pellagra comes from the Italian *pelle*, meaning skin, and *agro*, meaning rough. The backs of the hands are most noticeably affected, and the sunlight-exposed skin of the neck may show a broad band of scaliness called Casal's necklace. Both worsen in the spring and summer months, when sunshine is prolonged. Glossitis also develops, the buccal mucosa becomes inflamed, and the patient complains of a sore tongue and mouth. Digestive disturbances arise and gradually progress to persistent diarrhea. Weakness and depression develop. Later apprehension, headache, and dizziness also occur, but depression is the main mental effect. Eventually paralysis becomes incapacitating, and infection takes its final toll.

The body is able to synthesize some niacin from the amino acid tryptophan in the diet. Tryptophan thus acts as a provitamin, but in this conversion 60 mg of tryptophan are required to produce 1 mg of niacin. Maize, or Indian corn, is low in tryptophan, while rice contains somewhat more. It is for this reason that undernourished rice eaters seldom develop pellagra while undernourished maize eaters often do. The nicotine of cigarette smoke is not converted to the vitamin. Pellagra is extremely responsive to treatment; 100 mg of niacin cause the glossitis and stomatitis to subside and the mental depression to clear in 24 hours. The vitamin is abundant in yeast, liver, meat, and legumes. An intake of only 12 mg/day is sufficient to prevent pellagra. Occasional cases of this disease are still seen in the Near East, South Africa, and parts of Southeastern Europe.[10]

**Vitamin K deficiency**
Vitamin K is a naphthoquinone, isolated by Dam in 1935, who observed that a deficiency caused bleeding and named the substance *Koagulation vitamin*. It is abundant in food and is also formed by bacteria in the intestine, so that a deficiency is almost always due to a disease process rather than a dietary lack. The vitamin is necessary for the production of prothrombin, and its lack may be discovered by determining the prothrombin level in the blood. When the prothrombin level is low, bleeding occurs spontaneously and is often evident in the gums, skin, and mucous membranes. Since vitamin K is fat-soluble, the conditions with which it is associated are biliary obstruction, impaired assimilation (malabsorption syndromes, persistent diarrhea, ileojejunal fistula), and inadequate production (as when antibiotics are used to eliminate the vitamin-producing bacteria from the gut). A deficiency of vitamin K is especially likely in the first and last of these conditions because biliary obstruction often requires surgical intervention while antibiotics are commonly used to cleanse the intestine of bacteria before such operations.

In one other circumstance is a deficiency of vitamin K frequently seen. In the first few days after birth, the newborn may not have sufficient bacteria in the intestine to produce the vitamin, and widespread bleeding occurs. This condition, known as hemorrhagic disease of the newborn, is prevented by giving supplements of vitamin K to the mother prior to birth.

## OVERNUTRITION

Malnutrition includes overnutrition as well as deficiency states, and in highly developed countries overnutrition is a much greater threat to the national health than is undernutrition. This is attributable both to an abundance of food and to a tendency toward inactivity as a result of mechanization. Although the intestine regulates the absorption of minerals such as calcium and iron, it has no mechanism for controlling the absorption of carbohydrates, proteins, and fats. When caloric intake exceeds energy expenditure, therefore, the excess energy is stored as adipose tissue, and this process eventually leads to obesity.

Obesity is the degree of adiposity that is inconsistent with good health. Although the definition is arbitrary and changing, the amount of body fat is most conveniently indicated by skin fold thickness, which is measured over the mid-upper arm or over the subscapular region. More often actuarial tables are used. These give height-weight relationships that are presumed to be ideal. Obesity is arbitrarily defined as the weight that exceeds this ideal by 20 pounds or more for a given height. In the United States 30 per cent of women and 40 per cent of men over 40 years of age are obese by this definition.[10] Obesity therefore exists in epidemic proportions in the United States.

Obesity is determined by the number of fat cells and the amount of fat they contain. The number is fixed in early age and may be genetically determined, since obesity occurs in 50 per cent of children when one parent is fat, and in 80 per cent when both parents are.[11] The maximum number of fat cells is established by the time of adolescence, and overfeeding prior to that time, either on the part of the mother during gestation or on the part of the infant during development, may also increase the total number of fat cells in the body. When this number is established, it does not change, and obesity that develops in later life is due to an increase of the amount of fat stored in each of the cells. The nutritional status of the adult may thus be determined by the earliest days of life as well as during intrauterine gestation.

Obesity shortens life. It is associated with diabetes, hypertension, and coronary heart disease. Overeating is attended by an increased level of insulin in the blood. With this, the islet cells of the pancreas undergo enlargement. Moreover, obesity often precedes the development of adult-onset diabetes. This suggests that diabetes in the adult may be due to prolonged stimulation of the insulin-producing islet cells of the pancreas with eventual exhaustion of them.[12] Whatever the mechanism, diabetes is four times more common in the obese than in the lean.[10]

The mechanism of hypertension is not clear, although it may be related to the increased capillary bed of the adipose tissue, the increased blood volume in those vessels, or vascular disease of the kidneys associated with diabetes and arteriolar nephrosclerosis. The increased blood volume of the obese translates into an increased stroke volume of the heart, which leads to dilation, hypertrophy, and congestive failure. Death from heart disease is much more common in persons who are obese and hypertensive than in normal individuals of the same age.[13]

Obesity is also associated with an elevated level of serum lipids. Especially important is the serum cholesterol, which tends to rise after the ingestion of animal fats (saturated fatty acids) as compared with the lowering effect of many vegetable oils (polyunsaturated fatty acids). Persons with high blood lipids also tend to have atherosclerosis, and this affects the coronary vessels as well as other arteries of medium size. Coronary atherosclerosis causes angina pectoris, myocardial infarction, and congestive failure—aspects that are more common when the blood lipids are high. The incidence of coronary heart disease in men 45 to 55 years of age was found to be six per 1,000 when the serum cholesterol was under 200 mg/dl. When the serum level rose to 260 mg/dl, however, the incidence of coronary heart disease rose to 15 cases per 1,000.[14] There is accordingly some association between obesity, serum lipids, and coronary heart disease even though the relationships among these factors are not altogether clear. Half of all deaths of men in America over the age of 50 are due to coronary heart disease.[10]

Obesity also impairs movement of the chest wall so that respiration becomes labored and respiratory infections become frequent. In extreme cases somnolence from carbon dioxide narcosis also develops. Cholelithiasis is more common in the obese than in the lean; the reason is not known. Mechanical stress is increased by obesity, and with it hernias tend to form, arthritis often worsens, and varicose veins become frequent. Fungal infections of the skin develop in the recesses of the folds of fat. Standing above all of these, however, is heart disease with coronary insufficiency, angina pectoris, myocardial infarction, hypertension, and congestive failure. Diabetes mellitus with hyperlipidemia is also prone to develop, and this advances the vascular disease of atherosclerosis.[15] Thus obesity with all its consequences, especially cardiovascular, is the great pandemic of the 20th century. It is the sweeping bane of the affluent society.

## REFERENCES

1. Passmore R, Robson JS: *A Companion to Medical Studies*, vol 1. Philadelphia: Davis, 1968

2. Winick M, Brasel JA, Velasco E, et al: Effects of early nutrition on growth of the central nervous system. In *The Infant at Risk, Birth Defects Annual Conference Series* (Bergsma D, ed), vol 10, p 29. Huntington, NY: National Foundation, 1974

3. VonMuralt A: *Lipids, Malnutrition, and the Developing Brain*, a Ciba Foundation Symposium. New York: Associated Scientific Publishers, 1972

4. Mayer J: *Human Nutrition.* Springfield, Ill: Thomas, 1972

5. Predmore RL: What role for the humanist in these troubled times? *BioScience* 18:691, 1968

6. Nuclear war: Federation disputes academy on how bad effects would be. *Science* 190:248, 1975

7. Gerber A, Raab AP, Sobel AE: Vitamin A poisoning in adults. *Am J Med* 16:729, 1954

8. Smith JD, Stanton LW, Kramer NC, et al: Nodular pulmonary calcification in renal failure, report of a case. *Am Rev Respir Dis* 100:723, 1969

9. Secrell WH, Haggerty JJ: *Food and Nutrition.* New York: Time-Life Books, 1967

10. Beeson PB, McDermott W: *Textbook of Medicine,* 14th ed, vol 2. Philadelphia: Saunders, 1975

11. Wilson ND, ed: *Obesity.* Philadelphia: Davis, 1969

12. Albrink MJ: Overnutrition and the fat cell. In *Duncan's Diseases of Metabolism* (Bondy PK, Rosenberg L, eds), 7th ed, pp 417-443. Philadelphia: Saunders, 1974

13. Mayer J: *Overweight.* Englewood Cliffs, NJ: Prentice-Hall, 1968

14. Damon A, Damon ST, Harpending HD, et al: Predicting coronary heart disease from body measurements of Framingham males. *J Chron Dis* 21:781, 1969

15. McLaren DS: The vitamins. In *Diseases of Metabolism* (Bondy PK, ed), 6th ed, pp 1280-1317. Philadelphia: Saunders, 1969

# 10

## ABNORMALITIES OF GROWTH

Growth disturbances include tissue alterations that are reactive, new growths that are genuine tumors, changes caused by carcinogenic agents, and the process of transformation, in which normal cells are converted to tumor cells.

### REACTIVE CHANGES

The first alteration of growth is failure of the structure to form, called aplasia. It affects paired organs such as the kidneys, adrenals, and testes, where lack of one member is not functionally important. The term agenesis has the same general meaning. Quite different, however, is hypoplasia, which is failure of the part to reach normal adult size. One kidney, for example, may be well formed but weigh only 60 gm compared with the normal weight of 140 to 160 gm. It has, incidentally, become customary to use the term hypoplasia in reference to bone marrow failure, but this is incorrect; that process is atrophy. Aplasia, agenesis, and hypoplasia are congenital malformations.

Atrophy is the regression in size, and usually function, of a part that has previously been normal in all respects. It is an extremely common abnormality of growth and affects a wide variety of tissues. It has physiologic and pathologic causes. Physiologic causes include regression of the thymus at the time of puberty, shrinkage of the uterus after the menopause, and a decrease in the size of many organs in old age.

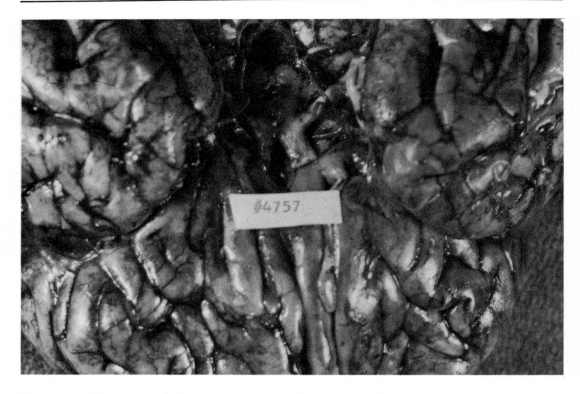

**Figure 10-1.** Disuse atrophy of left optic tract years after removal of left eye

Pathologic causes include pressure on cells, loss of blood supply, denervation of a part, absence of a trophic hormone, and simple disuse of the structure. Examples abound: the weakness and loss of muscle of the leg in a cast, the shrunken extremity that is paralyzed from poliomyelitis, and passive hyperemia of the liver, which distends the sinusoids, pushes against the hepatocytes, and causes disappearance of the cells in the centers of the lobules. Loss of blood supply, as in arteriolar nephrosclerosis, gradually causes the kidney to shrink and the surface to become granular as the nephrons succumb. In the weightlessness of space disuse is unavoidable; in one study, calf circumference was diminished after only three days.[1] In pituitary disease the absence of trophic hormones is reflected by shrinkage of the related part. In all these examples the individual cell undergoes au-

todigestion, large autophagic vacuoles form, and the result is often a small residual body containing lipofuscin that is eventually disposed of in the reticuloendothelial system. Whether physiologic or pathologic, therefore, atrophy is a gradual decrease of cell mass with a regression of organ size and a loss of functional capacity. The process is illustrated in Figure 10-1.

In the opposite direction are non-neoplastic alterations that increase the size of a part: hypertrophy and hyperplasia. Hypertrophy is enlargement of a part due to increase in the size of the existing cells. In contrast, is enlargement due to the proliferation of new cells. Hypertrophy is more common and is associated with increased function as well as size of the part. In earlier days this was evident in the blacksmith's arm, which was vigorously exercised over long periods. Today it is more likely to be seen in the arm of the professional tennis player or in the muscles of the weight lifter. These pronounced responses to strain also occur at internal sites; e.g., the left ventricle that pumps against the raised blood pressure of hypertension becomes thick, firm, and bulky. Histologic examination reveals enlargement of the muscle fibers and nuclei, and higher magnification reveals increases in the myofilaments and cell organelles as well.[2] Smooth muscle also participates; the wall of the intestine proximal to a site of stenosis similarly dilates, stretches, and thickens as the existing muscle cells enlarge. Any muscular tube in the body is subject to this alteration, including the gut, ureters, urinary bladder, and biliary channels. The process is not restricted to muscle, however. The removal of one kidney is followed by enlargement of the remaining member, and the injury of hepatic tissue occasions enlargement of the remaining cells for the purpose of coping with the additional stress.[2] Thus hypertrophy is a cellular adaptation to increased work load and results in enlargement of cells, an increase in the size of the part, and strengthened function to cope with the strain imposed.

Hyperplasia also connotes increase in size of the part, but it is due to an increase in the number rather than the size of cells. Hyperplasia is more a response to environmental conditions than an increase in functional capacity. For example, nodular hyperplasia of the prostate is likely a response to altered hormone balance in the elderly man; it provides no additional function and, indeed, may impose a serious handicap by compressing the prostatic urethra (see Figures 16-3 and 16-4). The skin, when subjected to repeated trauma, responds by increasing the number of cells at that site so that a physiologic response—a callus—is evident. When the trauma ceases, however, the reaction subsides. Hyperplasia is thus to be distinguished from neoplasia, which is a process of cell proliferation that is independent of functional stimuli.

There is a further non-neoplastic change, in which a cell of one type reverts to a cell of another type. The process is called metaplasia, and most examples are the conversion of columnar cells to squamous cells. This change has two causes: chronic inflammation and insufficiency of vitamin A. In the endocervical canal persistently affected by chronic inflammation, squamous metaplasia is especially frequent. At other sites, particularly the bronchi, chronic inflammation also occasions squamous metaplasia, and this alters the ciliary activity of the mucosa so that the sweeping function of the surface is diminished. The chronically inflamed bronchi in bronchiectasis regularly show squamous metaplasia (see Figure 12-5). Lack of vitamin A also causes the conversion of columnar mucosal surfaces to the squamous type, as seen in the lacrimal, salivary, bronchial, and pancreatic ducts as well as in the urinary tract, where roughening and keratinization may provide the nidus for stone formation. Stones may form in the renal pelves, ureters, or urinary bladder. When the stimulus for this metaplastic change is removed, the mucosal cells revert to normal. Thus metaplasia does not progress to neoplasia.

In addition to the foregoing, there is an intermediate state in which epithelial changes are neither absolutely non-neoplastic nor certainly preneoplastic. Several varieties of this intermediate stage are described and a confusing array of terms is used to identify them: epithelial atypism, basal cell hyperactivity, anaplasia, dyskaryosis, dyskeratosis, atypia, and atypical epithelial hyperplasia. The points of difference among them are indistinct. In sorting these conditions, it is helpful to understand that histologic differences in epithelial patterns are subjective interpretations made by different observers. It might be expected, therefore, that diagnoses made by different individuals independently examining the same tissues would be nonuniform, and there is some evidence of this.[3] To avoid confusion and the controversies of terminology, this book includes all of the intermediate stages, if they are in fact different, under the term *dysplasia*. Dysplasia is an epithelial change that may extend through the mucosa and consists of nuclear enlargement, hyperchromatism, slight increase of mitotic figures, and disarrangement of the orderly pattern. The process is reversible and may revert to normal or progress to a genuine neoplastic change with the formation of an invasive tumor.[4] There are no reliable criteria for predicting which course will be followed.[5] The topic must therefore be set aside, leaving specific questions to the experienced morphologist, but with the recognition that there is a stage between the non-neoplastic alteration and the preneoplastic change that is ill-defined and imprecise. Its existence is recognized, but it is not well understood.

### NEOPLASIA

Neoplasia is the process of tumor formation. A tumor is a focal growth of heritable nature that is harmful to the host. Tumors may be divided into two groups according to their behavior: benign and malignant. Benign tumors do not invade adjacent tissues, do not spread to distant sites, and are curable by local excision. Moreover, they are more common than malignant tumors and tend to arise at an earlier age.[6]

### Benign tumors

Benign tumors have six characteristics: They tend to grow slowly, their margins are smooth and sharply defined, their cell patterns resemble the tissue of origin, their textures are soft or resilient, they remain localized to their sites of origin, and their constituent cells are uniform without pronounced variation in size, shape, or mitotic activity. Benign tumors are named by adding the suffix "oma" to the tissue of origin. There are thus fibromas, osteomas, chon-

dromas, lipomas, angiomas, and myomas, all of which arise from connective tissue or mesodermal structures. Benign tumors of epithelial surfaces are called adenomas when a glandular pattern is formed, and papillomas when the surface is covered by squamous epithelium. Papillomas are common on skin, while adenomas form on internal structures such as colonic mucosa, bronchial surfaces, and ducts of various glands. Adenomas may be modified according to special features such as colloid secretion, cyst formation, or frond production. There are thus colloid adenomas, cystadenomas, and papillary adenomas.

Since benign tumors remain localized and grow slowly, their effects tend to be comparatively slight. Nevertheless, structural and physiologic effects may occasionally cause harmful consequences. For example, angiomas discolor the skin and may produce disfiguring cosmetic effects, lipomas of the subcutaneous tissue may deform a surface, and tumor mass alone, even when small, may obstruct a duct or channel. Myomas of the uterine wall compress veins and cause excessive bleeding during the menstrual period, while large tumors of the same kind may interfere with pregnancy. A tiny papilloma of the urethra may obstruct the passage of urine, while a pedunculated adenoma of the ileum may cause intestinal obstruction by invaginating the wall into its own lumen, a process called intussusception (see Figure 13-16). When a tumor arises in an endocrine gland, effects due to hormonal secretion follow. Thus adenomas of the anterior pituitary secrete growth hormone and cause gigantism in children and acromegaly in adults. In the same way, parathyroid tumors cause osteoporosis from the secretion of parathyroid hormone, and islet cell tumors of the pancreas cause hyperinsulinism with hypoglycemic attacks and unconsciousness. Benign tumors are therefore not altogether innocuous. They are more common than malignant tumors and do not discharge toxic substances into the blood, compete for metabolic products, or often undergo malignant transformation. They stop growing at a certain stage, and their effects are due more to their site and size than to unrestrained growth.

## Malignant tumors

Malignant tumors are also characterized by six gross and microscopic characteristics: They grow more rapidly than benign tumors, they enlarge by tissue invasion so that their margins are serrated rather than smooth, their cells are nonuniform and anaplastic, their texture is hard, central necrosis is common, and metastasis to distant sites eventually takes place. Thus malignant tumors, which are collectively known as cancers, invade locally and metastasize distantly.

Although the rate of growth of most cancers is relatively rapid, some are extremely slow. Moreover, it is likely that many years are required for the malignant transformation to take place and for the tumor to become clinically evident. Thus malignant neoplasia is a gradual process, accelerating in the clinical phase and causing death 18 months to three years after clinical appearance in most patients.

Serration of the margin is due to fingerlike processes that extend into the adjacent normal tissue. It is this crablike aspect that gave rise to the term cancer. Anaplasia is a

set of microscopic features that equate with malignancy and include irregularity of nuclear size, increased numbers of mitotic figures, abnormal mitotic figures, abnormal cell arrangements, and failure of adjacent columnar cells to retain their normal parallel alignment, called loss of polarity. Hardness is common in cancer, but not uniformly, and it comes from the tendency of tumor cells to stimulate dense fibrous connective tissue. This process, called desmoplasia, produces a characteristic texture, especially in the breast, that permits physical detection by screening procedures such as mammography. Lastly, metastasis, or distant spread, is a characteristic of malignant tumors although some, such as basal-cell cancer of the skin and the primary cancers of the brain, invade locally but seldom spread away from their sites of origin. There are accordingly several variations from the usual behavioral characteristics of most cancers.

Classification of cancers reveals that there are about 100 distinct types.[7] These may be separated into four main subtypes (Table 10-1).

Malignant tumors of epithelial cells are called carcinomas. They are considerably more common than all the others, and they arise from tissues of ectodermal and endodermal origin. Common examples are squamous-cell carcinoma of the skin and lungs and adenocarcinoma of such internal organs as the pancreas and colon.

The second group consists of the lymphomas, which are solid tumors that arise in lymphoid structures such as the lymph nodes, spleen, and, less frequently, the lymphoid deposits of the lungs and mucosa of the ileum and colon. The lymphomas compose about 6 per cent of the total, and Hodgkin's disease makes up about half this number. Since the others are less distinct, they are simply referred to as non-Hodgkin's lymphomas.

The third group consists of the leukemias, which arise in cells of the reticuloen-

Table 10-1.

## Subtypes of cancer

| Group | Incidence |
| --- | --- |
| Carcinoma | 85% |
| Lymphoma | 6% |
| Leukemia | 4% |
| Sarcoma | 2% |
| Miscellaneous | 3% |

dothelial system: the liver, spleen, lymph nodes, and bone marrow. The leukemias produce free circulating tumor cells in the blood. The tumor cells are like those that normally circulate, although many are often immature and, in the acute forms of the disease, blast cells may predominate. The laboratory evidence of the condition is therefore the increased number of circulating cells and the increased proportion of them that are immature. The leukemic cells invade solid tissues, but this invasion is widespread and unlike the focal solid growths of metastatic carcinoma. Both the lymphomas and the leukemias arise in tissues of mesodermal origin.

Table 10-2. _____

### Estimated incidence of cancer in the United States for 1980*

| Male | | |
| --- | --- | --- |
| Lung | 85,000 | (22%) |
| Prostate | 66,000 | (17%) |
| Colon/rectum | 55,000 | (14%) |
| Urinary | 36,500 | (9%) |
| Leukemia/lymphoma | 33,500 | (9%) |
| Pancreas | 12,500 | (3%) |

| Female | | |
| --- | --- | --- |
| Breast | 108,000 | (27%) |
| Uterus | 54,000 | (14%) |
| Colon/rectum | 43,000 | (15%) |
| Lung | 32,000 | (8%) |
| Leukemia/lymphoma | 28,100 | (7%) |
| Urinary | 15,900 | (4%) |

*Excluding nonmelanoma skin cancer and carcinoma in situ.

The least common are the solid tumors of mesodermal origin, which compose about 2 per cent of the total and are called the sarcomas. They arise in bone, cartilage, adipose tissue, skeletal muscle, and fibrous connective tissue. They are highly malignant as a rule, tend to spread by direct vascular invasion, and are named by adding "sarcoma" as a suffix to the tissue of origin, e.g., fibrosarcoma, leiomyosarcoma, osteosarcoma, chondrosarcoma.

There is finally a small group of unusual or rare tumors, often of mixed composition, that are difficult to classify. They arise from such structures as brain, testis, thymus, and pineal.

Malignant tumors are both common and serious. Second only to cardiovascular disease, cancer is the most common cause of death in the United States. It was estimated that 765,000 new cases of cancer would be diagnosed in the United States in 1979[8]—many causing pronounced discomfort, prolonged disability, economic adversity, and death in significant numbers in all decades of life. The sites of origin vary with sex and age. In children of either sex, leukemia, lymphomas, and tumors of the central nervous system are relatively common. In adults frequency varies according to sex. Table 10-2 shows the estimated incidence of malignant tumors according to site and sex in 1980.[9] It may be seen that cancer in men arises most frequently in the lung, colon, and prostate, while in women the most common sites are the breasts, uterus, and colon.

The effects of cancers are devastating when compared with those of benign tumors. The reason is that cancers are relentlessly progressive and constantly invade and erode into vessels and ducts to cause hemorrhage, necrosis, and obstruction of vital parts. Cancers of the intestine, for example, ulcerate the surface, invade the vessels to cause hemorrhage, stimulate connective tissue growth to cause obstruction, penetrate the wall to cause perforation, and lead to abscess formation or diffuse peritonitis. Cancers of the skin similarly invade, ulcerate, and deform. Moreover, these are only the local effects; cancers also spread, or metastasize, so that secondary sites of tumor growth take root, and each of these continues the process of invasion with all the consequences of obstruction, hemorrhage, necrosis, and perforation.

In addition to the local effects, there are general effects of an obscure nature. For example, anemia develops early in cancers that bleed, but late in other cancers, for reasons that are not clear. Cancers do not produce toxins that kill; they usurp nutrients instead, and this causes cachexia and invites infection. Moreover, the necrosis of the tumor impairs metabolism and occasions thrombosis, bleeding, and simple organ failure.

The clinical manifestations of all these effects vary greatly. Nevertheless, there are common systemic manifestations: weakness, anorexia, inanition, lassitude, · and loss of weight. Added to these are the main symptoms that relate to the site of the lesion, such as hoarseness from cancer of the larynx, convulsions from a tumor of the brain, fracture of a bone from unexpected metastatic disease, and a change of bowel habit from a cancer of the colon.

The clinical diagnosis of cancer may be suspected from these characteristic manifestations. The absolute diagnosis, however, requires histologic examination of the tumor. Biopsy, or the surgical removal of a portion of the tumor, is thus the procedure that secures the diagnosis. This is done through incision into the tissue, as in the breast, or puncture with a hollow needle so that a minute cylinder of tumor is removed, as with cancer of the prostate or liver. Cytologic examination of fluid from the region of the tumor or from scrapings of the tumor surface is less reliable and should be used as a detection procedure rather than a diagnostic one. The blood may also be examined for substances produced by the tumor, such as $\alpha_1$-fetoprotein from cancer of the liver or acid phosphatase from bony metastases of cancer of the prostate. Neither, however, constitutes a specific and absolute diagnosis. The blood may also be sieved in the laboratory for circulating tumor cells and although these are often found, the cells do not specify the site of the primary lesion, or whether the cancer is still localized and therefore probably curable. Most circulating tumor cells succumb without establishing foci of metastatic growth.

When the tumor tissue is prepared for histologic examination, its nature is determined according to the cell type, resemblance to the tissue of origin, and degree of anaplasia. Now an additional estimate is undertaken: the degree to which the tumor resembles the normal tissue from which it arose. This is the process of grading, and it results in a modifier that indicates the differentiation of the tumor. The tumor is noted as well differentiated when it closely resembles the tissue from which it arose, and as poorly differentiated when it does not. It may also show no differentiation and hence be registered as undifferentiated. The reason for this practice is that well-differentiated tumors tend to grow more slowly and spread less rapidly than tumors with little or no differentiation. The practice is not altogether successful, however, because grading is subjective and therefore inclined to be nonuniform, and the differentiation of a tumor is often irregular so that the site of the sample affects the outcome of the judgment. It is nevertheless true that well-differentiated cancers offer a better outlook than poorly differentiated ones, other factors being equal.

Although the diagnosis is established by histologic examination, there is no certain way to determine whether the tumor has spread away from its primary site. This occurs by invasion and metastasis, and it is important because metastatic disease often spells incurability. At the invasive margins of the primary tumor, aggressive cancer cells penetrate into vascular spaces, chiefly lymphatic, in which they become embolic and are swept in the current to regional lymph nodes. The afferent lymph channels enter about the periphery of the node, so that the first metastatic deposit is likely to be found just under the capsule. Later, after the tumor cells have grown in the lymphatic tissue, emboli of cancer cells emerge in the efferent channels that issue from the hilum of the node. The pattern of spread of the primary cancer is not altogether predictable, although nearby regional lymph nodes tend to be involved first. For example, cancer in the upper outer quadrant of the breast tends to metastasize to the axillary nodes, cancer of the lung spreads to the mediastinum, and tumors of the intestine are first found in the mesenteric nodes close to the primary site.

Metastatic carcinomas usually spread in the lymphatics, but some favor the venous route. This applies especially to carcinoma of the kidney, which invades the renal vein, extends into the inferior vena cava, and may then grow as a solid tumor thrombus that reaches the right atrium. Another example of venous invasion is primary carcinoma of the liver, which grows into venous branches within that organ but nevertheless tends not to spread widely outside the liver. A third example is carcinoma of the prostate, which tends to spread to the spine and brain through the vertebral veins of Batson.[10] Sarcomas, although uncommon as a group, often spread through veins rather than through lymphatics.

Carcinomas also penetrate directly onto serous surfaces, where tumor cells are discharged to cause widespread seeding. For example, carcinoma of the bronchus may spread to the surface of the lung so that tumor cells are discharged into the pleural fluid and are implanted widely on the visceral and parietal parts. Similarly, extension of bronchogenic carcinoma may reach the pericardium. In the peritoneum, carcinoma of the body or tail of the pancreas may pro-

duce massive implantation of tumor cells.

Some routes of spread are uncommon. One is penetration of cancer cells into arteries. Whether this is due to the musculoelastic nature of the arterial wall or the recurring pulsations of the vessel is not known. Nevertheless such penetration is seldom seen. Another uncommon route of spread is from mucosa to mucosa in the intestinal tract. Thus carcinoma of the esophagus or stomach does not spread by implanting tumor cells in the ileum or colon, and carcinoma of the cecum does not discharge tumor cells that implant in the mucosa of the descending or sigmoid colon. Nor does one cancer usually metastasize to another cancer in the same patient, although exceptions are known.[11] Lymphatic and venous channels are the main routes of metastasis for carcinomas.

After spread into lymphatic vessels the tumor cells are carried as emboli in the vascular current to two large vascular sieves: the liver and lungs. These two organs are accordingly the most common sites of metastatic disease. Other organs that provide favorable sites for metastases are the kidneys, adrenals, brain, and bone marrow. Although the patterns of spread are not predictable, cancer of the lung frequently metastasizes to one or both adrenals; they appear to be a site of special predilection.

The phenomenon of metastasis is poorly understood. What is the mechanism that allows an invading tumor cell to break away from the primary site and float free in the current of lymph or venous blood? Two possibilities that may induce cell separation are the concentration of calcium on the tumor cell surface, which is lower than on normal cells, and the quality of the desmosome, an intracellular organelle that holds normal cells together and may be weak, absent, or imperfectly formed in tumor cells.[12, 13] Once the tumor cell has broken free, there is still the question why metastatic deposits form in some tissues, such as the liver, lungs, kidneys, adrenals, bone, and brain, much more frequently than in others, such as the spleen, heart, and skeletal muscle. The difference may be that if the tumor cells progress to the capillaries of the organ, metastasis is likely, but if they cannot extend that far because of obstruction in the arterioles, metastatic growth is unlikely.[14] Thus the finding of circulating tumor cells in the blood does not necessarily mean that metastatic disease has already become established.

Once the tumor has been diagnosed, the question of treatment arises. The objective is to ablate all of the tumor since it must be taken as a premise that any surviving deposits will continue to grow and the tumor will sooner or later recur. Moreover, treatment should be administered as early as possible because cancers eventually spread away from their sites of origin and cure is then much harder to achieve. Finally, it is evident that clinical examination of the primary cancer will often not be sufficiently precise to determine whether the tumor has already metastasized to regional lymph nodes or to distant sites. From these considerations the principle of treatment naturally emerges: ablation of the primary tumor and the largest amount of surrounding expendable tissue at the earliest convenient time. Fulfilling this principle provides the highest prospect for cure because there is no way to exceed the largest amount of surrounding expendable tissue and there is no way to do it before the earliest convenient time.

Local treatment is applied to those cancers that are accessible and can be detected while they are still limited to the site of origin. Examples are carcinomas of the breast, lung, colon, and kidney. In each of these the widest excision at the earliest time is the method of choice. It is to be realized, however, that the term "expendable tissue" is subjective and judgmental: The surgical procedure cannot be so radical as to jeopardize the recovery of the patient, but it also cannot be so conservative as to

allow recurrence from tumor left in expendable tissue. The extent of the procedure, therefore, necessarily requires the judgment of the surgeon. Moreover, individual circumstances affect this judgment. For example, a frail, elderly woman with an apparently localized cancer of the breast might be treated less radically than a robust, younger woman with the same lesion.

Although this principle of treatment is valid for all unicentric cancers that appear to be localized, surgery is not the only effective modality of therapy. Radiation is sometimes used instead; the important example in which it is often preferred is carcinoma of the uterine cervix. In this instance the cancer is frequently identified while it is still localized and lies entirely within the field that can be exposed to intensive ionization. All portions of the tumor that lie within the cancerocidal range of the ionizing rays are thus ablated. Results are comparable to those of surgical extirpation.[15]

The method and extent of treatment are determined partly by staging—estimating the spread of the cancer from clinical examination of the patient. Staging is notoriously inaccurate. The error tends to be underestimating rather than overestimating, and the degree of error is about 30 to 40 per cent.[16,17] Nevertheless staging is perceived as serving two needs: to give some estimate of the requirements of optimal therapy and to identify cases of equal spread that may be treated by different methods so that a comparison of results will reveal the superior method. Neither point of reasoning, in my judgment, is sound.

For example, clinical evidence may suggest that a cancer of the breast has not yet spread to the axilla, but morphologic examination of the axillary contents refutes this impression. Therefore, in order to give the patient the highest prospect for cure, it is necessary to follow the stipulations of the principle of treatment and remove the largest amount of expendable tissue rather than select a smaller extirpation on the basis of clinical staging, which has so often proved inaccurate.

Staging is also used to identify cases of equal spread for comparison of results after different methods of treatment. However, this proposition has not succeeded in the case of several common cancers. The reason is that clinical staging is extremely inaccurate and the difference in therapeutic accomplishments of the respective methods is extremely slight. There is accordingly no plausible prospect that such an analysis will ever succeed.[18]

Although surgery and radiation are the main therapeutic modalities for cancers that appear to be localized, chemical treatment is of use when metastatic disease has already developed. The useful agents include hormones, antibiotics, and cytostatic compounds that interfere with mitotic division, including antimetabolites, plant alkaloids, and alkylating agents. Several of these antineoplastic drugs are also useful in the treatment of lymphomas (Table 10-3). The greatest success has been realized with methotrexate for the treatment of choriocarcinoma, in which cure appears to have been achieved.[19] Chemotherapy is also added to ablative treatment for apparently localized tumors such as cancer of the breast in the realization that minute metastases cannot be detected clinically and, if present, may be more vulnerable to chemotherapeutic agents when small than when large.[20] It is too early to tell whether this rationale will be proved correct. When chemotherapy is used, survival rates no longer turn entirely on local factors, and comparisons for the purpose of identifying superior methods then become valid.

Regardless of the method of treatment, success depends on identifying the tumor while it is still localized, or on the rate at which the tumor spreads away from its site of origin. Therefore tumors that are superficial, easily evident to clinical examination, and comparatively slow to spread are attended by the best results. Examples include cancers of the skin, breast, rectum, and uterine cervix. On the other hand, cancers that are internal and clinically obscure and tend to spread at an early time are attended by poor results. Examples include carcinomas of the esophagus, stom-

Table 10-3.

## Chemotherapy of cancer

| Class | Agent | Tumor |
| --- | --- | --- |
| Hormones | Estrogen | Cancer of prostate |
| | Cortisone | Leukemia |
| Alkylating agents | Nitrogen mustard | Hodgkin's disease |
| | Cyclophosphamide | Leukemia |
| Antimetabolites | 6-Mercaptopurine | Leukemia |
| | 5-Fluorouracil | Leukemia |
| | Methotrexate | Choriocarcinoma |
| Plant alkaloids | Vincristine | Lymphoma |
| | Vinblastine | Lymphoma |
| Antibiotics | Dactinomycin | Wilms's tumor |

ach, lung, and pancreas. From these two categories of tumors it may be seen that the distribution of the cancer is the main reason for the success or failure of treatment. This is the equivalent of saying that the rate of survival marks the delineation between those cancers that have spread and those that are still localized at the time of treatment. Thus survival rates turn mainly on the biologic behavior of the cancers, i.e., their aggressiveness or tendency to spread, rather than on the methods of treatment applied to them. This behavioral characteristic of the various cancers is known as biologic predeterminism.[21]

Although much progress has been made, chemotherapy for the treatment of cancer is largely palliative and, until more effective agents are found, it is likely that radiation and surgical extirpation will remain the principal methods of curative therapy.

## CARCINOGENESIS

The topic of carcinogenesis is extremely complex because there are so many different kinds of cancer, so many different agents that induce cancer, and so many mechanisms by which the malignant transformation may take place. Nevertheless, it is established that malignant tumors are induced by four main agents: chemicals, viruses, radiation, and hereditary factors. After reviewing these it will be necessary to consider the mechanisms by which the carcinogenic transformation takes place. Possibilities for which there is some evidence include membrane alterations, cytoplasmic changes, nuclear injuries, and immunologic adjustments.

### Chemicals

Chemical agents known to induce cancer include the polycyclic hydrocarbons, aromatic amines, azo dyes, nitroso compounds, plant alkaloids, and certain inorganic materials, including metals and plastics. All except the plant alkaloids are syn-

thetic substances. Altogether, over 100 chemicals have been reported to produce tumors in humans or other animals, and it is widely estimated that 60 to 90 per cent of cancers are caused by environmental factors, mostly chemical.[22]

Although cancer was originally presumed to be an unavoidable disease, it first occurred to Sir Percivall Pott in 1775 that its cause might be an environmental agent. In England at that time, boys and young men were hired to climb into chimneys to sweep out the soot with brooms. The soot impregnated their clothes and became lodged in the rugose folds of the scrotal skin. After a long latent period, scrotal "soot warts" formed and became invasive, spreading into the testicles, up the spermatic cords, and into the abdomen. Pott was the first to grasp the relationship between the soot and the cancer. This observation had immediate and lasting consequences. The immediate consequence was to prevent the disease: Within three years of Pott's observation, daily bathing was recommended and the condition failed to develop in those who followed this suggestion.[23] The lasting consequence was that the search for chemical carcinogens was begun, a search that continues today.

Pott's observation was not acted upon experimentally, however, until 1915, when Yamagiwa and Ichikawa produced cancers by painting coal tar on the ears of rabbits.[24] These Japanese investigators were accordingly the first to produce cancer by experimental means. Kennaway examined coal tar for carcinogenic compounds and identified the polycyclic hydrocarbons, especially benzo[a]pyrene and certain derivatives of anthracene, in 1955.[25] Among the latter was 3-methylcholanthrene, the most potent carcinogen so far known. These agents cause carcinoma when painted on the skin, sarcoma when injected subcutaneously, and carcinoma of the intestine when ingested by mouth.[26]

Polycyclic hydrocarbons are found in

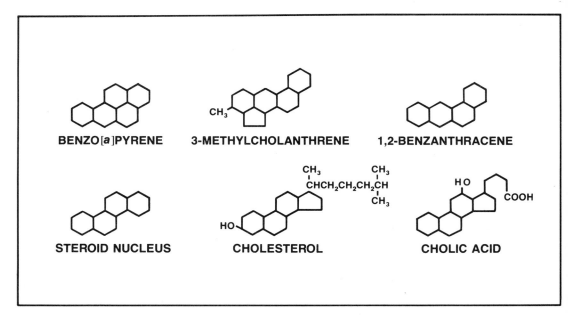

**Figure 10-2.** Similarity of ring structures of normal and carcinogenic compounds

tars, oils, and soot, or in their combustion products. About 1 $\mu$g of benzo[a]pyrene is present in the smoke of 100 cigarettes. This amount is so small as to make it unlikely that lung cancer associated with smoking is due solely to this substance.[27] It may be pointed out, however, that benzo[a]pyrene and other hydrocarbons are also present in coal gas, smoked food, and the exhaust fumes of gasoline engines. It may further be noticed that the structures of these compounds are similar to those of certain normal biologic materials (Figure 10-2). This suggests that carcinogenic activity within the body may arise from small changes within normal compounds. This possibility has not, however, been verified by experimental means.[27]

A second category of chemical carcinogen was identified by Yoshida in 1931. It was an azo dye with the structure shown in Figure 10-3. The dye caused carcinoma of the liver in experimental animals. This finding was of more than academic interest because at that time the dye was being used to color margarine to look like butter for human consumption. The dye was accordingly named "butter yellow" and the practice was promptly stopped. No cancers of the liver in humans have been attributed to it. Since then it has been realized that the experimental dose used by Yoshida was extremely high and the animals were subsisting on a deficient diet. Correction of the diet lessened carcinogenic effect.[27]

Aniline is a synthetic dye produced in the manufacture of rubber and electrical cables. In 1895 a German surgeon named Rehn noticed that dye workers developed cancer of the urinary bladder. The condition became known as aniline cancer. The cause was eventually found to be a derivative of $\beta$-naphthylamine, an intermediate product of aniline metabolism. In the body $\beta$-naphthylamine yields 2-amino-1-naphthyl, which is conjugated with glucuronic acid in the liver and passes through the kidney in a harmless state. However, the bladder mucosa normally contains a glucuronidase that cleaves away the glu-

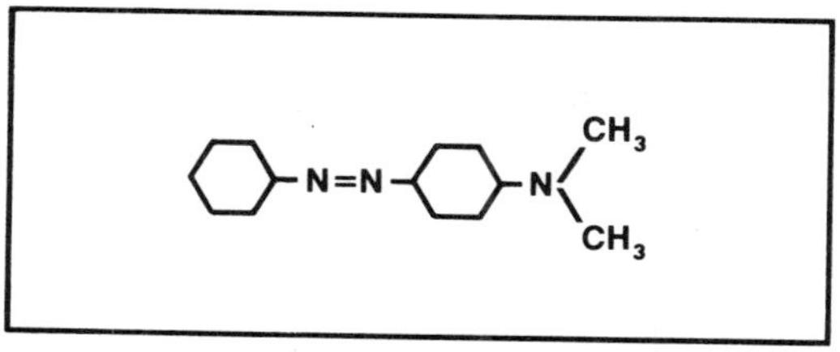

**Figure 10-3.** Dimethylaminoazobenzene (butter yellow)

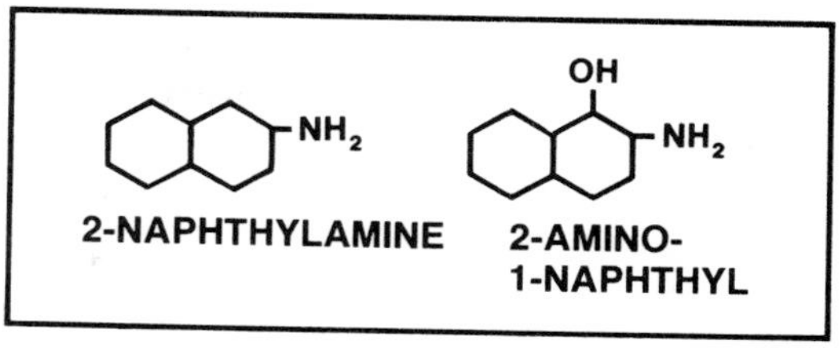

**Figure 10-4.** Compounds affecting bladder mucosa

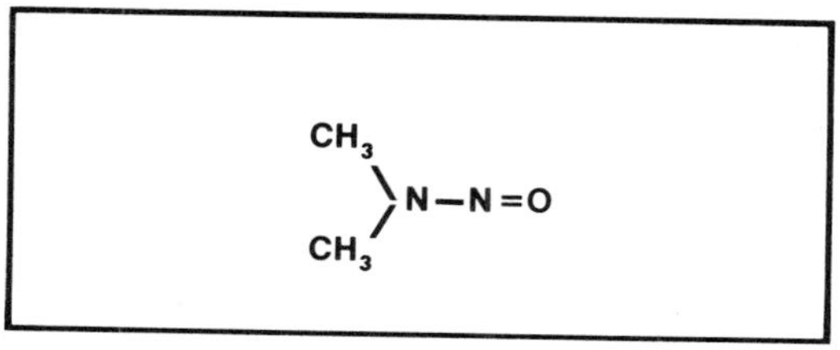

**Figure 10-5.** Dimethylnitrosamine

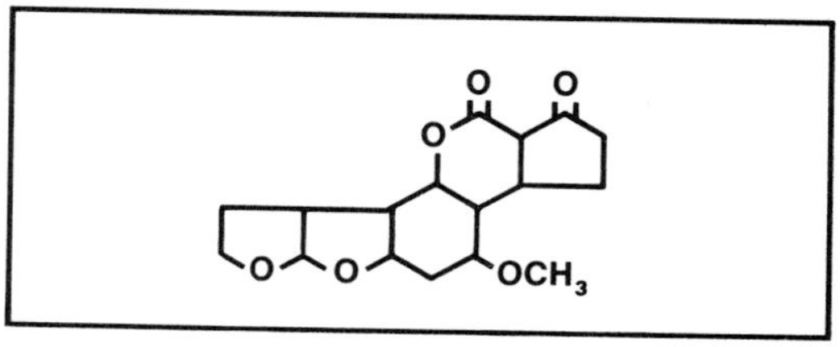

**Figure 10-6.** Aflatoxin

curonic acid and leaves the 2-amino-1-naphthyl residue. It is this substance in contact with the bladder mucosa that causes the cancer, and it is this mechanism that explains why the carcinogenic effect is limited to the urinary bladder. Other agents, including benzidine, are also carcinogenic for human uroepithelium.[28] The average latent period for the development of the cancer is 16 months.[27] The structural similarity of the aniline compounds is shown in Figure 10-4.

Dimethylnitrosamine was first produced as an industrial solvent but was found to cause hemorrhagic necrosis of the liver in animals. Subsequently, small amounts in the diets of experimental animals induced cancer of the liver and tumors of other organs, including the lung, esophagus, stomach, kidney, and urinary bladder. The danger of nitrosamines in the environment thus became evident.

The formula for these compounds is shown in Figure 10-5, in which $(R)_2N$ is the amine and $N=O$ is the nitroso component.

Nitrosamines are formed from two precursors, amines and nitrous acid. The amines are produced in the intestine from the digestion of protein. Nitrous acid is formed from nitrites, which are food preservatives, and from nitrogen dioxide and nitric oxide, which are products of oil, coal, and gas combustion. Amines are bound to nitrous oxide in the intestine and spontaneously in the atmosphere. Nitrosamines are also formed in cigarette smoke and are present in the exhaust fumes of cars. Of the 50 common nitrosamine compounds, dimethylnitrosamine is especially potent and acts as a hepatic carcinogen.[29] The use of nitrosamines as meat preservatives is now regulated by law.

Although no human cancers have yet been attributed specifically to nitrosamines, the common use of these chemicals in industrial processes and the high incidence of cancer in urban and industrial centers suggests the possibility of their causal involvement. Moreover, the precursors of these compounds are so abundant that their eradication from the environment is virtually impossible.

Alkaloids are complex, alkali-like organic bases produced chiefly by plants. Many are of medical importance, e.g., morphine (poppy), strychnine (nux vomica seeds), cocaine (coca leaves), quinine (cinchona bark), and nicotine (tobacco leaves and roots). In isolated form alkaloids are colorless crystals with a characteristically bitter taste. It has been suggested that the bitterness is the plants' protective mechanism against animal predation.

*Senecio* is the genus of a plant of worldwide distribution that has over 100 species. The name comes from the Latin *senex,* meaning "old man," and is derived from a tuft of soft white bristles that characterizes the plant. In the temperate zone a common variety is the weed known as ragwort *(Senecio jacobaea),* which produces a pyrrolizidine alkaloid. That the alkaloid is toxic to liver became evident when grazing livestock developed field poisoning and examination revealed hepatic disease. Subsequent experiments disclosed that the alkaloid is also a hepatic carcinogen. Such plants, moreover, are used for human consumption as herbal medicines in many parts of the world.[30] It is thus possible that the cause of Chiari's syndrome in South Africa is the eating of bread impregnated with *Senecio* seeds, and the cause of hepatic veno-occlusive disease in Jamaica is the drinking of "bush tea" made from *Senecio* plants. Both are associated with cancer of the liver. Cycasin is an alkaloid, produced by the nuts of *Cycas* palm trees, that is also a carcinogenic substance. It is thus evident that the *Senecio* and *Cycas* alkaloids are carcinogenic compounds, but it is not yet proven that they are the cause of hepatic cancer in humans.

Another pyrrolizidine alkaloid that may get into the diet is aflatoxin. It came to notice in 1960, when an epidemic struck the turkey-breeding industry in England and 100,000 poults died of hepatic disease. Investigation disclosed that the turkey feed was contaminated with the fungus *Aspergillus flavus*, which produces aflatoxin. Aflatoxin is an extremely potent hepatocarcinogen. This finding stimulated the search for aflatoxin in human diets. Cancer of the liver is common in parts of East Africa.[31] In that part of the world a favorite food is matoke, which is made of plantain bananas and is spiced with a sauce made of groundnuts (peanuts). The latter are sometimes contaminated with *A. flavus*. It is thus possible that aflatoxin contributes to the high incidence of hepatic cancer where groundnuts are eaten. The structure of aflatoxin is shown in Figure 10-6.

Most puzzling of all of the carcinogenic agents are the inorganic materials, including metals and plastics.[32] Carcinogenic metals include arsenic (skin), chromium (lung), and beryllium (bone). Others that induce cancers in experimental animals are cobalt, nickel, and zinc chloride. Plastics also cause cancer when implanted in rats for long periods. Bakelite in the form of discs was the first to be found to have this property, and thereafter thin films of many plastics, including polystyrene, polyvinylchloride, and polytetrafluoroethylene (Teflon), were found to have a tumor-inducing effect. Strands of silk, particles of quartz, and films of silver, tantalum, and stainless steel also induce experimental cancers. Although the mechanism of this effect is not clear, it appears less related to the release of free radicals into the tissue than to the physical form of the implanted material.[27] Whatever the mechanism, many more carcinogens probably remain to be identified.

A concluding aspect of chemical carcinogenesis is the geographic distribution of malignant disease. Although cancer is found in all human populations, there are striking regional differences that are attributable to various cultural practices. Examples include oral cancer in India from chewing betel nuts, lung cancer in the

United States from smoking cigarettes, and abdominal skin cancer in Asia from the application of hot stones to that area in order to keep warm. Other variations of common cancers are so striking as to implicate environmental factors. For example, cancer of the stomach is common in Chile, Iceland, and Japan, but not in the United States, where it is regressing. Esophageal cancer is common in South Africa and Iran but relatively infrequent in the United States. On the other hand, carcinoma of the colon is frequent in this country but uncommon in Africa and Asia. In China and Japan cancer of the oropharynx is extremely frequent while prostatic cancer is infrequent; the opposite is true in the United States. Cancers of the breast and uterine cervix also show pronounced regional differences.

**Table 10-4.**

## Oncogenic viruses

DNAviruses
  Papovavirus
    Benign tumors in animals
    Papillomas of the larynx in humans
    Verruca vulgaris (warts) in humans
  Adenovirus
    Ocular and respiratory infections
      in humans
    Experimental cancer in animals
  Herpesvirus
    Possibly Burkitt's lymphoma, cervical
      carcinoma, and nasopharyngeal
      carcinoma in humans
    Lymphoma, leukemia, and carcinoma
      in animals
  Poxvirus
    Skin infections in man
    Fibromas and fibrosarcomas in animals

RNAviruses
  Oncornavirus
    Suspect breast cancer, sarcoma, and
      acute lymphocytic leukemia
      in humans
    Lymphomas and leukemias in animals

These variations indicate that environmental factors, especially chemical carcinogens, play a large role in the cause of cancer. Further accounts of geographic variation have been detailed by Higginson.[33]

### Viruses

That a virus might cause cancer was long doubted because the disease neither appeared contagious nor resembled a viral infection. In 1908, however, Ellerman and Bang discovered a viral cause of leukemia in chickens, and in 1911 Rous found that chicken sarcoma is also caused by a virus. The question then arose: If viruses cause cancer in animals, why not in humans? Further interest in this question was stimulated by the finding of a mouse mammary tumor virus by Bittner in 1936 and of a mouse leukemia virus by Gross in 1951.

Viruses have seven to 20 genes, only a few of which are needed to transform a normal cell into a malignant cell. By contrast, mammalian cells contain over 2 million genes.[34] The viral core of DNA or RNA joins the nucleus of the host cell and directs it to produce more virions. In this process, normal animal cells are transformed into malignant tumor cells. The viruses that cause this transformation may be classified according to their core composition of DNA or RNA (Table 10-4).

Of the oncogenic DNAviruses, herpes has received especial attention. In 1964 Epstein and Barr discovered a virus in the tumor cells of Burkitt's lymphoma, and the possibility was raised that a viral cause of human cancer had finally been found. It was soon learned, however, that the Epstein-Barr virus (EBV) infects the majority of adults in all countries of the world. The infection occurs during childhood, with half the individuals remaining asymptomatic and the other half developing infectious mononucleosis. Nevertheless, patients with Burkitt's lymphoma are more often seropositive to herpes antibodies than are controls, and they may have eight to 10 times as much antibody as controls.[35] In addition, the tumor cells often show a highly specific translocation of chromosome 14 that is not seen in the lymphocytes of patients with infectious mononucleosis. The chromosomal alteration may be the factor that promotes the transformation of infectious mononucleosis cells to Burkitt's lymphoma cells. Another possibility is that the additional lymphoproliferative stimulus of superimposed malaria may promote this transformation. Either could account for the concept that Burkitt's lymphoma is an uncommon manifestation of a common disease, i.e., infectious mononucleosis. Whatever the explanation, it is not yet clear whether EBV is the cause of the cancer, the promoter of it, or just a harmless passenger within the tumor cells.

EBV is also associated with nasopharyngeal carcinoma, a tumor that is uncommon in the United States but extremely common in China. It may cause more suffering and death than any other human cancer.[36] The tumor consists of a mixture of invasive squamous cells and lymphoproliferative cells, although the latter are not regarded as malignant. It arises in young adults, occurs more often in men than in women, and affects especially the head and neck as does Burkitt's lymphoma. Antibodies against EBV are present more often in those affected than in controls. A striking difference, however, is that Burkitt's tumor is a lymphoma whereas the nasopharyngeal lesion is a carcinoma, and the virus is present in the lymphoid cells of the former while it occupies only the epithelial cells of the latter.[37] The role of Epstein-Barr virus in the pathogenesis of nasopharyngeal carcinoma is also uncertain.

Of more interest in the United States is the possibility that a herpesvirus is the cause of cancer of the uterine cervix. This is important because that cancer is common and such a disclosure would suggest the possibility of prevention by vaccination. The virus in question is herpesvirus homi-

nis (formerly h. simplex), of which there are two types. Type 1 (HVh-1) infects the oral mucosa, lives in equilibrium with its host cells, and causes cold sores or fever blisters when that equilibrium is upset. Type 2 (HVh-2) infects the genital mucosa. Antibodies to both form; HVh-2 antibodies are present in about 80 per cent of patients with cancer of the cervix, but in only about 30 per cent of controls. The antibody also has a high incidence in patients with carcinoma in situ. Cervical cancer patients report sexual intercourse with more different partners than do controls. These observations suggest a viral cause of the disease and indicate that cervical cancer could be regarded as a venereal infection. This view is still speculative, however, and the precise role of HVh-2 in causing cervical cancer remains to be clarified.[35]

The RNA viruses also cause malignant transformation of normal cells. In fact, they were the first to be discovered in the naturally occurring cancers of animals. The observers were Rous, Bittner, Gross, and Ellerman and Bang. The viruses they detected were found to be widespread in the animal kingdom, contain RNA, and cause cancer after long latent periods. They transform the infected cells and replicate at a steady rate, i.e., so many new viral particles per cell per hour. Within cells they are visible as C particles. Such viruses are implicated in human leukemia, sarcoma, and breast cancer. The evidence is both immunologic and visual, i.e., the presence of C particles in the neoplastic tissue. Whether such viruses act alone, are harmless passengers, or require conjunction with hormones or other substances is not known. Moreover, their mode of action as protoviruses or oncogenes may virtually preclude their detection.[34] The epidemiologic evidence of an infective agent is largely negative: Children born of leukemic parents bear no increased risk of the disease, studies of time-space clustering give more negative results than positive, and familial aggregation does not necessitate a viral cause. Although the implicating evidence is strong, it is also clear that no oncovirus has yet been proven to be the cause of any human cancer.

## Radiation

X-rays were discovered by Roentgen in 1895. The medical utility of this discovery was immediately grasped, and fluoroscopic examinations were soon widely used. Because the harmful nature of the rays was not known, physicians worked without shielding. By 1896 dermatitis of the hands, smarting of the eyes, and epilation of the skin had all been described. The first malignant tumor due to radiation was reported in 1902, a squamous-cell carcinoma of the hand. Within 15 years of Roentgen's discovery, 94 cases of skin cancer had been attributed to X-radiation.[38]

The term radiation also includes the particles emitted by radioactive isotopes, which were discovered in 1896 by Becquerel, as well as electromagnetic radiations, which are nonparticulate. Carcinogenicity is a property of all the particulate radiations, chiefly $\alpha$ and $\beta$ rays, as well as those electromagnetic radiations with wavelengths shorter than those of the visible spectrum. These include the ultraviolet, X, and $\gamma$ rays.

The evidence of the carcinogenicity of radiation is a litany of medical mistakes. This is understandable now because of the enthusiasm for the new diagnostic method, the long latent period between exposure and morbidity, and the slow realization that cancer is a consequence of the method. One of the first mistakes took place in the United States, where radium watch dial painters were allowed to wet their brushes with their lips; the radium was absorbed and sarcomas of the jaws developed after a latent period of 10 to 25 years. A more natural event occurred in the pitchblende miners of Central Europe, where radon was inhaled and $\alpha$-emitting isotopes were de-

posited on the bronchial mucosa; carcinoma of the lung frequently followed. Failure to realize the carcinogenic effect of radiation also permitted excessive exposure from medical use. For example, radiation of the mediastinum for enlargement of the thymus resulted in some cases of thyroid cancer years later. Pelvic irradiation for the treatment of menorrhagia was attended by subsequent leukemia and an increased incidence of intestinal cancers. X-irradiation of the spine for ankylosing spondylitis increased the incidence of chronic granulocytic leukemia in those patients. The examples are numerous: sarcoma at the site of treatment of non-neoplastic disorders, leukemia after the intravenous treatment of polycythemia rubra vera with radioactive phosphorus ($^{32}$P), carcinoma of the breast after irradiation for postpartum mastitis, and tumors of the liver after the injection of thorium oxide (Thorotrast) for angiographic studies. Even radiologic diagnostic examinations of pregnant women have given rise to an increased incidence of leukemia and other malignancies in their offspring.

In addition to these innocent mistakes, there is evidence from certain military adventures. After the atomic bombing of Hiroshima and Nagasaki, the incidence of leukemia in the exposed populations increased within five years, gradually declined thereafter, but still remains slightly above the prewar level. All types of leukemia except lymphocytic were represented. After a longer latent period carcinomas of the thyroid, breast, gut, and bronchial mucosa were also noted. Some years after the bombing of Japan another military event gave further evidence of the carcinogenicity of radiation. In 1954 an atmospheric atomic explosion allowed radioactive fallout to drift onto the Marshall Islands. In those inhabitants heavily exposed and under 10 years of age at the time, thyroid nodules developed eight to 16 years later in 80 per cent, whereas none had been present before the explosion. The topic of radiation carcinogenicity has been well reviewed by Upton.[38]

Because of these disclosures, certain protective measures became necessary. They represent a judgment of the benefits and risks of radiation. In general terms they include reducing the number, duration, and intensity of exposures and limiting the field exposed with shielding, especially of the gonads. Occupational whole-body exposure should not exceed a cumulative dose in rems (roentgen equivalents man) of five times the age of the worker beyond the age of 18. Thus a 28-year-old man should not have a cumulative dose that exceeds $10 \times 5$, or 50 rems. It is concluded that radiation is carcinogenic, that this effect is evident after high doses and long latent periods, and that protection is advisable whenever radiation is necessary.

## Heredity

That hereditary factors play a role in carcinogenesis cannot be doubted. The significance of the role of heredity, however, is uncertain. The reasons for this are that cancer may be many different diseases rather than only one, several genes may be affected, and the distinction between environmental effects and hereditary effects is extremely difficult to discern. Nevertheless it can be said that no general predisposition to cancer has been revealed by surveys of various human populations.[39]

Cancer does run in families, however, although usually not by simple mendelian laws. For example, the risk of cancer of the breast is three times greater for the sister of a woman with this disease than for a nonfamily member, and the risk rises to 50 times when both the mother and a sister have the cancer.[40] Increased incidence in family members is also seen with cancers of the stomach, colon, bladder, uterus, ovary, prostate, and thyroid, as well as with melanoblastoma, neuroblastoma, lymphoma, and leukemia.[41]

Although generalizations must suffice for most cancers, there are three malignant tumors that show inheritance by mendelian characters: familial polyposis, retinoblastoma, and xeroderma pigmentosum. All three are extremely uncommon. Familial polyposis is passed as a dominant autosomal trait. The colonic mucosa is normal at birth, adenomas arise after puberty, and the surface then becomes studded with hundreds of adenomas, one or more of which invariably undergo malignant transformation. Retinoblastoma is a malignant tumor of children that is also passed as a dominant autosomal trait. The genetic pattern becomes evident as therapeutic methods allow patients to survive into their reproductive years. Only about 40 per cent of patients, however, have the hereditary form of the disease.[42] Xeroderma pigmentosum is a recessive inborn metabolic error in which an enzyme necessary for the repair of DNA is missing. When skin is exposed to sunlight, ultraviolet radiation injures the DNA, which cannot be repaired because of the missing enzyme. The result is the formation of multiple skin cancers. The condition is thus a genetic state that predisposes to environmentally induced skin cancers.[43]

## TRANSFORMATION

The outstanding question in oncology is how the normal cell is transformed into a cancer cell. Certain observations bear on this process, although it is in no sense satisfactorily explained. First, transformation is a multistage process. This was revealed especially by Berenblum, who noted that a weak carcinogen applied to the skin of an experimental animal will not cause cancer until a second injury is applied later at the same site.[44] The first agent he called the initiator; the second, the promoter. No tumor is produced when the agents are applied in reverse order, and tumor production is independent of the interval between the application of the initiator and the promoter. Thus it became evident that the initiator causes an irreversible change in the tissue. Others have proposed more than two steps.[45] Knudson suggested a double-mutation model as in retinoblastoma, in which a second random mutation in the cell is required in addition to the autosomal defect already present in that cell from birth.[46] It is thus clear that the process requires more than one event for the transformation to take place and probably requires a series of incremental injuries to establish the irreversible change.

Second, the process takes a long time. In the early days of X-radiation, before harmful effects were known, the induction period for the onset of malignant tumor was 10 to 39 years.[38] Kinetic studies indicate that 25 years are required for an adenocarcinoma of the lung to attain a diameter of 2 cm.[47] How much of this time is due to transformation is not clear, but it is a gradual, multistage process and a long period usually passes between exposure to the carcinogen and the clinical appearance of the lesion.

Third, transformation is associated with membrane changes in the tumor cell. These are manifested by decreased adherence of one cell to another, loss of contact inhibition in cell culture, and increased permeability of the cell surface.[48] Whether these alterations cause the transformed state or are secondary to it is not known.

Fourth, the transformation may be due to an epigenetic change. This means that the genetic or chromosomal information is normal but the expression of that information is defective. Normally 90 per cent of the genetic information in a cell is repressed. Derepression of normal information allows the cell to behave abnormally. That behavior may be interpreted as a dedifferentiation of function. Thus malignant tumor cells produce fetal products such as $\alpha$-fetoprotein or carcinoembryonic antigen, or inappropriate adult products such as ACTH from carcinoma of the lung. In addi-

tion, tumor cells disclose structural dedifferentiation to the point where many are altogether undifferentiated. That these changes might be due to misuse of information rather than to abnormal information requires that the nucleus of a tumor cell be shown not to contain an irreversible injury. Transplantation of the nucleus of a frog carcinoma cell into the cytoplasm of an enucleated normal cell produces a normal tadpole.[49] Moreover, malignant human tumors rarely turn benign, as when a ganglioneuroblastoma matures or differentiates into a benign ganglioneuroma.[50] If the nucleus does not contain an irreversible injury, it is also necessary to show that the normal nucleus contains the potential for malignant behavior. This is indicated by the injection of scarlet red dye into the subcutaneous tissue of the rabbit. As a result, invasive epithelial growths develop but revert to normal when the dye is discontinued.[51] Since the dye could hardly carry new genetic information, it probably caused a temporary change in the expression of the normal nuclear information. Thus the normal nucleus carries the information necessary to establish the tumor cell, and the nucleus of the tumor cell is able to revert to normal behavior. The case for epigenetic transformation is made especially on these two counts. If this concept is true, it means hope for the treatment of cancer by reversing the transformation process rather than by the present technique of ablating the tumor cells after they have formed.

The predominant theory of transformation, however, is based on a somatic mutation in the genome of the cell. The evidence is indirect but compelling. For example, viruses cause cancer and they insert themselves into the nuclei of the tumor cells. Irradiation causes cancer and the ionizing rays are mutagenic. Most chemical carcinogens are also mutagens. The chromosomes of tumor cells are usually abnormal, although this is not constant from cell to cell except in chronic myeloid leukemia, in which 90 per cent of patients have the Philadelphia chromosome. The permanent and stable nature of the change that is passed onward from each cellular generation to the next strongly suggests a chromosomal mutation. The irreversible nature of the initiator effect in carcinogenesis also suggests a nuclear alteration. The clearly inherited nature of certain tumors, such as polyposis coli, retinoblastoma, and xeroderma pigmentosum, also signifies a permanent change in the genome of the cell. Moreover, many tumors are monoclonal, as revealed by X chromosome analysis of glucose 6-phosphate dehydrogenase.[52] All these data incline toward the conclusion that malignant transformation is due to a mutation in the genome of the somatic cell. That is the most logical mechanism for the initiation of a malignant tumor.

Finally, immune surveillance may play a role, not so much in the transforming process as in the recognition and destruction of cells that would otherwise progress to clinical cancers. In transformation the tumor cell generates surface antigens, the antigens are recognized by the immune system, and the tumor cells are destroyed. It is accordingly supposed that with advancing age the immune system declines, the process fails, and tumors appear. Observations compatible with this are the high frequency of malignant tumors in older age, the increased frequency of tumors in patients who have been immunosuppressed, and the frequency of tumors, 100 times greater than normal, in patients with primary immune deficiency diseases.[53,54] Despite these agreeable observations, however, the idea is questioned, largely on the basis of the high proportion of lymphomas in immunosuppressed patients as compared with the usual variety of tumors seen in a genetically heterogeneous population.[55] The mechanism of transformation is thus uncertain, the evidence is sketchy, and the interpretations are difficult. The cause of spontaneous cancer is unknown.

## REFERENCES

1. Page N: Weightlessness: A matter of gravity. *N Engl J Med* 297:32, 1977

2. LaVia MF, Hill RB Jr: *Principles of Pathobiology*, pp 59, 83, 193. New York: Oxford University Press, 1971

3. Villa Santa U: Diagnosis and prognosis in cervical dysplasia. *Obstet Gynecol* 38:811, 1971

4. Johnson LD, Nickerson RJ, Easterday CL, et al: Epidemiologic evidence for the spectrum of change from dysplasia through carcinoma in situ to invasive cancer. *Cancer* 22:901, 1968

5. Koss LG: Detection of carcinoma in the uterine cervix. *JAMA* 222:699, 1972

6. Peery TM, Miller FN: *Pathology*, 2nd ed, p 330. Boston: Little, Brown, 1971

7. What is cancer? What forms does it take? How does it kill? *Science* 183:1068, 1974

8. Silverberg E: Cancer statistics, 1979. *CA—Cancer J Clin* 29:6, 1979

9. Silverberg E: Cancer statistics, 1980. *CA—Cancer J Clin* 30:23, 1980

10. Batson OV: The vertebral vein system. *Am J Roentgenol* 78:195, 1957

11. Majmudar B: Metastasis of cancer to cancer: Report of a case. *Hum Pathol* 7:117, 1976

12. Coman DR: Mechanism of the invasiveness of cancer. *Science* 105:347, 1947

13. Robbins SL: *Pathologic Basis of Disease*, p 4. Philadelphia: Saunders, 1974

14. Coman DR, DeLong RP, McCutcheon M: Studies on the mechanism of metastasis. The distribution of tumors in various organs in relation to the distribution of arterial emboli. *Cancer Res* 1:648, 1951

15. Kardinal CB, Candy N, Rice W: Invasive carcinoma of the uterine cervix. *Mo Med* 72:685, 1975

16. Silverberg SG: Staging in the therapy of cancer of the breast. *Am J Clin Pathol* 64:756, 1975

17. DeVita VT, Canellos GP, Moxley JH: A decade of combination chemotherapy of advanced Hodgkin's disease. *Cancer* 30:1495, 1972

18. Smith JC: Interpreting the rate of survival in carcinoma. *Can J Surg* 18:129, 1975

19. Hertz R, Lewis J Jr, Lipsett MB: Five years' experience with chemotherapy of metastatic choriocarcinoma and related trophoblastic tumors in women. *Am J Obstet Gynecol* 82:631, 1961

20. Carbone PP: The role of chemotherapy in the

treatment of cancer of the breast. *Am J Clin Pathol* 64:774, 1975

21. MacDonald I: Biologic predeterminism in human cancer. *Surg Gynecol Obstet* 92:443, 1951

22. Research news. *Science* 183:940, 1974

23. Miller JA: Carcinogenesis by chemicals: An overview. G.H.A. Clowes memorial lecture. *Cancer Res* 30:559, 1970

24. Yamagiwa K, Ichikawa K: Experimental study of the pathogenesis of carcinoma. *J Cancer Res* 3:1, 1918

25. Kennaway E: The identification of a carcinogenic compound in coal-tar. *Br Med J* 2:749, 1955

26. Ackerman LV, del Regato JA: *Cancer*, 4th ed, p 20. St. Louis: Mosby, 1970

27. Badger GM: *The Chemical Basis of Carcinogenic Activity*. Springfield, Il: Thomas, 1962

28. Wendel RG, Hoegg UR, Zavon MR: Benzidine: A bladder carcinogen. *J Urol* 111:607, 1974

29. Magee PN, Barnes JM: Carcinogenic nitroso compounds. *Adv Cancer Res* 10:163, 1967

30. Schoental R: Toxicology and carcinogenic action of pyrrolizidine alkaloids. *Cancer Res* 28:2237, 1968

31. Korobkin M, Williams EH: Hepatoma and groundnuts in the West Nile District of Uganda. *Yale J Biol Med* 41:69, 1968

32. Bischoff F, Bryson G: Carcinogenesis through solid state surfaces. *Prog Exp Tumor Res* 5:85, 1964

33. Higginson J: Environment and cancer. *Practitioner* 198:621, 1967

34. Allen DW, Cole P: Viruses and human cancer. *N Engl J Med* 286:70, 1972

35. Research news. *Science* 183:1066, 1974

36. Wen CP: Nasopharyngeal cancer. In *China Medicine as We Saw It* (Quinn JR, ed). Washington, DC: Department of Health, Education, and Welfare Publication No. (NIH) 75-684, 1974

37. Klein G: The Epstein-Barr virus and neoplasia. *N Engl J Med* 293:1353, 1975

38. Upton AC: Physical carcinogenesis: Radiation-history and sources. In *Cancer, a Comprehensive Treatise* (Becker FF, ed), vol 1, p 391. New York: Plenum, 1975

39. Koller PC: In *Biology of Cancer*, 2nd ed, p 23. New York: Wiley-Interscience, 1975

40. Correa P: The epidemiology of cancer of the breast. *Am J Clin Pathol* 64:720, 1975

41. Harnden DG Jr: In *Scientific Foundations of Oncology*, p 188. Chicago: Year Book Medical Publishers, 1976

42. Knudson AG: Mutation and cancer: Statistical study of retinoblastoma. *Proc Nat Acad Sci USA* 68:820, 1971

43. Giannelli F: In *Scientific Foundations of Oncology*, p 476. Chicago: Year Book Medical Publishers, 1976

44. Berenblum I: A speculative review: The probable nature of promotive action and its significance in the understanding of the mechanism of carcinogenesis. *Cancer Res* 14:471, 1954

45. Wolman SR, Horland AA: Genetics of tumor cells. In *Cancer, a Comprehensive Treatise* (Becker FF, ed), vol 3, p 157. New York: Plenum, 1975

46. Knudson AG Jr: Heredity and human cancer. *Am J Pathol* 77:77, 1974

47. Garland LH, Coulson W, Wollin E: The rate of growth and apparent duration of untreated primary bronchial carcinoma. *Cancer* 16:694, 1963

48. Nicholson GL, Poste G: The cancer cell: Dynamic aspects and modifications in cell-surface organization. *N Engl J Med* 295:197, 253, 1976

49. McKinnel RG, Deggins BA, Labat DD: Transplantation of pluripotential nuclei from triploid frog tumors. *Science* 165:394, 1969

50. Dyke PC, Mulkey DA: Maturation of ganglioneuroblastoma to ganglioneuroma. *Cancer* 20:1343, 1967

51. Braun AC: Differentiation and dedifferentiation. In *Cancer, a Comprehensive Treatise* (Becker FF, ed), vol 3, p 5. New York: Plenum, 1975

52. Fialkow PJ, Klein G, Gartler SM, et al: Clonal origin for individual Burkitt tumors. *Lancet* 1:384, 1970

53. Hoover R, Fraumeni JF Jr: Risk of cancer in renal-transplant recipients. *Lancet* 2:55, 1973

54. Hersh EM, Gutterman JU, Mavligit GM: Cancer and host defense mechanisms. *Pathobiol Annu* 5:133, 1975

55. Melief CJM, Schwartz RS: Immunocompetence and malignancy. In *Cancer: a Comprehensive Treatise* (Becker FF, ed), vol 1, p 121. New York: Plenum, 1975

# PART II
# Systemic pathology

# 11

# CARDIOVASCULAR DISEASE

## CONGENITAL HEART DISEASE

Congenital heart disease is a gross structural abnormality of the heart or great vessels that is present at birth. The incidence is about eight per 1,000 live births and it is estimated that 25,000 infants with this condition were born in the United States in 1975.[1] Although many varieties exist, only three congenital defects of the heart and three of the great vessels are common, serious, and surgically correctable. Ventricular septal defect is the most common and represents about 30 per cent of the total. Congenital heart disease is equally frequent in blacks and whites.[1]

The heart is fully formed during the first trimester of gestation, and it is during this time that malformations develop. Maternal influences are important; German measles (rubella) during this time is attended by malformations of the ears, heart, teeth, and eyes.[2] Maternal influenza, tuberculosis, and toxoplasmosis may cause malformations, as may cortisone or cytotoxic agents given to the mother during this period. Regular measles (rubeola), poliomyelitis, and viral hepatitis do not cause congenital heart disease. However, such defects are about three times more common in the sibs of children with congenital heart disease than the incidence that is found at random.[2] The evidence therefore suggests that the cause of congenital heart disease is an interaction of genetic and environmental factors.

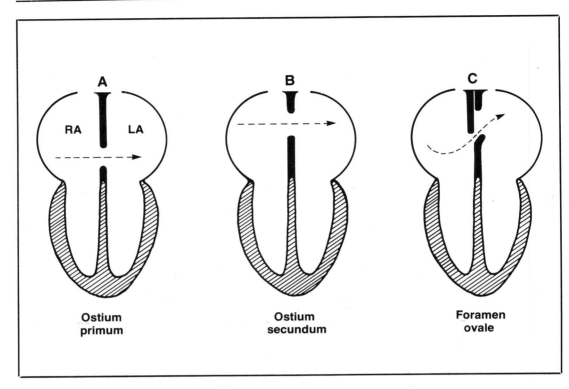

**Figure 11-1.** Formation of the interatrial septum

## Atrial septal defect

This defect is due to faulty development of the interatrial septum. Normal development is shown in Figure 11-1. First (A), the septum primum grows downward from above and divides the right atrium (RA) from the left atrium (LA), leaving open the ostium primum. In the first trimester the ostium primum closes and the ostium secundum opens (B). The ostium secundum becomes the foramen ovale. Later the septum secundum grows downward to cover most of the ostium secundum (C). During intrauterine life, placental blood passes through the ostium secundum or foramen ovale to enter the left atrium and thence the left ventricle and aorta. The flexible part during this time is the lower portion of the septum primum, which bends in accordance with the higher pressure in the right atrium (C). At birth the ductus arteriosus closes, the pulmonary vessels open, and blood passes from the right ventricle into the lungs. When blood enters the left atrium the pressure there rises above that in the right atrium, and the flexible portion of the lower part of the septum primum bends back toward the septum secundum and fuses with it to form the fossa ovalis.

Atrial septal defect is a persistent small or large opening in the partition between the two atria. It is more common in girls than in boys, and it imposes a left-to-right shunt so that cyanosis does not develop until late. The shunting of blood overloads the pulmonic circuit, and because of this the right ventricle undergoes hypertrophy and dilation, the pulmonary artery dilates, and pulmonary hypertension develops.

The clinical effects of this disturbance are foreseeable: A systolic murmur in the pulmonic area arises, chest X-ray discloses enlargement of the right ventricle, an electrocardiogram reveals right axis deviation, and the radiographic shadows of the pulmonary artery become conspicuous throughout the lung fields. The patient remains in reasonable health except for some dyspnea, however, and the life expectancy is 30 to 50 years. As the right ventricle fails, pressure rises in the right atrium, the shunt is reversed, and cyanosis appears as venous blood enters the systemic circuit. The condition is effectively treated by surgical closure so that neither atherosclerosis of the pulmonic vessels nor failure of the right ventricle develops.

In 2 to 5 per cent of patients with atrial septal defect, stenosis of the mitral valve is also present. This may be part of the congenital defect or it may be acquired later as a consequence of rheumatic disease. It may therefore occur at any age. It is known as Lutembacher's syndrome, and it worsens the atrial defect by impairing the outflow of blood from the lungs, which are already overloaded. Unless mitral valve replacement and closure of the atrial defect are performed, death takes place from right heart failure, pulmonary hemorrhage, or bacterial endocarditis.

### Ventricular septal defect

This abnormality is the most common of the congenital heart malformations and is known as maladie de Roger. It is a smooth, round, small or large defect usually located in the upper portion of the septum adjacent to the membranous part. It is due to failure of fusion of the upgrowing ventricular septum and the downgrowing atrial septum. The effect again is to produce a left-to-right shunt because of the higher pressure on the left side. Right ventricular hypertrophy, pulmonary hypertension, and atherosclerosis of the pulmonary arteries result. Clinically there are a harsh systolic "machinery" murmur, a thrill over the precordium, a globular cardiac outline from biventricular hypertrophy, prominent pulmonary ar-

teries on chest X-ray, and a "hilar dance" of the pulmonary vessels as observed on fluoroscopy. The outlook for the patient depends on the size of the opening. Small defects tend to close spontaneously in the first year of life from continued growth of the membranous portion of the interventricular septum or from attachment of the base of a tricuspid leaflet around the defect. Large defects may be closed surgically as soon as the child reaches a body weight of 30 to 40 pounds and is able to withstand the procedure. If this is not done, bacterial endocarditis is a hazard to life in addition to development of right heart failure. A small interventricular septal defect is shown in Figure 11-2. This was asymptomatic and was an incidental autopsy finding.

### Transposition of the great vessels

In the embryonic period the great single arterial channel that forms above the heart is the truncus arteriosus. Normally it divides into a pulmonary artery and aorta, which are twisted so that the pulmonary artery overlies the right ventricle and the aorta attaches to the left ventricle. If this twisting fails to take place, the two arteries come to overlie the wrong ventricles. Thus the right ventricle pumps blood into the aorta and it returns to the right atrium, right ventricle, and back into the aorta. On the other side, the left ventricle pumps blood into the pulmonary artery and that blood returns to the left atrium and thence to the left ventricle. Thus in transposition the systemic and pulmonic circulations are disconnected. Life is accordingly impossible, and cyanosis is pronounced at birth. Nevertheless, some infants barely survive because of two channels that allow for mixing of blood in the otherwise disconnected circuits. One is a small foramen ovale, and the other is a ductus arteriosus that may remain patent. Complicated as the task is, surgical correction of these defects is possible. Palliation is achieved by enlarging the

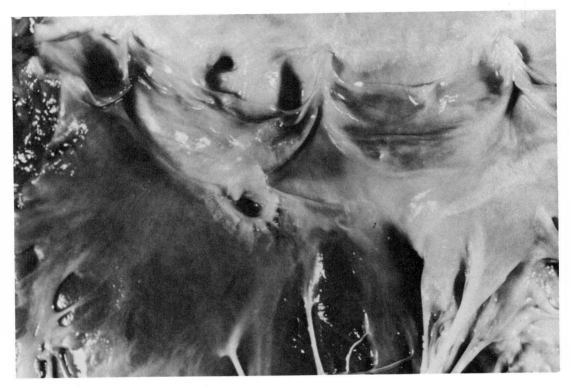

**Figure 11-2.** A small interventricular septal defect just below the right coronary cusp of the aortic valve

foramen ovale as described by Rashkind and Miller,[3] and definitive correction is later possible by the Mustard procedure, which is an interatrial transposition of venous return.[4]

### Tetralogy of Fallot

The tetralogy of Fallot is a common, correctable cardiac defect that accounts for 70 per cent of "blue (cyanotic) babies." The cause is unequal division of the truncus arteriosus so that the pulmonary artery is small and the aorta is large. That produces pulmonic stenosis and an aorta that opens over the right ventricle as well as the left. The aorta is thus said to be "overriding," and this causes an interventricular septal defect and contributes to thickening and dilation of the right ventricle. The four parts of the tetralogy are thus an overriding aorta, a ventricular septal defect, pulmonic stenosis, and right ventricular hypertrophy (Figure 11-3).

The consequences of the tetralogy are that the aorta receives blood from both ventricles, the lungs receive too little blood, and survival depends on the sum of blood delivered to the lungs through the pulmonary artery and the ductus arteriosus, which may remain patent. Seven clinical features characterize the condition: cyanosis from birth, systolic murmurs and thrills, a large cardiac outline, polycythemia from pulmonary hypoxia, retarded development, clubbing of fingers and toes, and dyspnea from air hunger. Unless the tetralogy is treated, the patient will succumb in childhood or adolescence from failure of the right ventricle or the development of intercurrent infection.

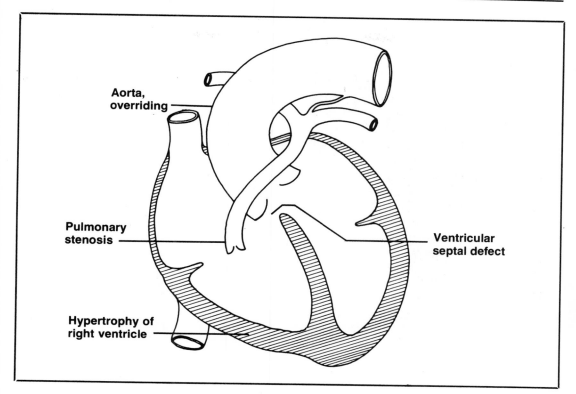

**Figure 11-3.** The tetralogy of Fallot

The purpose of treatment is to open up the supply of blood to the lungs in order to improve oxygenation. The Blalock procedure achieves this by anastomosis of the right subclavian artery to the right pulmonary artery. After this the blue baby turns pink, the dyspnea subsides, the polycythemia disappears, and somatic development resumes. Nevertheless, permanent satisfaction requires the definitive operation, which includes discontinuation of the Blalock shunt and surgical enlargement of the main pulmonary channel so that venous blood is able to reach the lungs normally.

A modification of the tetralogy is the Eisenmenger complex, in which pulmonic stenosis is slight or absent. This reduces the severity of the dysfunction and provides a better outlook because of the improved pulmonary circulation.

**Patent ductus arteriosus**

During intrauterine life most of the blood in the pulmonary artery bypasses the lungs by moving through the ductus arteriosus into the aorta. At birth or within one month thereafter, this channel closes and the pulmonic tissue is then supplied by the pulmonary artery and, to a much lesser extent, by the bronchial arteries. A ductus arteriosus that remains patent after the first month of extrauterine life is abnormal. The opening may be a large tubular connection or a small fenestration between two closely apposed vessels. The consequences of this opening become pronounced as the size increases; they include a left-to-right shunt so that cyanosis does not develop, high pressure in the pulmonic circuit, and, on that account, dilation and hypertrophy of the right ventricle as well as atherosclerosis of the pulmonary arteries. The conveyance of high pressure to the right ventricle is dependent on dilation of the pulmonary conus and valve ring.

Physical examination reveals a harsh systolic murmur that has a sawing or humming quality. There is also a thrill over the precordium and a collapsing pulse that is due to low diastolic pressure from runoff of the systolic thrust into the pulmonary vessels. Chest X-ray discloses prominent pulmonary arteries, and a catheter extended into the pulmonic artery reveals both abnormally high pressure and excessive oxygen saturation of the blood. The physical diagnosis is easily confirmed by the catheter studies.

Life may persist to the age of 40 years or even longer, but right heart failure eventually develops, and as the pressure in the right ventricle exceeds that of the aorta because of the increasing degree of failure, the shunt reverses and cyanosis appears as venous blood turns into the aorta. None of this is necessary, as surgical closure of the defect is highly successful.

**Coarctation of the aorta**

Coarctation is a constriction of the thoracic aorta that accounts for 6 per cent of all cardiovascular anomalies, is seen four times more often in males than in females, and occurs in a preductal and a postductal form. A diagram of the preductal form is shown in Figure 11-4.

In the preductal or infantile form, the ductus delivers blood to the descending aorta during intrauterine life. There is accordingly no need for anastomoses to develop that would connect the proximal aorta with the distal aorta, i.e., the portion distal to the constriction. At birth the ductus either closes or remains open. If it closes, the left ventricle fails because there are no collaterals to decrease the pressure in the proximal aorta or convey oxygenated blood to the lower parts of the body. The baby accordingly dies at birth or within two or

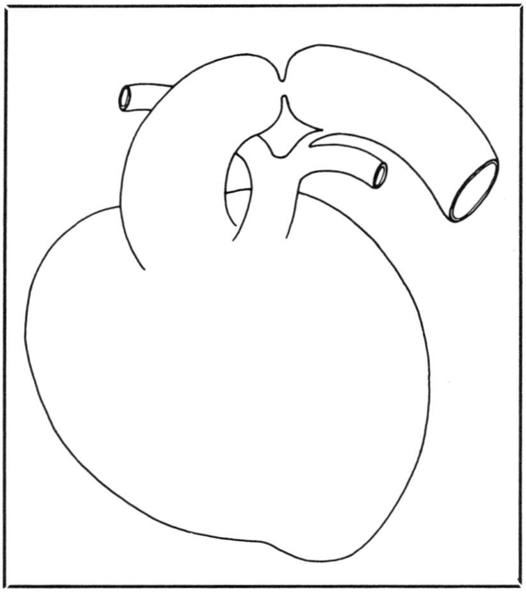

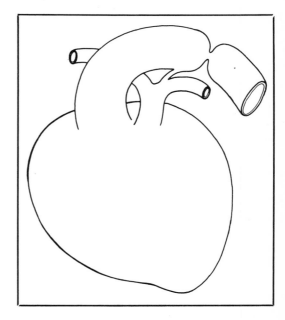

**Figure 11-4.** Preductal (infantile) coarctation. The constriction is proximal to the opening of the ductus into the aorta.

**Figure 11-5.** Postductal (adult) coarctation. The constriction is distal to the opening of the ductus into the aorta.

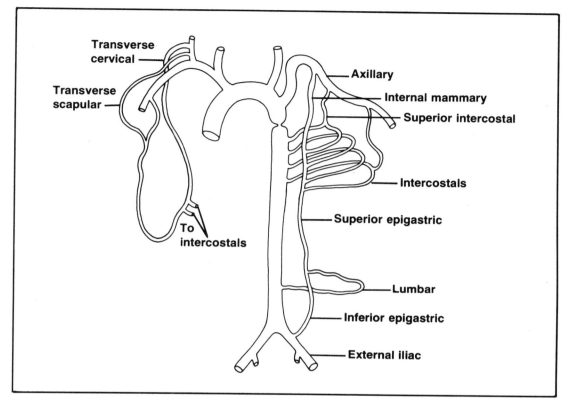

**Figure 11-6.** Collateral vessels of postductal coarctation

three days. If the ductus remains open, however, the hands are pink from oxygenated blood delivered by the upper aortic segment, and the feet are blue from unoxygenated blood delivered by the ductus and lower aortic segment. This differential cyanosis is characteristic of the preductal form of coarctation when the ductus remains open. Eventually the heart fails: the right ventricle because it cannot supply enough blood for the lungs and lower body at the same time, and the left ventricle because it has no collaterals to let off the pressure from the constricted upper segment.

The postductal or adult form of coarctation is altogether different (Figure 11-5). The constriction tends to be slight. The ductus closes at birth. As the infant develops and the aorta grows, however, the con-

striction does not change so that the stenosis gradually becomes more pronounced. As this constriction increases, collaterals develop that deliver blood from the upper to the lower segment. Chief among these are the intercostal arteries, which become thick and tortuous and run along the inner lower surfaces of the ribs. Pulsations of these tortuous vessels cause erosion of the bone so that "notching" of the undersurfaces of the ribs is a characteristic radiographic feature of the condition. A schematic diagram of these collateral vessels is shown in Figure 11-6.

The effects of postductal constriction develop gradually and include hypertrophy of the left ventricle, a loud systolic murmur over the precordium and midback, and hypertension in the upper extremities. The

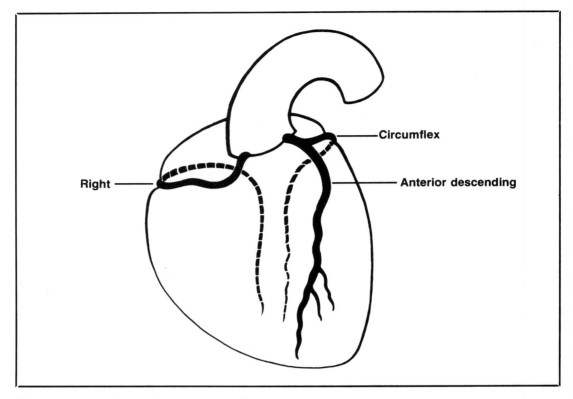

**Figure 11-7.** The three main coronary arteries

hypertension produces headache, dizziness, nosebleeds (epistaxis), and nervousness. The lower extremities, in contrast, tend to be hypotensive, pale, cold, weak, and underdeveloped. Cyanosis is absent because pulmonary oxygenation is unimpaired and the blood is proceeding along its "normal" routes.

Without treatment of postductal coarctation, the average lifetime is 40 years, although there is much variation according to the degree of the constriction and the adequacy of the collaterals. Causes of death include dissecting aneurysm of the proximal segment, bacterial infection of the constriction with perforation, cerebral hemorrhage from persistent hypertension, and congestive failure of the heart. All of these are avoidable by surgical correction of the constriction.[5]

## CORONARY ARTERY DISEASE

Heart disease is the leading cause of death in the United States. It affects 28 million Americans, causes 1 million deaths each year, and accounts for approximately 30 per cent of the total mortality in the United States annually.[6] Of the various forms, coronary artery disease is the most important, far surpassing hypertensive, valvular, or congenital heart disease. The pathologic process causing this enormous amount of illness is atherosclerosis, which occurs in medium-sized vessels throughout the body and especially in the coronary arteries.

The reason for this pandemic is not altogether clear. The process, however, is associated with six major risk factors: age, sex, hypercholesterolemia, hypertension, cigarette smoking, and diabetes. Atherosclerosis increases as age advances, is more pronounced in men than in women, especially before the menopause, and is accelerated by hypertension. Less certain risk factors are obesity, inactivity, and personality type.[7] The most powerful predictor of risk, however, is the blood level of cholesterol. The normal value is 200 to 220 mg/dl. It is determined by the total calories in the diet and the proportion of them that come from cholesterol or saturated fatty acids, as found in animal fat.[8] When the blood level of cholesterol exceeds 250 mg/dl, the risk of coronary heart disease rises sharply. When saturated fatty acids are fed to animals, the blood cholesterol rises and atherosclerosis develops. When the diet is changed to unsaturated fatty acids, as found in vegetable and fish oils, the cholesterol level declines and the pathologic process regresses. Moreover, in vegetarians, who have a negligible intake of saturated fatty acids, both the blood cholesterol and the incidence of coronary disease are reduced.[9] In fact, in vegan children, the blood cholesterol is 30 to 40 mg/dl lower than the norm.[10] The evidence is accordingly strong that diet is an essential factor in the causation of hypercholesterolemia, which is associated with atherosclerosis and coronary heart disease. How high blood cholesterol causes atherosclerosis is discussed in the section on diseases of the aorta.

The coronary arteries consist of a right and a left main vessel, with the left dividing into an anterior descending and a circumflex branch (Figure 11-7). There are also intercoronary anastomoses that develop as needed, and small thebesian vessels that open directly onto the endocardial surfaces of the ventricles.[11] The atherosclerotic process in a coronary artery (Figure 11-8) consists of an accumulation of lipid-laden macrophages, fragmentation of the internal elastic lamina, extracellular accumulation of cholesterol, and focal fibrosis of the plaque, which, in Figure 11-8, obstructs about two-thirds of the lumen.

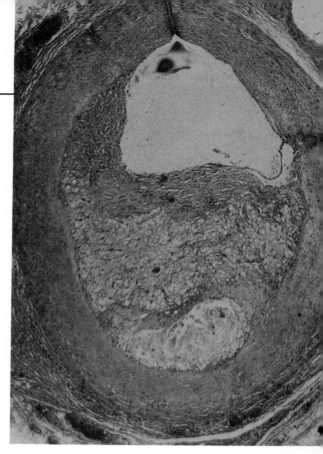

**Figure 11-8.** Atherosclerosis of a coronary artery

The pathologic process begins with a lipid streak, which progresses to a fibrous plaque and then becomes a complicated lesion. The complicated lesion includes intramural hemorrhage, focal calcification, or ulceration of the intima. Any combination of these may be present, and all cause some degree of stenosis of the lumen. This process is irregularly distributed and seldom diffuse. Moreover, it does not affect the coronary branches beyond those in the epicardial adipose tissue.[12] The consequences of this process are eddying of the current, which abrades the endothelium, release of clotting factors from ulceration of the surface, and closure of the lumen from hemorrhage beneath a plaque, which dislodges it into the lumen of the vessel. On any of these accounts thrombosis tends to develop. These events take place mainly in the first 6 cm of the main coronary arteries. The result is coronary heart disease, manifested by angina pectoris, congestive failure, and myocardial infarction.

Angina pectoris consists of pain in the chest, usually brought on by exercise, that is often referred to the left arm, less frequently to the left neck, and occasionally to both sides of the neck or the right arm. It is due to atherosclerotic stenosis of the coronary arteries associated with an increased need for oxygen, as brought on by exercise or emotional stress. The diagnosis requires pain of this type unassociated with anatomic or electrocardiographic evidence of permanent injury to the myocardium.

Congestive failure is due to a deficiency of the cardiac pump and is regarded as "forward" or "backward." Forward failure is attributed to hypoxia of the endothelium of the vessels ahead of the pump, so that vascular permeability develops, the tissues become waterlogged, and the body compensates by hypervolemia. Backward failure is attributed to damming up of blood in the vessels behind the pump, so that hydrostatic pressure rises and the tissues become waterlogged on this account. Perhaps both forward and backward failures occur simultaneously. Pump failure takes place because coronary atherosclerosis deprives the heart muscle of oxygen, focal myocytolysis develops, and patchy fibrosis of the myocardium follows. This impairs contractility of the ventricular wall. Subsequent events are most easily understood in terms of backward failure. As the left ventricle empties incompletely, blood accumulates and dilation follows. The heart compensates for this by hypertrophy and tachycardia. Eventually decompensation develops and the increased pressure of the left ventricle is transmitted to the left atrium and thence to the capillaries of the lung. The high hydrostatic pressure in the pulmonary capillaries causes edema of the lungs. Rales are heard clinically, and pleural effusions form. Erythrocytes enter the alveoli by diapedesis, macrophages then phagocytize them, and hemosiderin appears. Coughing from edema of the lungs follows, along with expectoration of "rusty" sputum from hemosiderin-laden macrophages. Eventually pulmonary fibrosis develops; this is then known as brown induration. The pressure is then conveyed to the right ventricle, which also dilates and becomes hypertrophic. As the tricuspid ring stretches, the pressure enters the right atrium and is then transferred to the systemic veins. This decompresses the pulmonary circuit and initiates right heart failure, which is characterized by hepatomegaly, congestive splenomegaly, ascites formation, and dependent edema.

Myocardial infarction is focal coagulation necrosis of the heart muscle. It occurs mainly in men over 45 and women over 55. It is six times more common in men than in premenopausal women, but only 1.5 times more common in men than in postmenopausal women. Myocardial infarction accounts for about 20 per cent of all deaths in the United States.[6]

The clinical events include a prodrome consisting of vague precordial distress that often lasts for some weeks before the onset of the infarction. The onset occurs about as frequently at sleep or rest as during exertion.[12] It is a dramatic event, consisting of sudden, agonizing, viselike substernal pain that radiates down the left arm. The skin is cool, moist, ashen, and sometimes cyanotic. The patient experiences anxiety, faintness, nausea and vomiting, and occasionally dizziness. The blood pressure drops, and the pulse is fast and weak. Sweating, pallor, and dyspnea develop. The ECG reveals a characteristic elevation of the ST segment, and within hours there follow fever, leukocytosis, and a rise in serum enzymes that leak out of the damaged muscle cells. These include especially lactate dehydrogenase (LDH) and creatine phosphokinase (CPK).

The enzymes that leak from the injured cells into the interstitium are for the most part denatured. Some, however, reach the coronary veins or cardiac lymphatics to enter the general circulation, from which they are cleared at various rates by the reticuloendothelial system. The main enzymes useful in the diagnosis of myocardial infarction are CPK and LDH. Serum glutamate-oxaloacetate transaminase and hydroxybutyrate dehydrogenase are less useful.[13] CPK, which is found in myocardium, brain, and skeletal muscle, rises in the serum four to eight hours after infarction, peaks at 24 hours at five to 10 times above normal, and subsides within the following five days. LDH, which is present in virtually all tissues, rises at 12 to 24 hours, peaks at day 3 at two to three times above normal, and subsides by day 10. Both are measured by their effects on substrates. Diagnostic usefulness, however, is improved by measurement of the different molecular forms (isoenzymes) of CPK and LDH. CPK has three isoenzymes: MM, found in skeletal muscle; BB, found in brain; and a hybrid, MB, which is virtually specific for myocardium. Separation of the isoenzymes is performed by electrophoresis, and the presence of an MB band of CPK is the single most sensitive enzyme determination for detecting a myocardial infarct.[14] LDH has five isoenzymes, and an elevation of total LDH with an increase of isoenzyme 1 over isoenzyme 2 is characteristic of infarction of the heart. Taken together, these two enzymes with their isoenzymes, measured within 48 hours of the presumed infarction, are highly accurate in the diagnosis of myocardial necrosis.

The infarct almost always occurs in the left ventricle. The two most common sites are the anterior wall and adjoining two-thirds of the interventricular septum (anteroseptal) and the posterior wall and adjacent one-third of the ventricular septum (posteroseptal). The infarct may, of course, also occur in the lateral wall of the left ventricle, at any level from base to apex. Since the process is dynamic, the infarct may be at any of the stages of recent necrosis, organizing repair, or old fibrosis. In many infarcts no thrombus of a coronary artery is found and only pronounced atherosclerosis with marked stenosis is present. When a thrombus is identified, it regularly occurs in the first portion of a main vessel; the coronary sites include the anterior descending branch of the left (50 per cent), the main right (35 per cent), and the circumflex branch of the left (15 per cent).

What is seen at autopsy depends on when the patient died. When the interval is eight to 10 hours after onset, no gross or microscopic changes are evident. At 24 hours the cut surface of the muscle is dry and pale, and microscopically there are loss of striations and a light infiltration of segmented granulocytes at the site of injury. By seven to 10 days the necrosis is fully developed, leukocytic infiltration with neutrophils is pronounced, and small numbers of macrophages are present. The cut surface at this time is pale yellow with a hemorrhagic margin. Thinning of the muscle wall is also evident. This appearance is shown in Figure 11-9 (see color section, p C-1). By the second week the margins of the infarct become pallid, and microscopically there are fewer neutrophils, more macrophages, some hemosiderin, a few capillary buds at the margin, and a scattering of fibroblasts. By week 3 fibroblastic ingrowth is conspicuous, collagen is evident, and capillary formation is well developed. At four to six weeks the process subsides: The leukocytes disappear, vascularity decreases, a scar forms, and the site contracts. By two to three months nothing is left but a dense, white, fibrous scar.

Myocardial infarction was originally presumed to be difficult to diagnose, impossible to treat, and the cause of sudden death.[15] Moreover, it was widely presumed to be due to thrombosis of a coronary artery. The evidence for this is impressive; thrombi are often found in the artery serving the infarcted site, and ligature of a coronary artery in a dog causes an infarct in the tissue supplied by that vessel. Never-

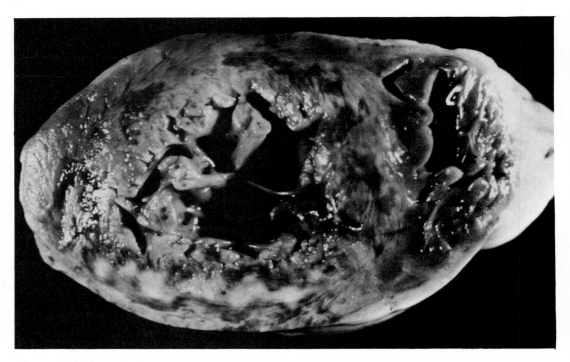

**Figure 11-9.** Cut surface of recent infarct (pallid zone), seven to 10 days after onset. Also shown in color section, p C-1.

theless, it has been reported that the incidence of thrombi in cases of myocardial infarction is extremely variable, that the frequency of thrombi increases with the survival time of the patient, and that the local conditions in the region of the infarct are conducive to thrombus formation.[12, 16] On these accounts, Roberts and Buja proposed that the arterial thrombi are consequences of the infarction process.[12] Subsequently Erhardt and colleagues injected fibrin tagged with a radioactive marker into the circulation of patients as soon as possible after the clinical onset of the infarction. They reasoned that if thrombi cause infarcts, the fibrin could only adhere to the outside of the thrombus, but if infarcts cause thrombi, the fibrin should be evenly mixed within the thrombus. When the experiment was performed, the radioactive tag was for the most part mixed within all parts of the thrombus.[17] Credibility was

thus given to the idea that infarcts may cause thrombi.

The obvious question remains: If coronary thrombi do not cause infarcts, what does? The constant finding is that more than 75 per cent stenosis is present in at least two of the three main arteries in cases of infarction.[12] The question may therefore be rephrased: What causes barely adequate oxygenation to become inadequate oxygenation? It is experimentally demonstrable that catecholamines lead to myocardial necrosis, and this has been extrapolated to suggest that environmental stress may be the cause of myocardial necrosis.[18] A clinical example may be the father who has a heart attack and dies within hours after learning that his son has been killed in war. In this connection, Sodi-Pallares of the Heart Institute of Mexico has said, "The heart is not alone in the body." It is subject to metabolic effects, and it is especially responsive to thyroxine, insulin, and catecholamines. Sodi-Pallares regards coronary thrombi as secondary events, and aims therapy at the metabolic causes of infarction rather than at thrombi as the cause of those infarcts (personal communication).

It is thus evident that the pathogenesis of myocardial infarction is still uncertain. The spectrum of possibilities includes coronary atherosclerosis, coronary thrombosis, and metabolic disturbances of the myocardium. The truth will eventually be learned. Meanwhile it is interesting to observe the transition from the earliest days of hopeless disregard, barely 60 years ago, to the middle period of confidence in pathogenesis, and to the present, when metabolic effects bid to become known as the root cause of myocardial disease.

Regardless of the mechanism, certain consequences follow the development of the infarct. About 15 per cent of patients die within 48 hours of onset.[12] Most of the remaining 85 per cent recover, and white, fibrous scars form in the ventricular wall. A much smaller proportion of patients develop any of five major complications: mural thrombus, ventricular aneurysm, rupture of the interventricular septum, rupture of a papillary muscle, and rupture of the wall of the ventricle.

Necrosis stimulates acute inflammation so that an infarct lying just below the endocardium evokes fibrin over the surface. This is soon the site of deposition of platelets, leukocytes, red cells, and more fibrin to form a mural thrombus. Such a thrombus is dynamic, organizes by capillary and fibroblastic ingrowth, and gradually is transformed into a thick, white scar of the endocardium (Figure 11-10). Particularly bulky thrombi undergo yellowish-gray central (puriform) degeneration, and others break off solid fragments that embolize, especially to the brain, spleen, and kidneys. It is embolic potential that makes mural thrombi important.

In the infarction process, dead muscle is

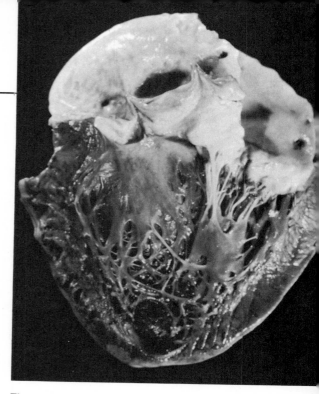

**Figure 11-10.** Mural thrombus of endocardium at apex of left ventricle

carried away by macrophages and the wall becomes thin because muscle cells do not replicate. Survival is possible even when the infarct is large, if interarterial anastomoses have developed before the onset of the infarct. In these circumstances the ventricular wall may become extremely thin and bulge outward to form a ventricular aneurysm (Figure 11-11). Ventricular aneurysms usually fill with mural thrombi so that embolism and congestive failure often result, the latter from an insufficiency of contracting muscle.

When the necrosis is transmural and extends through the interventricular septum, that septum may rupture. In this event blood is pumped into the right ventricle with every systole, and congestive failure becomes suddenly overwhelming. When the necrosis affects the base of a papillary muscle, rupture may take place so that a mass of muscle floats in the ventricular current on the tether of a tendinous cord. The clinical manifestations include a new, harsh murmur together with the abrupt onset of fulminant congestive failure.[19] A ruptured

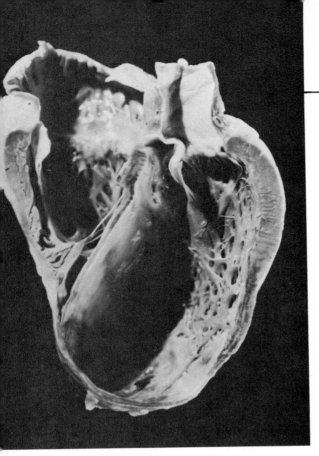

**Figure 11-11.** Aneurysm of left ventricle

papillary muscle is shown in Figure 11-12. Finally, the necrosis may cause rupture of the ventricular wall so that blood is thrust into the pericardial sac. This is often not an abrupt event because the channel is not straight, open, and large, but small and tortuous. Nevertheless, the pericardial sac is not distensible, the extravasated blood is not compressible, and soon the heart is unable to expand in diastole. Heart failure from cardiac tamponade is the result.

Before 1940 the treatment of coronary artery disease was entirely symptomatic. Surgical treatment was then tried, and early procedures, especially by Beck and Leighninger[20] and by Vineberg,[21] included abrasion of the epicardium to induce new vessel formation, attachment of adjacent tissue to the epicardium for the same purpose, and implantation of the internal mammary artery into the myocardium so that oxygenated blood could reach the inadequately vascularized heart muscle. Al-

though these methods gave occasional promise, the overall results were not impressive. In the late 1950s, however, Sones perfected catheterization of the coronary arteries so that the injection of a radiopaque medium could reveal the site and degree of the arterial stenosis. This development was followed approximately 10 years later by the procedure of Favaloro, who resected a segment of the patient's saphenous vein and transplanted it to the heart, connecting one end to the aorta and the other to the coronary artery distal to the constriction. These historical events have been reviewed by Bordley and Harvey.[22] The aortocoronary bypass procedure immediately became popular and was soon in use for the prevention of coronary thrombosis. About 85 per cent of patients gain symptomatic improvement of their angina, and about 70 per cent gain complete relief. Moreover, the operative mortality is often under 5 per cent, and the vein graft remains patent in about 70 per cent. Nevertheless, it is not established that life is prolonged beyond what is achieved by medical treatment, and for this reason the procedure is most suitable for patients whose angina is refractory to medical management.[23,24] It is important to keep in mind that the symptomatic relief from the operation is independent of the progress of the underlying disease, and it is necessary to persist in the control of the risk factors associated with atherosclerosis of the coronary arteries.

## VALVE DISEASE

Although the major diseases of the heart are coronary, hypertensive, and congenital, valve disease is nevertheless of great importance because the process tends either to destroy the valve with insufficiency or to convert it into a fibrous ledge with stenosis. The principal types of valve disease are rheumatic, infective, and noninfective. Rheumatic valvulitis is now disappearing because of prevention through the use of antibiotics. Antibacterial agents have also dramatically changed the outlook for infective (bacterial) endocarditis. Noninfective endocarditis is sterile and does not harm the valve although it may give rise to embolic phenomena. Although fairly frequent, it is of less importance than the others because it usually occurs as a secondary event in debilitated patients with terminal disease.

## Rheumatic heart disease

Rheumatic fever is an inflammatory disease of granulomatous nature associated with a streptococcal infection, usually of the upper respiratory tract, that begins in youth, recurs over months to years, and affects primarily connective tissue, especially of the heart, joints, and skin. It affects the sexes equally, it is more apt to occur in temperate zones, and the onset tends to be in children between the ages of 5 and 15 years. Its incidence is decreasing because of the control of streptococcal infection by antibiotic agents.

Acute rheumatic fever has four main clinical aspects: arthritis, subcutaneous nodules, chorea, and carditis. The arthritis affects mainly large joints, such as the knees or elbows, which become hot, red, swollen, and painful. The inflammatory process has the unique feature of migrating from one joint to another, so that it flares up and subsides spontaneously at different sites. The subcutaneous nodules form connective tissue, usually about joints, and measure 1 to 2 cm in diameter. The nodules are painless and subside spontaneously after a few weeks. Chorea minor, or Sydenham's chorea, is a slow, purposeless, or writhing (athetoid) movement of the hands associated with a slight, transient meningoencephalitis. The words "minor" and "Sydenham's" distinguish it from Huntington's chorea, which occurs in adults, progresses to dementia, and is inherited as a mendelian dominant trait. The clinical evi-

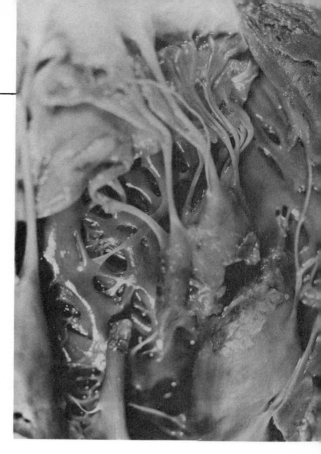

**Figure 11-12.** Rupture of a papillary muscle of the left ventricle

dence of cardiac involvement includes enlargement of the heart, development of a murmur, the presence of dysrhythmia, elongation of the PR interval on the electrocardiogram, and congestive failure as manifested by dependent edema and rales throughout the lungs. Leukocytosis is present, and the serum antistreptolysin O titer is usually elevated. The importance of these various manifestations is indicated by the statement that the joint lesions attract immediate attention by the pain they cause, the movements of chorea are not likely to escape notice, but it is the cardiac lesion that shortens life.

Rheumatic disease appears to be an immune condition mediated by an antigen-antibody interaction. This is supported by the sequence of events: a streptococcal infection that posits the antigen, a free period of two to five weeks during which antibody develops, and a clinical onset that is

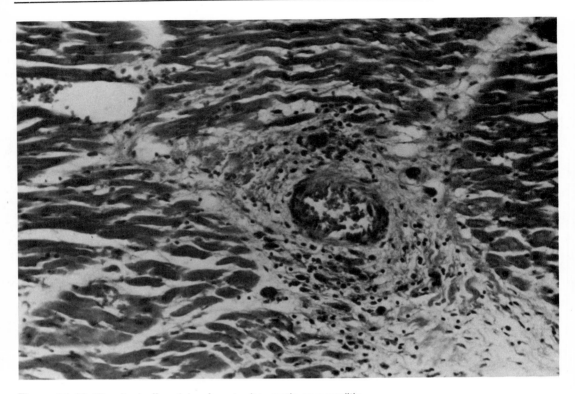

**Figure 11-13.** The Aschoff nodule of acute rheumatic myocarditis

attributable to the interaction of the antibody with the antigen. The organisms are β-hemolytic streptococci, and the infection takes place in the tonsils, throat, or elsewhere in the upper respiratory tract. It is to be emphasized that the effects of the bacteria are not direct; the rheumatic lesions are sterile. Two mechanisms for the development of this condition are postulated: The bacterium-produced antigen may be similar in some way to the cardiac structure so that the antibody reacts with both, or the antigen produced at the infected site diffuses into the circulation and attaches to the myocardium, where the antibody reacts with it. Whichever mechanism applies, it is evident that rheumatic fever is a poststreptococcal hypersensitivity disease.

The process in the heart is a pancarditis; i.e., it affects all portions. The main lesions of the acute phase are fibrinous pericardi-tis, interstitial myocarditis, and acute verrucous endocarditis. All are sterile. The pericarditis is nonspecific. The myocarditis is characterized by more or less discrete collections of lymphocytes and macrophages in intermuscular connective tissue septa adjacent to blood vessels. Occasional multinucleated giant cells are present. Minute foci of fibrinoid necrosis also develop at these sites. This lesion, the Aschoff nodule (Figure 11-13), is specific for rheumatic myocarditis. As the process subsides, foci of scarring between muscle bundles are left. Verrucous endocarditis affects mainly the left side of the heart—the mitral and aortic valves. The verrucae occur on the atrial surface of the mitral valve on the margin of closure adjacent to the free border, and in a row something like a string of beads. Each consists of a minute mound of loosely structured connective tissue often covered with a cap of fibrin and permeated lightly with lymphocytes and a few segmented granulocytes. The firm, sessile attachment of the verrucae precludes embolism. On the aortic valve the verrucae occur on the margins of closure of the ventricular surfaces. The valves are not affected equally; mitral and aortic involvement together occurs in 40 per cent, the mitral valve alone in 40 per cent, the aortic alone in 10 per cent, and others, including the tricuspid and infrequently the pulmonic, in the remaining 10 per cent.

As the inflammation at these sites subsides, nothing may be left other than a fine, slight vascularity of the cusps or leaflets together with small, fibrous, intercommissural adhesions (Figure 11-14). When bouts of streptococcal infection recur, however, over the course of several years the connective tissue builds up and the mitral leaflets gradually become thick, stiff, fibrotic ledges that are well vascularized. The commissures are drawn together, and the chordae tendineae are fused, shortened, and thickened so that the valve orifice becomes markedly stenotic. The small opening is likened to a buttonhole or fish mouth (Figure 11-15). The consequence, of course, is obstruction of the passage of blood through the heart so that the left atrium dilates. Dilation may be so pronounced as to compress portions of the left lung and indent the esophagus as well. The latter may be seen by a barium swallow. Hydrostatic pressure backs up into the pulmonary capillaries, edema with rales follows, and eventually brown induration of the pulmonary tissue develops. When the increased pressure extends to the pulmonary artery, the right ventricle dilates and hypertrophy causes thickening of the wall of that chamber, which is known as cor pulmonale. Eventually the tricuspid ring stretches, the pressure is conveyed into the systemic veins, and right heart failure follows.

Stenosis is also the main lesion of the aortic valve. With recurrent infection, the con-

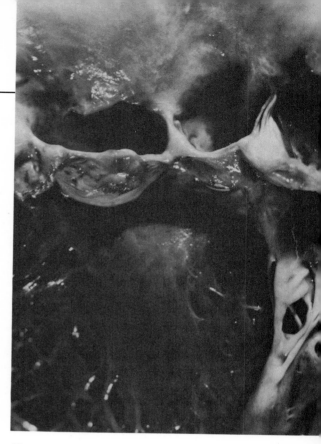

**Figure 11-14.** Subcommissural adhesions from previous rheumatic aortic valvulitis

nective tissue between the cusps forms a shelflike ledge so that the lumen is gradually reduced and hypertrophy of the left ventricle develops. With these changes there are a systolic ejection murmur over the aortic area and the gradual development of congestive failure.

The fibrosis may progress to massive nodular calcification with pronounced stenosis. The nodules appear on the aortic and ventricular sides of the aortic cusps. The unopened aortic surface is shown in Figure 11-16. This condition is regarded as a separate entity because the cause is not certain. Although Karsner and Koletsky attributed the lesion to progression of the rheumatic disease,[25] Roberts cited congenital bicuspid valve as a frequent cause,[26] and Peery made the case for chronic bacterial endocarditis, especially that due to *Brucella*.[27] Whatever the reason for this pronounced

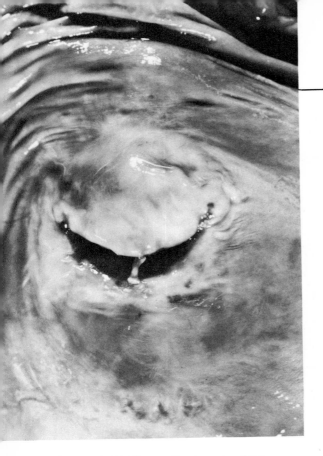

**Figure 11-15.** Rheumatic stenosis of the mitral valve with "fish mouth" opening

deformity, it occurs four times more often in men than in women, death occurs at the age of about 60 years, and the cause is congestive failure that follows pronounced hypertrophy of the left ventricle. The extremely narrow orifice causes a thrill over the aortic area, a harsh systolic murmur transmitted to the neck, and a low pulse pressure from impediment to the systolic thrust. In about one-third of cases there is an associated calcification of the anulus of the mitral valve.

The outlook for the patient with rheumatic valve disease depends on the valve affected, the number of recurrences, the degree of stenosis, and the cardiac reserve. Generally, however, one-third of patients die within five years after the onset of the process, another one-third die between five and 10 years, and the remaining one-third succumb between 10 and 20 years. The most frequent cause is congestive heart failure, although some die of a conduction disturbance, a bacterial infection of a damaged valve, or a mycotic aneurysm in such structures as brain or kidneys. All these consequences are avoided through the use of antibiotics. If the valve disease does develop, however, valve replacement is surgically practicable.

### Bacterial endocarditis

Bacterial endocarditis is an infection of the heart valves. It occurs equally in males and females and affects mainly the mitral leaflets and aortic cusps. The condition is extremely important because it causes valve destruction with congestive failure, thromboembolism with vascular obstruction, and septic emboli with disseminated infection.

Concepts of valvular disease have changed in recent decades.[28] It was not until the second decade of this century that rheumatic disease was distinguished from bacterial infection of the heart valves. It was then realized that bacterial endocarditis occurs most often on valves that have previously been damaged by congenital or rheumatic disease. In the fifth decade of this century antibiotics became available; their use changed the course of the bacterial infections and prevented development of the rheumatic process. Thus bacterial endocarditis is now seen perhaps 60 per cent of the time in patients over 50 with normal heart valves.

There are two forms of bacterial endocarditis, acute and subacute. Their pathogenesis may be different. In acute endocarditis infection with an invasive organism develops at some site distant from the heart. Transient or persistent bacteremia arises. In the meantime, turbulence about a previously damaged valve, especially from rheumatic fever, causes blood to rush from a high-pressure chamber to a low-pressure sink, e.g., from the aorta to the left ventricle, or from the left ventricle to the left atrium. This, in turn, causes traumatic denudation of the endothelium on the

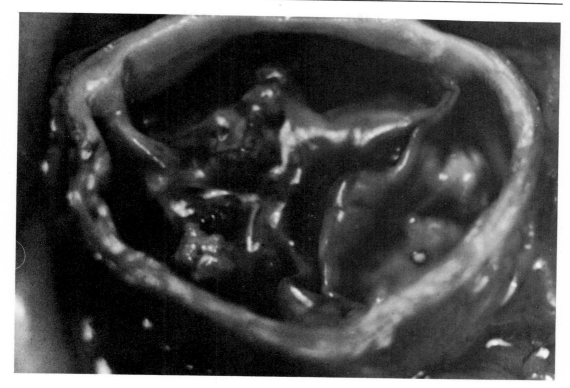

**Figure 11-16.** Top view of unopened aortic valve distorted by calcific aortic stenosis

sink side of the constriction. The circulating bacteria then invade the denuded tissue: the ventricular surface of the aortic valve or the atrial surface of the mitral valve. Platelets and fibrin adhere to this focus so that an infected thrombus or vegetation forms.[29]

In subacute endocarditis the situation is somewhat different. The turbulence and valve denudation are the same. At the denuded site platelets and fibrin attach to form a sterile thrombus. Minor trauma to tissues normally harboring noninvasive bacteria, such as teeth, urinary tract, or gut, causes transient bacteremia. If agglutinating antibodies are circulating, clumps of the noninvasive organisms attach to the thrombus and colonize within it. Thus the subacute form does not require a focus of infection with invasive organisms but depends on

the presence of agglutinating antibodies to posit the noninvasive bacteria in the valve thrombus. Without the agglutinins, the bacteria are too bland or too few in number to invade the sterile thrombus.[29] This concept of the pathogenesis of subacute bacterial endocarditis was introduced by Angrist and Okra in 1963.[30]

Acute bacterial endocarditis is caused especially by *Staphylococcus aureus*; *Streptococcus pyogenes*, *S. pneumoniae*, and *Neisseria* organisms are much less common.[31] The thrombus that builds up on the valve is bulky, friable, and loosely attached. An example on the mitral valve is shown in Figure 11-17. The thrombus or vegetation is composed of masses of fibrin, clusters of platelets, neutrophilic leukocytes, necrotic cellular debris, and colonies of bacteria. A scanning histologic view of

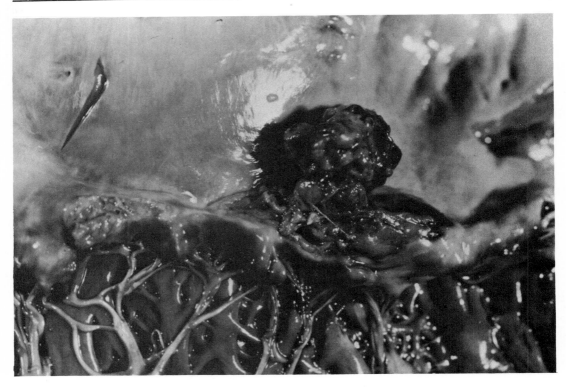

**Figure 11-17.** Acute bacterial endocarditis of the mitral valve. The vegetation is septic and loosely attached; the leaflet has been perforated near the site of attachment.

such a septic thrombus on the aortic valve is shown in Figure 11-18. The septic thrombi or vegetations invade and destroy the valve so that tearing or perforation follows (Figure 11-19; see color section, p C-1). On the mitral valve the process may extend to the chordae tendineae, which rupture. Valvular insufficiency then develops and fulminant congestive failure follows. In addition, emboli from the loosely attached vegetations cause vascular obstruction and infarction, especially in the spleen, kidneys, and brain. Since the emboli are septic, disseminated infection also arises. In the myocardium, which is embolized through the coronary arteries, the discrete foci of acute inflammation are known as Bracht-Wächter bodies. Abscesses, of course, may also develop. Acute peri-

carditis, pyelonephritis, and meningitis are septic complications of the infected emboli.

The patient who suffers from acute bacterial endocarditis experiences a rapidly progressive, overwhelming infection. It begins with high fever, shaking chills, and pronounced fatigue. There follow loss of weight and pallor from hypochromic anemia, which may become pronounced. A neutrophilic leukocytosis of 10,000 to 20,000 is usual. The blood culture is positive for the causative circulating organism. Murmurs develop, become harsh, and change rapidly as the valve destruction proceeds. Without treatment the course is rapidly progressive, and death may occur in as little as two weeks. The cause is fulminant heart failure, widespread embolization, or disseminated infection.

Subacute bacterial endocarditis is most often caused by *Streptococcus viridans*, although some cases are due to microaerophilic streptococci or *Staphylococcus epidermidis*. The mitral and aortic valves are mainly affected, and the inflammation proceeds slowly so that a reparative process attempts to keep pace. Nevertheless, valve destruction gradually develops, followed eventually by congestive failure, myocarditis, and mycotic aneurysms, especially of the brain.

Loss of appetite, low-grade fever, and slowly developing anemia may be the only clinical manifestations. However, there may be no fever. There may also be no leukocytosis, and no murmur. Moreover, if a murmur appears, it may be constant instead of changing. The clinical diagnosis is therefore sometimes difficult. If the condition is not recognized and treated, life expectancy is on the order of several months

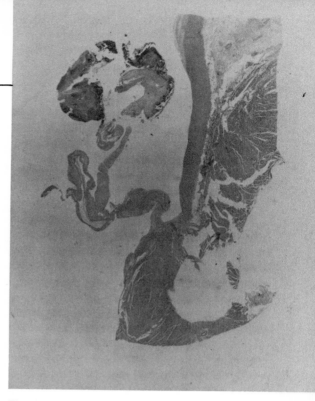

**Figure 11-18.** Septic vegetation of aortic valve. The central part of the cusp is necrotic and perforated.

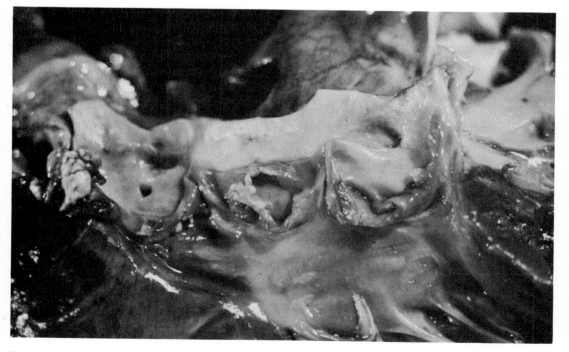

**Figure 11-19.** Destruction of aortic cusps by acute bacterial endocarditis (same valve as shown in Figure 11-18). Also shown in color section, p C-1.

to a year. The cause of death is gradually progressive heart failure complicated by embolization, especially to the spleen, kidneys, and brain. Disseminated infection tends to be infrequent because of the low invasiveness of the organism.

Clinical manifestations in both acute and subacute forms that were previously ascribed to microembolism include petechiae of the skin, buccal mucosa, and conjunctivae as well as punctate hemorrhages of the pads of the fingers and toes (Osler's nodes), the palms and soles (Janeway lesions), and the retinae (Roth's spots). In this same category is the so-called embolic glomerulonephritis, which is associated with microscopic hematuria. All of these signs are now uncommon, they are associated with a high level of circulating antibody, and they are now attributed to a focal hypersensitivity vasculitis.[29]

In the past, acute bacterial endocarditis was uniformly fatal. It is still a condition of guarded outlook, in part because of poor diffusion of antibiotics into the nonvascularized septic vegetations. On the other hand, subacute bacterial endocarditis, which formerly also had an extremely high mortality, may now be cured in nearly all cases when the condition is recognized early and treated appropriately. This therapeutic improvement has been an important achievement in medical care.

## Nonbacterial endocardiosis (endocarditis)

In debilitated patients, often in a state of terminal disease, sterile thrombi tend to form on the mitral and aortic valves. These remain sterile, perhaps because of insufficient agglutinating antibodies that would otherwise posit organisms from the transient bacteremias that occur in normal persons. The condition in which this is most frequent is mucinous adenocarcinoma, regardless of the site of origin. It also occurs, although less frequently, in pneumonia, congestive heart failure, pyelonephritis,

and glomerulonephritis. The clinical evidence of a valve disorder may be masked by the terminal disease; when it is not, the clinical features may mimic bacterial endocarditis with fever, leukocytosis, murmurs, and emboli. The blood culture yields no organism, however, and histologic examination of the vegetation discloses a bland accumulation of fibrin and platelets without leukocytes, colonies of bacteria, or destruction of the underlying valve tissue (Figure 11-20). The clinical manifestation of this condition, as might be expected, is embolization with bland infarction of such organs as the spleen, kidneys, or brain. Since the condition is noninflammatory, it should be termed nonbacterial endocardiosis rather than nonbacterial thrombotic endocarditis, which is commonly used.

In summary, four main types of valvular disease exist. All affect mainly the mitral leaflets and aortic cusps. Rheumatic endocarditis proceeds from noninfected verrucae to massive fibrosis with pronounced stenosis of both left heart valves. Acute bacterial endocarditis needs nothing more than a denuded valve surface and bacteremia with an invasive organism. The septic thrombus or vegetation destroys the valve, causing acute insufficiency, and follows a septic, rapidly progressive course with fulminant heart failure, embolic obstruction of arteries, and foci of inflammation within the heart and throughout many organs. Subacute endocarditis begins silently, smolders along, may be difficult to diagnose, and eventually causes valve destruction with congestive failure and septic infarcts of spleen, kidneys, or brain. The most common "endocarditis" is the sterile thrombotic endocardiosis that develops in the debilitated patient, does not destroy the valve, but does give off emboli causing widespread bland arterial obstructions. These four forms of valvular disease account for almost all examples of endocarditis, and, whether infected or not, they are characterized by cardiac failure, dissemi-

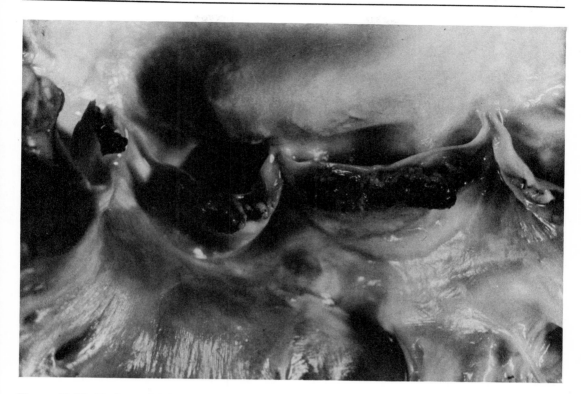

**Figure 11-20.** Nonbacterial thrombotic endocardiosis of aortic valve

nated infection, thrombotic disease, or some combination of all three of these clinical manifestations.

## DISORDERS OF THE PERICARDIUM, MYOCARDIUM, AND ENDOCARDIUM

### Pericardium

Diseases of the pericardium are often classified according to cause. This is not altogether satisfactory because a single agent may evoke different reactions, and the specific cause may not be known until cultures are made or tissue sections are examined. It is therefore preferable to classify the disorders according to their gross features; the diagnosis is evident on first inspection, and subsequent determination of etiologic agents does not affect the original judgment. Considered in this way, the main significant abnormalities of the pericardium are effusion, hemorrhage, acute inflammation, and fibrosis. Fibrosis may be focal, obliterative, or constrictive.

The pericardial sac normally contains less than 50 ml of clear, pale yellow, watery fluid. It has a lubricating function by separating the visceral and parietal layers. When the amount of fluid exceeds 100 ml, an effusion exists. This is also known as hydropericardium. The frequent causes are congestive heart failure and hypoalbuminemia, especially as seen with chronic renal disease. Radiation in excess of 4,000 rad is another cause.[32] There is no reaction to the fluid, and it is clinically silent unless the amount is so great that the heart is compressed and diastolic filling is impaired. This amount is extremely variable; if the accumulation is rapid, the constricting amount is much less than when it is slow. When accumulation is slow, however,

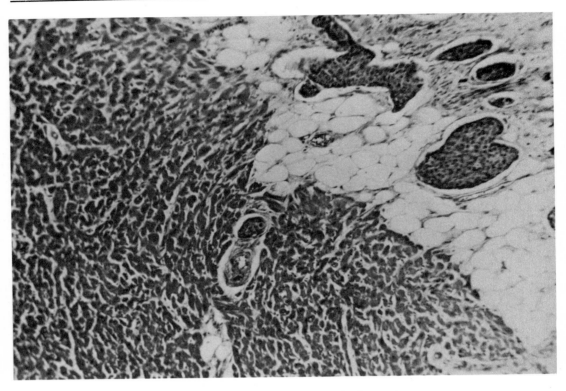

**Figure 11-21.** Metastatic carcinoma in lymphatics of epicardial adipose tissue

many times the normal maximum volume may fail to cause constriction. Effusions are usually 200 to 400 ml. They tend to be blood-tinged when the cause is an underlying infarct of the myocardium, and frankly bloody when due to metastatic disease in the epicardium. Chylous (milky) effusions are rare.[33] Metastatic carcinoma in the epicardium is shown in Figure 11-21.

Hemopericardium results from ventricular rupture after myocardial infarction, from traumatic perforation of the heart wall, or from extension of a dissecting aneurysm into the pericardial sac. Cardiac tamponade usually results; i.e., diastolic filling is prevented and the circulation fails. The amount of blood in the sac, which often clots to form a solid mass, is usually 300 to 500 ml. An unopened pericardial sac filled with blood from a ventricular rupture is shown in Figure 11-22.

Acute pericarditis has many causes. When it is fibrinous and sterile, common causes are uremia, acute rheumatic fever, and myocardial infarction. Why uremia should cause fibrin to form on the epicardium is not known. The surface of the heart is dull rather than smooth and glistening, and the epicardium is roughened by minute, pale yellow, elastic adhesions that are friable and scrape away easily from the surface. A microsection is shown in Figure 11-23. The clinical manifestations are scant, although a friction rub may be heard, at least until the fluid accumulation separates the visceral and parietal layers. The reaction evidently subsides without deformity although focal fibrous adhesions between the two layers may result.

Acute pericarditis may also be infective and purulent. This is usually associated with widespread fulminant infection, especially of the lungs, pleura, and mediastinum. The organisms reach the pericardium by hematogenous spread except when the cause is a perforating injury or rupture of a myocardial abscess. The most common organism is the staphylococcus. Gram-negative bacilli, often coliform organisms, are also found, and fungi may be isolated from patients who are immunosuppressed or otherwise debilitated. Grossly the entire surface of the sac is roughened by a thick, shaggy mat of pale yellow fibrin with varying amounts of fluid exudate. The clinical features are fever, chest pain, and a friction rub. Fluid can be detected in the sac by echocardiography and, in addition, by a globular outline of the heart on chest X-ray. Aspiration of the sac is necessary to establish the purulent nature of the process and the specific organism causing it.[34] The outlook for the patient is poor because of the fulminant, widespread nature of the accompanying infection.

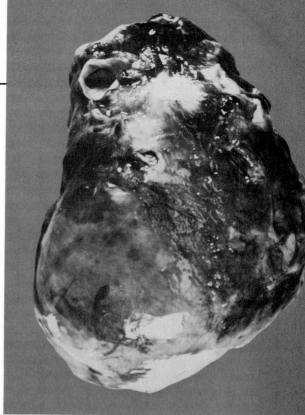

**Figure 11-22.** Hemopericardium with unopened pericardial sac. The patient died of cardiac tamponade.

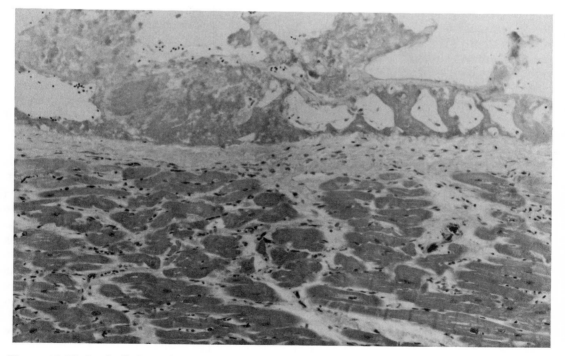

**Figure 11-23.** Sterile fibrin on the surface of the epicardium

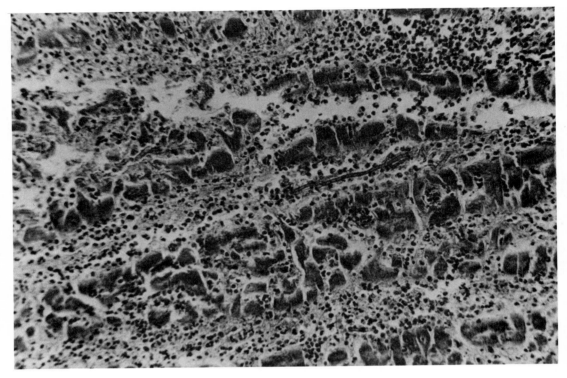

**Figure 11-24.** *Aspergillus* myocarditis

Inflammations subside, usually through the process of organization, which involves the development of granulation tissue. As the granulation tissue turns to scar, fibrous adhesions form. When these are focal in the pericardial sac, they are of little consequence. When they are widespread, the sac may be obliterated. No functional disturbance develops, however, unless the scar becomes thick and circumferential and contracts; then constrictive pericarditis results. The term is a misnomer because the inflammatory process has completely subsided by that time; the connective tissue is dense, frequently hyalinized, and cell-poor. Calcification may develop and be focal or widespread. A better term is therefore constrictive fibrosis of the pericardium with or without calcification.

The cause is a previous episode of purulent disease or an ongoing connective tissue disorder such as lupus erythematosus, scleroderma, or rheumatoid arthritis. It may occur in chronic renal disease, although the mechanism is not clear, and as a postirradiation event in the treatment of Hodgkin's disease or mediastinal lymphoma.[35] Gradually the heart is bound down and compressed so that atrial filling is slowed and ventricular output is reduced. The pulse pressure is therefore diminished and venous blood backs up, especially into the systemic circulation. The clinical feature is distention of the neck veins with increased venous pressure but without enlargement of the heart. The heart is small and quiet, being unable to dilate or undergo hypertrophy. Hepatomegaly also develops, and ascites without peripheral edema is characteristic. The electrocardiogram reveals low voltage in the QRS complex. Once the diagnosis is made, relief is pro-

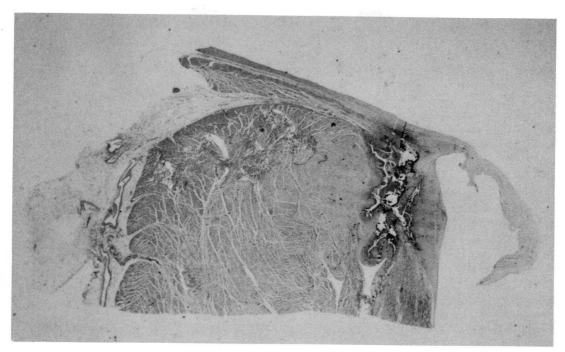

**Figure 11-25.** Subjacent to the attachment of the mitral leaflet, which extends to the right, is a rheumatoid nodule with central necrosis and marginal granulomatous inflammation.

vided by pericardiectomy, which loosens the binding constriction.

## Myocardium

Cardiomyopathy is the term for those disorders of the heart that are not due to coronary, valvular, hypertensive, congenital, or pulmonary disease.[36] Some are inflammatory, some are noninflammatory, and some are infiltrative. The inflammatory cardiomyopathies are mainly those associated with overwhelming infections, immunosuppression, or bacterial endocarditis. The myocardial involvement is secondary, and nearly every organism has been isolated. Bacteria, viruses, rickettsiae, spirochetes, and fungi have been found. The histologic appearance of *Aspergillus* myocarditis is shown in Figure 11-24.

In addition to cardiac involvement secondary to overwhelming infection, systemic diseases—especially rheumatic fever, rheumatoid disease, and sarcoidosis—frequently affect the heart. The Aschoff nodule is the specific chronic granulomatous lesion of rheumatic fever (see section on valvular disease). In rheumatoid arthritis the heart is involved in about 3 per cent of patients.[37] The granulomas microscopically resemble the subcutaneous nodules of rheumatoid disease, and they are found in the epicardium, myocardium, and valves. Most frequently, however, the rings of attachment of the mitral and aortic valves are affected. The granulomas are large and display central necrosis with a margin of fibrinoid change and a periphery of palisaded fibroblasts along with lymphocytes and frequent plasma cells. The large size, central necrosis, and absence of Aschoff bodies distinguish the lesion from rheumatic disease. Figure 11-25 illustrates such a nodule underlying the attachment of a mitral leaflet. Conduction disturbance, valve dysfunction, and occasionally congestive failure are clinical consequences that depend on the site of the lesions.

Sarcoidosis also affects the heart. Heart involvement is found in about 20 per cent of patients with this disease who are examined at autopsy.[38] Although no area of the heart is immune, the left ventricle is most often involved, especially the upper part of the interventricular septum, the papillary muscles, and the free wall. The granulomas are small, firm, and pale gray. Massive scarring of the free wall with transmural fibrosis may occur in the absence of coronary artery disease. When the heart is involved, granulomas are also found in the lymph nodes, lungs, liver, and spleen. The clinical effects, however, are mainly cardiac, and consist of sudden death, conduction disturbances, congestive failure, and recurrent pericardial effusions. The course in patients with extensive cardiac sarcoidosis is not prolonged, and sudden death may be the first manifestation of the disease.[39]

In noninflammatory cardiomyopathy the heart may be dilated or hypertrophic. The former, which is idiopathic, is characterized by dilation of both ventricles, mural thrombi of the right and left ventricles and atrial appendages, and foci of endocardial fibrosis that may be due to the organization of previous mural thrombi. The hearts are heavy, averaging 600 gm in one study, and also dilated so that the left ventricular thickness is often less than 1.5 cm.[38] The texture of the muscle is flabby, and histologic examination reveals only slight interstitial fibrosis with hypertrophy of some cells and atrophy of others. The arrangement of the fibers is normal. There is no inflammation of the myocardium, and the coronary arteries are widely patent. These findings are constant whether or not the patient gives a history of chronic alcoholism. Chest pain is not a clinical feature. The functional effects are inadequate ventricular contraction, decreased stroke volume, and progressive heart failure.

The hypertrophic form of cardiomyopathy is also idiopathic. It was first noted in 1958 by Teare, who described nine patients.[40] He called the condition asymmetrical hypertrophy of the heart. Subsequently it became known in the United States as idiopathic hypertrophic subaortic stenosis while in England it was termed hypertrophic obstructive cardiomyopathy. Obstruction is absent more often than present, however, and for this reason Roberts recommended the simpler term hypertrophic cardiomyopathy.[38] The main morphologic features are disproportionate hypertrophy of the ventricular septum, a chaotic disarray of the muscle fibers in the hypertrophic part, normal or small ventricular cavities, and dilated right and left atria. The first two changes are evident at birth; the rest evidently develop later. Thus the ventricular wall is thick and the ventricular cavities are small. The condition is one of a "muscle-bound" heart with ventricular hypercontractility, rather than a dilated, flabby heart with hypocontractility.

Thickening of the ventricular septum is most pronounced in the midportion. This is said to cause the anterior leaflet of the mitral valve to impinge on the endocardium of the ventricular septum with each systole. The results are focal fibrosis of the endocardium, thickening of the anterior leaflet, and obstruction of the outflow of blood from the left ventricle. It is not certain, however, that the obstruction is the main cause of the morbidity or mortality of the condition.[41] The aortic valve is normal.

Hypertrophic cardiomyopathy occurs in families, affects the sexes equally, and is transmitted as an autosomal dominant characteristic. Sporadic cases are uncommon. Although it is not rare, the true incidence of the condition is not known, mainly because so many individuals with this condition tend to be asymptomatic. Most patients feel well but develop a systolic mur-

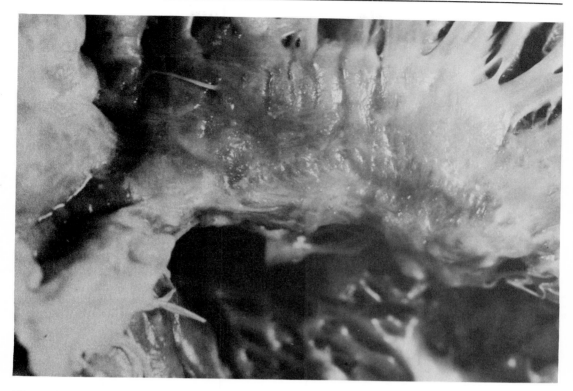

**Figure 11-26.** Granular translucent amyloid deposits in the posterior leaflet of the mitral valve

mur around age 20; symptoms begin at a mean age of 30, and disability develops at about age 35. The symptoms are dyspnea, excessive fatigue, palpitations, and chest pain that responds poorly to nitroglycerin. Syncope is present in 20 to 30 per cent.[42] Physical examination reveals a systolic murmur. The cardiac outline on chest X-ray is usually normal. The diagnosis may be made by echocardiography alone. Although the course is extremely variable, Ross and colleagues have pointed out that sudden death is a hallmark of the condition.[42] Eight of Teare's nine patients died in this way. Older patients usually go on to develop congestive failure.

The principal example of infiltrative cardiomyopathy is amyloidosis. It is frequent, slight, and of no clinical significance in patients over 60 years of age. In this form it is referred to as "senile amyloidosis." In younger patients extensive deposits occasionally develop in association with chronic inflammatory disease (secondary amyloidosis) and in the absence of such disease (primary amyloidosis). In both, deposits in other organs are frequent although rarely the heart alone is involved. The amyloid may occur in any part of the heart, including the coronary arteries, conduction system, and myocardial nerves. It is grossly evident in the endocardium, however, especially the atria (Figure 11-26), where it is visible as firm, granular, pale yellowish-gray translucent deposits. The endocardial involvement does not cause valvular dysfunction.[43] Amyloid is also grossly evident in the myocardium, not as visible focal deposits but as a firm, rubbery, noncompliant ventricular wall. The myocardial involvement causes

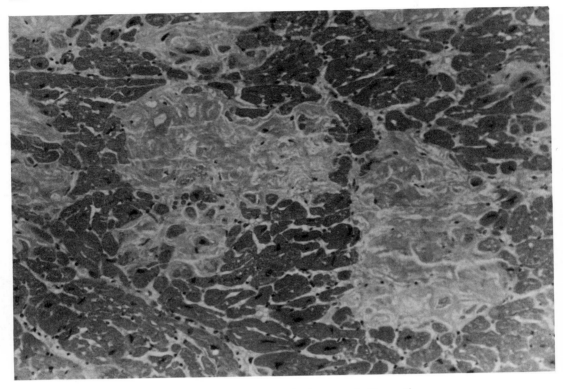

**Figure 11-27.** Acellular amyloid surrounding and replacing muscle fibers of the heart

conduction disturbance, low-voltage electrocardiographic tracings, and congestive failure. The clinical diagnosis is weak without the last two of these features. The myocardial deposits are patchy or diffuse and impair the contractility of the muscle. The histologic appearance is illustrated in Figure 11-27.

The congestive failure is unresponsive to digitalis, and it is characterized by slow cardiac filling at high venous pressure with greatly reduced left ventricular contraction. The condition is referred to as the "stiff heart syndrome."[44] The atrial chambers are dilated, but the ventricular cavities are small unless other disease is present. Amyloidosis thus joins hypertrophic cardiomyopathy and constrictive pericarditis as a cause of congestive failure without dilation of the ventricular cavities.

## Endocardium

Aside from valvulitis, which is a form of endocardial disease, two other conditions—atrial myxoma and fibroelastosis—deserve mention. Both are uncommon.

Atrial myxoma is the most common primary tumor of the heart.[45] It is a condition of adults, affecting women more often than men, that arises in the 30- to 60-year age group. It occurs three times more often in the left atrium than in the right. The tumor is smooth and ovoid (Figure 11-28). Some tumors are sessile, but most are attached to the endocardium by a pedicle. The surface is pale yellowish-gray mottled with light brown. The cut surfaces are pale gray, wet, and translucent. There are no laminations as are seen on the cut surface of a mural thrombus. Histologic examination reveals cell-poor myxoid tissue in which small numbers of endothelial cells, fibroblasts, macrophages, and smooth muscle cells may be identified. From this composition, Ferrans and Roberts interpreted the lesion as a benign tumor of multipotential mesenchymal cells.[46]

Although dyspnea is the most common symptom, the clinical presentation is in the form of embolization, mitral obstruction, or constitutional symptoms.[47] Emboli are frequent, and this event in a young adult without bacterial endocarditis should bring the clinical diagnosis to mind. The bulky tumor may block the mitral aperture and simulate mitral stenosis. However, syncopal attacks are also frequent and are relieved by a change of position as the pedunculated mass falls away from the mitral orifice. Constitutional manifestations include fever, anemia, and weight loss, possibly from hemorrhage and necrosis within the lesion. There is no history of rheumatic disease, hemoptysis does not occur, and the electrocardiogram is nondiagnostic. A chest X-ray may or may not show enlargement of the left atrium. Congestive failure gradually develops. The symptomatic period to the time of diagnosis is about one year. Surgical removal of the tumor effects cure.

Endocardial fibroelastosis is a diffuse thickening of the left ventricular surface with a dense, pale gray layer of fibrous and elastic tissue. The primary form is idiopathic and occurs mainly in infants and children. Postulated causes include fetal hypoxia and fetal myocarditis, especially due to maternal mumps, with passage of the virus across the placenta to the developing fetus.[48] The secondary form of the disorder is associated with congenital anomalies, cardiac irradiation, valve disease, and viral infections. The anomalies include aortic stenosis, coarctation of the aorta, hypoplasia of the aorta, and abnormalities of the left coronary artery. The primary and secondary forms have the same gross appearance (Figure 11-29). Microscopically, however, Fishbein and associates found the elastic

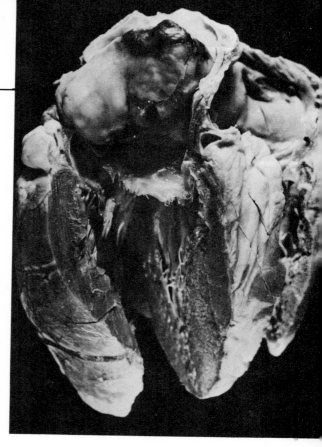

**Figure 11-28.** Myxoma of left atrium attached just above anterior leaflet of mitral valve

fibers to be larger in the primary form.[49] Whatever the cause, the endocardium is covered by a thick blanket of rigid, nearly white connective tissue that stiffens the wall and impairs the contractility of the muscle. The mitral valve is often affected, but the other endocardial surfaces are usually spared.[50] The muscle subjacent to the fibroelastic layer is not remarkable. In infants congestive failure may be fulminant and cause death within the first year of life. In adults the symptomatic period is longer and failure is less abrupt.

## VASCULAR DISEASE

The vascular system is composed of arteries, veins, capillaries, and lymphatics. Diseases affect arteries and veins. Arteries are subdivided by size into the aorta, medium-sized vessels, and arterioles.

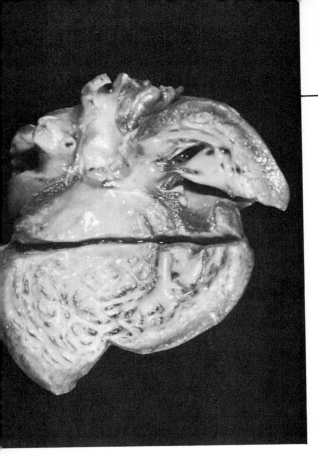

**Figure 11-29.** Endocardial fibroelastosis

## Aorta

Four main conditions affect the aorta: atherosclerosis, dissecting aneurysm, syphilis, and nonspecific aortitis. Each is distinct, and all have life-threatening complications. Atherosclerosis is by far the most common, nonspecific aortitis is uncommon, and syphilitic aortitis is now becoming rare.

At the outset it should be understood that the term arteriosclerosis is generic; it encompasses the processes of atherosclerosis, Mönckeberg's medial calcification, and arteriolar hyalinization. Atherosclerosis affects the aorta and medium-sized vessels, Mönckeberg's calcification is clinically silent and occurs principally in the elderly, and arteriolar hyalinization is common and associated with nephrosclerosis and essential hypertension. It is atherosclerosis that is so important; it is the chief cause of death in the United States. Along with cancer, it is the greatest unsolved problem in medicine. Holman and colleagues put the pro-

cess in context: "While mental disease is our greatest socio-economic problem, cancer our greatest enigma, arthritis our greatest crippler, and accidents our greatest disgrace, atherosclerosis is our greatest killer."[51] And to this Boyd added, "It kills by diminishing the blood supply to a vital organ, in particular the heart, the brain, and the kidneys."[52]

The process begins with the migration of smooth muscle cells from the tunica media of the aorta through the fenestrae of the internal elastic lamina to the intima, where they become phagocytic and distended with lipids.[53] The lipids are rich in cholesterol, and the lesion is a sessile, slightly raised focus of pale yellow discoloration that is known as a lipid or fatty streak. It is present in the aorta of virtually every child by the age of 10 years. From then on to the age of 25, the extent of intimal involvement increases to about 40 per cent.[53] These observations suggest that measures to prevent atherosclerosis must be undertaken early in life to be effective.

The second lesion consists of the fibrous plaque, in which elastic fibers, collagen bundles, and proteoglycans (mucopolysaccharides) are added to the focus of cell proliferation and lipid deposition. The result is an opaque, slightly raised, pale gray focus covered with a fibrous cap that tends to be located around the ostia and branches of the vessel. The fibrous plaque appears at the age of about 20 years.[54] It is widely presumed but not altogether certain that the fibrous plaque is a progression from the fatty streak.

The final stage is the complicated lesion—a fibrous plaque altered by ulceration, hemorrhage, calcification, or thrombosis. The fibrous plaques and complicated lesions are more pronounced in the abdominal aorta than elsewhere. The three lesions of atherosclerosis, ordinarily considered to occur in sequence, are thus the lipid streak, the fibrous plaque, and the complicated lesion. Whether or not they occur in sequence, the histologic features include proliferation of smooth muscle cells that become phagocytic, deposition of lipids inside and outside cells, and accumulation of collagen bundles, elastic fibers, and proteoglycans. The consequences of this process are stenosis of the lumen, weakening of the wall, and thrombosis. Atherosclerosis of the aorta is shown in Figure 11-30.

The central question in atherosclerosis is the pathogenic mechanism by which the process develops. Originally Virchow proposed that injury to the endothelium allows lipids to seep into the intima, but Rokitansky believed that thrombi form on the surface so that organization of the thrombus with central degeneration produces the fibrous plaque.[55] These two theories stood apart for years. In 1949 the Rokitansky hypothesis was re-emphasized by Duguid.[56] The contending ideas were brought closer together, however, by the disclosure through electron microscopy that the smooth muscle cells of the aortic media migrate into the intima and not only proliferate but also become macrophages that phagocytize lipids. The distinction between the thrombotic and lipid theories of atherogenesis was further blurred by the finding that platelets, which aggregate at the site of endothelial injury, release a mitogenic factor that stimulates smooth muscle cells from the media to proliferate.[57]

An attempt was made to reconcile all these observations under a single hypothesis called the response-to-injury mechanism of atherogenesis.[53] This envisages an endothelial injury with ulceration that will heal if not repeated. The injury is presumably caused by viruses, bacteria, the endotoxins from bacteria, carbon monoxide or other chemicals from cigarette smoke, circulating cholesterol in excess, antigen-antibody complexes, and the shear stress of hemodynamic forces, especially in the presence of hypertension.[57] When the injury is repeated, platelets aggregate at the site, a mitogenic factor is released, and smooth muscle

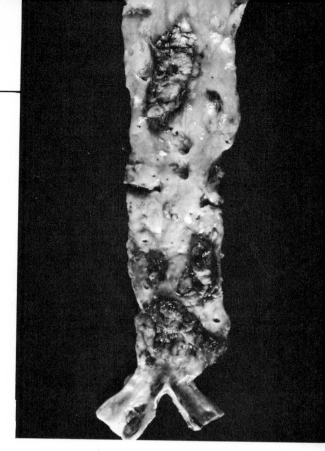

**Figure 11-30.** Atherosclerosis of aorta with intimal ulceration and mural thrombus formation

cells migrate into the intima, proliferate, and phagocytize lipoproteins rich in cholesterol. The smooth muscle cells also produce collagen, elastin, and proteoglycans.[58] Thus the lipid streak progresses to the fibrous plaque, and, with repeated injury coupled to the reaction of repair, the fibrous plaque progresses to the complicated lesion.[59] The atherogenic process is interpreted as a reaction to injury.

In 1973 Benditt and Benditt proposed a second, genuinely different pathogenic mechanism known as the monoclonal theory.[60] In females only one X chromosome is active; it may be the X chromosome from either the father or the mother. The X chromosome codes for the glucose 6-phosphate dehydrogenase (G6PD) enzyme. G6PD has two distinguishable isoenzymes, one determined by the maternal X and the other by the paternal X. It is therefore possible to culture tissue cells, study the G6PD isoenzymes, and determine whether the cultured cells are from a single parent (monoclonal, with one isoenzyme) or from both parents (diclonal, with both isoenzymes). Using this method, many normal tissues, including smooth muscle cells from the aortic wall, were found to be diclonal, whereas certain benign tumors were found to be monoclonal. The cells from atherosclerotic lesions were also monoclonal. The Benditts therefore proposed that atherosclerosis is due to proliferation of smooth muscle cells in the manner of a benign tumor, and that some environmental injury, such as a virus or chemical, transforms the cells into a proliferating monoclonal colony. This suggested mechanism of pathogenesis has stimulated much interest.

Whichever mechanism is eventually found to be true, there are nevertheless certain risk factors that correlate with the clinical manifestations of atherosclerotic disease. The clinical manifestations are angina pectoris, myocardial infarction, sudden death, stroke, and peripheral vascular disease. The risk factors that correlate with these manifestations are age, sex, high blood cholesterol, hypertension, diabetes mellitus, and cigarette smoking.

The atherosclerotic process advances with age. Lipid streaks increase rapidly through the ages of 8 to 18, fibrous plaques begin to form at about age 20, and complicated lesions become more pronounced in older persons. Atherosclerosis is thus a lifelong process. The lesions are more pronounced in men and postmenopausal women, in whom female hormones are either absent or greatly diminished. The reasons for this apparent protective effect of female hormones are not clear.[54]

The strongest risk factor, next to age and sex, is hypercholesterolemia. The blood level of cholesterol is determined by the intake of total calories, animal fats (saturated), and cholesterol. Animals given a diet rich in cholesterol develop atherosclerosis. Human populations with a high consumption of animal fat have a higher incidence of atherosclerotic disease than populations on a diet rich in vegetable (polyunsaturated) fats.[57] In the United States, where the population is relatively affluent, the normal blood cholesterol is 200 to 220 mg/dl and one-third of the adult population is hyperlipidemic, with a blood level above 250 mg/dl.[10] Most of this is due to overeating; only a small part is due to a heritable metabolic disorder such as familial hyperlipidemia, in which clinical manifestations of atherosclerosis arise at age 20 to 30. In countries where economic standards are low, the blood level of cholesterol is under 150 mg/dl and atherosclerotic disease is scarce to absent.[61] It is also virtually absent in populations subject to poor nutrition, as in war or famine.[62] Therefore it is evident that atherosclerosis is associated with hyperlipidemia, and the level of blood cholesterol is a powerful index of the risk of the disease.

Hypertension is also associated with atherosclerosis, and especially with cerebrovascular disease. The mechanism may be separation of the connections between the endothelial cells by hemodynamic stress, increased filtration of plasma rich in lipoproteins through the intimal surface, or increased work load of the underlying smooth muscle cells. Atherosclerosis is also a major health hazard for diabetics, who have a higher than normal level of blood lipids. This, however, does not account for the increased risk of the disease.[54] Nor is it attributable to thickening of the basement membranes of capillaries. Neither insulin nor oral hypoglycemic agents protect from this increased risk. Finally, cigarette smoking augments the atherosclerotic process and probably contributes to terminal thrombotic events as well. Carbon monoxide is suspected of being the harmful component that injures the endothelial cell. This is not certain, however, as cigarette smoke contains 3,000 identified chemicals and probably more that are not identified. The number of possibly harmful substances is thus great. Less well supported as risk factors are obesity, personality type, a sedentary life, and the mineral content of drinking water.[62]

It is tempting to suppose that atherosclerosis might be prevented or reversed by treating hypertension, discontinuing smoking, and lowering the intake of cholesterol, saturated fatty acids, and a high-calorie diet. There is some evidence that such measures may be helpful. They do decrease the level of cholesterol in the blood. Walker reported a decrease of 25 per cent in the mortality from coronary disease in American men under 55 years of age.[63] This was associated with a decrease in the consumption of tobacco and animal fats as well as an increase in the use of vegetable oils. In hyperlipidemic patients, Buchwald and colleagues lowered blood cholesterol by 40 per cent through ileal bypass operations.[64] This method is not suitable for all patients, however, and it was not established that the atherosclerotic lesions regressed in the same measure as the blood cholesterol.

Finally, an elevated serum level of high-density lipoproteins (HDL) is associated with a low rate of atherosclerotic disease.[65] Chylomicrons, very-low-density lipoproteins, and low-density lipoproteins have the opposite effect and are associated with an increased risk of atherosclerosis. It is thought that HDL facilitate the transport of lipids from tissue deposits to the liver, where catabolism and excretion take place. Whatever the explanation, it is evident that HDL may have a role in the treatment of hyperlipidemia and perhaps atherosclerotic disease as well.

Whatever the future may hold for treatment or prevention, it is necessary in the present to be concerned with the complications of the atherosclerotic process. In the aorta these include atheroembolism, thromboembolism, thrombosis, and aneurysm formation. When the intima over an

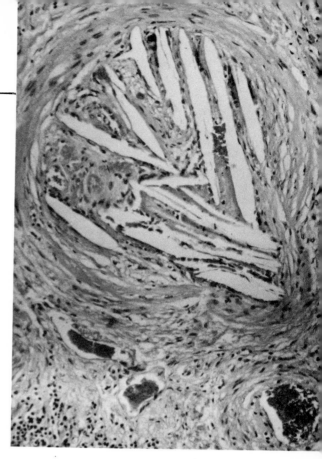

**Figure 11-31.** Acicular (needle-like) cholesterol crystals in organized thrombus of intrarenal artery

atheromatous plaque ulcerates, the pultaceous debris is released and carried in the vascular current to embolic sites. The sites are manifold and so are the clinical manifestations, including the "small stroke" syndrome, transient blindness, sudden hypertension, purple toes, and abdominal pain with bloody stool from infarction of a segment of gut. The variety of clinical manifestations is so wide that cholesterol embolism is referred to as the "great masquerader."[66] The most frequent clinical event, however, is renal disease with unexplained failure. This may be spontaneous but more often follows abdominal trauma, aortic surgery, or cardiac catheterization via the femoral artery. Cortical infarcts may form in the kidney, but often only acicular (needle-like or slitlike) crystals of cholesterol in thrombi of the interlobular arteries are seen (Figure 11-31).

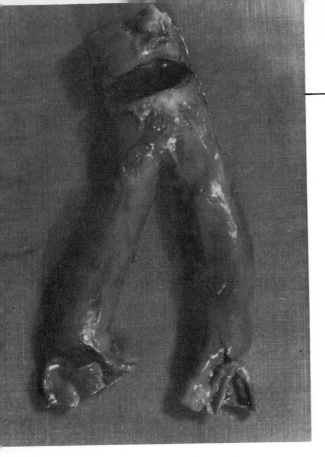

**Figure 11-32.** Total thrombosis of abdominal aorta with extension into iliac bifurcation

Thrombi on ulcers of the aorta may dislodge to become embolic, especially to the legs. Such thromboemboli may also impinge on the aortic bifurcation. These "saddle emboli" can arise from the left ventricle after myocardial infarction, or from the left atrial appendage in cases of atrial fibrillation. The saddle embolus of the aortic bifurcation causes agonizing pain of sudden onset in the legs that is associated with pallor, loss of pulses in the lower extremities, and, unless relieved by embolectomy, ischemic necrosis of the feet.

Since atherosclerosis is most pronounced in the abdominal aorta, thrombi tend to form at that site and may occlude the lumen (Figure 11-32). As the process is gradual, collaterals form, and the compensatory routes may be so effective that the patient is asymptomatic.[67] Middle-aged men may develop the Leriche syndrome: atrophy and weakness of the legs, absence of pulses, intermittent claudication, and failure to maintain an erection because of insufficient blood to fill the corpora spongiosa of the penis. Without surgical treatment the claudication increases and ischemic necrosis of the feet gradually develops.

The main complication of atherosclerosis of the aorta is aneurysm formation. It is saccular, affects the abdominal portion, and lies between the ostia of the renal arteries and the iliac bifurcation. It occurs in middle and old age, more frequently in men than in women, and regularly ruptures as the advancing process continues to weaken the wall. The aneurysms measure up to 15 cm in diameter, fill with laminated thrombi, and project in an anterior direction, often inclining toward the left (Figure 11-33). The clinical indications of rupture include sudden, often excruciating midabdominal pain that may be referred to the lower back or into one or both groins, also nausea, vomiting, weakness, and fainting. Signs include pallor, sweating, tachycardia, and a tender, pulsatile mass in the abdomen. The aneurysm usually contains calcium in the wall so that the most useful diagnostic procedure is a lateral X-ray of the abdomen. Curved lines of calcium in the region of the palpable mass can be seen. Diagnosis is urgent because survival depends on immediate resection with implantation of a prosthetic device.

Rupture of such aneurysms occurs in four particular places: the retroperitoneum, the peritoneal cavity, the inferior vena cava, and the duodenum. Retroperitoneal rupture is the most frequent, and since the soft tissue has to be split apart to make room for the hematoma, a period of relative cardiovascular stability precedes exsanguination. With rupture into the peritoneal cavity, however, shock is sudden, profound, and unrelenting. There are also an abdominal bruit, renal failure, hepatic dysfunction, edema of the extremities, and various degrees of lethargy and confusion.

Perforation into the inferior vena cava creates a giant arteriovenous fistula that is manifested by fulminant congestive heart failure. The least frequent site of rupture is into the duodenum, which crosses over the top of the aneurysmal wall. Sudden massive vomiting of bright red blood signals the event.

**Dissecting aneurysm.** A dissecting aneurysm is a split in the wall of the aorta in a plane between the inner two-thirds and outer one-third of the media (Figure 11-34). This occurs in the age range of 40 to 70 years, six times more frequently in men than in women, and usually in individuals who are hypertensive. The process tends to begin in the thoracic portion with a transverse tear just above the aortic valve (Figure 11-35). Less often the intimal tear is at the ligamentum arteriosum, and occasionally no tear is discovered. The hemorrhage progresses through the thoracic portion

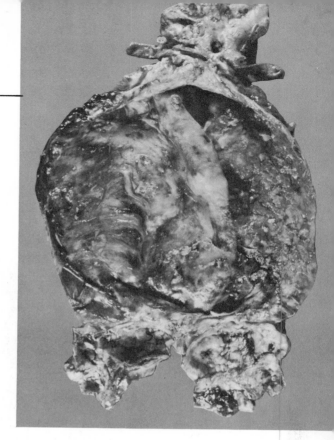

**Figure 11-33.** Saccular aneurysm of abdominal aorta

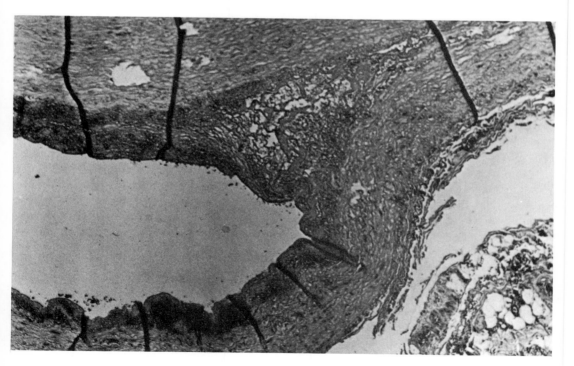

**Figure 11-34.** Hemorrhagic split of aortic wall. Adventitia (below) and lumen (above) are not visible.

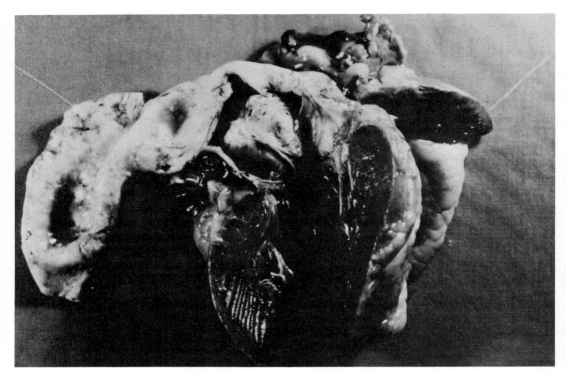

**Figure 11-35.** Transverse tear of dissecting aneurysm just above aortic valve

and distally so that about one-third reach the iliac bifurcation. Short extensions into the walls of the aortic branches—e.g., carotids, celiac, renal, lumbar, iliac, and femorals—are frequent.

The clinical manifestations include a sudden, severe, stabbing pain in the chest that is often associated with shock and collapse. The diagnosis is evident from five clinical features: The pain radiates to the interscapular region and shifts downward (caudally) as the dissection proceeds; radiographs show a characteristic widening of the mediastinum; the electrocardiogram is negative for infarction; the blood pressure is often asymmetrical in the extremities; and compression of the aortic branches causes a spectrum of changes including coma, confusion, hemiplegia, paralytic ileus, anuria, paresthesias, weakness, and paralysis.

Within a few hours to a few days the aneurysm ruptures, most frequently into the pericardium, causing cardiac tamponade, and less frequently into the mediastinum or a pleural space, causing hemothorax and atelectasis. Infrequently the aneurysm ruptures back into the normal lumen, producing a double-barrel aorta; only this form is compatible with long survival. Some patients are amenable to surgical therapy, but most are treated medically with the main effort directed toward reducing the hypertension.[68]

Although the cause of dissecting aneurysm is not known, it is not atherosclerosis. The aneurysm may occur in youth, when advanced atherosclerosis is uncommon; it begins in the ascending portion, where atherosclerosis is slight; and it is infrequent in the abdominal portion, where atherosclerosis is pronounced. Erdheim attributed the condition to intramural foci of necrosis, which he termed "cystic medionecrosis." It is now supposed that these foci form, the vasa vasorum proliferate in a reparative attempt, and hemorrhage begins within the foci from rupture of the vasa vasorum. Why the foci of necrosis should form is not clear, although the lesion may be produced by β-aminopropionitrile, which is present in the seeds of sweet pea plants, genus *Lathyrus*. The lathyrogenic agent in sweet pea meal causes dissecting aneurysms in turkeys, which are inordinately susceptible to the lesion. The lathyrogenic agent appears to act on the ground substance, medial musculature, and elastic tissue of the aorta. The relationship of this agent to the human disease, however, is not known.

**Syphilitic aortitis.** Cardiovascular syphilis is primarily an aortic disease. It affects the thoracic portion, which undergoes fragmentation of the elastica, vascularization and fibrosis of the media, chronic inflammation of the entire wall, and miliary gumma formation in the adventitia (Figure 11-36). These processes weaken the wall so that aneurysms form. The aneurysms are saccular, occur in the thoracic portion, fill with mural thrombi, and push against bone and soft tissues (Figure 11-37). Thus displacement of the esophagus causes dysphagia, pressure on the recurrent laryngeal nerve causes hoarseness, and attachment to the bronchi causes a tracheal tug that is synchronous with the heartbeat. Compression of the pulmonary artery causes overwork of the right ventricle, and erosion of the sternum or bronchus is associated with rupture onto the skin or into the airways. Untreated aneurysms usually rupture within two years of the clinical diagnosis.

The aortitis gradually extends toward the heart so that it eventually encounters the cusps of the aortic valve and the ostia of the coronary arteries. The coronary arteries often become stenosed, especially when the ostia are above the sinuses of Valsalva.

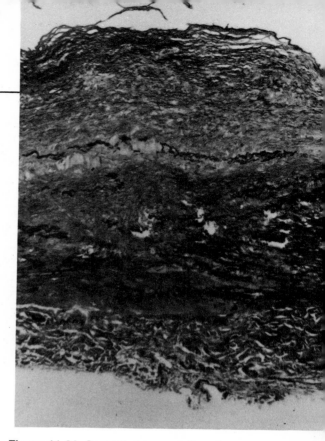

**Figure 11-36.** Syphilitic fragmentation of elastica in media of aortic wall

The process does not extend beyond the ostia. The consequences of the stenosis are angina pectoris, exertional dyspnea, and pronounced congestive failure. A case is recorded in which both ostia were occluded; the heart evidently survived on oxygenated blood reaching the myocardium through the thebesian vessels.[69]

When the inflammatory process reaches the aortic cusps, the commissures are sealed to the wall and the free borders roll outward toward the ventricle. These changes cause an insufficiency of the valve, manifested by dilation and hypertrophy of the left ventricle as well as by a harsh diastolic murmur that replaces the second heart sound. Since the insufficiency lowers the diastolic pressure, a collapsing pulse develops. Also called a Corrigan or water-hammer pulse, it is clinically evident by pulsatile blanching of the retinae and nail beds. When the abnormality is pronounced, even the patient's bed may be noted to

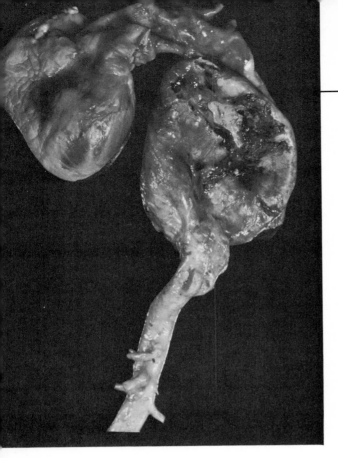

**Figure 11-37.** Syphilitic saccular aneurysm of thoracic aorta

develop. The intima is greatly thickened with granulation tissue, and histologic examination reveals rich infiltration with lymphocytes, plasma cells, and multinucleated giant cells. Corticosteroids are effective in controlling the progress of the inflammation. Otherwise most patients recover spontaneously within two years, although the affected vessel may be converted to a fibrous cord.[70]

In 1908 Takayasu described a pronounced, nonspecific inflammation of the arteries of the aortic arch that progresses to thrombosis. As this happens the radial pulses disappear, and the condition was later dubbed pulseless disease. It affects young women and is worldwide in distribution; any part of the aorta may be affected. The aortic stenosis that results has been called an "atypical coarctation."[71] Two-thirds of the patients have systemic manifestations that include malaise, fever, night sweats, anorexia, and loss of weight. Localizing signs often indicate ischemia to the head or arms. The cause is unknown.

## Medium-sized arteries

Arteries of medium size include the cerebral, coronary, mesenteric, splenic, renal, femoral, and popliteal vessels. These are affected mainly by atherosclerosis, which has been described. Two other conditions affect these vessels and small arteries as well. The first is polyarteritis nodosa. It is a rare, focal arteritis characterized by fibrinoid necrosis and a transmural exudate in which eosinophils are conspicuous. The wall is focally destroyed and the result is thrombosis with infarction or aneurysm formation with rupture. The patients are adults, more often men than women, and most are hypertensive. Any organ system may be involved, most frequently the skin, kidneys, and testes. The clinical signs are extremely varied. Diagnosis is secured by biopsy of skin nodules, sore skeletal muscles, or, especially, testicular tissue.[72] The condition appears to be a hypersensitivity

shake in synchrony with the heartbeat. Death is often abrupt, caused by unsustained filling of the coronary circulation. The four main lesions of cardiovascular syphilis are thus aortitis, saccular aneurysms of the thoracic portion, stenosis of the coronary arteries, and insufficiency of the aortic valve.

**Nonspecific aortitis.** Two conditions are associated with nonspecific inflammation of the aorta: giant-cell arteritis and pulseless disease. Both affect medium-sized arteries as well, and neither has a known cause. Giant-cell arteritis affects both sexes, usually after the age of 65, and the vessels to the head tend to be involved. Although the condition was originally termed "temporal arteritis," it was soon found that many vessels, including the aorta, are affected. Pain in the neck and shoulders is common, and throbbing temporal pain or blindness may

disease of arteries.[73] The clinical course is gradually progressive, although adrenal steroids induce remission. When death occurs it is often attributable to renal failure, intestinal hemorrhage, or congestive heart failure.

In 1908 Buerger described an acute exudative inflammation of arteries, especially of the lower extremities, that occurs almost exclusively in men under 35 years of age who are heavy cigarette smokers. The inflammation spreads to veins and nerves and is known as Buerger's disease or thromboangiitis obliterans. The vessels become thrombosed, and all of the structures are bound up in connective tissue as the process organizes. Ischemia develops, and necrosis of the toes or feet follows. The process is extremely painful. In the lower extremities the ischemia does not advance proximally above the knees. The upper extremities occasionally show ischemia. The condition is considered rare. All races are affected, the cause is unknown, and amelioration of symptoms is achieved by the cessation of smoking.[74]

## Veins

The two main processes affecting veins are inflammation and dilation. Phlebitis develops whenever veins are close to an infectious process. Septic thrombi then form and, as these become embolic, dissemination of bacteria follows. This occurs about the face, often from boils, and septic thrombosis of the cavernous sinuses results. A brain abscess located close to the sagittal or other dural sinus has the same effect, although in this instance the emboli are carried to the lungs. In the veins of the legs thrombi may form and cause swelling and tenderness. This is associated with venous stasis and endothelial injury. It is also frequent after surgical operations. The calf veins are affected first, and the condition is known as phlebothrombosis. With infection, however, and spread to the deep veins, the venous obstruction becomes more pronounced and the seriousness of pulmonary emboli, which are infected, becomes greater. If all the deep veins are thrombosed, cyanosis occurs and ischemic necrosis impends. Injection of a contrast medium into a distal vein may reveal the site of obstruction. The risk of pulmonary embolism may justify ligation of the inferior vena cava or insertion of a filter into it. Otherwise bed rest, anticoagulants, leg elevation, and antibiotics are helpful.

In middle age the veins of the legs dilate. This separates the valve cusps from each other so that a taller column of blood rests on the next lowermost valve. As the pressure increases, the process advances, and as the dilation becomes pronounced, the vessels elongate, bulge, and become tortuous. Thrombi may form but emboli are not common. Ischemia, however, causes ulceration of the skin of the lower legs, and these "stasis ulcers" may be intractable. The reason for the venous dilation is not altogether clear, although the high frequency in athletes and parous women suggests that sustained pressure may play a significant role. Esophageal varices and varicocele are described elsewhere.

## REFERENCES

1. Brinsfield DE, Plauth WH Jr: Clinical recognition and medical management of congenital heart disease. In *The Heart* (Hurst JW, ed), 4th ed, p 831. New York: McGraw-Hill, 1978

2. Campbell M: Causes of malformations of the heart. *Br Med J* 2:895, 1965

3. Rashkind WJ, Miller WW: Creation of an interatrial septal defect without thoracotomy. *JAMA* 196:991, 1966

4. Mustard WT: Successful two-stage correction of transposition of the great vessels. *Surgery* 55:469, 1964

5. Kirklin JW, Pacifico AD: Surgical treatment of congenital heart disease. In *The Heart* (Hurst JW, ed), 4th ed, p 939. New York: McGraw-Hill, 1978

6. Kolata GB, Marx JL: Epidemiology of heart disease: Searches for causes. *Science* 194:509, 1976

7. Glass DC: Stress, behavior patterns, and coronary disease. *Am Scientist* 65:177, 1977

8. Glueck CJ, Mattson F, Bierman EL: Diet and coronary heart disease: Another view. *N Engl J Med* 298:1471, 1978

9. Sacks FM, Castelli WP, Donner A, et al: Plasma lipids and lipoproteins in vegetarians and controls. *N Engl J Med* 292:1148, 1975

10. Glueck CJ, Connor WE: Diet and atherosclerosis: Past, present and future. *West J Med* 130:117, 1979

11. Bloor CM: Functional significance of the coronary collateral circulation. A review. *Am J Pathol* 76:561, 1974

12. Roberts WC, Buja LM: The frequency and significance of coronary arterial thrombi and other observations in fatal myocardial infarction. *Am J Med* 52:425, 1972

13. Gann D, Cabello B, DiBella J, et al: Optimal enzyme test combination for diagnosis of acute myocardial infarction. *South Med J* 71:1459, 1978

14. Galen RS: The enzyme diagnosis of myocardial infarction. *Hum Pathol* 6:141, 1975

15. Osler W: *Modern Medicine*, vol 4, *Diseases of the Circulatory System*, p 559. Philadelphia: Lea & Febiger, 1908

16. Hellstrom HR: Coronary artery stasis after induced myocardial infarction in the dog. *Cardiovasc Res* 5:371, 1971

17. Erhardt LR, Unge G, Boman G: Formation of coronary arterial thrombi in relation to onset of necrosis in acute myocardial infarction in man. A clinical and autoradiographic study. *Am Heart J* 91:592, 1976

18. Eliot RS, Clayton FC, Pieper QM, et al: Influence of environmental stress on pathogenesis of sudden cardiac death. *Fed Proc* 36:1719, 1977

19. Smith JC: Rupture of papillary muscle of the heart. *Circulation* 1:766, 1950

20. Beck CS, Leighninger DS: Coronary heart disease treated by operation. *Arch Surg* 85:383, 1962

21. Vineberg A: Revascularization of the right and left coronary artery systems. Internal mammary artery implantation, epicardiectomy and free omental graft operation. *Am J Cardiol* 19:344, 1967

22. Bordley J III, Harvey AM: *Two Centuries of American Medicine*. Philadelphia: Saunders, 1976

23. Buccino RA, McIntosh HD: Aortocoronary bypass grafting in the management of patients with coronary artery disease. *Am J Med* 66:651, 1979

24. Murphy ML, Hultgren HN, Detre K, et al: Treatment of chronic stable angina. *N Engl J Med* 297:621, 1977

25. Karsner HT, Koletsky S: *Calcific Disease of the Aortic Valve*. Philadelphia: Lippincott, 1947

26. Roberts WC: Anatomically isolated aortic valvular disease. *Am J Med* 49:151, 1970

27. Peery TM: Brucellosis and heart disease. Etiology of calcific aortic stenosis. *JAMA* 166:1123, 1958

28. Pomerance A: Pathology and valvular heart disease. *Br Heart J* 34:437, 1972

29. Weinstein L, Schlesinger JJ: Pathoanatomic, pathophysiologic and clinical correlations in endocarditis. *N Engl J Med* 291:832, 1122, 1974

30. Angrist AA, Okra M: Pathogenesis of bacterial endocarditis. *JAMA* 183:249, 1963

31. Weinstein L: "Modern" infective endocarditis. *JAMA* 233:260, 1975

32. Roberts WC, Spray TL: Pericardial heart disease: A study of its causes, consequences, and morphologic features. *Cardiovasc Clin* 7:11, 1976

33. Naef AP: Primary chylopericardium and its surgical treatment. *Dis Chest* 30:160, 1956

34. Klacsmann PG, Bulkley BH, Hutchins GM: The changed spectrum of purulent pericarditis. An 86 year autopsy experience in 200 patients. *Am J Med* 63:666, 1977

35. Hirschmann JV: Pericardial constriction. *Am Heart J* 96:110, 1978

36. Roberts WC, Ferrans VJ: Pathologic anatomy of the cardiomyopathies. Idiopathic dilated and hypertrophic types, infiltrative types, and endomyocardial disease with and without eosinophilia. *Hum Pathol* 6:287, 1975

37. Roberts WC, Kehoe JA, Carpenter DF, et al: Cardiac valvular lesions in rheumatoid arthritis. *Arch Intern Med* 122:141, 1968

38. Roberts WC: Cardiomyopathy and myocarditis: Morphologic features. *Adv Cardiol* 22:184, 1978

39. Roberts WC, McAllister HA, Ferrans VJ: Sarcoidosis of the heart. A clinicopathologic study of 35 necropsy patients (Group I) and review of 78 previously described necropsy patients (Group II). *Am J Med* 63:86, 1977

40. Teare D: Asymmetrical hypertrophy of the heart in young adults. *Br Heart J* 20:1, 1958

41. Criley JM: The bottom line syndrome—Hypertrophic cardiomyopathy revisited. *West J Med* 130:350, 1979

42. Ross J Jr, Shabetai R, Curtis G, et al: Nonobstructive and obstructive hypertrophic cardiomyopathies—University of California, San Diego, School of Medicine, and the San Diego Veterans Administration Medical Center (specialty conference). *West J Med* 130:325, 1979

43. Buja LM, Khoi NB, Roberts WC: Clinically significant cardiac amyloidosis. Clinicopathologic findings in 15 patients. *Am J Cardiol* 26:394, 1970

44. Chew C, Ziady GM, Raphael MJ, et al: The functional defect in amyloid heart disease. The "stiff heart" syndrome. *Am J Cardiol* 36:438, 1975

45. Prichard RW: Tumors of the heart. Review of the subject and report of one hundred and fifty cases. *Arch Pathol* 51:98, 1951

46. Ferrans VJ, Roberts WC: Structural features of

cardiac myxomas. Histology, histochemistry, and electron microscopy. *Hum Pathol* 4:111, 1973

47. Nasser WK, Davis RH, Dillon JC, et al: Atrial myxoma. I. Clinical and pathological features in nine cases. *Am Heart J* 83:694, 1972

48. St Geme JW, Davis CWC, Noren GR: An overview of primary endocardial fibroelastosis and chronic viral cardiomyopathy. *Perspect Biol Med* 17:495, 1974

49. Fishbein MC, Ferrans VJ, Roberts WC: Histologic and ultrastructural features of primary and secondary endocardial fibroelastosis. *Arch Pathol Lab Med* 101:49, 1977

50. Moller JH, Lucas RV Jr, Adams P Jr, et al: Endocardial fibroelastosis. A clinical and anatomic study of 47 patients with emphasis on its relationship to mitral insufficiency. *Circulation* 30:759, 1964

51. Holman RL, McGill HC Jr, Strong JP, et al: The natural history of atherosclerosis. *Am J Pathol* 34:209, 1958

52. Boyd W: *A Textbook of Pathology*, 8th ed, p 576. Philadelphia: Lea & Febiger, 1970

53. Ross R, Glomset J, Harker L: Response to injury and atherogenesis. *Am J Pathol* 86:675, 1977

54. McGill HC Jr: Risk factors in atherosclerosis. *Adv Exp Med Biol* 104:273, 1978

55. McMillan GC: Atherogenesis: The process from normal to lesion. *Adv Exp Med Biol* 104:3, 1978

56. Duguid JB: Pathogenesis of arteriosclerosis. *Lancet* 2:925, 1949

57. Mustard JF, Packham MA, Kinlough-Rathbone R: Platelets, thrombosis, and atherosclerosis. *Adv Exp Med Biol* 104:127, 1978

58. Ross R, Glomset JA: The pathogenesis of atherosclerosis. *N Engl J Med* 295:369, 1976

59. Woolf N: The origins of atherosclerosis. *Postgrad Med J* 54:156, 1978

60. Benditt EP, Benditt JM: Evidence for a monoclonal origin of human atherosclerotic plaques. *Proc Nat Acad Sci USA* 70:1753, 1973

61. Wissler RW: The progression and regression of atherosclerotic lesions. *Adv Exp Med Biol* 104:77, 1978

62. Strong JP, Eggen DA, Tracy RE: The geographic pathology and topography of atherosclerosis and risk factors for atherosclerotic lesions. *Adv Exp Med Biol* 104:11, 1978

63. Walker WJ: Changing United States life-style and reclining vascular mortality: Cause or coincidence? *N Engl J Med* 297:163, 1977

64. Buchwald H, Moore RB, Varco RL: The partial ileal bypass operation in treatment of the hyperlipidemias. *Adv Exp Med Biol* 63:221, 1975

65. Gordon T, Castelli WP, Hjortland MC, et al: High density lipoprotein as a protective factor against coronary heart disease. The Framingham study. *Am J Med* 62:707, 1977

66. Darsee JR: Cholesterol embolism: The great masquerader. *South Med J* 72:174, 1979

67. Smith JC: Review of thrombosis of abdominal aorta and report of two asymptomatic cases. *Med Ann DC* 41:673, 1972

68. DeBakey ME, Henly WS, Codley DA, et al: Surgical management of dissecting aneurysms of the aorta. *J Thorac Cardiovasc Surg* 49:130, 1965

69. Moritz AR: Syphilitic coronary arteritis. *Arch Pathol* 11:44, 1931

70. Lande A, Berkmen YM: Aortitis. Pathologic, clinical and arteriographic review. *Radiol Clin North Am* 14:219, 1976

71. Nakao K, Ikeda M, Kimata S, et al: Takayasu's arteritis. Clinical report of eighty-four cases and immunological studies of seven cases. *Circulation* 35:1141, 1967

72. Dahl EV, Baggenstoss AH, DeWeerd JH: Testicular lesions in periarteritis nodosa, with special reference to diagnosis. *Am J Med* 28:222, 1960

73. Alcaron-Segovia D: The necrotizing vasculitides. A new pathogenetic classification. *Med Clin North Am* 61:241, 1977

74. Van der Stricht J, Goldstein M, Flamand JP, et al: Evolution and prognosis of thromboangiitis obliterans. *J Cardiovasc Surg* 14:9, 1973

# 12

## RESPIRATORY DISEASE

### THE NORMAL RESPIRATORY SYSTEM

Certain normal features are useful in understanding pulmonary disease. The lungs normally weigh about 300 to 400 gm. The right main bronchus is more nearly vertical than the left, so that aspiration occurs more often in the right lower lobe than elsewhere. There are three lobes on the right and two on the left, and these are divided into 18 bronchopulmonary segments. The lungs have a double arterial supply, the pulmonary artery and the bronchial arteries, which arise from the upper thoracic aorta. Surfaces proximal to the vocal cords are covered with squamous mucosa; distal to this the mucosa is pseudostratified, columnar, and ciliated. The bronchial walls include mucous glands, goblet cells, and smooth muscle in addition to the ciliated mucosal cells. Bronchioles smaller than 1 mm in diameter have no cartilage. The alveoli are lined by membranous (type I) and granular (type II) pneumocytes. Type I cells constitute 90 per cent of the total, and their function is gas exchange. Type II cells produce a surfactant that prevents the air sacs from sticking together. Alveolar walls also have elastic fibers. Apertures in the walls of the air sacs, known as the pores of Kohn, may contribute to the spread of bacteria in pulmonary infections.

The tidal volume is 500 ml, the total volume is 4,000 ml, and the residual volume is about 1,200 ml. Gas exchange requires intact alveolar walls so that collapse of pul-

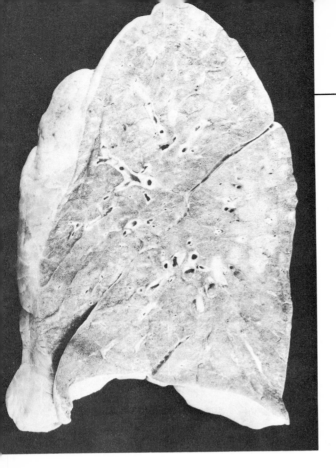

**Figure 12-1.** Bronchopneumonia with pale patches of exudate in the upper lobe and upper portion of the lower lobe

monary tissue (atelectasis), decrease of alveolar surface (emphysema), compression of lung tissue (pleural fluid, chest deformity, kyphoscoliosis), or neuromuscular disorder (myasthenia gravis) impairs respiratory function. Cyanosis appears when 5 gm of circulating hemoglobin are reduced (nonoxygenated). If cyanosis is relieved by nasal oxygen, a pulmonary cause is suggested; if not, a cardiac shunt with venous blood bypassing the lungs is indicated.

## INFLAMMATIONS

### Pneumonia

Pneumonia means inflammation of the lung. It implies more than bronchitis or pleuritis, however, and more than a light scattering of leukocytes in the air sacs, which is known as pneumonitis. Pneumonia is evidenced pathologically by a thick cellular exudate in a significant proportion of the alveoli. Pneumonia affects normal adults but is seen most often in the newborn, the elderly, and those weakened by other diseases. It occurs in a lobar form, which is now uncommon, and in a lobular form (bronchopneumonia), which is extremely common. In the lobar form the exudate extends over an entire lobe or lung. It is a diffuse process now restricted largely to alcoholics and those who are ill and unattended. Bronchopneumonia, in contrast, is patchy in distribution (Figure 12-1). One main classification of pneumonia is thus based on the distribution of the exudate.

Pulmonary inflammation is a dynamic process that progresses through four stages: hyperemia, red hepatization, gray hepatization, and resolution. Although these stages occur in all pulmonary inflammations, they are most easily observed in lobar pneumonia, in which at least an entire lobe is affected. In the stage of hyperemia the lung is large, wet, heavy, and dark purplish-red. Sections reveal a boggy, red cut surface from which a thin, yellowish-pink exudate easily flows. A few leukocytes are present in the alveoli, and bacteria are numerous. In one to two days the appearance changes: The exudate becomes massive and leukocytes, packed in the alveoli, replace the edema fluid. As this happens, the lung on section becomes moist and firm. Strands of fibrin may appear on the pleura. This is the stage of red hepatization, a term derived from the consistency of the tissue, which resembles that of liver. It lasts two to four days and is followed by the stage of gray hepatization, in which the lung is extremely heavy and the cut surfaces are dry, gray, and granular. Microscopically the alveoli are now filled with fibrin and the leukocytes are undergoing degeneration. Bacteria are no longer present. The pleura is covered with a conspicuous layer of pale yellow, friable fibrin. This lasts four to eight days and then transforms into resolution. In this stage leukocytic enzymes dissolve the fibrin, macrophages carry away the debris, frothy fluid occupies the air sacs, and the tissue returns to a spongy softness. This requires perhaps a week, after which the hyperemia subsides, the edema disappears, and the tissue is restored to normal. It is to be understood that the transition from one stage to the next is gradual, and that the use of antibiotics interferes with the natural progression of these stages. It is nevertheless noteworthy that in lobar pneumonia the alveoli often remain intact and the recovered lung is remarkably normal.

The clinical manifestations include tachypnea, pleuritic chest pain, and cough with the production of purulent sputum. A shaking chill heralds the onset. Examination reveals fever, cyanosis, rales, and diminished breath sounds over the affected part. A pleural friction rub may develop. Diagnostic aids include a gram stain of the sputum, a blood culture, a leukocyte count with differential, and a chest X-ray to reveal the extent of the consolidation.

Five main organisms are the common causes of pneumonia: pneumococci, staphylococci, other streptococci, *Klebsiella*, and *Haemophilus*. In addition, mixed organisms are characteristic of aspiration pneumonia, in which inhalation of food, foreign bodies, or gastric contents takes place. Vomitus is aspirated especially by alcoholics, those who are unconscious, and those who have been anesthetized. The type of bacterial organism affects the nature of the inflammatory process. For example, *Streptococcus (Diplococcus) pneumoniae* tends to cause a lobar distribution of exudate. Staphylococcal pneumonia, however, is lobular (peribronchial) and tends to cause abscess formation. It is thus pustular in nature and patchy in distribution. Pneumonia due to other streptococci is uncommon, spreads rapidly, and quickly becomes bilateral and extensive. Destruction of pulmonary tissue with these organisms leads to

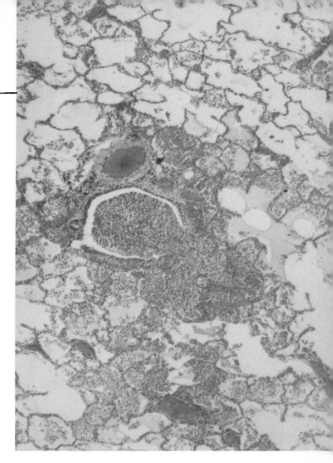

**Figure 12-2.** Necrotizing bronchitis with extension of exudate into peribronchial tissue

widespread scarring. *Klebsiella oxytoca (pneumoniae)* (Friedländer's bacillus) produces a mucoid exudate that clings to the finger as it is raised from the cut surface. It may thus be recognized grossly. This organism is also destructive so that abscess formation is frequent. The bacterium *Haemophilus influenzae* was identified by Pfeiffer in 1892. The influenza virus was discovered in 1933, although it had been suspected in the flu epidemic of 1918-1919.[1] Alone, the bacterium causes only a slight bronchitis, being an organism of low virulence. As a secondary invader with the influenza virus, however, it causes a necrotizing bronchitis that frequently progresses to bronchopneumonia (Figure 12-2). It is thus the combined effect of the two organisms that has accounted for the severity of the pulmonary reaction in the worldwide influenza pandemics.

As the various organisms affect the pulmonary tissue in somewhat different ways, the stage of resolution may be imperfect so that complications arise. Chief among these are abscess formation, bronchiectasis, bronchopleural fistula, empyema, and organization of the exudate. Abscesses are caused especially by type III pneumococci, *Klebsiella*, staphylococci, and, less frequently, hemolytic streptococci. The abscesses arise from necrosis of the exudate with breakdown of tissue so that an inflammatory margin forms and a fibrous capsule may develop. Perforation into a bronchus promotes spread, with clusters of abscesses forming around the bronchus. Perforation of the pleura leads to bronchopleural fistula formation. As the pleura is ruptured, bacteria enter the serous cavity and empyema, or pyothorax, develops. If the perforation is abrupt, the empyema tends to be large, the lung is compressed, and the entire pleural surface is affected so that obliterative fibrosis of the pleural cavity may result. On the other hand, if the pleural rupture is gradual, the empyema tends to be small, loculated, and walled off. The pneumonia may also damage the bronchial walls so that dilation follows and infection persists. Thus bronchiectasis arises. Mucus accumulates in the dilated passages, infection spreads to the adjacent pulmonary tissue, and scarring destroys the adjacent lung. Last, resolution may fail so that the exudate, instead of dissolving and disappearing, becomes organized and converted into granulation tissue. As this tissue matures, a broad, contracting scar replaces the affected part.

Pneumonia has many causes, ranging from dusts, fumes, and noxious gases to viruses, fungi, and even parasitic infestations. The most important include pulmonary inflammation with *Pneumocystis*, bird-transmitted organisms, *Mycoplasma* infection, cytomegalic disease, and fungal infections. *Pneumocystis carinii* is a protozoan that infects the lungs, especially in malnourished children and in adults with weak immune defenses, terminal disease, or cancer under therapy. The organism is demonstrable in the sputum. It evokes a widespread but slight chronic inflammation in which plasma cells are numerous. Only the lungs are affected.[2] The frequency of death depends on the primary condition that allowed the secondary pulmonary infection to develop.

The bird-transmitted infections are caused by chlamydial organisms that reach the lung by inhalation of dried excrement of infected birds.[3] The conditions include psittacosis (parrots, parrakeets) and ornithosis (ducks, pigeons, turkeys, chickens). The illnesses are febrile with headache, leukopenia, and pneumonia in which mononuclear cells predominate. Both types respond to antibiotics, and the mortality is low. A minute bacterium, *Mycoplasma pneumoniae*, causes an influenza-like respiratory syndrome that only occasionally progresses to pneumonia. The organism was discovered by Eaton and colleagues in 1944 and was isolated by Chanock et al in 1962.[4,5] Formerly called primary atypical pneumonia, the condition is characterized by edema and widespread hyaline membranes within the alveoli so that it resembles diffuse alveolar damage rather than exudative pneumonia.[6] Cytomegalic inclusion disease occurs in infants and in adults with immunologic impairment. It is associated with other "opportunistic" pulmonary organisms such as *Pneumocystis* and fungi.[7] Given normal immunologic status, the reaction is more nearly a pneumonitis than a genuine pneumonia. The diagnostic finding is an intranuclear inclusion within macrophages or desquamated alveolar cells. The inclusions may also be found in the cells or the urinary sediment. *Mycoplasma* and cytomegalic infections are thus caused by organisms of low virulence, most often in persons who are weakened by other disease.

Fungal organisms also infect the lung. The mycotic diseases are especially histoplasmosis, coccidioidomycosis, cryptococcosis, and actinomycosis. *Histoplasma capsulatum* infects millions of Americans, causes a subclinical illness or transient respiratory distress, and leaves only the evidence of a positive skin test and focal calcification of lung and perihilar lymph nodes. In sporadic cases, however, the minute organisms proliferate in the tissues of the reticuloendothelial system: the liver, spleen, lymph nodes, and bone marrow. As these tissues are overwhelmed, anemia, leukopenia, and thrombocytopenia develop. Amphotericin B and rifampicin are effective in treating the infection.[8]

Coccidioidomycosis is due to inhalation of *C. immitis* in dust. The condition is endemic in the western and southwestern United States. Ordinarily it causes a self-limited respiratory distress that subsides in one to two weeks. Uncommonly the organisms escape control, proliferate by endosporulation, and cause widespread abscess formation, especially in the lungs, with frequent spread to the meninges (Figure 12-3). The condition is difficult to treat.[9]

The worldwide fungus *Cryptococcus neoformans*, also known as *Torula histolytica*, causes infection affecting the lungs and brain. At both sites granulomatous inflammation develops, and cavities may form in the pulmonary tissue. The organism, which has a clear capsule that aids in its identification, may be found in the lungs and cerebrospinal fluid. The progress of the disease is slow, and death may end a progressive illness of several months' or years' duration.[10] Mucormycosis also affects the lungs and brain; it is mainly a hospital-acquired infection, principally in diabetics and immunosuppressed patients. Pulmonary tuberculosis is described in the section on chronic granulomatous disease in Chapter 5.

Actinomycosis, caused by *Actinomyces israelii*, is an infection of worldwide distribution that occurs in three forms: cervicofacial, intestinal, and pulmonary. The organisms are normally present in the intesti-

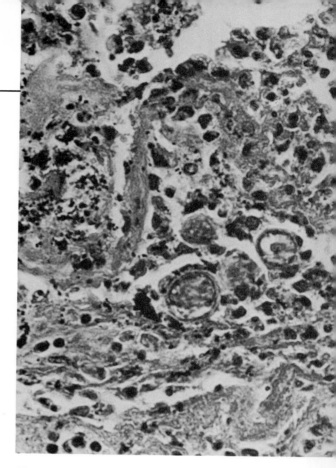

**Figure 12-3.** Sporules of *Coccidioides* in margin of pulmonary abscess

nal tract.[11] In the cervicofacial form, infection from a tooth socket causes abscesses about the jaw that frequently form fistulae to the skin. The condition is chronic but usually not fatal. In the intestinal form, the organism reaches the tissue through an inflamed appendix or colon. Local abscesses and fistulae to the skin develop. The organisms are also carried in the portal veins to the liver, where coalescing abscesses form. The pulmonary infection develops from aspirated organisms and is also characterized by abscess formation. At all sites pus from the draining fistulae contains colonies of organisms that are recognizable to the unaided eye as pale yellow "sulfur" granules.

## Bronchiectasis

Bronchiectasis is an inflammatory dilation of the bronchi. It occurs mainly in the verti-

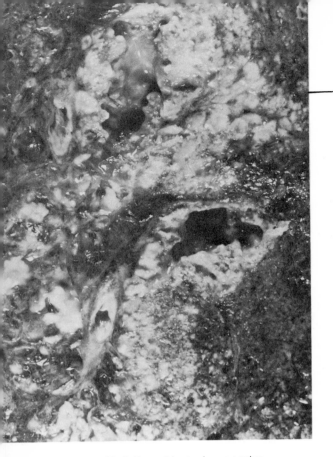

**Figure 12-4.** Bronchiectasis; saccular dilations of bronchi filled with mucopus

cal tubes of the lower lobes. The inflammation evokes hypersecretion of mucus, squamous metaplasia of the ciliated mucosa, and weakening of the wall so that the lumen dilates. All this impairs the clearance mechanism so that pools of stagnant mucus accumulate. Infection of the mucus perpetuates the bronchitis. The patient is thus faced with a chronic infection, a failing bronchial system, and a spoilage of mucus in his lungs. He accordingly loses weight, develops anemia and chest pain, and complains of dyspnea with intractable cough, worse in the mornings, that produces massive amounts of greenish-yellow, foul-smelling sputum.

Approximately half the cases of bronchiectasis are secondary to bronchopneumonia. Other causes are obstructions of the bronchi from tuberculous lesions or bronchogenic carcinomas. Some result from pulmonary fibrosis due to pneumoconiosis. A congenital form, usually localized to one lobe, is seen in children. The condition may also be a consequence of mucoviscidosis. The bronchial dilations are usually cylindrical but may be fusiform or saccular. Cords of viscous mucus occupy the lumens (Figure 12-4). In addition to squamous metaplasia of the mucosa, microscopic examination reveals chronic inflammation, hyperplasia of mucous glands, and highly vascularized granulation tissue that replaces much of the wall (Figure 12-5). In this granulation tissue anastomoses form between the bronchial and pulmonary arteries.[12] Pneumonia develops in the peribronchial alveoli. The overlying pleura undergoes fibrosis with obliteration of the pleural space. Complications include bronchopleural fistula, empyema, pulmonary hemorrhage, and hypertrophy of the right ventricle with eventual right heart failure.

### Lung abscess

Abscesses of the lungs are caused by inhaled septic debris, by obstruction of a bronchus, especially by carcinoma, by pneumonia when caused by staphylococci or *Klebsiella*, and by septic thromboemboli from the systemic veins. In addition, amebiasis may invade the lung from the liver by direct penetration of the diaphragm after having ascended in the portal veins from the colon to the hepatic tissue. The clinical events depend on the size and location of the abscess, although cough, fever, and leukocytosis are usual. The virulence of the organism and the resistance of the host determine whether the abscess will enlarge, cross an interlobal fissure, rupture into a vein or bronchus, or perforate the pleura with inflammation of that space and empyema formation. A fibrous wall tends to form around the pulmonary defect as the inflammation subsides. When the wall obstructs a bronchus permanently, bronchiectasis is likely to form. Aspiration abscesses from portions of teeth, necrotic fragments of tonsil, or carious debris from

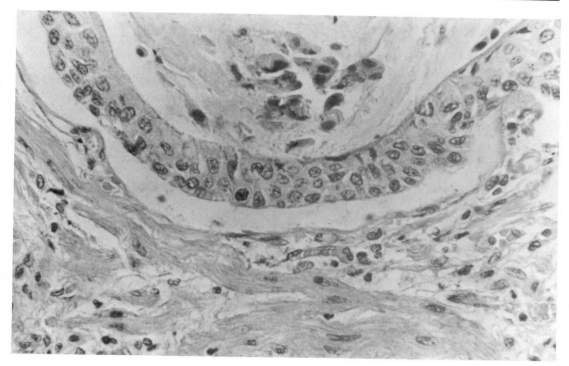

**Figure 12-5.** Squamous metaplasia of bronchial mucosa in bronchiectasis

periodontal disease are most apt to arise in the right lower lobe. Otherwise the abscesses are distributed according to the position of the patient—e.g., standing or supine—at the time of aspiration.

## CIRCULATORY DISTURBANCES

### Passive hyperemia and edema

Slowing of the circulation, usually from failure of the heart, causes the capillaries of the lung to become engorged with blood. The vessels are dilated, the hydrostatic pressure is raised, and a few red cells enter the alveoli by the process of diapedesis. Macrophages phagocytize the erythrocytes, disassemble the hemoglobin, and become pigmented with hemosiderin, forming the so-called heart failure cells. As this condition persists, more pigment accumulates and fibroblasts begin to proliferate in the interstitial tissue. As a result, brown induration develops and the lung becomes pigmented, fibrous, and tough.[13] When the rise in hydrostatic pressure is abrupt and pronounced, the alveoli fill with clear fluid from the intravascular compartment and pulmonary edema forms. The process may be so fulminant that death from respiratory failure occurs within 20 minutes of the onset.[14] The usual cause is myocardial infarction or cardiac dysrhythmia.

### Thromboembolism

Thrombi form in the deep veins of the calves and, less frequently, in the large veins of the groin or pelvis, in conjunction with major trauma, childbirth, obesity, myocardial infarction, or congestive heart failure.[15] The process is phlebothrombosis; it is noninflammatory, the thrombi are sterile, and the attachment to the endothelium is weak so that dislodgement is fre-

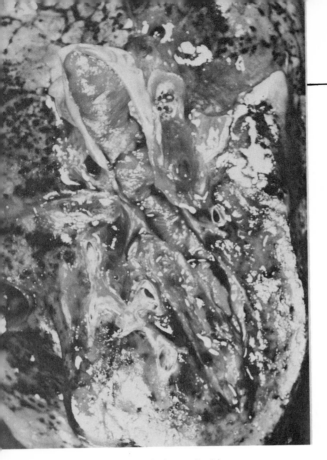

**Figure 12-6.** Embolus coiled in pulmonary artery

quent.[16] Homans' sign, i.e., pain in the calf on dorsiflexion of the foot, indicates the presence of such deep vein thrombi. Dislodgement allows the thrombus to become an embolus. It then passes with the current to the next site of vascular narrowing, which is in the lungs. If the thrombus is large, owing to its formation in the iliofemoral veins, it often becomes coiled and may impinge on the bifurcation of the pulmonary artery to form a "saddle" embolus. In this event death occurs within minutes because of right heart failure. If the embolus is smaller, impaction takes place wherever the diameter of the vessel is no longer able to accommodate the floating mass (Figure 12-6). Emboli are most often small and multiple. The process is common, the clinical diagnosis is often missed , and recovery with anticoagulant therapy is the rule.[17]

Most pulmonary emboli fail to cause infarction, probably because the pulmonary

tissue is nourished by two arterial systems and the bronchial arteries preserve the viability of the injured part. Infarcts are prone to form, however, when passive hyperemia of the pulmonary tissue exists. Even in this event, the embolus is often present in the hilar region and the infarct is small and peripheral in the pulmonary tissue. A wedge shape is usual, with the base toward the pleura. The size rarely exceeds 5 cm. The tissue is hemorrhagic and dark red with a swollen pleural surface over which fibrin forms. When the embolus is infected, the infarct progresses to abscess formation. Most, however, undergo organization so that a scar gradually develops and the overlying pleura is depressed from the adjacent normal surface. If the embolus is large, death may occur without an infarct. Otherwise the patient experiences sudden collapse, air hunger, and shock. There may also be cyanosis, chest pain, distended neck veins, and hemoptysis. Perhaps 20 per cent survive the initial event and then deteriorate over a period of several days.[16] If the embolus is small, there may be only sudden dyspnea with unilateral chest pain that disappears or gradually progresses to congestive failure. The clinical diagnosis is aided by lung scanning with radioisotopes that show a focal defect of vascular supply.

### Pulmonary hypertension

Pulmonary hypertension may be caused by increased blood flow (interatrial or interventricular septal defects), by increased venous pressure (mitral stenosis, left ventricular failure), by vascular obstruction (microemboli, sickle cells, polyarteritis, lymphangitic carcinoma), or by vascular destruction (emphysema, diffuse fibrosis). In all these the vessels show some changes, especially hypertrophy of the arteriolar musculature with hyperplasia of the endothelial cells. Such cases, which constitute the vast majority, are regarded as secondary pulmonary hypertension; the cause is known and the vessels show some degree of stenosis. Primary pulmonary hypertension is much less common and exists when the pulmonary arterioles reveal stenosing lesions but the cause is not evident. Such cases tend to arise in young women, the course is relentlessly progressive, and death occurs from right heart failure. The condition may be attributed to miliary emboli with organization and gradual obstruction of the small arteries.[18] More often, no vascular obstruction is seen; in this event, injection studies reveal disappearance of small peripheral nonmuscular arteries.[19] The cause of this change is not known.

## OBSTRUCTIVE AIRWAY DISEASE

Airway obstruction may be caused by an aspirated chunk of food, carcinoma of the vocal cords, a foreign body in the trachea, or an abundant exudate that fills the passage. Food can be dislodged by the Heimlich maneuver—a sharp compression of the abdomen that lifts the diaphragm and forces air upward against the bolus.[20] Scar formation in the trachea as a consequence of pressure cuff necrosis may also cause stenosis of that channel. These conditions also occur in the main bronchi. The consequences of these obstructions include focal overdistention of air sacs (emphysema), collapse of the affected part (atelectasis), infection of the alveoli (pneumonia), and septic dilation of the bronchi distal to the obstruction (bronchiectasis). The infectious process may go on to abscess formation in the lung and rupture of the pleura with infection in that space (empyema).

Atelectasis is airlessness of the lung. It may be congenital, from failure of expansion at birth, or acquired from collapse later in life. It is usually focal but may affect all lobes. The acquired types are absorptive and compressive. When a bronchus is blocked, no air enters the tissue distal to the obstruction, and the air remaining in that tissue is gradually absorbed. Conversely, fluid in the pleural space may compress the pulmonary tissue so that it becomes airless even though the bronchial channels are widely patent. When a pathologic process in the lung perforates the pleura, air rushes into that negative pressure cavity and the lung collapses. Such pulmonary processes as cancer, pleural bleb, or lung abscess may do this. The air in the pleural space constitutes a pneumothorax. If the opening in the pleura is small, healing takes place and the air is absorbed. If the opening is large, the lung remains collapsed and the pressure in the pleural space equates with the atmospheric pressure. In this open pneumothorax, the mediastinum bulges toward the abnormal side. When the pleural opening allows air to enter but not escape from the pleural space, the pressure there may exceed that of the atmosphere because of coughing or forceful inspiration. In this tension pneumothorax, the mediastinum is pushed so that it bulges toward the normal side. Both atelectasis and pneumothorax are noninflammatory conditions unless bacterial infection complicates the situation.

### Asthma

Asthma is respiratory distress due to intermittent attacks of bronchial constriction. In the extrinsic type the constriction is due to inhaled antigens such as pollens, dusts, and animal dander. In the intrinsic type the reaction is set off by infection, exercise, emotional disturbance, or changes in temperature or humidity. Intrinsic asthma is more common than the extrinsic type, although most patients have a combination of the two. In extrinsic asthma a specific IgE antibody is formed to an antigen. The antibody attaches to the bronchial mucosa so that exposure to the antigen causes an antigen-antibody reaction in the bronchial wall. As a result, mast cells release histamine, which causes the bronchial constriction. The pathogenesis of the intrinsic form is less clear.[21] Pathologic changes in both include thickening of the bronchial basement

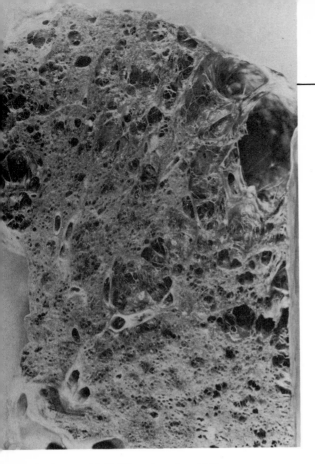

**Figure 12-7.** Chronic pulmonary emphysema

membrane, hypertrophy of the bronchial musculature, and obstruction of the lumens by plugs of mucus. The bronchial wall is inflamed with segmented granulocytes, of which a conspicuous proportion are eosinophils. In addition, the bronchial mucus may disclose Charcot-Leyden crystals, which are eosinophilic granules, and Curschmann spirals, which are coils of mucous fibers. Hyperinflation of the lung may occur, but emphysema is rare.[22]

### Bronchitis

Chronic bronchitis with emphysema is the most common of all pulmonary disorders. Bronchitis is presumed to exist when the patient has persistent cough with sputum production for at least three months in two consecutive years.[23] Although the condition is serious, patients tend not to seek help until dyspnea develops. Purulent spu-

tum signifies advanced disease. The responsible organisms are most often pneumococci and *Haemophilus influenzae*.

Bronchial infection is related to atmospheric pollutants; the condition is prevalent in urban areas, especially in industrial regions, and the highest incidence is seen in cigarette smokers. In the United States population of about 220 million there are 50 million to 60 million cigarette smokers.[24] The bronchi on histologic section show enlargement of mucous glands, replacement of ciliated cells with goblet cells, and hypertrophy of the bronchial smooth muscle, apparently induced by spasm. The degree of the process may be estimated from the thickness of the mucous glands in the bronchial wall.[25] The bronchial lumens fill with mucus. This accumulation overwhelms the cilia, the mucous raft is not propelled upward, and infection develops in the stagnant secretions. Pneumonia follows in the parabronchial alveoli, and distortions from scar formation lead to air trapping and the development of emphysema.

### Emphysema

Emphysema is an enlargement of air sacs with destruction of alveolar walls.[26] It is important because it is the most common chronic disease of the lungs and causes gradually progressive respiratory distress. It is associated with cigarette smoking and

**Table 12-1.**

### Classification of emphysema

| |
| --- |
| Widespread |
|    Centrilobular |
|    Panlobular |
| |
| Localized |
|    Parabronchial |
|    Paracicatricial |

chronic bronchitis. It is more common in men than in women, and the clinical onset is most often in the sixth decade.[26] There are four anatomic types. Focal emphysema is generally of slight clinical importance and is occasioned by bronchial obstruction or scar formation that alters respiratory structure and traps air within discrete foci of pulmonary tissue. The main types associated with crippling airway disease are the centrilobular and panlobular varieties. In both, the lungs are large and the lesions are widespread. Not to be construed as emphysema is the small-lung atrophy of old age, in which there is no destruction of pulmonary tissue, or the overinflation of pulmonary lobes in infancy, which is due to a congenital absence of bronchial cartilage. In the small-lung atrophy of old age, both lungs are affected and the condition does not become clinically significant.[27] A simple classification of emphysema is presented in Table 12-1.

Large-lung emphysema is characterized by voluminous lobes that fail to collapse after death. The tissue is "pillowy" and sections reveal coarse porosity from coalescence of alveolar clusters to form sizable spaces (Figure 12-7). Balloon-like chambers subjacent to the pleura are called bullae, and similar, smaller spaces are termed blebs. Classification of large-lung emphysema is based on the lobule, the functional unit of pulmonary tissue. In the centrilobular form the alveolar destruction is localized to the centers of the lobules, leaving the periphery intact. In the panlobular form the destruction is uniform throughout the lobules. In 1952 Gough pointed out that these forms of the disease are unrelated.[28] The centrilobular form is more common than the panlobular form, the upper lobes are predominantly affected, and carbon pigment is localized to the margins of the dilated sacs[29] (Figure 12-8). Panlobular emphysema is less frequent, more widely distributed throughout all the lobes, and less discretely pigmented. Moreover, the cen-

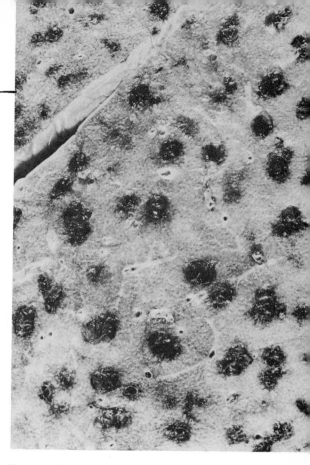

**Figure 12-8.** Centrilobular emphysema with discoloration by carbon pigment

trilobular form is attributed to ectasia of the respiratory bronchioles whereas the major segmental bronchi are implicated in the panlobular form.[30] Both forms of emphysema, however, have the same clinical manifestations.[31] The microscopic features include a lacy alveolar pattern with thin walls, large air sacs, and thick arterioles with hypertrophic walls.

The pathogenesis of emphysema is not altogether clear. The condition does not arise in glassblowers or players of wind instruments. It is associated with smoking and bronchitis. Pigment deposition and inflammation appear to destroy the elastic tissue in bronchioles so that they collapse on expiration, when the alveolar pressure is high. Difficulty in exhaling is thus the dominant clinical feature. How smoking destroys the alveoli and bronchioles is the question. Smoking brings forth macrophages in the alveoli. Macrophages contain proteolytic enzymes, including elastase, in their lysosomes. Niewoehner and associates suggested that the macrophages release lysosomal enzymes, especially elastase, that destroy elastic tissue in alveolar walls and bronchioles. With this, emphysema gradually develops.[32]

Normally the elastic tissue of the lung is protected by protease inhibitors that nullify the effect of proteases released from macrophages in the pulmonary alveoli. The main inhibitor is $\alpha_1$-antitrypsin; it is a single polypeptide of mol wt 54,000, produced solely by the liver, that circulates in several body fluids and covers the surfaces of the pulmonary airways.[33] $\alpha_1$-Antitrypsin is the main constituent of the protease inhibitor (Pi) system. It is controlled by at least 26 codominant alleles, designated by letters of the alphabet. Normal persons have middle-alphabet alleles (M), with extension in the "proximal" direction as the amount increases (B) and in the "distal" direction as the amount decreases (Z). Thus PiMZ signifies a heterozygote with a reduced amount of inhibitor, and PiZZ registers a homozygote with virtually none. Carriers (Z heterozygotes) are present in 4 to 5 per cent of the population.[34] It is of incidental interest that the substitution of a single amino acid in the polypeptide chain (lysine for glutamic acid) converts the normal structure (M) to the abnormal structure (Z). The abnormal inhibitor cannot escape from the cytoplasm of hepatocytes, and accumulates there in the form of periodic acid-Schiff (PAS)-positive globules that resist diastase digestion, which distinguishes them from glycogen. Without inhibitor, elastase from alveolar macrophages is free to destroy elastic tissue in the lung, with the consequent development of emphysema. Not more than 10 per cent of clinical emphysema is due to this cause. However, such a mechanism should come to mind whenever emphysema develops in a non-smoker, in a patient under 30 years of age,

or in several members of the same family.[35] In PiZZ patients liver disease, especially cirrhosis, may develop in infancy, although the mechanism of this is not known.[34]

Clinical manifestations of emphysema begin when 30 per cent of the lung parenchyma is destroyed.[23] Difficulty in exhaling begins; the patient cannot get air out of his/her chest. This is followed by cough with sputum and later by dyspnea at rest. A hunched posture develops and the chest expands, with an increase in the anterior-posterior dimension. There is loss of weight and flattening of the abdomen, which emphasizes the thickness of the chest, and the patient sits on the edge of his chair, using his secondary muscles of respiration. The face is wizened, the expression is anxious, and nicotine stains may be evident on the fingers. If the emphysema is pronounced but the bronchitis is slight, gas exchange is sufficient and the patient may be characterized as a "pink puffer." On the other hand, if the bronchitis is pronounced and gas exchange is impaired, cyanosis with right heart failure develops and the patient could be called a "blue bloater." Either way, emphysema reveals three characteristic radiographic changes: hyperlucent lung fields, a narrow mediastinum, and a low, flat diaphragm in an elongated chest. The expiratory dyspnea is relentless, and respiratory acidosis with coma may develop, or a bleb or bulla may rupture with collapse of the lung. In addition, hypertrophy of the right heart occurs in advanced cases, and this is attributed to thinning of the vascular bed and contracture of the remaining arterioles from hypoxia. Pulmonary or right heart failure eventually causes death.

**Other conditions**
If the alveolus is presumed to be an airway, four other conditions should be considered obstructive airway diseases. They are diffuse alveolar damage, alveolar proteinosis, idiopathic pulmonary hemosiderosis, and Goodpasture's syndrome.

Diffuse alveolar damage is an umbrella term that covers a group of conditions previously known as desquamative interstitial pneumonia, adult respiratory distress syndrome, congestive atelectasis, traumatic wet lung, and idiopathic interstitial fibrosis. The last has also been known as the Hamman-Rich syndrome. The main causes of diffuse alveolar damage are shock and oxygen therapy. Shock is associated with hemorrhage, burns, trauma, fractures, coma, sepsis, and abdominal surgery. Other causes include smoke inhalation, viral pneumonia, kerosene poisoning, irradiation, and such cytotoxic agents as busulfan, the bleomycins, and cyclophosphamide.[6] Oxygen therapy is an especially important cause because of its frequent use. Diffuse alveolar damage develops after 14 hours of 70 per cent nasal oxygen, and after two to six days at a concentration of 40 per cent. One week after exposure, interstitial fibrosis is likely to develop.

The clinical manifestations of diffuse alveolar damage are tachypnea and gasping respirations. Hypoxemia develops. The chest X-ray shows diffuse mottling, suggestive of edema, that transforms into coarse, nodular densities. These are, however, reversible if the inciting agent can be removed. Grossly the lungs are firm, wet, and heavy. The changes are uniform and bilateral. Under the microscope there are alveolar edema, fibrin filaments covering the alveolar walls, and proliferation of septal lining cells that accumulate within the air sacs. Unless resolution takes place, these changes go on to diffuse induration of all lobes with extensive interstitial fibrosis. Death results from gradually worsening respiratory failure.

For reasons unknown, some adults develop a noninflammatory, evenly distributed accumulation of lipid-rich proteinaceous material within the air sacs of both lungs. The onset is gradual with cough and dyspnea accompanied by a copious, gelatinous, yellow sputum. The signs include rales, di-

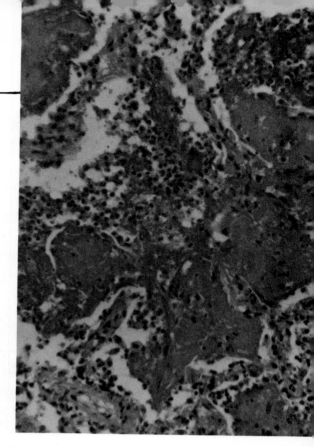

**Figure 12-9.** The intra-alveolar colloid accumulation of alveolar proteinosis

minished breath sounds, and occasional clubbing of the fingers. Radiographs show fine diffuse mottling throughout both lung fields, and in the laboratory neutrophilic leukocytosis and high serum lactate dehydrogenase are found. Grossly the lungs are heavy, the pleura is smooth, and the pulmonary tissue has the consistency of soft rubber. Sections reveal a colloid-like material within the alveoli that is PAS-positive and devoid of inflammation (Figure 12-9). It is not clear whether the material within the alveoli is normal and the pulmonary clearance mechanism is at fault, or whether the lining cells of the alveoli are secreting an abnormal material that suppresses the normal clearing process.[36] Golde and colleagues suggested that the pulmonary environment is abnormal and that the macrophages of the lung are adversely affected on this account.[37] Regardless of the mechanism, therapy consists of pulmonary la-

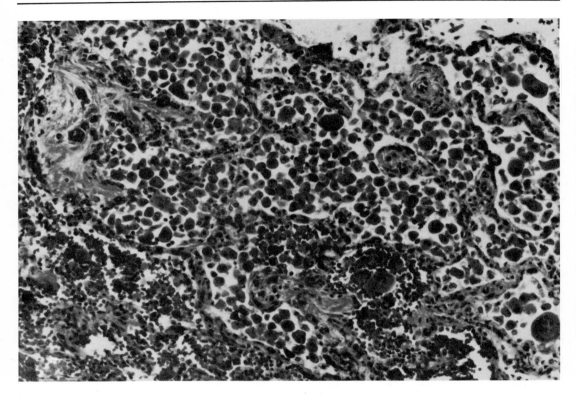

**Figure 12-10.** Hemosiderin-filled macrophages of idiopathic pulmonary hemosiderosis

vage. Some patients recover spontaneously while others, even though treated, succumb to progressive respiratory failure.

Goodpasture's syndrome is an immunologic disorder affecting the lungs and kidneys. It arises spontaneously, most often in young men, and the first sign is hemoptysis that may be slight or pronounced. The sputum contains hemosiderin-laden macrophages and chest X-ray discloses perihilar mottling that tends to fan outward. Hypochromic anemia is frequent. Rapidly progressive glomerulonephritis then develops, with conspicuous hematuria and proteinuria. Death follows from pulmonary hemorrhage or renal failure.

The lungs are large and heavy with hemorrhage in the tissue and macrophages in the alveoli. The kidneys are large and soft. Sections reveal fibrinoid necrosis of the glomeruli that progresses to crescent formation and fibrosis. It is supposed that an antigenic similarity exists between the basement membranes of the glomerular and pulmonary capillaries so that an antibody to either binds at both sites.[38] Steroids have been used with some success, and reversal of the pulmonary lesion has taken place after nephrectomy.

Idiopathic pulmonary hemosiderosis is a distinct clinicopathologic entity of unknown cause that resembles the pulmonary phase of Goodpasture's syndrome. Four out of five patients are children, and adult victims are under 30 years of age. There is spontaneous pulmonary bleeding with hemoptysis, X-ray changes, anemia, hemosiderosis of the lungs, and eventually pulmonary fibrosis. Dyspnea and cyanosis develop, weight loss follows, and death occurs from massive hemorrhage or right heart failure.[39] The pulmonary tissue shows brown induration, desquamation of alveolar lining cells, and masses of brown macrophages filled with hemosiderin (Figure 12-10). Although the cause is unknown, Mathew and colleagues found antibodies attached to glomerular membranes in a kidney biopsy from a patient with normal renal function.[40] They accordingly suggested that idiopathic pulmonary hemosiderosis may be the pulmonary component of Goodpasture's syndrome.

## PNEUMOCONIOSES

The inhalation of dust is unavoidable. However, the body provides four mechanisms to prevent dust from reaching the lungs. The first is a nasal channel only 1 mm wide between the inferior turbinate and nasal septum, through which inspired air must pass. This warms, moistens, and filters the incoming air. The second mechanism is the "mucous raft," which is propelled over the bronchial surface by cilia of the mucosa at the rate of 2.5 mm/minute. This sheet of mucin propels dust upward and removes about 60 per cent on the first day. The third mechanism is the phagocytic activity of macrophages, which engulf 30 per cent of inspired dust and remove it by expectoration or swallowing over the next several days. The remaining 10 per cent is carried out in the lymphatics to be disposed of in the reticuloendothelial system. These mechanisms may be overwhelmed, and whether or not pulmonary disease develops is determined by three conditions: the nature of the dust, the size and concentration of the particles together with the period of exposure, and the presence or absence of other lung disease.[41] Although particles above 40 $\mu$m in diameter are removed in the nasopharynx, pulmonary retention increases as particle size decreases, and 90 per cent of inhaled particles under 5 $\mu$m reach the alveolar ducts or air sacs.[42]

About 100 years ago Zenker combined *pneumo*, meaning "lung," with *konis*, meaning "dust," to form the word *pneumoconiosis*. This is the generic term for the effect of inhaled particles on pulmonary tissue. A wide variety of particles is, of course, inhaled. Some are inert, others are fibrogenic, some predispose to tuberculosis, and some evoke immune reactions. Moreover, one is associated with both carcinoma of the lung and mesothelioma of the pleura. The inert dusts are cement, gypsum (calcium sulfate in plasterboard), and pure carbon. The harmful dusts include coal dust, silica, asbestos, and beryllium. Inhaled animate bodies, including spores and vegetable fibers, are also toxic to pulmonary tissue.

### Anthracosis

Anthracosis is due to the inhalation of soot. It causes black discoloration of pulmonary tissue and is especially noticeable in the lungs of urban dwellers. Most of the carbon particles are filtered out in the nasopharynx, but some reach the alveoli and are engulfed there by macrophages. Deposition takes place in tissue, especially those parts least affected by respiratory movement, i.e., adjacent to blood vessels and bronchi, the subpleural region, and the tissue immediately adjoining scars. The pure pigment is inert, causing neither inflammation nor fibrosis, and for this reason anthracosis is not associated with impairment of health unless emphysema is also present.[42] Although the carbon particles are regarded as innocuous, carcinogens adsorbed onto them could increase the risk of lung cancer.

### Coal workers' pneumoconiosis

Coal workers are exposed to dust that consists of coal, kaolin, mica, and silica in varying proportions. The silica content is usually extremely slight. The dust calls forth macrophages in the alveoli that phagocytize the particles and move them to the respiratory bronchioles, and thus to the mu-

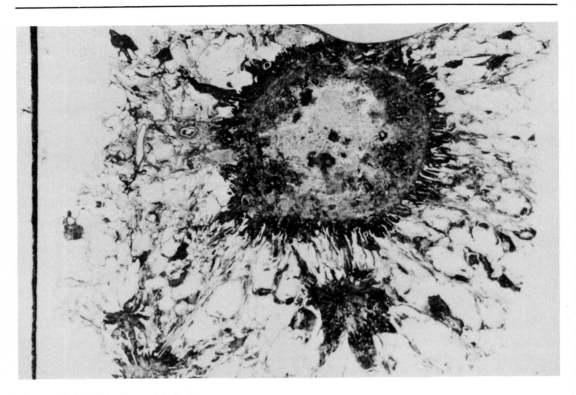

**Figure 12-11.** Silicotic nodule in lung

cociliary escalator, whence they are disposed of by swallowing or expectoration. When the exposure persists, this clearance mechanism may be overwhelmed, and death of the macrophages in the alveoli releases enzymes that stimulate fibroblasts to proliferate. A focus of fibrosis with black discoloration and slight alveolar wall breakdown, known as a "coal macule," arises. This is the primary lesion of coal workers' pneumoconiosis. The macules measure up to 0.5 cm in diameter and tend to arise in the upper lobes of both lungs. This simple form of the disease produces neither signs nor symptoms. With continued exposure, however, the condition advances to the complicated form of progressive massive fibrosis. In this form fibrosis and pigmentation are extensive. The process is poorly delineated, however, so that the rubbery induration becomes widespread and is alto-gether different from the discrete nodules of silicosis. The black, fibrous masses encroach on both arteries and veins and gradually destroy them. Paracicatricial emphysema may develop. Associated tuberculosis is rare. As more and more tissue is affected, exertional dyspnea and cough with black sputum arise. Pain and hemoptysis are rare. The physical signs are those of consolidation of the pulmonary tissue and they progress to hypertrophy of the right ventricle with cor pulmonale and congestive failure. Thus simple coal workers' pneumoconiosis does not progress to disabling emphysema although emphysema may be associated with the complicated form of the disease.[43] Studies indicate that only about 10 per cent of working miners have the simple form of the disease and about one-third of these advance to progressive massive fibrosis.[41]

## Silicosis

Silica is released into the air wherever rock is cut. Therefore exposure takes place in the mining of gold, copper, tin, anthracite coal, and especially granite, which is 20 per cent quartz (silicon dioxide). Sandblasters, stonemasons, and pottery workers are also exposed. The harmful particles are composed of silicon dioxide ($SiO_2$), which is the cause of nodular fibrosis of pulmonary tissues, and they measure 0.5 to 5 $\mu$m in diameter. Particles under 3 $\mu$m are especially fibrogenic.[41]

Why silicon dioxide causes fibrosis is not altogether clear. One notion is that silicic acid, released by hydrolysis of $SiO_2$, is the fibrogenic substance. Another possibility is that the silicon particles combine with protein to form an antigen and the pulmonary fibrosis is evoked by the reaction of antibody with it. It has also been suggested that the silica particle is phagocytized by a membranous pneumocyte that ruptures, spilling phospholipid, and the phospholipid stimulates the nodular fibrosis. Which of these suggested pathogenic mechanisms is correct is not clear.[42]

The incubation period for silicosis is 10 to 15 years. Symptoms include progressive dyspnea, dry cough, and chest pain. Chest X-ray discloses a fine reticulation that progresses to gross nodularity. The gross characteristic is firm, round, dense, fibrous nodules that are distributed throughout the pulmonary tissue and within the hilar lymph nodes. Subpleural nodules cause firm, fibrous adhesions of the surface. Black speckling of the nodules is due to carbon pigment, which is frequently present (Figure 12-11). Microscopically there are multinucleated giant cells at the margins of the nodules, and examination under polarized light reveals the silica granules. Complications include advancing emphysema, bronchiectasis, and, less often, cor pulmonale. Of more importance is pulmonary tuberculosis, which is frequent. Silicosis does not predispose to lung cancer.[42]

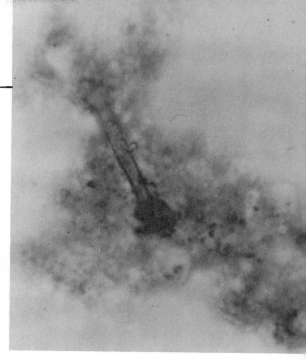

**Figure 12-12.** Asbestos filament forming "bamboo body"

## Asbestosis

Asbestos consists of magnesium-calcium silicate fibers that are found in rock and measure up to 2 cm in length. The fibers are valuable because of their intrinsic qualities of spinnability, tensile strength, and heat resistance. They are accordingly useful in the production of gaskets, brake linings, conveyor belts, and insulation materials. In fact, it is estimated that there are over 3,000 uses for asbestos fibers.[41] The production of asbestos rose from 500,000 tons in 1935 to 5 million tons in 1965. Three-quarters of the world's supply comes from asbestos-containing rock in Canada; the remainder comes mainly from South Africa and Russia.

The incubation period is 20 to 30 years.[41] The inhaled fibers are large, with an average length of 50 $\mu$m, so that they impact in bronchioles and do not reach the alveoli or the hilar lymph nodes. The fibers become encrusted with a golden, hemosiderin-containing protein that causes a beaded appearance with "drumstick" ends. These ferruginous bodies, sometimes called "bamboo bodies," are characteristic of asbestosis (Figure 12-12). The fibers cause a

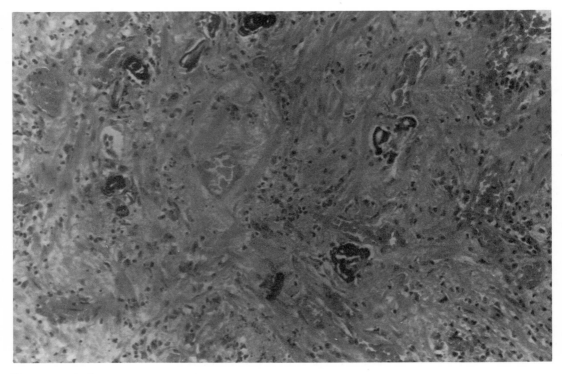

**Figure 12-13.** Conchoidal bodies of berylliosis in fibrotic pulmonary tissue

chronic granulomatous inflammation with widespread pulmonary fibrosis. The fibrosis extends to the pleural space, which becomes obliterated. The patient experiences dyspnea, rales, finger clubbing, reduced vital capacity, and X-ray shadows throughout the lung fields.[44] The complications are bronchiectasis, cor pulmonale, and occasionally pulmonary tuberculosis. Bronchogenic carcinoma and pleural mesothelioma are also caused by asbestos fibers, the former condition much more frequently than the latter.[45]

**Berylliosis**

Beryl is a crystal composed of beryllium, silicon, and aluminum oxide. Beryllium is a light, strong, hard, heat-resistant metal. It is therefore useful in the fabrication of space capsules, fishing rods, furnace bricks, guidance systems, and brake linings

for jet airplanes.[46] Inhalation of beryllium fumes causes an acute, nonspecific pneumonitis with hyperemia and edema of the lungs. The alveoli contain fibrin, macrophages, and a few segmented granulocytes. Granulomas and inclusion bodies are absent. Although the acute reaction usually subsides, death may occur in as little as two weeks.[42] Chronic exposure causes noncaseating granulomas throughout the lungs that bear a close resemblance to sarcoidosis. However, there are no cystic bone changes, ocular involvement, or uveoparotid fever. The lungs disclose interstitial fibrosis, pleural thickening, and noncaseating granulomas in which three inclusions are often present: conchoidal (Schaumann) bodies, asteroid bodies, and acicular clefts encrusted with calcium. Conchoidal bodies (Figure 12-13) are the most frequent. Similar granulomas may be found in the skin,

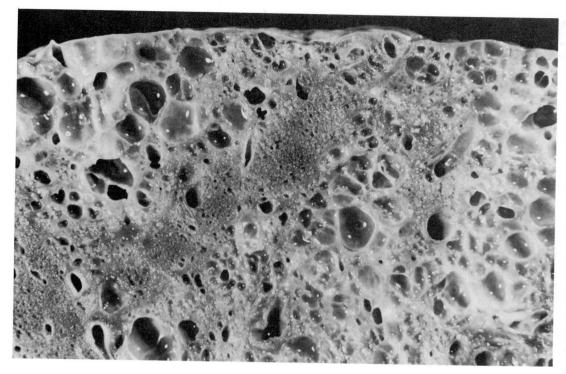

**Figure 12-14.** Honeycomb lung, the nonspecific end stage of many pulmonary diseases

liver, kidneys, skeletal muscles, and extrathoracic lymph nodes.

Patients experience lassitude, shortness of breath, and loss of weight. Chest X-rays disclose bilateral infiltrations. Adrenal steroids relieve the respiratory symptoms but do not change the histologic reaction.[46] Carcinoma does not tend to develop, and tuberculosis is infrequent.

### Bagassosis

Bagasse is the fibrous residue of sugarcane after the juice has been pressed out. Prior to 1922 bagasse was destroyed by burning. It was found, however, that bagasse could be used for insulation, and after 1922 it was saved for this purpose. Workers who process bagasse for the production of insulating materials develop, over a period of several weeks, a hypersensitivity pneumonia that may progress to interstitial fibrosis with emphysema and bronchiectasis. This is bagassosis.

The condition occurs in the southern United States, Cuba, and India. The first case was described in 1941. Clinically there are dyspnea, cough with sputum that may be blood-streaked, fever, and widespread mottling of the lung fields as seen on chest X-ray. The tissue reveals interstitial inflammation, multinucleated giant cells, and accumulations of intra-alveolar foam cells. Although no fungi or bacteria are consistently isolated from the pulmonary tissue, each gram of bagasse contains millions of fungal spores of many species. It is not known whether the pulmonary reaction is due to the cellulose fibers, to the fungal spores, or to a hyperimmune state. Whatever the cause, about half of individuals with bagassosis develop antibodies to extracts of bagasse.[42]

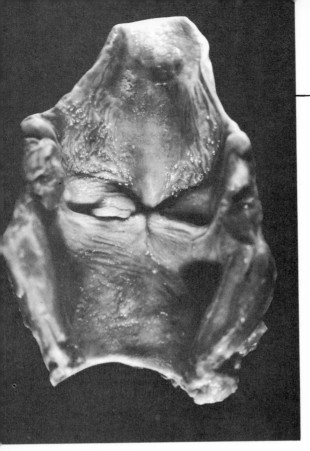

**Figure 12-15.** Papilloma of the left vocal cord

## Byssinosis

*Byssos* is the Greek word for flax. Workers who blow and card raw cotton develop cough, tightness in the chest, and an asthma-like wheezing known as byssinosis. It occurs on Monday mornings, after the workers have been away from the mill over the weekend. It is therefore also known as "Monday morning fever." The pulmonary changes are chronic bronchitis with moderate emphysema and focal squamous metaplasia of the bronchial mucosa. Specific rounded dust particles are present in the tissue; they are covered with a protein coat and measure up to 10 $\mu$m in diameter.[42] The condition is due to a histamine-releasing agent present in cotton dust that causes bronchoconstriction. Antihistaminics relieve the respiratory symptoms.

## Farmer's lung

Many sporeforming organisms grow in moldy hay, grain, or silage. After these materials have dried, handling them gives rise to clouds of dust containing spores. Chief among these are two actinomycetes that induce a pulmonary hypersensitivity state.[42] The sera of exposed patients agglutinate antigens made from these organisms. Clinically there are dyspnea, fever, sweating, and dry cough followed by loss of weight and widespread mottling of the lung fields on radiographic examination. The lungs show acute interstitial pneumonia with bronchiolitis, vasculitis, and sarcoid-like granulomas. Later, pulmonary fibrosis may develop with cystic changes and pulmonary hypertension.[47] The condition is thus a pulmonary hypersensitivity state that causes interstitial granulomatous pneumonitis.

In summary, the principal particle dusts are carbon, silica, asbestos, and beryllium, while the main diseases due to animate structures or vegetable fibers are bagassosis, byssinosis, and farmer's lung. This selection is arbitrary; there are, of course, many other pollutants that cause pulmonary reactions. Nevertheless, in terms of frequency and seriousness, these are the most important. With the exception of pure carbon, most cause an acute phase with nonspecific pneumonitis, and a chronic phase with granulomatous inflammation proceeding occasionally to massive fibrosis that is diffuse or nodular. "Honeycomb lung" with extensive fibrosis and air sac dilation is the end-stage result of many of these conditions (Figure 12-14). The clinical features of the chronic phase often require one to three decades for development. Foreign bodies, sometimes unique, are frequently identifiable in the affected tissue. The usual complications of these vast changes in pulmonary structure are emphysema, bronchiectasis, and abscess formation. The special complications are tuberculosis, which is often associated with silicosis, and cancer of the lung or pleura, which occasionally accompanies asbestosis. It is thus evident that the reactions of the lungs to pollutants in the air form a special consideration of pulmonary pathology.

## TUMORS OF THE RESPIRATORY TRACT

### Larynx

The common tumor of the larynx is papilloma of the vocal cords, which is a fibrous polypoid projection covered with an intact squamous mucosa (Figure 12-15). It tends to arise in singers and is curable by local excision. The uncommon tumor is the carcinoma, which may be intrinsic and arise from the vocal cords, or extrinsic and arise from the epiglottis, pyriform sinus, or arytenoepiglottic folds. The intrinsic cancer is four times more common than the extrinsic tumor. Both are usually squamous. The intrinsic lesion causes hoarseness early and is curable by irradiation or surgical excision of the affected tissue (Figure 12-16). Extrinsic cancers tend to spread widely and are therefore more difficult to cure.

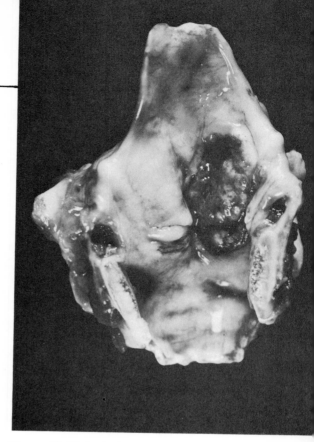

**Figure 12-16.** Intrinsic carcinoma of the larynx

### Lung

Most tumors of the lung are carcinomas. They account for 40 per cent of all male cancer deaths and are therefore the most common fatal cancer in men.[48] Moreover, the incidence is rising rapidly. In 1950 the incidence of lung cancer in men was 20/100,000; it rose to 43/100,000 by 1967.[49] The corresponding figures for women were 4.5 in 1950 and 7.5 in 1967. Over this same period there was no change in the incidence of carcinomas of the colon, breast, prostate, or pancreas. The American Cancer Society predicted 112,000 new cases of lung cancer in 1979.[50]

Lung cancer is probably caused by cigarette smoking and atmospheric pollutants, including asbestos particles. The risk of lung cancer is five to 15 times greater in smokers than in nonsmokers, and the incidence correlates with the rate of smoking, the habit of inhaling, and the duration of

the practice.[49] Smoking causes deciliation of the bronchial mucosa and atypical hyperplasia of the underlying reserve cells.[51] These changes regress when smoking is stopped. There are other respiratory oncogens, including ferric oxide and nitrosourea, which cause lung cancer in hamsters when instilled into the trachea,[52] and it should not be overlooked that approximately 10 per cent of patients with lung cancer are not smokers.

Soot is a product of incomplete combustion; gasoline and diesel engines are among the chief offenders. Polycyclic hydrocarbons, including benzo[a]pyrene, are absorbed onto the particles. Cigarette smoke contains benzo[a]pyrene as well as several other oncogenic agents.[53] Inhaled soot particles are normally removed by ciliary action of the bronchial mucosa or by macrophages that phagocytize the particles. In smokers, however, the soot particles lie stationary on the deciliated surface so that

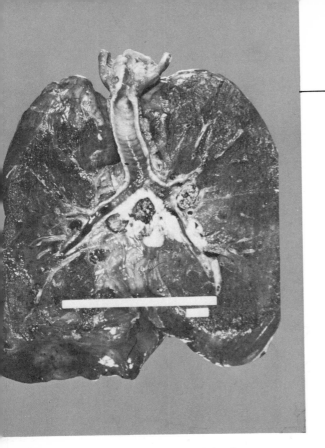

**Figure 12-17.** Hilar site of origin of squamous-cell bronchogenic carcinoma

**Bronchogenic carcinoma.** Squamous-cell carcinomas are associated with cigarette smoking and are estimated to be about four times more common in men than in women.[50] The cancers arise from basal or resting cells of the bronchial mucosa. Grossly the tumors appear in the distal trachea or main bronchi (Figure 12-17). At these sites the mucosa is raised, nodular, pale gray, and firm over a region that often measures about 1 cm in diameter (Figure 12-18; see color section, p C-2). The tumor projects into the lumen, which becomes obstructed, and into the bronchial wall, which becomes fixed. Necrosis then develops within the center of the neoplastic mass. Pulmonary tissue distal to the bronchial obstruction undergoes emphysema or atelectasis as well as pneumonitis, bronchiectasis, and sometimes pulmonary abscess formation. The abscess, discovered by chest X-ray, is occasionally the first clinical indication of the cancer. The tumor spreads to the carina and hilar lymph nodes as well as the scalene nodes, which provide a convenient site for biopsy and diagnosis. Spread then continues to adjacent structures, including the mediastinum, pericardium, and pleural surfaces. The tumor may compress or invade vessels and cause the superior vena caval

the mucosa is exposed to the carcinogens on the particles.[54] Squamous metaplasia, atypical hyperplasia, dysplasia, carcinoma in situ, and invasive carcinoma may then develop at these sites. The time interval between the beginning of smoking and the clinical onset of cancer is 20 to 40 years.[52]

Examination of 1,218 cases of carcinoma of the lung revealed the distribution of types shown in Table 12-2.[55] The undifferentiated variety is composed of about half large-cell and half small-cell (oat-cell) tumors. The bronchial adenomas are misnamed; although most grow slowly, metastatic disease eventually develops and the tumors are genuinely malignant. The categories of Table 12-2 suggest discrete divisions within this classification. It should be understood that a considerable number grow in a "mixed pattern."[55] Nevertheless, it is evident from these figures that most carcinomas of the lung arise in the bronchi and are squamous.

**Table 12-2.**

## Incidence of various types of carcinoma of the lung

| Type | | Proportion |
|---|---|---|
| Bronchogenic carcinoma | | 93% |
| Squamous | 70% | |
| Undifferentiated | 20% | |
| Adenocarcinoma | 10% | |
| Bronchial "adenoma" | | 5% |
| Alveolar cell carcinoma | | 2% |

syndrome. Metastasis is especially frequent to the adrenals and, in decreasing frequency, to the liver, brain, bones, and kidneys.

Microscopically the squamous tumors are identified by an arrangement in solid sheets with focal whorls of keratohyalin and intercellular bridges between adjoining cell borders. The doubling time of the tumor cells is approximately four months, so that about nine years are required for the tumor to reach a diameter of 2 cm.[56]

Undifferentiated carcinomas also arise in the hilar region and bear a relationship to cigarette smoking. They are evenly divided between large-cell cancers, including the giant-cell carcinoma, and small-cell tumors, including the oat-cell carcinoma. Although both are devoid of recognizable tissue pattern and are hence undifferentiated, the giant-cell cancers are characterized by multinucleated tumor cells, and the oat-cell cancers by tumor cells in which the cytoplasm is scant and the nuclei are round and deeply basophilic. The cells are approximately twice the size of lymphocytes. Both spread rapidly and are accordingly difficult to cure. Oat-cell cancers, however, are extremely radiosensitive. The large-cell undifferentiated cancers are presumed to arise from basal or resting cells of the bronchial mucosa; the small-cell cancers reveal neurosecretory granules when sections are examined under the electron microscope, and are thought to be of neuroendocrine nature, belonging to the amine precursor uptake and decarboxylation system.[57] For this reason oat-cell tumors often cause clinical syndromes due to inappropriate hormone production.[58]

Adenocarcinomas occur equally in men and women, are not associated with smoking, and tend to arise at the periphery of the lung and occasionally subjacent to scars of the pleura (Figure 12-19). They are characterized histologically by simulated gland formation. Growth tends to be slow compared with other bronchogenic cancers,

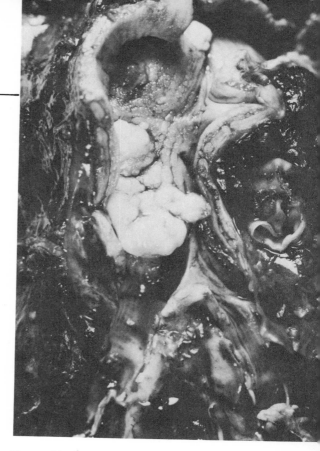

**Figure 12-18.** Bronchogenic carcinoma. Also shown in color section, p C-2.

and it is estimated that the doubling time of adenocarcinomas is on the order of seven months. This rate extrapolates to 25 years for the tumor to reach a size of 2 cm.[56] The cancer is thought to arise from basal cells of the bronchial mucosa, although origin in the mucous glands of the bronchial wall is also possible.

The bronchogenic carcinomas produce a variety of secretions, including hormones, enzymes, antigens, and polypeptides, that are collectively known as marker substances. These include adrenocorticotrophic hormone, chorionic gonadotrophin, parathyroid hormone, serotonin (5-hydroxytryptamine), insulin, and growth hormone. The only hormones not produced by the bronchogenic carcinomas are thyrotrophin, gastrin, and erythropoietin.[58] This wide variety of marker substances is explained by various degrees of liberation of gene expression (derepression) in the cancer cells. $\alpha$-Fetoprotein is produced in

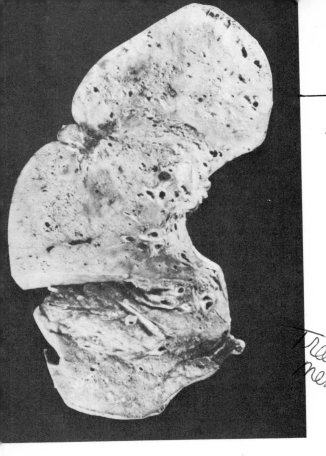

**Figure 12-19.** Although not grossly evident, a carcinoma underlies the indented scar at the periphery on the left upper border of the cut surface.

*Post test*

*Treatment*

Bronchogenic carcinoma develops between the ages of 40 and 70 years. The squamous and undifferentiated cancers are related to smoking and are more frequent in men than in women. Symptoms average seven months in duration before hospitalization.[4] The most common complaint is cough, followed, in decreasing frequency, by loss of weight, pain in the chest, and shortness of breath. Anorexia, weakness, and lassitude also develop. Chest X-ray discloses the lesion, and cytologic examination of the sputum may confirm the diagnosis. Biopsy of a scalene lymph node may reveal the tumor type.

A staging system for cancer of the lung is accepted, but the accuracy is uncertain. Accuracy is critical because the purpose of staging is to establish parity within different series that are treated by different methods, and unless staging is accurate, it is of little use.[61]

Although radiotherapy is helpful, especially for the treatment of oat-cell carcinoma, surgical excision of the entire lesion is the only hope of cure. That hope, unfortunately, is slight. Benfield estimated that of 100 cases of lung cancer, 75 will be nonresectable on clinical grounds, 10 of the remainder will be found incurable after mediastinoscopy, and three more will be found nonresectable by thoracotomy. Of the 12 remaining, one patient will die of the surgical procedure and two will succumb to metastatic disease within five years after therapy. A five-year survival rate of 9 per cent results.[59]

The reason for this discouraging outlook is that the tumors tend to be clinically silent, they often spread rapidly, and patients procrastinate in seeking medical care. For example, Carbone found with 200 patients that the symptomatic period to the time of hospitalization was 46 weeks, the hospital time required to establish the diagnosis was an additional four weeks, and the interval between diagnosis and death was about six weeks.[48] Moreover, Carr and

about 7 per cent of patients with bronchogenic carcinoma, and the carcinoembryonic antigen in 75 to 85 per cent.[58] Although the fetal antigens are not specific for an individual tumor type, the marker substances may nevertheless be used as a screen for subclinical disease and as an indication of metastatic spread.

Screening for lung cancer by chest X-rays has not proved effective. Not only it is expensive, but the cancers must exceed 1 cm in diameter to be visible,[48] and immediate treatment of those tumors that have been identified has not improved the rate of survival.[59] It appears less costly and more effective to persuade smokers to quit, although this effort has not met with success.[59] Recent refinements of staining techniques suggest that cytologic screening may permit identification of bronchial tumors before metastasis develops.[60]

Mountain found that staging was useless for oat-cell cancers because of their rapid spread.[62] The extent of spread as estimated by clinical staging was, however, the major determinant of survival in the remainder of the patients. Combinations of chemotherapy and preoperative radiation were found by Benfield to extend the survival time of patients by several months, although the proportion of patients who succumbed was unchanged over those who received no preoperative therapy.[59]

**Bronchial adenoma.** Bronchial adenomas occur under the age of 40 years, equally in men and women, and represent the respiratory component of the intestinal carcinoid. The tumors are composed of small, basophilic neuroendocrine cells that grow in solid sheets without mitotic figures. Only a few show cytoplasmic argentaffin granules. The tumor arises in the hilar region and extends as an oval projection into the bronchial lumen (Figure 12-20). The surface is covered with intact mucosa. The rate of growth is slow, and tissue infiltration tends to be slight although metastasis to regional nodes eventually develops. There are two consequences. The first is emphysema or atelectasis in the tissue distal to the blocked airway, with the later development of pneumonia, bronchiectasis, or pulmonary abscess. The second is the secretion of serotonin, which causes the carcinoid syndrome: intermittent attacks of wheezing, cyanosis, facial flushing, and diarrhea. Surgical excision of the tumor may cure, and the survival rate at five years exceeds 90 per cent.[63]

**Alveolar cell carcinoma.** Alveolar cell carcinomas arise in the periphery of the pulmonary tissue and are characterized by tall columnar cells that line the alveolar margins in a single layer. The tumor cells produce a clear pink mucin that fills the air sacs and is expectorated abundantly. The

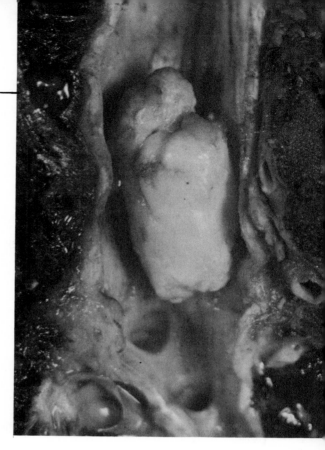

**Figure 12-20.** Bronchial adenoma extending into lumen

alveolar walls remain intact—a distinctive feature. The tumor eventually spreads to the mediastinal lymph nodes. Patients experience productive cough, progressive dyspnea, and occasionally cyanosis. The cancers occur equally in men and women and tend to grow slowly, but the cure rate is nevertheless low. The condition is uncommon, and the fatal course lasts two to three years.[64]

**Others.** Lymphosarcoma and fibrosarcoma of the lung as well as mesothelioma of the pleura are extremely uncommon. Mesothelioma coats the pleura with a thick, solid, pale gray tumor mass that fixes the lung to the pleura, mediastinal surface, and diaphragm. Carcinoma of the lung and mesothelioma of the pleura have both been linked causally to exposure to asbestos particles.[65]

# REFERENCES

1. Spencer H: *Pathology of the Lung*, 2nd ed, p 204. New York: Pergamon Press, 1968

2. Hughes WT: *Pneumocystis carinii* pneumonia. *N Engl J Med* 297: 1381, 1977

3. Schachter J: Chlamydial infections. *N Engl J Med* 298:490, 1978

4. Eaton MD, Meikeljohn G, von Herick W: Studies on etiology of primary atypical pneumonia: filterable agent transmissible to cotton rats, hamsters, and chick embryos. *J Exp Med* 79:649, 1944

5. Chanock RM, Hayflick L, Barile MF: Growth on artificial medium of an agent associated with atypical pneumonia and its identification as a PPLO. *Proc Nat Acad Sci USA* 48:41, 1962

6. Katzenstein AA, Bloor CM, Liebow AA: Diffuse alveolar damage—The role of oxygen, shock, and related factors. *Am J Pathol* 85:210, 1976

7. Spencer H: *Pathology of the Lung*, 2nd ed, p 221. New York: Pergamon Press, 1968

8. Kitahara M, Kobayashi GS, Medoff G: Enhanced efficacy of amphotericin B and rifampicin combined in treatment of murine histoplasmosis and blastomycosis. *J Infect Dis* 133:663, 1976

9. Stevens DA, Levine HB, Deresinski SC: Miconazole in coccidioidomycosis. *Am J Med* 60:191, 1976

10. Hammerman KJ, Powell KE, Christianson CS, et al: Pulmonary cryptococcosis: Clinical forms and treatment. *Am Rev Respir Dis* 108:1116, 1973

11. Brown JR: Human actinomycosis. A study of 181 subjects. *Hum Pathol* 4:319, 1973

12. Liebow AA, Hales MR, Lindskog GE: Enlargement of bronchial arteries and their anastomoses with pulmonary arteries. *Am J Pathol* 25:211, 1949

13. Robin ER, Cross CE, Zelis R: Pulmonary edema. *N Engl J Med* 288:239, 1973

14. Fleischner FG: The butterfly pattern of acute pulmonary edema. *Am J Cardiol* 20:39, 1967

15. Kakkar VV: Deep vein thrombosis. *Circulation* 51:8, 1975

16. Hume M, Sevitt S, Thomas DP: *Venous Thrombosis and Pulmonary Embolism*. Cambridge, Mass: Harvard University Press, 1970

17. Dalen JE, Albert JS: Natural history of pulmonary embolism. *Prog Cardiovasc Dis* 17:259, 1975

18. Blount GS Jr: Primary pulmonary hypertension. *Mod Concepts Cardiovasc Dis* 36:67, 1967

19. Anderson EG, Simon G, Reid L: Primary and thrombo-embolic pulmonary hypertension: A qualitative pathological study. *J Pathol* 110:273, 1973

20. Heimlich HJ, Hoffmann KA, Canestri FR: Food-choking and drowning deaths prevented by external subdiaphragmatic compression. *Ann Thorac Surg* 20:188, 1975

21. Turner-Warwick M: On observing patterns of airflow obstruction in chronic asthma. *Br J Dis Chest* 71:73, 1977

22. Spencer H: *Pathology of the Lung*, 2nd ed, p 715. New York: Pergamon Press, 1968

23. Pratt PC, Kilburn KH: A modern concept of the emphysemas based on correlations of structure and function. *Hum Pathol* 1:443, 1970

24. Gori GB: Low-risk cigarettes: A prescription. *Science* 194:1243, 1976

25. Reid L: Measurement of the bronchial mucous gland layer: A diagnostic yardstick in chronic bronchitis. *Thorax* 15:132, 1960

26. Thurlbeck WM: Pulmonary emphysema. *Am J Med Sci* 246:332, 1963

27. Millard M: Lung, pleura and mediastinum. In *Pathology* (Anderson WAD, Kissane JM, eds), 7th ed, p 1067. St. Louis: Mosby, 1977

28. Gough J: The pathology of emphysema. *Postgrad Med J* 41:392, 1965

29. Wyatt JP, Fischer VW, Sweet H: Centrilobular emphysema. *Lab Invest* 10:159, 1961

30. Wyatt JP, Fischer VW, Sweet HC: Panlobular emphysema: Anatomy and pathodynamics. *Dis Chest* 41:239, 1962

31. Mitchell WS, Silvers GW, Goodman N, et al: Are centrilobular emphysema and panlobular emphysema two different diseases? *Hum Pathol* 1:433, 1970

32. Niewoehner DE, Kleinerman J, Rice DB: Pathologic changes in the peripheral airways of young cigarette smokers. *N Engl J Med* 291:755, 1974

33. Morse JO: Alpha₁-antitrypsin deficiency. *N Engl J Med* 299:1045, 1099, 1978

34. Talamo RC: Alpha-1-antitrypsin deficiency. *Johns Hopkins Med J* 142:67, 1978

35. Williams WD, Fajardo LF: Alpha-1-antitrypsin deficiency; a hereditary enigma. *Am J Clin Pathol* 61:311, 1974

36. Ramirez RJ: Pulmonary alveolar proteinosis. Treatment by massive bronchopulmonary lavage. *Arch Intern Med* 119:147, 1967

37. Golde DW, Territo M, Finley TN, et al: Defective lung macrophages in pulmonary alveolar proteinosis. *Ann Intern Med* 85:304, 1976

38. Pollak VE, Mendoza N: Rapidly progressive glomerulonephritis. *Med Clin North Am* 55:1397, 1971

39. Soergel KH, Sommers SC: Idiopathic pulmonary hemosiderosis and related syndromes. *Am J Med* 32:499, 1962

40. Mathew TH, Hobbs JB, Kalowski S, et al: Goodpasture's syndrome: Normal renal diagnostic findings. *Ann Intern Med* 82:215, 1975

41. Wyatt JP: Occupational lung diseases and inferential relationships to general population hazards. *Am J Pathol* 64:197, 1971

42. Spencer H: *Pathology of the Lung*, 2nd ed, p 452. New York: Pergamon Press, 1968
43. Morgan WKC, Lapp NL: Respiratory disease in coal miners. *Am Rev Respir Dis* 113:531, 1976
44. Murphy RLH, Ferris BG Jr, Burgess WA, et al: Effects of low levels of asbestos. *N Engl J Med* 285:1271, 1971
45. McDonald AD, Harper A, El Attar OA, et al: Epidemiology of primary malignant mesothelial tumors in Canada. *Cancer* 26:914, 1970
46. Freiman DG, Hardy HL: Beryllium disease. *Hum Pathol* 1:25, 1970
47. Seal RME, Hapke EJ, Thomas GO, et al: The pathology of the acute and chronic stages of farmer's lung. *Thorax* 23:469, 1968
48. Carbone PP: Lung cancer: Perspective and prospects. *Ann Intern Med* 73:1003, 1970
49. Robbins SL: *Pathologic Basis of Disease*. Philadelphia: Saunders, 1974
50. Silverberg E: Cancer statistics, 1979. *CA—Cancer J Clin* 29:6, 1979
51. Auerbach O, Hammond EC, Kirman D, et al: Effects of cigarette smoking on dogs. II. Pulmonary neoplasms. *Arch Environ Health* 21:754, 1970
52. Harris CA: Cause and prevention of lung cancer. *Semin Oncol* 1:163, 1974
53. Wynder LL, Hoffman D: Tobacco and tobacco smoke. *Semin Oncol* 3:5, 1976
54. Kotin P, Falk HL: The role and action of environmental agents in the pathogenesis of lung cancer. I. Air pollutants. *Cancer* 12:147, 1959
55. Galofre M, Payne WS, Wooner LB, et al: Pathologic classification and surgical treatment of bronchogenic carcinoma. *Surg Gynecol Obstet* 119:51, 1968
56. Garland LH, Coulson W, Wollin E: The rate of growth and apparent duration of untreated primary bronchial carcinoma. *Cancer* 16:694, 1963
57. Gould VE, Yannopoulds AD, Sommers SC, et al: Neuroendocrine cells in dysplastic bronchi: Ultrastructural observations and quantitative analysis of secretory granules and the Golgi complex. *Am J Pathol* 90:49, 1978
58. Primak A: The production of markers by bronchogenic carcinoma: A review. *Semin Oncol* 1:285, 1974
59. Benfield JR: Current and future concepts of lung cancer. *Ann Intern Med* 83:93, 1975
60. Nasiell M, Kato H, Auer G, et al: Cytomorphological grading and Feulgen DNA-analysis of metaplastic and neoplastic bronchial cells. *Cancer* 41:1511, 1978
61. Smith JC: The inertia of tradition. *Surg Gynecol Obstet* 145:905, 1977
62. Carr DT, Mountain CF: The staging of lung cancer. *Semin Oncol* 1:229, 1974
63. Okike N, Bernatz PE, Woolner LB: Carcinoid tumors of the lung. *Ann Thorac Surg* 22:270, 1976
64. Decker HR: Alveolar-cell carcinoma of the lung (pulmonary adenomatosis). *J Thorac Surg* 30:230, 1955
65. Borow M, Conston A, Livornese L, et al: Mesothelioma following exposure to asbestos: A review of 72 cases. *Chest* 64:641, 1973

# 13

# DISEASES OF THE DIGESTIVE TRACT

The intestinal tract begins at the vermilion border of the lips and extends to the squamocolumnar junction of the anus. It is a tortuous tube with various dilations and outpouchings. Many disease states affect this internal conduit. Only the main abnormalities, beginning at the mouth, are considered here.

## MOUTH

Carcinoma of the lip is the most common primary malignancy of the head and neck.[1] It may be thought of as the "95 per cent disease" because that is the approximate frequency of four of its features: occurrence in males, occurrence on the lower lip, squamous cell type, and occurrence on either side of the midline. An indurated ulcer in the midline should bring to mind the possibility of a chancre. The cancer occurs most often in the 50s and 60s, and usually in persons such as farmers who are exposed to sunlight much of the time. The etiologic importance of cigarette and pipe smoking is not clear.[1] The lesion is treated by irradiation or surgical resection. Survival depends on the extent of spread at the time therapy is applied. Most cancers are well differentiated so that regional metastasis is minimal. Five-year survival rates are on the order of 80 to 90 per cent when the cancer is well differentiated.

Carcinoma of the tongue was studied by Flamant and colleagues, who examined 904 cases.[2] These occurred in men nearly seven

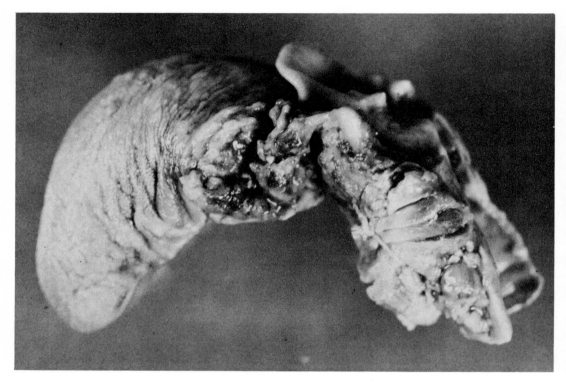

**Figure 13-1.** Carcinoma on posterolateral margin of tongue

times more often than in women, the average age was 59 years, and most of the tumors were squamous. The lesions appear as indurated ulcers, more frequently in the movable portion of the tongue than at the base. Four-fifths of cancers on the movable portion arise on the lateral margins (Figure 13-1). Alcohol, tobacco, and abrasively carious teeth may be etiologic factors. Implanted irradiation or hemiglossectomy with or without dissection of cervical lymph nodes is the method of treatment. Outlook depends on the extent of spread; for clinically localized tumors the five-year rate of survival in the series of Jeppsson and Lindstrom was 64 per cent.[3]

Tumors also arise in the salivary glands. Most occur in the parotid, and about 70 per cent are benign.[4] Women are affected more often than men, and the average age is 47 years. The tumor is at first small, firm, and freely movable, appearing in front of and just below the ear. Little or no discomfort for months to years is characteristic. In one series of 119 tumors, the average period from onset to diagnosis was four years.[5] Grossly the tumor is firm, pale gray, and sharply defined (Figure 13-2). Microscopically the growth is composed of a mixture of squamous cells, islands of cartilage, clusters of glands, and masses of myxoid tissue. On this account the lesion is termed a "mixed tumor," which is suitably descriptive, although "polymorphous adenoma" has been proposed.[5] This unusual composition also confounds any clear understanding of histogenesis. Removal is fraught with two difficulties: damage to the facial nerve, which runs close to the tumor mass, and incomplete removal because of tumor

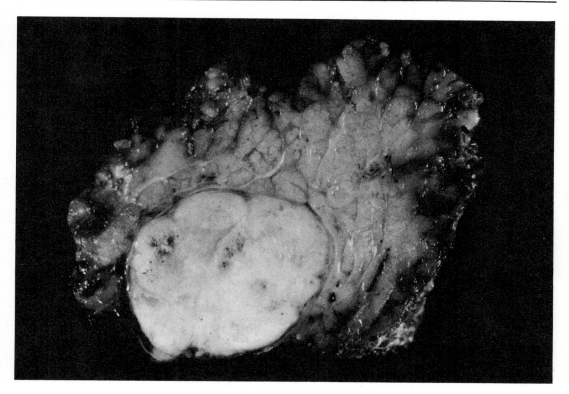

**Figure 13-2.** Cut surface of mixed tumor of parotid

nodules outside the capsule that are too small to be seen grossly. On this account, wide excision is recommended.[6] Although malignant transformation occasionally occurs, cure is usually achieved.

In about 30 per cent of patients the preauricular mass is malignant. Mucoepidermoid carcinoma is by far the most frequent although malignant mixed tumors, acinic cell carcinomas, adenocarcinomas, and adenoid cystic carcinomas (cylindromas) also occur.[7] These tend to appear a decade later than mixed tumors, the clinical duration preceding diagnosis is shorter, and the tumors are smaller, averaging 3.8 cm in diameter in one series.[5] Pain, paralysis of one side of the face, and enlargement of cervical lymph nodes suggest the diagnosis. Radical parotidectomy with or without irradiation is required for cure. The five-

year rate of survival was 41 per cent in the series of Molnar and colleagues.[5]

One tumor of the jaw deserves special notice. It is the ameloblastoma (adamantinoma) that arises in a tooth socket, usually in the region of the lower molars. The tumor occurs more often in women than in men. The average age in one series was 37 years, and two-thirds of the patients were under 40 years of age.[8] The cause is not known, although the tumor is occasionally preceded by a dentigerous cyst. Clinical manifestations include swelling, followed by pain and the occasional development of a draining sinus. X-ray examination reveals a coarsely trabeculated cystlike structure with sharp margins that destroys bone. The gross cut surface is shown in Figure 13-3. The histologic pattern consists of nests, islands, and cords of columnar epi-

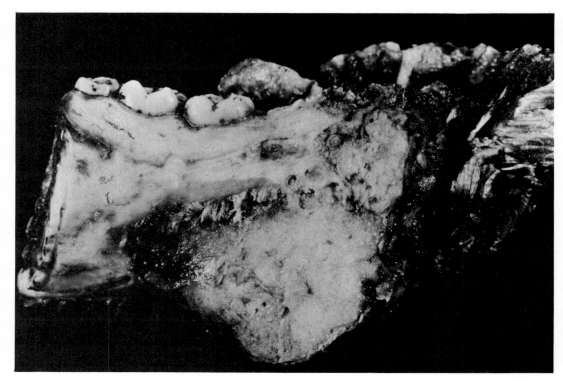

**Figure 13-3.** Cut surface of ameloblastoma (adamantinoma) of jaw

thelial cells separated by sparse amounts of fibrous connective tissue (Figure 13-4). About half these tumors show foci of squamous metaplasia. The tumor is not malignant, but it is locally destructive and will recur unless widely excised.

## ESOPHAGUS

The main pathologic changes in the esophagus are congenital anomalies, inflammations, diverticula, chemical burns, varices, and malignant tumors.

In the beginning the trachea and esophagus are a single tube in the mediastinum that divides longitudinally to form two separate, parallel channels. Failure of that division may leave an absent midsection of the esophagus with one or both of the separated segments connected to the trachea. The anomaly thus consists of an atresia of the esophagus with or without a tracheo-esophageal fistula. Usually the upper segment ends in a blind pouch so that the newborn salivates excessively, gags when fed, and shows a cul-de-sac of the upper segment on X-ray examination after a barium swallow. In addition, a fistula to the trachea is often present. The varieties of configuration are many and include no fistula, upper fistula, double fistula, and lower fistula. Of these, by far the most common is a blind upper pouch and a lower tracheal fistula (Figure 13-5). When the barium swallow reveals a blind upper pouch, the presence of a lower fistula is indicated if air is visible in the stomach on a radiograph of the abdomen. Although the anomaly can be corrected by surgical treatment, low birth weight, other anomalies, and collapse of the lung from the operation cause the mortality to range from 35 to 45 per cent.[9, 10]

In an examination of the esophagi from 1,000 autopsies, Postlethwait and Musser found acute inflammation in 27 per cent and chronic slight inflammation in 76 per cent.[11] Acute esophagitis may be due to streptococci, diphtheria organisms, or monilial infections. Of more importance are chemical burns, which occur most often in children and are usually due to accidental swallowing of lye. Of 71 patients, 85 per cent were 1 to 5 years of age and lye was the corrosive agent in 95 per cent.[12] Pain is severe although there is no immediate mortality. Emergency treatment consists of drinking orange juice or dilute vinegar. In the first few hours there is mucosal necrosis, after 48 hours bacterial invasion is common, and by six weeks the epithelium is replaced.[13] The significance of the injury, however, is the development of a stricture from contraction of granulation tissue in the healing process. This expected result may be discernible as early as two weeks after the injury. It is usually present in the proximal third and is treated by periodic bouginage. When constriction is untreated, "spillover" disease tends to develop: Ingested food backs up into the esophagus, spills over the epiglottis, and is aspirated into the bronchi and lungs. The results are pneumonia, bronchiectasis, and lung abscess. A second complication is the development of carcinoma at the stricture site. This occurred in seven of 200 patients (3.5 per cent), and the average age was 35 years, whereas the usual age for carcinoma of the esophagus is 50 to 65 years.[14, 15]

Chalasia is the term for a loose sphincter of the lower esophagus. Achalasia is purposeless contractions of the esophagus and failure of the lower sphincter to relax. This vitiates the directional effect of peristalsis and creates a functional obstruction of the lower sphincter so that the lumen undergoes marked dilation and the wall becomes hypertrophic. The condition affects only the esophagus. The cause is not known although it has been observed in some pa-

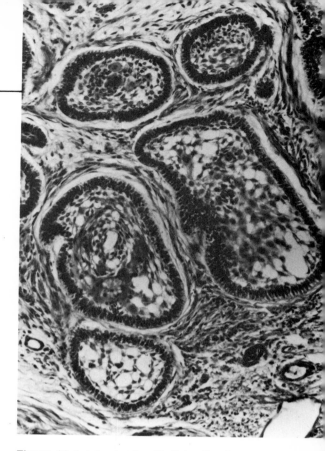

**Figure 13-4.** Islands of epithelial cells of ameloblastoma of the jaw with central degeneration forming cystlike structures

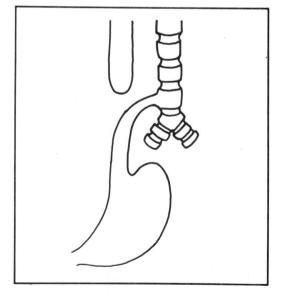

**Figure 13-5.** Usual configuration of atresia of esophagus with lower segment forming tracheoesophageal fistula

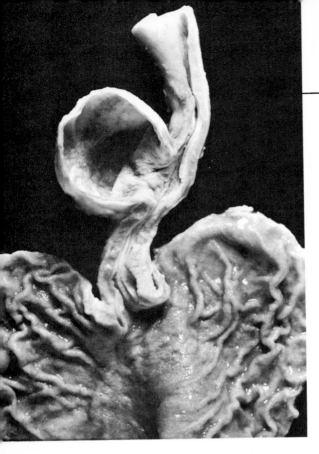

**Figure 13-6.** Large traction diverticulum of esophagus. Also shown in color section, p C-2.

tients that ganglion cells of the myenteric plexus are few or absent.[16] Both sexes are affected, the average age at clinical onset is 46 years, and the symptoms are difficulty in swallowing, regurgitation, weight loss, and epigastric pain. The average duration of symptoms in one series of 269 patients was eight years.[17] Radiographic study reveals a cone-shaped dilation of the lumen that narrows toward the cardia. Without treatment spillover disease develops. Prompt relief is obtained by the Heller operation, which consists of a single longitudinal muscle-splitting incision through the unrelaxed sphincter. Carcinoma is a rare complication of achalasia.[18]

There are two main diverticula of the esophagus: a pulsion outpouching at the proximal end on the posterior surface and a traction outpouching in the middle on the anterior surface. According to Lahey and Warren, the distinction between pulsion and traction diverticula was made by Zenker and Ziemssen in 1877.[19] The upper lesion is also known as a Zenker or pharyngoesophageal diverticulum. It occurs more often in men than in women, and is attributed to weakening of the wall so that the mucosa and submucosa protrude through a muscle defect in the posterior surface of the pharynx. The weakness occurs between the inferior constrictor of the pharynx and the transverse fibers of the cricopharyngeal muscle. It is presumed to be congenital.[20] Over the years the small pouch enlarges and gradually forms a true diverticulum that hangs down between the esophagus in front and the prevertebral fascia behind. Further enlargement causes obstruction of the esophagus by indentation from the posterior surface. The condition tends to occur in the elderly.[21] Clinical manifestations are dysphagia, regurgitation, foul breath, a gurgling sound in the neck, and nocturnal paroxysms of choking. X-ray studies confirm the diagnosis. Without treatment malnutrition, aspiration, and pulmonary infections tend to develop. Hemorrhage, perforation, and malignant transformation, however, do not occur. Surgical treatment consists of diverticulectomy for patients under 60 and diverticulotomy for patients over this age.[22]

Traction diverticula occur at the level of the tracheal bifurcation on the anterior surface of the esophagus in the region of the hilar lymph nodes. It is presumed that healing of tuberculous nodes causes fibrous attachment to the wall so that contraction of the connective tissue pulls the wall outward and forms the diverticulum. In my experience, however, diverticula occur without such nodal attachments. The evaginations tend to be small, food does not accumulate in them, and no treatment is required as they are ordinarily asymptomatic and of no clinical consequence. A large traction diverticulum is shown in Figure 13-6 (see color section, p C-2).

Several conditions impede the passage of portal blood through the liver. Chief among these is cirrhosis. Others include tumor compression of the portal vein and thrombosis of that vessel at the hilum of the liver (porta hepatis). When the portal blood meets this obstruction, alternative pathways develop to allow that blood to reach the caval system and thus return to the right heart. Although there are several of these portacaval anastomoses, the chief one involves the submucosal veins of the esophagus (Figure 13-7). These dilate as portal blood is diverted to the coronary vein of the stomach, submucosal veins of the esophagus, and azygos system, which empties into the superior vena cava. In this process the esophageal veins become markedly dilated, the walls are poorly supported, and such trivial events as coughing, which raises venous pressure, or the abrasion of poorly masticated food, cause rupture. The varices tend to be clinically silent until they rupture. The mortality of the first hemorrhage is about 75 per cent.[23] The reason for this high frequency of death is not only massive bleeding; cirrhotic livers are often decompensated, coagulopathy is common in cirrhotic patients, hepatic coma is frequent, and prerenal azotemia may develop.[24] In addition, the surgical treatment of esophageal hemorrhage carries a considerable mortality by itself. Varices of the esophagus are therefore extremely important lesions.

A significant proportion of cirrhotic patients have peptic ulcers of the stomach or duodenum, and these also cause upper gastrointestinal hemorrhage. The physician is faced with the question of determining the site of the bleeding. A palpable spleen, a firm, enlarged liver, and the absence of epigastric tenderness favor the esophagus as the site of the hemorrhage.[23]

The common benign tumor of the esophagus is the leiomyoma. It usually measures less than 1 cm in diameter and is of only incidental interest. The important tumor of

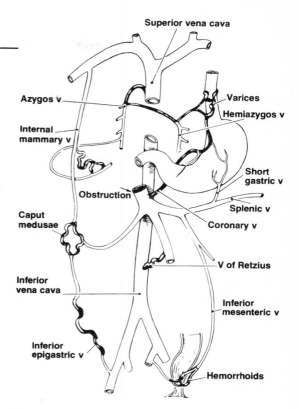

**Figure 13-7.** Portacaval anastomoses following obstruction of portal flow through the liver, usually from cirrhosis (after a drawing by J. Wyman)

the esophagus is the squamous-cell carcinoma. Its frequency is about three cases per 100,000 population in the United States.[25] It occurs in men two to six times more often than in women, and the average age is 60 years.[26, 27] Symptoms include dysphagia, loss of weight, pain, and regurgitation. These are gradual in onset and the symptomatic period is usually less than six months.[28] X-rays indicate the diagnosis, which is confirmed by esophagoscopy.

Squamous cancers arise in the upper, middle, and lower esophagus in the proportions of approximately 2:5:3.[25] At the cardia, however, adenocarcinomas are common, and it is not always evident whether they are tumors of the esophagus or extensions from a cancer of the stomach. Origin in ectopic gastric glands is also possible. The squamous cancers are well differentiated. All ulcerate the mucosa and gradually

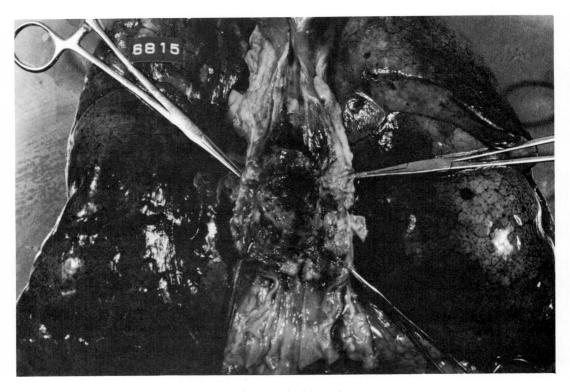

**Figure 13-8.** Advanced squamous-cell carcinoma of midesophagus

cause obstruction from fungation into the lumen or invasion and fixation of the wall. By the time of diagnosis, most measure 5 to 7 cm in length and have already invaded adjacent structures so that total resection is precluded.[25] For this reason treatment by resection or irradiation provides an outlook that has been described as the "triumph of hope over experience."[29] The five-year survival rate is usually under 10 per cent. The cancer spreads to the aorta and pericardium and especially to the trachea, with the frequent formation of a tracheoesophageal fistula. Metastasis to the lungs and mediastinal lymph nodes is common. Death is due to metastatic disease and respiratory failure. An advanced carcinoma is shown in Figure 13-8, and a tracheoesophageal fistula is illustrated in Figure 13-9.

Although the cause of this cancer is not known, striking variations in frequency suggest a strong environmental or dietary influence. It is common in France, Japan, India, Iran, and Puerto Rico. Within different communities of Africa the variation is as great as 200 per cent.[30] Moreover, in the Transkei of South Africa, the cancer emerged from virtual nonexistence to epidemic proportions in a period of 25 years.[25] These differences may be due to smoking and nutritional deficiency, which appear to be the major risk factors. Tobacco smoke contains several carcinogens, and the risk to smokers is two to six times that to nonsmokers. The effect, however, is independent of the form, whether cigars, cigarettes, or pipes. Nutritional deficiency is endemic in parts of the world and is the main effect in patients with the Plummer-Vinson syndrome,* who also have an in-

*Anemia, dysphagia, glossitis, and congenital weblike strictures of the esophagus.

creased incidence of esophageal cancer. Alcohol appears to potentiate the carcinogens of tobacco smoke, although the mechanism of this effect is not known. Alcohol also is associated with faulty dietary habits so that it contributes to nutritional deficiency. Therefore alcohol increases the risk of esophageal cancer even though it contains no carcinogens and is not itself carcinogenic. Perhaps for this reason the effect of alcohol is independent of the form in which it is consumed. The topic has been essayed by Wynder and Mabuchi.[31] Other associated conditions include achalasia, lye stricture, betel chewing, and reflux esophagitis with extension of columnar mucosa into the lower portion (Barrett's esophagus).[32],[33]

## STOMACH

Inflammation is a common lesion of the stomach. Acute gastritis is a recurrent condition due to many causes, frequently dietary indiscretions and abuse of alcohol. The clinical manifestations are dyspepsia and "sour stomach." Healing is prompt. Acute necrotizing gastritis is due to strong acids or alkalis often taken for suicidal purposes; the mucosa sloughs and hemorrhage is prominent if not massive. Chronic gastritis occurs in atrophic and hypertrophic forms. Atrophic gastritis is characterized by loss of parietal cells with thinning of the wall and effacement of the rugal pattern. It increases with age and is associated with hypoacidity. Atrophic gastritis is also invariable in pernicious anemia, affecting all of the fundus so that achlorhydria results. In this form there is failure to secrete intrinsic factor, which prevents the absorption of vitamin $B_{12}$ so that megaloblastic (pernicious) anemia results. An immune reaction is thought to cause this lesion since antibodies to parietal cells develop in most patients.[34] Atrophic gastritis is also a precursor of carcinoma of the stomach.[35] In the hypertrophic form of gastritis the mucosa is thick, hyperacidity may or may not

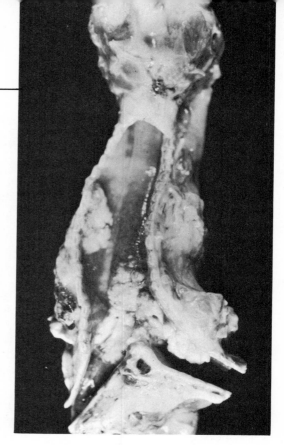

**Figure 13-9.** Extension of esophageal carcinoma into trachea with tracheoesophageal fistula

be present, and the surface has a cobblestone appearance (Figure 13-10). It is sometimes associated with excessive secretion of protein and is then known as Menetrier's disease.[25] Hypertrophic gastritis seems to be decreasing in frequency.

Stress ulcers of the stomach are small, round, multiple, shallow, and black from the effect of acid. They occur anywhere in the stomach, heal rapidly, and leave no scars. There are many causes, including head injuries, which occasion hyperacidity, and uremia and stressful situations, which do not. Stress ulcers also tend to occur with the use of cortisone. Bleeding may result, but stress ulcers do not lead to chronic peptic ulcers.

Peptic ulcers occur wherever acid and pepsin are present: the stomach, duodenum, postoperative gastrojejunal stoma, lower esophagus from reflux, and Meckel's

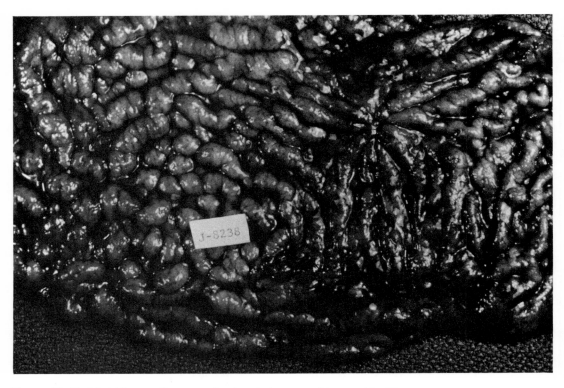

**Figure 13-10.** "Cobblestone" mucosa in chronic hypertrophic gastritis. The stellate scar of a small, healed ulcer is present in upper portion at right.

diverticulum, where ectopic gastric glands are often present. Over 98 per cent arise in the stomach or duodenum, in a ratio of the former to the latter of about 1:7. Peptic ulcers are single, round, seldom over 2 cm in diameter, and almost always occur in the antral portion, usually on the lesser curvature. The walls are steep, the bases are clean, and the margins are level with the surrounding mucosa. A chronic peptic ulcer of the stomach is shown in Figure 13-11. Histologic examination of the base reveals a layer of necrotic debris, a layer of leukocytic exudate, and a zone of granulation tissue beneath which dense fibrous scar tissue forms. Acute ulcers may penetrate quickly and are then complicated by massive hemorrhage or, less frequently, perforation with peritonitis. Chronic ulcers are complicated by extensive scarring that ra-

diates in a stellate pattern and constricts the stomach, occasionally to form an hourglass configuration, or by stenosis of the pylorus with dilation, vomiting, and electrolyte imbalance. Malignant transformation is regarded as extremely infrequent, with an incidence of less than 1 per cent.[36] Without these complications, chronic gastric ulcers heal by mucosal regeneration over the denuded base. A healed ulcer is shown in Figure 13-12.

Although peptic ulcers of the stomach or duodenum are extremely common, the cause is unknown. It is popular to suppose that the gastric mucosa defends itself against self-digestion by the production of a film of protective mucus and that the acid-pepsin mixture attempts to overcome this protective effect. Ulcers of the duodenum, which occur mainly in the first 2 cm beyond

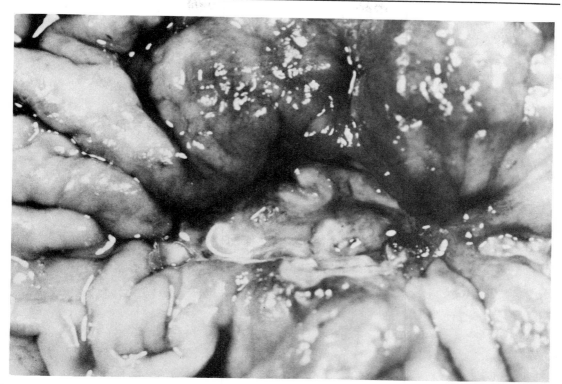

**Figure 13-11.** Chronic ulcer of stomach

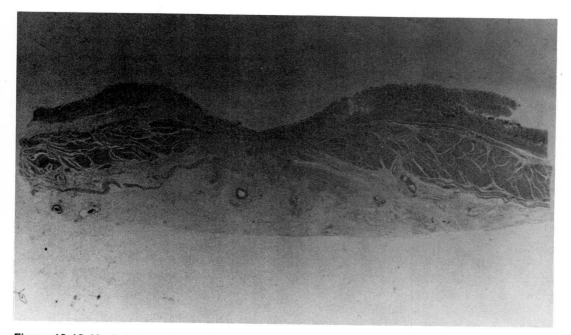

**Figure 13-12.** Healed ulcer of stomach

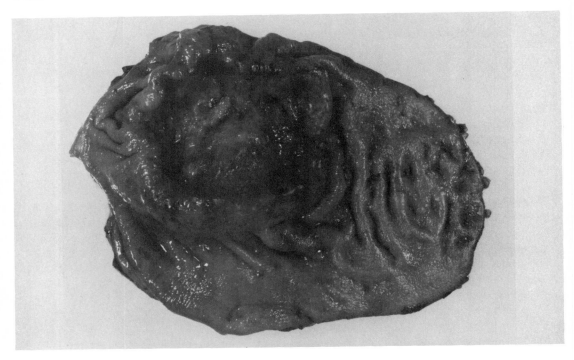

**Figure 13-13.** Adenocarcinoma of stomach

the pyloric ring, are associated with hyper-acidity, but gastric ulcers occur in patients without an excess of acid. The cause is simply not known, although gastric ulcers do not form in achlorhydric patients and vagotomy, which reduces acid production, has a healing effect. Clinical features are piercing midepigastric pain, an X-ray defect of the gastric wall, and occult blood in the stool. Moreover, the pain of gastric ulcer is subdued by food gradually, whereas the pain of a duodenal ulcer is immediately relieved by food or antacid and recurs some hours after eating. Therapeutic measures include a bland diet, drugs to block the effect or reduce the secretion of acid, vagotomy, and partial gastrectomy.

The only significant tumors of the stomach are adenomas, leiomyomas, and carcinomas. The first two are small, uncommon, and covered with intact mucosa. Both tend to be clinically silent although adenomas occasionally undergo malignant transfor-

mation and leiomyomas occasionally ulcerate and bleed.

The important stomach tumor is cancer of the mucosa. It occurs in later life, twice as often in men as in women. Most arise in the pyloric antrum on either curvature, and some ulcerate and infiltrate the wall while others fungate prominently into the lumen. Mixed patterns also occur (Figure 13-13). Most are adenocarcinomas, often well differentiated. Least frequent is the undifferentiated cancer in which the tumor cells spread widely in the wall to cause fibrosis of the submucosa and muscularis. A "leather bottle" configuration results. Called linitis plastica, it presents as a stiff, uniformly thickened gastric wall over which the mucosa is mostly intact. A stain for mucin reveals the cancer cells, which usually have a "signet ring" pattern.

Clinical manifestations of all gastric cancers include anorexia, epigastric distress, loss of weight, anemia, and blood in the stool, usually occult. The tumor cells are often spread beyond resectability by the time clinical signs appear. Such spread precludes cure, and the five-year rate of survival after total gastrectomy is on the order of 10 per cent.[35] Metastasis takes place to the regional lymph nodes and liver, followed by the lungs, brain, and bones. Bilateral ovarian metastases form Krukenberg's tumor; spread to the lower peritoneal reflection forms Blumer's shelf, and spread to the left supraclavicular fossa forms Virchow's node. Virchow's node, however, is not specific for gastric cancer. The usual postgastrectomy survival period is 12 to 18 months.

The remarkable aspect of gastric cancer is its decline in incidence over the past 40 to 50 years. The age-adjusted mortality rate for males declined from 28/100,000 in 1930 to 9.7 in 1967.[35] By 1974, the number was approximately seven in 100,000.[37] Moreover, this decline is not worldwide; the incidence remains especially high in Japan, Chile, Iceland, and Finland. More than half of all male cancer deaths in Japan are due to gastric cancer. The tumor occurs more often in lower socioeconomic groups, more often in patients with blood group A, and more often in patients with pernicious anemia and atrophic gastritis than in others.[35] In addition, there is a slight familial aggregation although it is not known whether this is a genetic or environmental effect. Studies of dietary habits, geographic differences, racial migrations, soil composition, and precursor conditions have failed to reveal the cause of this cancer or the reason for its declining incidence in the United States.

## ILEUM

The major lesions of the small intestine are obstructions, inflammations, vascular disturbances, and malabsorptive states. Minor lesions include ulcers, diverticula, and tumors. These will be considered more or less in order of progression from the proximal to the distal small intestine.

Ulcers of the distal duodenum or proximal jejunum are characteristic of the Zollinger-Ellison syndrome. The syndrome, identified in 1955, consists of a fulminating ulcer diathesis, marked gastric hypersecretion, and a non-$\beta$-cell tumor of the islets of the pancreas.[38] The tumors, which are small, often multiple, and not infrequently malignant, secrete gastrin, which stimulates parietal cell hyperplasia of the gastric mucosa and causes excess acid production, often 10 to 20 times normal. The ulcers are usually multiple, often intractable, and unusually located. The islet tumors presumably consist of $\delta$ cells although this is not altogether clear.[39] Nevertheless, gastrin is secreted and the tumors are "ulcerogenic." Two years after the syndrome was first reported, pronounced diarrhea and hypokalemia were added as frequent aspects of the clinical condition. These are probably due to excessive acid that inhibits pancreatic enzyme activity.[40] Treatment consists of total gastrectomy, after which the malignant tumors may stop progressing or may even regress.[39]

Diverticula affect the duodenum and midileum. Duodenal diverticula are present in the second portion and are large with wide ostia so that food tends not to be retained and clinical disturbance is rare.[41]

Meckel's diverticulum is a blind cul-de-sac 10 to 12 cm in length located on the antimesenteric side of the small intestine approximately 100 cm proximal to the ileocecal junction.[42] It is a remnant of the omphalomesenteric duct, which normally disappears by the eighth week of gestation when the fetus begins to be nourished by the placenta rather than by the yolk sac. The tip of the diverticulum may contain ectopic gastric glands and, less frequently, pancreatic tissue. Peptic ulcers occasionally form on this account. More often, the ileum becomes entangled so that intestinal obstruction develops. Other consequences

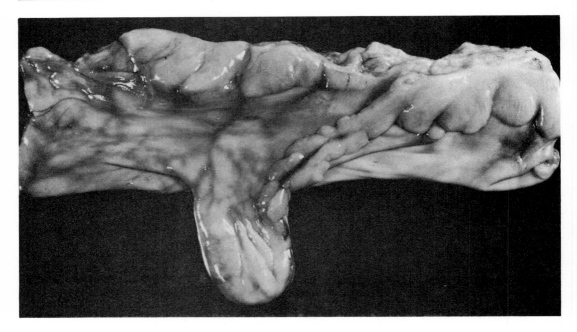

**Figure 13-14.** Meckel's diverticulum of midileum

include bleeding, abdominal tenderness, pain in the midabdomen, and, rarely, perforation from a peptic ulcer. A characteristic diverticulum is shown in Figure 13-14. In addition to the blind pouch, a fibrous strand may extend from the tip to the umbilicus, and rarely a patent omphaloenteric fistula exists.

Intestinal disturbances tend to develop because of the mobility of the small intestine. This portion of the gut is 20 feet long, attached to a wide mesentery, and covered by a smooth, wet, glistening surface. Moreover, the ileum pulses with peristaltic thrusts at more or less regular intervals. For these reasons this slippery, flexible tube tends to work itself into places that cause obstruction. One of these is the scrotum. When the testes migrate from the abdomen to the scrotum, the passageway may remain open as an inguinal canal into which a loop of ileum becomes extended. An indirect hernia forms as the loop of gut emerges through the internal inguinal ring, passes medially down the canal, and pro-

jects into the scrotum through the external inguinal ring. If the projection takes place through the external ring only, the hernia is direct. In either case the veins are compressed, the arteries pump blood into a stagnant chamber, and the edema that follows prevents return of the bowel loop to the peritoneal cavity. It is thus incarcerated. Unless relieved, the hemorrhagic wall will undergo necrosis and the intestine will become strangulated and rupture.

A second mobility disturbance is volvulus, in which a loop of intestine becomes twisted on its mesenteric root. At the twisted site the veins are again compressed, the arteries, under higher pressure, remain open, and a blood-filled loop of gut forms. In this sac (Figure 13-15) fluid accumulation is immense, and the tissue, deprived of circulation, undergoes necrosis and sooner or later bursts.

A third mobility lesion is intussusception, in which a portion of bowel wall invaginates into its own lumen to produce an obstruction of the intestine (Figure 13-16).

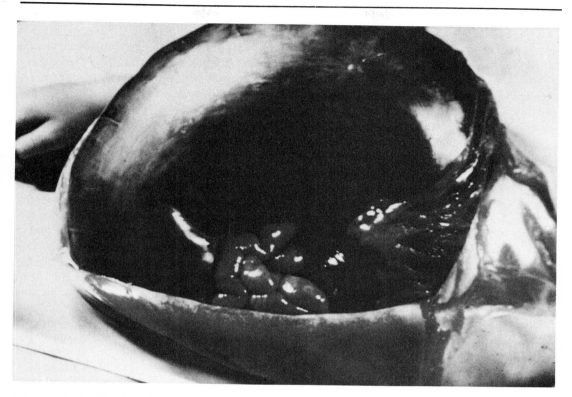

**Figure 13-15.** Volvulus of ileum

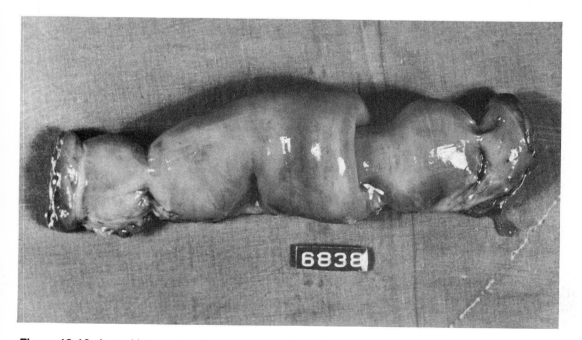

**Figure 13-16.** Agonal intussusception, showing configuration of the deformity

This occurs often in children, usually in boys under the age of 5 years. The cause is not evident. The sites are mainly ileoileal or ileocecal. In adults some mass attached to the wall appears to drag the margin inward in the direction of the fecal stream to produce the abnormality. The masses may consist of a submucosal lipoma, a mucosal adenoma, a polypoid malignant tumor, or even an invaginated Meckel's diverticulum.[43] In all these instances the veins become compressed, the circulation is impaired, and nonviability of the tissue impends as the obstruction forms.

The most frequent mobility disturbance is kinking or knotting of an intestinal loop around a fibrous adhesion of the peritoneum. In a series of 465 cases of small-bowel obstruction, 69 per cent were due to such adhesions, most of which were postsurgical.[44] Moreover, the obstructions may occur months to years after the operations. Talc in the peritoneum from surgeons' gloves is one cause that is altogether preventable. Unless operative treatment is instituted early, the mortality is high from electrolyte imbalance, cardiorespiratory complications, sepsis, and pronounced loss of fluid into the lumen of the obstructed segment.

The symptoms of intestinal obstruction from these mechanical causes are pain in the abdomen, often of abrupt onset, that recurs in paroxysms synchronous with the peristaltic waves. Moreover, the pain tends to escalate with each successive paroxysm. Nausea, vomiting, leukocytosis, and sometimes fever also occur. Auscultation of the abdomen reveals high-pitched peristaltic sounds, or borborygmi. Shock follows unless the obstruction is relieved, and peritonitis develops if the intestine ruptures.

Vascular disturbances of the ileum also cause intestinal obstruction, especially mesenteric thrombosis and embolism. Emboli are associated with atrial fibrillation or recent myocardial infarction with mural thrombi of the endocardium or atrial appendage. In 67 of the 136 patients studied by Ottinger and Austen, however, no vascular occlusion was identified.[45] The patients are old and the early clinical sign is severe pain in the abdomen, often of sudden onset, that is steady, persistent, and poorly localized. The abdomen discloses few physical signs.[46] The presentation is thus altogether different from the noisy borborygmi and recurring paroxysms of mechanical obstruction. Both emboli and thrombi tend to block the superior mesenteric artery close to its junction with the aorta. Venous thrombi also cause infarction, especially when associated with cirrhosis and portal hypertension. The affected bowel turns dark purple from the presence of stagnant blood, the mucosa undergoes necrosis, and the lumen fills with a bloody transudate. Vomiting and bloody diarrhea often follow. Leukocytosis is pronounced, and the serum amylase rises. As the necrosis extends to the muscularis, perforation impends and peritonitis threatens. Unless early resection of the necrotic segment or embolectomy is performed, the outlook is poor. Of the 136 patients of Ottinger and Austen, only 11 survived, a mortality rate of 92 per cent.[45]

Hemorrhagic necrosis of the intestine also occurs in conjunction with heart failure and shock from any cause. The circulatory disturbance of shock centers on intravascular fibrin formation with hemorrhages and necrosis of tissue.[47] Large segments of gut may be affected; the mucosa shreds, the lumen contains blood, and ulcers form. The condition is termed hemorrhagic enteropathy, and it is distinguished from other vascular disturbances by the localization of the thrombi to the venous system; arteries and arterioles are unaffected. Moreover, the large arteries and veins are patent, and it is presumed that vasospasm is a pathogenic mechanism.[48] Ming pointed out that the condition is probably due to a conglomeration of microinfarcts of the mucosa secondary to a markedly decreased blood flow.

He counseled that vasopressors may be harmful.[49] The clinical manifestations may be obscured by the cardiac disease or the cause of the shock.

From the foregoing it may be concluded that mechanical obstruction of the intestine is associated with sudden onset, escalating paroxysms of pain, borborygmi, and rapid progression with the development of necrosis and perforation. When the obstruction is vascular the circulation is weak, the abdomen is silent, and the pain tends to be steady and persistent. If the obstruction is high in the abdomen, in the duodenum or jejunum, vomiting begins early, the vomitus is bile-stained, and the abdomen shows little distention. If the obstruction is low, however, the vomiting is late in onset, the material is light brown with fecal odor, and abdominal distention is pronounced. It is thus possible from examination of the patient to gain some idea of the nature of the obstruction and its probable cause. If there is a risk in treatment, it is waiting too long before surgical investigation is undertaken, regardless of the cause of the obstruction.[50]

A number of inflammatory diseases of the ileum have essentially disappeared from the United States because of hygienic improvements, preventive measures, diagnostic advances, and effective treatment. Among these are typhoid fever, cholera, tuberculosis, and potassium chloride ulcers. Unmoved by these advances, however, is regional enteritis, the premier inflammatory disease of the small intestine. It is a chronic recurring granulomatous inflammation especially of the terminal ileum. It affects mostly young adults; 60 per cent of cases occur between the ages of 10 and 25 years.[51] It is characterized by ulceration and fibrosis of segmental distribution that penetrate to the mesentery, regional lymph nodes, and adjacent tissues with frequent fistula formation.

Regional enteritis was recognized as an entity by Crohn, Ginzburg, and Oppenheimer in 1932.[52] The cause is not known. The

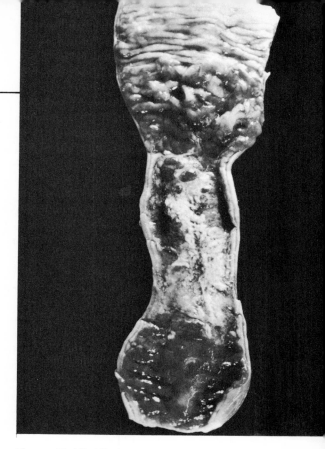

**Figure 13-17.** Affected segment of distal ileum in regional enteritis. Also shown in color section, p C-3.

condition begins with abdominal pain, often in the right lower quadrant, associated with cramps, constipation, or diarrhea. The patient also experiences anorexia, nausea, vomiting, and loss of weight. Over half have blood in the stool. Remissions are spontaneous, and exacerbations may be associated with emotional stress. Contrast X-rays show a narrow "string sign" through the affected part and a wide "skip area" in the unaffected portions. Grossly the bowel wall is thick and stiff with an ulcerated, hyperemic mucosal surface (Figure 13-17; see color section, p C-3). Microscopically there is massive fibrosis of the submucosa with occasional granulomas bearing a resemblance to sarcoidosis.

The clinical consequences of this persistent inflammatory lesion are poor nutrition, loss of weight, and malabsorption. Anatomically, fistulae form to the bladder, skin, or, more often, adjacent loops of bowel. Further consequences are perforation, peritonitis, abscess formation, stenosis, and hemorrhage. The hemorrhage may be life-threatening. Cancer occurs, but it is extremely infrequent.[53]

The area of the absorptive surface of the small intestine is approximately 100 times greater than the body surface. This is due to the extending effect of the plicae circulares, the mucosal villi, and the microvilli, of which there are 300 to 500 atop each epithelial cell.[40] Carbohydrates, folic acid, iron, and amino acids are absorbed in the duodenum and jejunum. Nearly all lipids are absorbed in the first 100 cm of ileum. It is in the lower small intestine that bile acids and vitamin $B_{12}$ are absorbed.[54] For absorption to take place, the stomach must secrete acid, which indirectly activates the pancreas, the pancreas must deliver digestive enzymes, and the bile must flow into the intestine so that fats are emulsified. Failure of absorption, or malabsorption, is therefore due principally to gastric abnormalities, biliary dysfunction, or pancreatic disease. In fact, most cases result from gastric resection.[55] A long list of conditions may be assembled under these three mechanisms as the possible explanation for malabsorption in a given individual. Two other mechanisms should also be kept in mind. One is an insufficiency of absorptive surface, and the other is dysfunction of a sufficient surface. An example of insufficiency is regional enteritis with a jejunocolic fistula so that the ileal mucosa is bypassed. Dysfunctions include widespread ulceration of the mucosa, as in regional ileitis, and primary abnormalities of the surface, such as gluten enteropathy (nontropical sprue, celiac disease) or Whipple's disease.

The commonest presentation of malabsorption is diarrhea, loss of weight, and macrocytic hypochromic anemia.[54] The outstanding characteristic, however, is steatorrhea, which results from failure to absorb lipids. The stool is copious, and the normal excretion of 5 gm of fat per day rises to 25 gm. On this account the stool floats and becomes yellow, glistening, and greasy. Bacterial effects also include the production of organic acids from carbohydrates, which make the stool frothy and liquid, and the reduction of protein to indoles and amines, which impart a foul odor to it. Steatorrhea is accordingly unmistakable; the stool is liquid, copious, yellow, frothy, glistening, foul, and it floats.

In the diagnosis of malabsorption, the history ordinarily gives evidence of disease of the stomach, pancreas, or biliary tract. Regional enteritis is usually obvious. Less apparent, however, are gluten enteropathy and Whipple's disease. In gluten enteropathy the mucosal cells of the ileum lack an enzyme needed to metabolize gluten, which is a component of flour. Gluten contains gliadin, a protein harmful to the mucosa. The harm is reflected by increased shedding of the epithelial cells, at up to six times the normal rate, and by acceleration of new cell production in the basal crypts. New cell production is insufficient to keep up with cell loss, and as a result the mucosa gradually becomes atrophic and flat. Exactly how gliadin causes this reaction is not altogether clear.[56] The clinical onset occurs from infancy to middle age, and the diagnosis is established by peroral biopsy of the ileal mucosa. The characteristic finding is absence of villi together with an increased rate of mitotic activity in the basal crypt cells. Clinical and histologic improvement result from diet modification.

Whipple's disease is rare. It affects men eight times more often than women, the median age is 44 years, and the presenting complaints are usually steatorrhea and arthralgia.[57] It was described in 1907 by Whipple, who suggested the term "intestinal lipodystrophy."[58] He did this because the autopsy examination of his patient revealed a thick, coarse ileal mucosa whose surface had changed from a velvety texture to a nubbly appearance. The lamina propria and mesenteric lymph nodes were engorged with lipid-distended macrophages. Later, dispersion of the macrophages to virtually all organ systems was found, especially the endocardium and joints. The macrophages take the periodic acid-Schiff (PAS) stain. The one tissue always involved, however, is the ileal mucosa, and the diagnosis is secured by peroral biopsy of that tissue; no other condition causes PAS-positive macrophages to accumulate in the lamina propria of the ileum. Patients regularly used to die from malabsorption and a gradually worsening nutritional state. It was subsequently discovered that bacilli infect the lamina propria and that clinical and histologic remission is induced by tetracycline therapy. Whipple's disease is thus regarded as a bacterial infection even though the bacilliform organism has not been cultured and the disease has never been experimentally reproduced.[59]

The epithelium of the ileum consists of four cell types: absorptive, mucous, Paneth, and Kulchitsky. Paneth cells are limited to the ileum and are characterized by red supranuclear granules. Their function is unknown. Kulchitsky cells are found throughout the intestinal tract and are recognizable by their red infranuclear granules. These cells give rise to carcinoids, the most common tumors of the small intestine. They occur in either sex at any age, most often in young adults. Carcinoids also occur in the appendix, colon, and rectum. In the ileum the tumors are firm, round, and movable in the submucosa and measure up to 2 cm in diameter. The cut surfaces are pale yellow. Microscopically the carcinoid cells are uniformly round, small, and without mitotic activity. They do have an affinity for silver stains, however, and for this reason carcinoids are also known as argentaffinomas. The cells secrete serotonin (5-hydroxytryptamine), which is carried in the portal blood to be inactivated by monoamine oxidase in the liver. Carcinoids also metastasize to mesenteric lymph nodes and

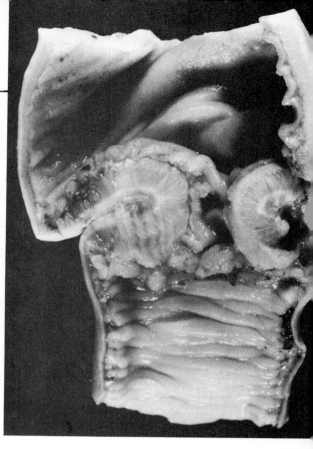

**Figure 13-18.** Carcinoid of ileum causing stenosis. Note dilation of the lumen and hypertrophy of the wall proximal to the tumor.

liver, where serotonin is further produced. When the total amount exceeds the inactivating capacity of the monoamine oxidase, serotonin passes into the systemic circulation to cause the carcinoid syndrome. This consists of 5- to 10-minute paroxysms of facial flushing with cyanosis, asthma-like wheezing from bronchoconstriction, hypotension, and watery diarrhea. In the systemic circulation the serotonin is degraded to 5-hydroxyindoleacetic acid (5-HIAA), which is excreted in the urine. A positive test for 5-HIAA in the urine in a patient with the carcinoid syndrome thus establishes the diagnosis. It is evident that the syndrome cannot be diagnosed until metastatic disease has developed. Fortunately, prolonged survival is frequent, and pharmacologic agents are helpful in controlling the symptoms.[60] A carcinoid is illustrated in Figure 13-18.

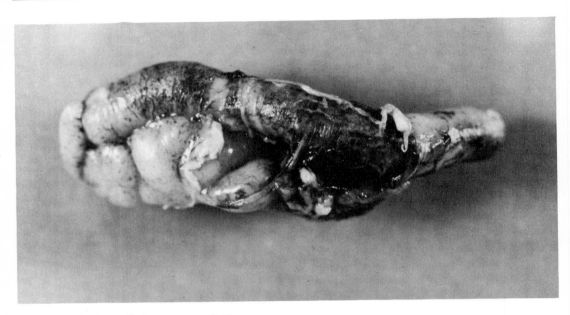

**Figure 13-19.** Acute fibrinous appendicitis

## APPENDIX

The principal lesion of the appendix is inflammation. It occurs in either sex at any age, but most frequently in young adults, especially men. The cause is obstruction of the lumen, usually by a fecalith or by hyperplasia of the abundant submucosal lymphoid tissue. Less frequent causes are seeds, parasites, or a carcinoid tumor. Secretions in the blocked lumen accumulate, the mucosa ulcerates, and infection of the wall develops. This is manifested by an acute exudative transmural inflammation with hyperemic vessels of the serosa and fibrin over the surface (Figure 13-19). Without relief of the obstruction, the wall ruptures. The common complications are a periappendiceal abscess or diffuse acute suppurative peritonitis. Less frequent is acute inflammation of the portal vein (pylephlebitis) from septic emboli that may cause thrombosis of that vessel or scattered abscesses throughout the liver. Septicemia is then possible. Rarely the lumen is obstructed without inflammation, leaving a dilated chamber that gradually fills with mucoid secretions (mucocele). Chronic appendicitis does not exist.

The patient with acute appendicitis experiences nausea and vomiting, followed by periumbilical discomfort that gradually shifts to the right lower quadrant of the abdomen. This is accompanied by localized tenderness, fever, leukocytosis, and neutrophilia. Prompt removal of the appendix is necessary to avoid complications.

## COLON

The colon has a dual function. The proximal part absorbs water while the distal part stores stool. Moreover, the proximal part to the midtransverse colon is supplied by the superior mesenteric artery, which is large, while the distal colon from the midtransverse portion on is supplied by the inferior mesenteric artery, which is small. These two aspects have a bearing on the lesions that affect this portion of the gut.

Hirschsprung's disease is a segmental absence of ganglion cells from the rectosig-

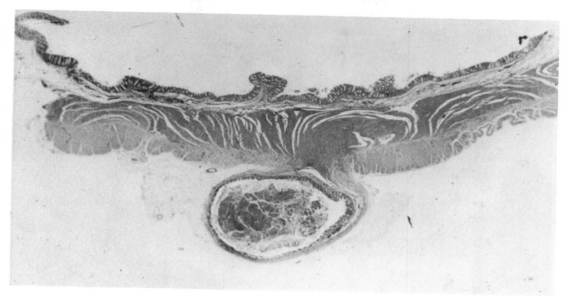

**Figure 13-20.** Diverticulum of colon

moid that impairs the passage of stool so that the colon dilates, the abdomen swells, and the bowel movements may be so infrequent as to occur only once in several weeks. The absence is congenital, and both the submucosal and myenteric plexuses are affected.[61] The condition is found most often in the first year of life but is also seen in adults. Additional manifestations include colicky abdominal pain, periods of watery diarrhea, vomiting, anorexia, weight loss, fetid breath, hypochromic anemia, and explosive borborygmi.[62] The abdominal enlargement may be so great as to push the diaphragm upward and cause respiratory disturbance. A barium enema establishes the megacolon, and biopsy reveals the ganglionic absence. Fecal impaction is common. Bowel function is restored by operative removal of the aganglionic segment and anastomosis of the descending colon to the anal portion.

Diverticula constitute the most common lesion of the colon. They are rare under 40 years but increase from 5 per cent of patients at age 50 to 50 per cent of patients at age 90.[63] The sigmoid and descending portions are most often affected. The diverticula are saccular, measure about 0.5 cm in diameter, and tend to be aligned in rows on either side of the tenia coli. They consist of mucosa only, covered by peritoneum if they lie next to the free surface, or by adipose tissue if they lie within the mesentery. The configuration of a diverticulum is shown in Figure 13-20.

The lumens contain fecal material that becomes fixed and inspissated because the necks are narrow and there is no muscle in the walls to contract and empty the sacs. Abrasion from the inspissated debris causes ulceration, which is followed by inflammation, perforation, and peritonitis if the sac lies close to the surface, or by pericolic abscess if the sac is embedded in mesenteric adipose tissue. It is unusual for more than three or four diverticula to be inflamed at once.[64] The sacs are mucosal extrusions between bands of circular muscle at points of presumed weakness where vessels penetrate the wall to nourish the mucosa.[65] On this account inflammation of

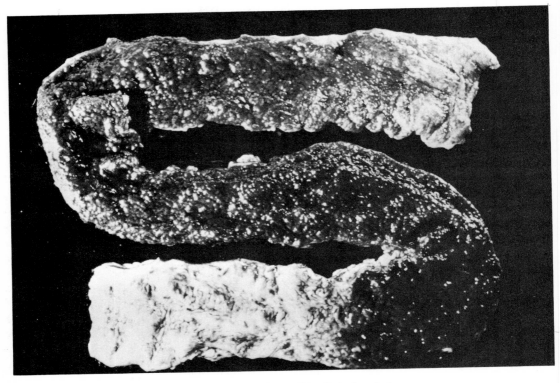

**Figure 13-21.** Mucosal surface in chronic ulcerative colitis. Only the dark, hyperemic portion is affected. Also shown in color section, p C-3.

the diverticula may affect the vessels so that hemorrhage becomes pronounced. Other complications include pericolic fibrosis with stenosis of the colon, fibrous adhesions of the peritoneum, and fistula formation to adjacent viscera.

Although all these consequences are possible, diverticula are clinically silent in most patients. The main symptoms, when present, are irregularity of bowel habit and intermittent pain in the left lower quadrant of the abdomen. Barium studies reveal the sacs but do not disclose whether they are the cause of the symptoms. Morson contended that diverticula are due to a disorder of muscle function with greatly increased tone,[64] and Painter and Burkitt regarded them as a deficiency disease.[66] The deficiency is one of fiber in the diet. With adequate fiber the stool is bulky and

soft and passes quickly. In economically developed countries, however, where diverticular disease is endemic and low-residue diets are customary, the stool transit time is long, the colonic wall shows segmentation, and the mucosa herniates through the muscle bands. There is no agreement on the cause of diverticulosis.

Except for bacillary and amebic dysentery, four main ulcerative diseases affect the colon: ulcerative colitis, granulomatous colitis, ischemic enterocolitis, and drug-induced necrosis of the mucosa. The premier condition is chronic ulcerative colitis. The condition affects young adults of either sex, pursues a chronic intermittent course often lasting for decades, and tends to develop serious complications. It is a superficial exudative inflammation that begins in the rectosigmoid and progresses proximally for varying distances; about one-third of cases affect the entire colon and extend to the ileocecal junction. The process commences with microabscesses of the mucosa that enlarge, coalesce, and spread to form elongated ulcer streaks. Between the ulcers are protuberant islands of remaining mucosa that form pseudopolyps. The mucosal surface is shown in Figure 13-21 (see color section, p C-3). The external muscle layers contract to shorten the colon and thicken the wall. The proximal margin of involvement is poorly defined. The disease has no pathognomonic feature, although ulcerative colitis may be distinguished from Crohn's disease of the colon by absence of skip areas, of mesenteric node involvement, of fistula formation, and of granulomas in the wall. In addition, granulomatous colitis rarely affects the rectosigmoid whereas ulcerative colitis almost invariably does. Nevertheless, distinction between the two conditions is sometimes impossible.[67]

Patients experience a sudden or gradual onset of diarrhea with a characteristic mixture of blood, pus, and mucus in the stool. With this there are fever, anorexia, loss of weight, and colicky pain in the abdomen. Although the diarrhea may persist for long periods, the course tends to be intermittent with remissions that are spontaneous and exacerbations that are frequently precipitated by emotional stress. The cause is not known; it has been thought to be infection, allergy, autoimmunity, psychosomatic disorder, nutritional deficiency, or enzyme defect, among others.[67]

Extracolonic manifestations are a feature of the disease. A minority of patients have ankylosing spondylitis, sacroiliac disturbance, or peripheral arthritis. In addition, pericholangitis and chronic active hepatitis are often seen. Complications include toxic dilation of the colon, pronounced hemorrhage through the rectum that may be exsanguinating, and carcinomatous transformation of the mucosal epithelium in the pseudopolyps. The carcino-

mas may be multiple and are difficult to diagnose because of the irregularity of the mucosal surface caused by the ulcerative disease. Cancer is most likely when the disease begins in childhood, affects the entire colon, and lasts more than 10 years. Under these circumstances prophylactic colectomy is sometimes deemed advisable.

The colonic mucosa is vulnerable to ischemia, uremia, and low blood pressure. Uremia and low blood pressure occur with all the conditions that cause shock. Ischemia is due to atherosclerosis, thrombosis, or atheromatous emboli within the mesenteric arteries, causing ulceration of the mucosa. Since the causative conditions are common, ischemic colitis is a frequent lesion although it is often only a terminal aspect of a main disease process. Broad stretches of mucosa are ulcerated, the margins are hemorrhagic, and the centers become dark greenish-brown from conjunction with stool. Extension into the ileum is frequent. The lesion is illustrated in Figure 13-22. A light, exudative inflammation underlies the denuded surface, and recent and organizing thrombi are present in the small vessels of the submucosa. The clinical manifestations tend to be obscured by the main disease, and death ordinarily precludes the development of complications.

Infrequently certain antibiotics cause a unique lesion of the colon with a characteristic mushroom-shaped focus of necrosis, streamers of leukocytes, and hypersecretion of mucus (Figure 13-23). The lesion is limited to the colon, always affects the rectum, and can be diagnosed by proctoscopic examination.[68]

The main tumors of the colon are polypoid adenomas, villous adenomas, and adenocarcinomas. Polypoid adenomas are the most frequent, occurring in 10 per cent of the adult population and increasing as age advances.[69] Most arise in the left colon, especially in the sigmoid and rectum. Most measure less than 1 cm in diameter and consist of a globular mass of epithelial cells

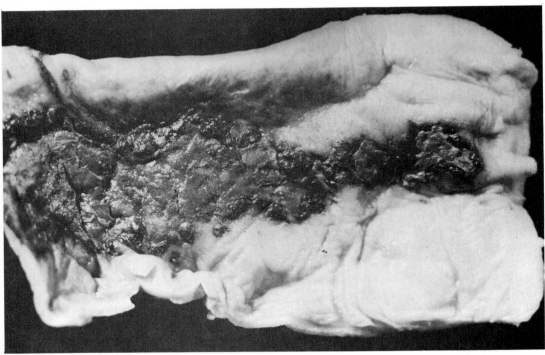

**Figure 13-22.** Ischemic colitis with mucosal ulceration

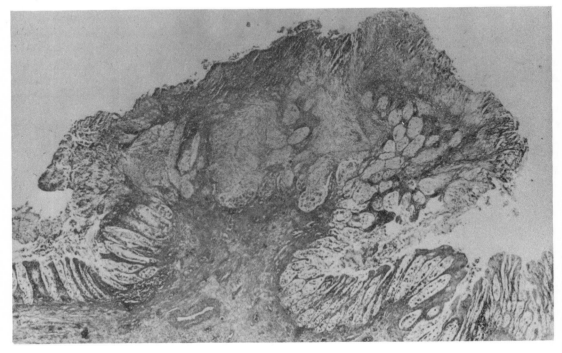

**Figure 13-23.** The mushroom or volcano configuration of ulcers associated with antibiotics, especially clindamycin

mounted on a narrow pedicle covered with normal mucosa (Figure 13-24). The epithelial cells reveal large, hyperchromatic nuclei that occupy most of the cytoplasm. Mitotic figures are frequent, but polarity is preserved. Focal malignant change is identified in 5 per cent, and this increases with the size of the adenomas so that it is seen in two-thirds of those over 2 cm in diameter.[70] If the muscularis mucosae is not invaded, there is no risk of metastasis (Figure 13-25).[69] Most adenomas are clinically silent although bleeding may occasionally occur. Diagnosis is aided by fiberscopy; all should be removed.

A related condition is familial polyposis, which is inherited in the mendelian pattern of an autosomal dominant. It is characterized by hundreds of polypoid adenomas that cover the surface of the colon from cecum to rectum (Figure 13-26). The mucosa is normal until after puberty, when the tumors begin to develop. Most are diagnosed by the age of 25. Without treatment one or more of the tumors will become malignant within 15 years of the diagnosis. Since this transformation is inevitable, prophylactic colectomy is warranted.

In the Peutz-Jeghers syndrome the lips, buccal mucosa, and digits display foci of melanin pigmentation that are associated with polypoid structures in small numbers anywhere in the intestinal tract from the esophagus to the rectum. The lesions are hamartomas (tumor-like masses of normal tissue) and are not given to malignant transformation.[69]

Villous adenomas are large, single, sessile growths that arise almost exclusively in the rectosigmoid. The surface is papillary and may resemble a carpet covering the entire circumference of the wall (Figure 13-27). On microscopic examination 20 to 50 per cent disclose focal adenocarcinoma, and about 30 per cent have invaded beyond resectability by the time of diagnosis.[71] Both sexes are affected, the average age is 63, and the clinical symptoms include

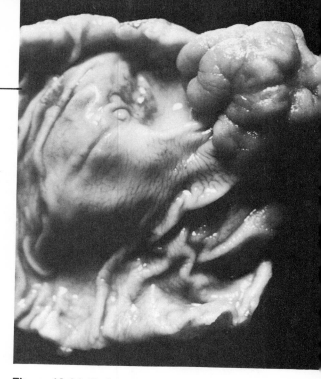

**Figure 13-24.** Pedunculated adenoma of colonic mucosa

**Figure 13-25.** Fibrous stalk of pedunculated adenoma with tuft of hyperplastic epithelial cells, no malignant transformation, and intact muscularis mucosae.

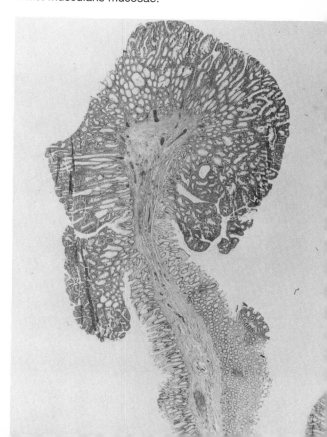

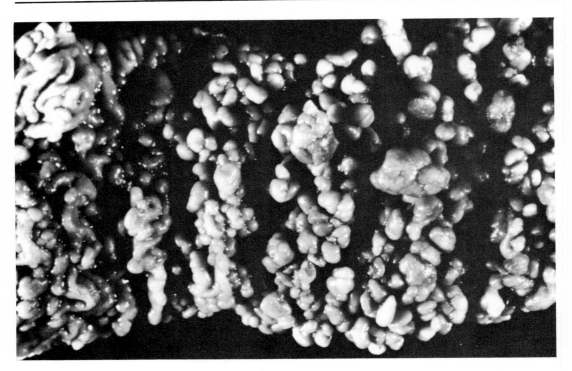

**Figure 13-26.** Pedunculated adenomas of familial polyposis

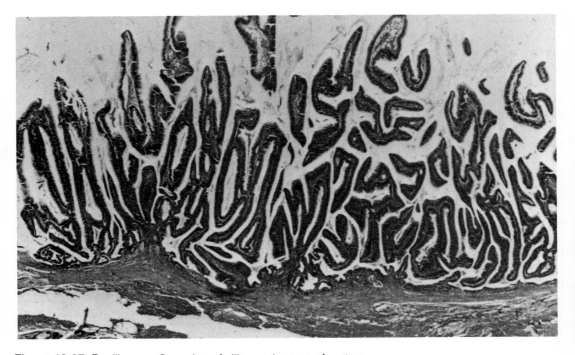

**Figure 13-27.** Papillary configuration of villous adenoma of rectum

mucous discharge, rectal bleeding, and painful defecation. Secretions from the tumor may be so great as to cause dehydration, hyponatremia, and hypokalemia. Intrarectal excision is ordinarily sufficient treatment.

Carcinoma of the colon is second in frequency only to cancer of the lung in men and cancer of the breast in women. It comprises 13 per cent of all human cancers in the United States; it was estimated that 100,000 individuals would develop this tumor in 1978, with half this number succumbing to it.[72] Men and women are equally affected; two-thirds of cases occur after age 50, the average age being 67 years.[73]

Seventy-five per cent of all intestinal cancers arise in the sigmoid colon, rectum, or anus.[73] Those on the left side of the colon encircle the lumen, invade the wall, and ulcerate the mucosa. On this account the clinical signs are abdominal pain, gross blood in the stool, and a change of bowel habit that progresses to obstruction of the lumen. A carcinoma of the descending colon is illustrated in Figure 13-28 (see color section, p C-4). On the right side the lumen is large, the wall is distensible, and the stool is semiliquid. Moreover, right colonic cancers tend to fungate into the lumen rather than encircle the wall. Therefore the clinical manifestations of right colonic cancers are usually abdominal pain, a palpable mass, and occult blood in the stool associated with hypochromic microcytic anemia. Unexplained anemia of this kind should prompt an investigation of the cecum or right colon. The period from symptomatic onset to diagnosis in the series of Irvin and Greaney was 5.3 months.[74] Carcinomas of the rectum cause bleeding, tenesmus, and a sense of incomplete evacuation.[75] Nearly all are well-differentiated adenocarcinomas, although a few produce an excess of colloid and some are undifferentiated. Diagnostic procedures include digital examination, sigmoidoscopy, barium studies, fiberoptic endoscopy, and biopsy.

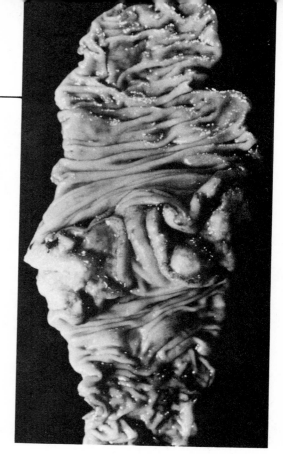

**Figure 13-28.** Encircling or "napkin ring" carcinoma of descending colon. Also shown in color section, p C-4.

Colonic cancers gradually invade the wall, extend into the mesentery, and spread to the regional lymph nodes (Figure 13-29). Distant metastases then arise; the most common sites are the liver, lungs, bone, and brain. Of these, the liver is overwhelmingly the most frequent.[76] Death is due to perforation of the colon with peritonitis or to obstruction of the lumen with inanition and terminal infection.

In 1932 Duke classified colonic cancers according to their depth of spread. Group A tumors are confined to the wall of the colon, group B have spread to the mesentery, and group C have metastasized to the regional lymph nodes. Prognosis becomes worse as the tumor spreads. For example, in the series of Corman et al the survival rate for group A was 84 per cent, dropping to 65 per cent for group B and to 36 per cent for group C.[77]

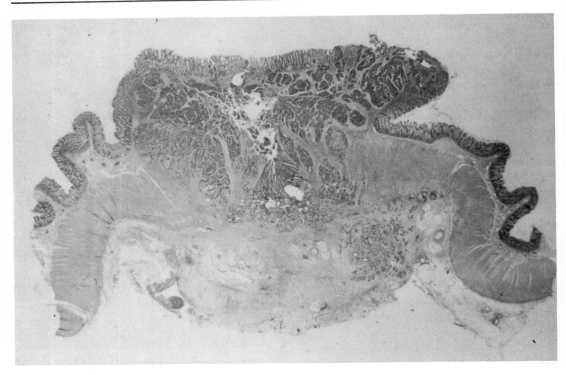

**Figure 13-29.** Spread of carcinoma through wall and into subjacent fibroadipose tissue of mesentery

The traditional treatment is colectomy, often by abdominoperineal resection. This operation was initiated by Miles in 1908. More recently Cole identified tumor cells in the venous drainage from the tumor site, and Turnbull introduced ligation of the vascular pedicle before touching the tumor in order to minimize spread from operative manipulation.[76] The five-year rate of survival has reached a stable level of about 40 per cent for all patients.[78] It is accordingly evident that earlier recognition might be expected to provide improved results. The screening procedure of least cost, slightest inconvenience, and acceptable reliability is the guaiac-impregnated filter paper (Hemoccult) test. This test has therefore been recommended as a routine office procedure.[78] It is especially important because colonic carcinomas tend to be clinically silent in their early stages, and 15 to 25 per cent have hepatic metastases at the time of surgical treatment.[79] Although these cancers often produce carcinoembryonic antigen that may be identified in the serum, the test is not specific for the tumor and it is therefore not suitable as a screening method. It may be used to monitor treatment, however, as an indication of recurrence or metastatic disease.[75]

Carcinomas of the colon are not especially radiosensitive. Nevertheless, for certain selected cases, Papillon reintroduced the method of contact radiation.[80] When the tumor was low-lying, well differentiated, and clinically localized to the rectal wall without induration of the pararectal lymph nodes, Papillon applied 10,000 to 15,000 rad directly to the cancer in four treatments. The procedure requires no anesthesia and is done on an outpatient basis. This method avoids hospitalization, a major operation fraught with significant mortality, and the need for a lifelong colostomy. These are important advantages. The results have been encouraging: a 72 per cent five-year rate of survival.[80] In considering this treatment it should be kept in mind that colectomy is superior to radiotherapy only when some of the tumor has spread outside the tissue ablated by the radiation but not outside the tissue ablated by the surgery. Otherwise both methods equally fail or equally succeed. Patients with this precise distribution of tumor are surely scarce, and it should be borne in mind that this proportion is probably smaller than the operative mortality of the surgical procedure. For selected patients, therefore, a reasonable case can be made for the radiation method.

Four conditions predispose to carcinoma of the colon: polypoid adenomas, villous (papillary) adenomas, familial polyposis, and chronic ulcerative colitis. All have been described above. It had generally been presumed that most cancers of the colon arise in polypoid adenomas until this dogma was challenged in 1958 by Spratt and colleagues.[81] Castleman and Krickstein later voiced the same view.[82] All these authors believed that most cancers arise de novo from nonadenomatous mucosa. Morson, however, disputed this view and asserted that most colonic cancers evolve through the adenoma-malignant change sequence.[70] Moreover, Fenoglio and Lane emphasized two "fundamental facts": Minute intramucosal carcinomas are rare while malignant changes in polypoid adenomas are common.[83] The mechanism of origin of colonic cancer remains unsettled.

Epidemiologic considerations are also of interest. The incidence of colonic cancer is greater in the United States than in some countries of Africa.[84] This and other geographic comparisons indicate a strong environmental influence. Burkitt suggested a noxious metabolite produced in the bowel by the effect of bacteria on sterols or bile acids. Both these substances have chemical structures not unlike those of known carcinogens (see ring structures shown in Figure 10-2). Burkitt pointed out that colonic cancer is a disease of economically developed countries, where low-residue diets cause slow transit time that allows carcinogens to contact the mucosa over comparatively long periods. In contrast, colonic cancer is infrequent in countries where high-residue diets are eaten that produce rapid transit times, which minimize contact of stool with the mucosa. Geographic differences might be explained in this way. Although this argument is persuasive, it has recently been discovered that a chemical, dimethylhydrazine dihydrochloride, causes cancer of the colon when injected into mice but not when given by mouth.[85] The possibility that nonenteric carcinogens may cause colonic cancer is thus also extant.

## REFERENCES

1. Wurman LH, Adams GL, Meyerhoff WL: Carcinoma of the lip. *Am J Surg* 130:470, 1975

2. Flamant R, Hayem M, Lazar P, et al: Cancer of the tongue. A study of 904 cases. *Cancer* 17:377, 1964

3. Jeppsson PH, Lindstrom J: Cancer of the tongue. *Acta Oto-laryngol* 75:314, 1975

4. Woods JE, Chong GC, Beahrs OH: Experience with 1,360 primary parotid tumors. *Am J Surg* 130:460, 1975

5. Molnar L, Ronay P, Dobrossy L: Mixed tumors of the parotid gland. *Oncology* 25:143, 1971

6. Bardwil JM: Tumors of the parotid gland. *Am J Surg* 114:498, 1967

7. Spiro RH, Huvos HG, Strong EW: Cancer of the parotid gland. A clinicopathologic study of 288 primary cases. *Am J Surg* 130:452, 1975

8. Mehlisch DR, Dahlin DC, Masson JK: Ameloblastoma: A clinicopathologic report. *J Oral Surg* 30:9, 1972

9. Cozzi F, Wilkinson AW: Esophageal atresia. *Lancet* 2:1222, 1967

10. Romsdahl MM, Hunter JA, Grove WJ: Tracheoesophageal fistula and esophageal atresia. Surgi-

cal management and results at a university hospital. *J Thorac Cardiovasc Surg* 52:571, 1966

11. Postlethwait WW, Musser AW: Changes in the esophagus in 1,000 autopsy specimens. *J Thorac Cardiovasc Surg* 68:953, 1974

12. Hardin JC Jr: Caustic burns of the esophagus. A ten year analysis. *Am J Surg* 91:742, 1956

13. Buford TH, Webb WR, Ackerman L: Caustic burns of the esophagus and their surgical management. A clinico-experimental correlation. *Ann Surg* 138:453, 1953

14. Bigger IA, Vincent PP: Carcinoma secondary to burn of the esophagus from ingestion of lye. *Surgery* 28:887, 1950

15. Bigelow NH: Carcinoma of the esophagus developing at the site of lye stricture. *Cancer* 6:1159, 1953

16. Misiewicz JJ, Waller SL, Anthony PP, et al: Achalasia of the cardia: Pharmacology and histopathology of isolated cardiac sphincteric muscle from patients with and without achalasia. *Q J Med* 38:17, 1969

17. Ellis FH Jr, Kiser JC, Schlegel JF, et al: Esophagomyotomy for esophageal achalasia: Experimental, clinical, and manometric aspects. *Ann Surg* 166:640, 1967

18. Sariyannis C, Mullard KS: Esophagomyotomy for achalasia of the cardia. *Thorax* 30:539, 1975

19. Lahey FH, Warren KW: Esophageal diverticula. *Surg Gynecol Obstet* 98:1, 1954

20. Clagett OT, Payne WS: Surgical treatment of pulsion diverticula of the hypopharynx: One-stage resection in 478 cases. *Dis Chest* 37:257, 1960

21. Ellis FH Jr, Schlegel JF, Lynch VP, et al: Cricopharyngeal myotomy for pharyngo-esophageal diverticulum. *Ann Surg* 170:340, 1969

22. Trible WM: The surgical treatment of Zenker's diverticulum: Endoscopic vs external operation. *South Med J* 68:1260, 1975

23. Orloff MJ: The complications of cirrhosis of the liver. *Ann Intern Med* 66:165, 1967

24. Conn HD: The prognosis and management of bleeding esophageal varices. *Ann NY Acad Sci* 170:345, 1970

25. Min SC: *Tumors of the Esophagus and Stomach. Atlas of Tumor Pathology*, fasc 7. Washington, DC: Armed Forces Institute of Pathology, 1973

26. Gunnlaugsson GH, Wychulis AR, Roland C, et al: Analysis of the records of 1,657 patients with carcinoma of the esophagus and cardia of the stomach. *Surg Gynecol Obstet* 130:997, 1970

27. Kay S: A ten year appraisal of the treatment of squamous cell carcinoma of the esophagus. *Surg Gynecol Obstet* 117:167, 1963

28. Leon W, Strug LH, Brickman ID: Carcinoma of the esophagus. A disaster. *Ann Thorac Surg* 11:583, 1971

29. Rambo VB, O'Brien PH, Miller XM III, et al: Carcinoma of the esophagus. *J Surg Oncol* 7:355, 1975

30. Annotation: œsophageal cancer in Africa. *Lancet* 2:1178, 1969

31. Wynder EL, Mabuchi K: Cancer of the gastrointestinal tract. Etiological and environmental factors. *JAMA* 226:1546, 1973

32. Naef AP, Savary M, Ozello L: Columnar-lined lower esophagus: An acquired lesion with malignant predisposition. *J Thorac Cardiovasc Surg* 70:826, 1975

33. Stephen SJ, Uragoda CG: Some observations on esophageal carcinoma in Ceylon, including its relationship to betel chewing. *Br J Cancer* 24:11, 1970

34. Castle WB: Current concepts of pernicious anemia. *Am J Med* 48:541, 1970

35. Lilienfeld A: Epidemiology of gastric cancer. *N Engl J Med* 286:316, 1972

36. Jordan GL Jr: Decreasing incidence of carcinoma of the stomach. *Am J Surg* 116:407, 1968

37. Silverberg E: Cancer statistics, 1977. *CA—Cancer J Clin* 27:26, 1977

38. Zollinger RM: Islet cell tumors and the alimentary tract. *Am J Roentgenol* 126:933, 1976

39. Case Records of the Massachusetts General Hospital: Hypercalcemia and diarrhea in a 38-year-old woman. *N Engl J Med* 294:37, 1976

40. Medical Grand Rounds: Malabsorption. *South Med J* 67:211, 1974

41. Juler GL, List JW, Stemmer EA, et al: Perforating duodenal diverticulitis. *Arch Surg* 99:572, 1969

42. DeBartolo HM Jr, van Heerden JA: Meckel's diverticulum. *Ann Surg* 183:30, 1976

43. Felix EL, Cohen MH, Bernstein AD, et al: Adult intussusception; case report of recurrent intussusception and review of the literature. *Am J Surg* 131:758, 1976

44. Laws HL, Aldrete JS: Small bowel obstruction: A review of 465 cases. *South Med J* 69:733, 1976

45. Ottinger LW, Austen WG: A study of 136 patients with mesenteric infarction. *Surg Gynecol Obstet* 124:251, 1967

46. Mackenzie RL, Provan JL: Recognition and management of embolism to the superior mesenteric artery. *Can Med Assoc J* 111:1207, 1974

47. McGovern VJ: Shock. *Pathol Annu* 6:279, 1971

48. Freiman DG: Hemorrhagic necrosis of the gastrointestinal tract. *Circulation* 32:329, 1965

49. Ming SC: Hemorrhagic necrosis of the gastrointestinal tract and its relation to cardiovascular status. *Circulation* 32:332, 1965

50. Skinner DB, Zarins CK, Moossa AR: Mesenteric vascular disease. *Am J Surg* 128:835, 1974

51. Janowitz HD, Sachar DB: New observations in Crohn's disease. *Annu Rev Med* 27:269, 1975

52. Crohn BB, Ginzburg L, Oppenheimer GC: Regional ileitis: A pathologic and clinical entity. *JAMA* 9:1323, 1932

53. Frank JD, Shorey BA: Adenocarcinoma of the small bowel as a complication of Crohn's disease. *Gut* 14:120, 1973

54. Cooke WT: Common problems of malabsorption. *Practitioner* 216:637, 1976

55. Toffolon EP, Goldfinger SE: Malabsorption following gastrectomy and ileal resection. *Surg Clin North Am* 54:647, 1974

56. Spiro HM: *Clinical Gastroenterology*, p 432. Toronto: Macmillan, 1970

57. Perara DR, Weinstein WM, Rubin CE: Small intestinal biopsy. *Hum Pathol* 6:157, 1975

58. Whipple GH: A hitherto undescribed disease characterized by deposits of fat and fatty acids in the intestinal and mesenteric lymphatic tissues. *Bull Johns Hopkins Hosp* 18:382, 1907

59. Maizel H, Ruffin JM, Dobbins WO III: Whipple's disease: A review of 19 patients from one hospital and a review of the literature since 1950. *Medicine* 49:175, 1970

60. Welch JP, Malt RA: Management of carcinoid tumors of the gastrointestinal tract. *Surg Gynecol Obstet* 145:223, 1977

61. Ehrenpreis T: Megacolon and megarectum in older children and young adults. *Proc R Soc Med* 60:799, 1967

62. Metzger PP, Alvear DT, Arnold QC, et al: Hirschsprung's disease in adults: Report of a case and review of the literature. *Dis Colon Rectum* 21:113, 1978

63. Simonowitz D, Paloyan D: Diverticular disease of the colon in patients under 40 years of age. *Am J Gastroenterol* 69:69, 1977

64. Morson BC: Pathology of diverticular disease of the colon. *Clin Gastroenterol* 4:37, 1975

65. Hughes LE: Postmortem survey of diverticular disease of the colon. *Gut* 10:336, 1969

66. Painter NS, Burkitt DP: Diverticular disease of the colon: A deficiency disease of Western civilization. *Br Med J* 2:450, 1971

67. Wright R: Ulcerative colitis. *Gastroenterology* 58:875, 1970

68. Smith JC: Pseudomembranous colitis. A review. *Mo Med* 74:593, 1977

69. Rawson RW: Colonic polyps: Antecedent or associated lesions of large bowel cancer. *Semin Oncol* 3:361, 1976

70. Morson BC: Polyps and cancer of the large bowel. *West J Med* 125:93, 1976

71. Takolander RJ: Villous papilloma of the colon and rectum. *Acta Chir Scand Suppl* 473:10, 1977

72. Schein PS, Woolley PV III: Introduction. *Semin Oncol* 3:329, 1976

73. Rubin P: Current concepts in cancer. Cancer of the GI tract: Colon, rectum, anus. *JAMA* 231:513, 1975

74. Irvin TT, Greaney MG: Duration of symptoms and prognosis of carcinoma of the colon and rectum. *Surg Gynecol Obstet* 144:883, 1977

75. Woolley PV III: Clinical manifestations of cancer of the colon and rectum. *Semin Oncol* 3:373, 1976

76. Corman ML, Veidenheimer MC, Coller JA: Recent thoughts on the development of colorectal cancer. *Med Clin North Am* 59:347, 1975

77. Corman ML, Swinton NW, O'Keefe DD, et al: Colorectal carcinoma at the Lahey Clinic. 1962 to 1966. *Am J Surg* 125:424, 1973

78. Miller SF: Colorectal cancer: Are the goals of early detection achieved? *CA—Cancer J Clin* 27:338, 1977

79. Kardinal CG, Perry MC: Colorectal cancer—1977. *Mo Med* 74:675, 1977

80. Papillon J: Intracavitary irradiation of early rectal cancers for cure. *Am J Proctol* 26:37, 1975

81. Spratt JS, Ackerman LV, Moyer CA: Relationship of polyps of the colon to colonic cancer. *Ann Surg* 148:682, 1958

82. Castleman B, Krickstein HI: Do adenomatous polyps of the colon become malignant? *N Engl J Med* 267:469, 1962

83. Fenoglio CM, Lane N: The anatomic precursor of colorectal carcinoma. *JAMA* 231:640, 1975

84. Burkitt DP: Large bowel cancer: An epidemiologic jigsaw puzzle. *J Nat Cancer Inst* 54:3, 1975

85. Toth B, Malick L, Shimizu H: Production of intestinal and other tumors by 1,2-dimethylhydrazine dihydrochloride in mice. *Am J Pathol* 84:69, 1976

# 14

## DISEASES OF THE LIVER, BILIARY SYSTEM, AND PANCREAS

### THE LIVER

The liver normally weighs 1,200 to 1,600 gm and consists of a large right lobe, a small left lobe, and two comparatively small bulges on the undersurface, the caudate and quadrate lobes. It is suspended under the diaphragm by the falciform and triangular ligaments. It is covered by a thin, smooth Glisson's capsule. A double vascular supply—the portal vein and the hepatic artery—enters on the undersurface at the porta hepatis. The common bile duct also emerges from the liver at this site to deliver bile into the gallbladder and duodenum. About 1,500 ml of blood enter the liver each minute, somewhat more through the portal vein than the hepatic artery, and considerably more after eating than at rest.

The liver is composed of lobules that consist of columns of hepatocytes with intervening sinusoids. The venous and arterial blood mixes at the periphery of the lobules, passes down the sinusoids, and enters the central vein, which is the smallest branch of the outflow system. The central veins coalesce to form larger channels that emerge from the liver on the posterior undersurface to enter the inferior vena cava, penetrate the diaphragm, and flow into the right atrium of the heart. One surface of each hepatocyte faces a sinusoid; the opposite surface forms a groove that is the first portion of the biliary system. Bile formed in the hepatocyte is passed into the groove, from which it is propelled to the periphery

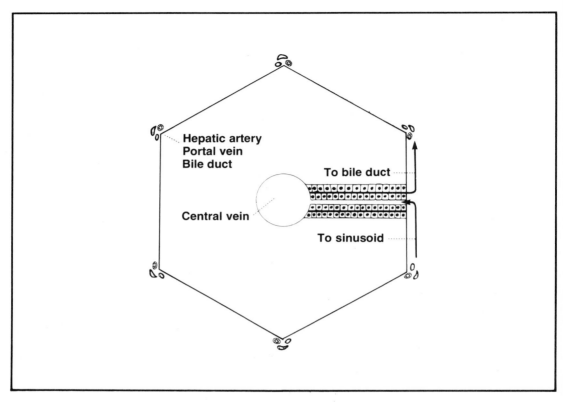

**Figure 14-1.** Diagrammatic structure of the hepatic lobule

of the lobule and thence into larger channels that eventually form the hepatic duct emerging at the porta hepatis. The periphery of the lobule thus consists of a triad of structures: the hepatic arteriole, the portal venule, and the bile ductule. It is interesting that as blood passes through the liver toward the heart, bile is secreted into channels with flow in the opposite direction—i.e., toward the porta hepatis—to emerge from the liver in the hepatic duct. The sinusoids are incompletely lined by macrophages called Kupffer cells, which extract particulate debris from the sinusoidal blood and thus convert the liver to a reticuloendothelial organ. A diagram of the hepatic lobule is shown in Figure 14-1.

The main pathologic processes of the liver are degeneration, necrosis, inflammation, circulatory disturbances, and tumor formation. Biliary obstruction is treated here as a separate process. In several important diseases a combination of processes is involved: Viral hepatitis combines inflammation and necrosis, and cirrhosis combines circulatory disturbance and inflammation. The various hepatic diseases are taken up according to these principal processes.

## Degenerations

The most common lesions of the liver are degenerative. They tend to be slight, diffuse, and reversible without residua. Chief among them are hydropic degeneration, steatosis, amyloidosis, and brown atrophy. Hydropic degeneration is due to cellular imbibition of water, which causes the cell to swell and the cytoplasm to take on a granular appearance. The nucleus is unaffected.

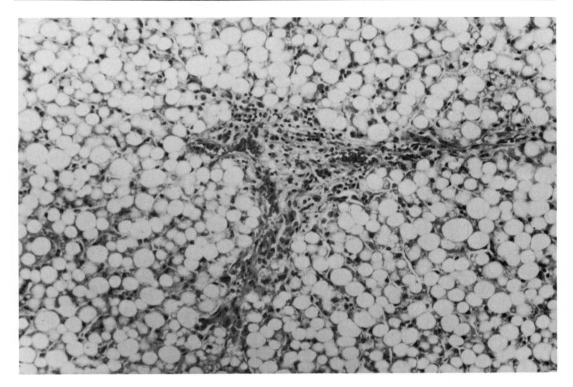

**Figure 14-2.** Steatosis of the liver. All the hepatocytes contain large, round globules of fat.

The liver enlarges, the capsule retracts on section, and the parenchyma bulges above the level of the cut. The condition is also known as cloudy swelling, albuminous degeneration, or parenchymatous degeneration. It accompanies anemia or fever regardless of the cause, but it is not manifested clinically. It subsides spontaneously.

Steatosis is the accumulation of lipid droplets in the cytoplasm of hepatocytes. The nucleus is pushed to the side, forming a signet ring configuration. The central cells of the lobules are affected first. Steatosis is associated with fever, anemia, undernutrition, and especially alcoholism. It may become pronounced, affecting the entire lobule (Figure 14-2). The liver enlarges, weighing as much as 6,000 gm, the cut surface is pale yellow, and droplets of fat appear on the cutting blade. The condition is

reversible and is not ordinarily evident as a clinical illness. However, a large, smooth, palpable liver and pain in the right upper quadrant occasionally occur. Jaundice and ascites seldom develop. Two consequences are possible: The steatosis progresses to portal cirrhosis or, especially when it is pronounced, causes sudden, unexpected death. The mechanism is not clear.[1]

Amyloidosis of the liver is more an infiltration than a degeneration. The process affects the liver in over half of cases, and hepatic involvement is about equal in the primary and secondary forms.[2] The hyaline material accumulates between the sinusoidal lining cells and the hepatocytes, so that the latter gradually succumb from increasing pressure. The process is uniform, and hepatomegaly develops. The capsule is smooth, the cut surface is pallid, and the

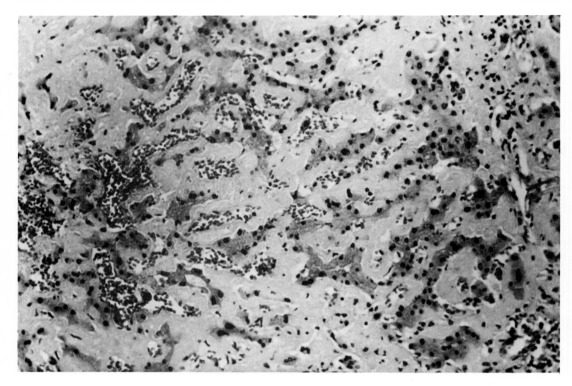

**Figure 14-3.** Amyloidosis of liver. Only remnants of the hepatic cells are evident.

tissue is firm with a rubbery texture. The clinical illness is dominated by the associated disease, although hepatomegaly and splenomegaly are frequent. Jaundice and ascites are unusual. Proteinuria is common because of the associated renal involvement. The diagnosis should be thought of in a patient with proteinuria, azotemia, anemia, and hepatomegaly. It is confirmed by needle biopsy. The histologic picture is shown in Figure 14-3. Death is seldom due to hepatic disease.

In old age and inanition visceral tissues undergo atrophy. In the liver atrophy is accompanied by the presence of an iron-free lipochrome pigment in the region of the nuclei of the hepatocytes. The liver thus becomes small and dark brown. The change is termed brown atrophy; it has no clinical significance.

## Circulatory disturbances

The two serious and frequent circulatory disturbances of the liver are chronic passive hyperemia, usually from heart failure, and centrilobular necrosis, usually from shock. Chronic passive hyperemia causes pericentral atrophy of hepatic cells that occasionally progresses to congestive "cirrhosis," whereas in shock centrilobular necrosis is due to hypoxia from low blood pressure and slow flow (Figure 14-4). Infarcts of the liver are uncommon because of the small size and tortuous path of the hepatic artery. They do occur, however, and atherosclerosis and aneurysms of the hepatic artery with or without thrombosis are the most frequent causes. The infarcts are usually small and clinical manifestations are limited to biochemical changes.[3] Hepatic infarction in cirrhosis is rare.

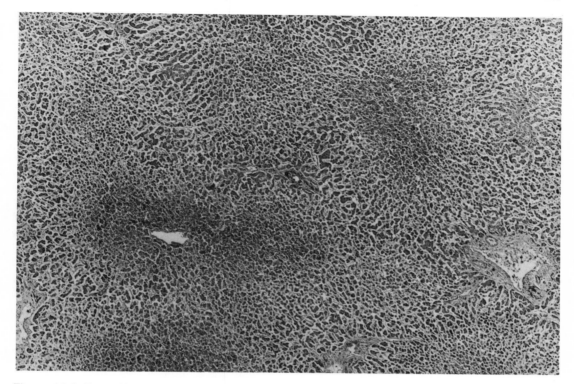

**Figure 14-4.** Central hemorrhagic necrosis associated with shock and underperfusion of the liver

Three other specific circulatory disturbances affect the liver. One is due to cirrhosis and is described separately. The others are an impediment to vascular inflow, known as the Cruveilhier-Baumgarten condition, and obstruction of vascular outflow, known as the Budd-Chiari syndrome.

Pego in 1833, Cruveilhier in 1835, and Baumgarten in 1907 described the condition now known as the Cruveilhier-Baumgarten disease.[4] It consists of a normal liver with portal hypertension and no evident cause. It is rare. Much more common is a similar situation in which the portal hypertension is due to cirrhosis. This is known as the Cruveilhier-Baumgarten syndrome. The clinical manifestations of both the disease and the syndrome, which reflect portal hypertension, include esophageal varices, occasional splenomegaly, occasional as-

cites, occasional hypersplenism (anemia, leukopenia, and thrombocytopenia), and canalization of the umbilical ligament with a caput medusae and a periumbilical venous hum. Less frequent causes of the syndrome include tumor compression of the portal vein and pylephlebitis with thrombosis of that vessel. In all these circulatory impairments the hepatic tissue survives on the oxygenated blood that is able to reach it through the hepatic artery.

The other main circulatory disturbance is obstruction of the outflow tract. The paradigm of this process is the Budd-Chiari syndrome, which was described clinically by Budd in 1845 and pathologically by Chiari in 1899.[5] The lesion Chiari described was endophlebitis of the hepatic veins of unknown cause. Today the cause in most cases still remains obscure.[6] Known causes include carcinoma of the liver, carcinoma of the kidney with a tumor thrombus in the vena cava at the hepatic vein juncture, and thrombosis from a myeloproliferative disease, especially polycythemia or, most recently, from the use of an oral contraceptive.[7,8] Veno-occlusive disease of the small hepatic veins from ingestion of pyrrolizidine alkaloids in bush tea causes the same syndrome.[9] The liver is large, smooth, purple, and blunt-edged. Sections reveal pronounced pericentral hyperemia with necrosis if the onset is abrupt and fibrosis if the illness is prolonged. The clinical features are hepatomegaly, abdominal pain, and massive recurrent ascites. Jaundice is slight or absent. Varices of the esophagus and dilation of periumbilical veins may develop. Progression to hepatic coma is gradual, and death is frequent.

**Necrosis**

Examination of the liver reveals that necrosis is zonal, affecting the same part of each lobule, or massive, affecting all lobules in one or more areas of the liver. Zonal necrosis is further observed to be central, peripheral, or in the intervening region, i.e., midzonal. The central zones of the lobules are the most vulnerable to toxins and circulatory changes. The two toxins associated with central necrosis are chloroform and carbon tetrachloride. The principal circulatory disturbances are shock and congestive heart failure. Both are important because of their frequency. Congestive failure of the right ventricle, as well as all conditions that impede the flow of blood out of the liver, causes increased pressure in the central veins of the lobules. The central veins dilate, the pressure is conveyed to the pericentral sinusoids, and the hepatocytes succumb to the pressure and disappear from this portion of the lobules. If the process is gradual, hyperemia becomes pronounced in the central portions and contrasts with the less affected peripheral portions, so that the nutmeg appearance is produced. Conditions impeding the flow of blood out of the liver include calcific stenosis of the aortic valve, rheumatic disease of the mitral valve, myxoma of the left atrium, vascular disease of the pulmonary vessels, right ventricular failure, insufficiency of the tricuspid valve, myxoma of the right atrium, and thrombosis or tumor compression of the hepatic veins. When the flow is impaired abruptly, as with shock, hypoxia is the main disturbance and pericentral necrosis develops (Figure 14-4). The liver is thus markedly affected by shock. If the patient survives the acute obstruction, or if the chronic obstruction is especially prolonged, pericentral fibrosis may develop. This fibrosis has been called cardiac or congestive cirrhosis, but it is not true cirrhosis because it is not progressive and regenerative nodules do not form.

Midzonal necrosis occurs with yellow fever, and the cytoplasm of some hepatocytes contains eosinophilic Councilman bodies, which are hyaline masses of an uncertain nature. Peripheral or periportal necrosis is characteristic of eclampsia and phosphorus poisoning.

Massive necrosis of the liver is caused by drugs, especially the antituberculous agent isoniazid[10] and the anesthetic agent halothane.[5] Viral infection of the liver also causes massive necrosis. In all of these the liver is limp, flabby, and so small that the weight is often reduced to 600 to 800 gm. The loss of tissue produces a finely wrinkled capsule. The cut surfaces are yellow from necrosis, red from hemorrhage, and green from the retention of bile. Viable islands of hepatic tissue undergoing regeneration produce large, pale gray masses on the cut surface while the necrotic zones are dark red and disclose loss of hepatocytes, collapse of stroma, and only scattered remnants of bile ducts. The cut surface appearance is shown in Figure 14-5 (see color section, p C-4). The clinical onset is abrupt, with liver failure and coma. The serum transaminase and bilirubin levels are ele-

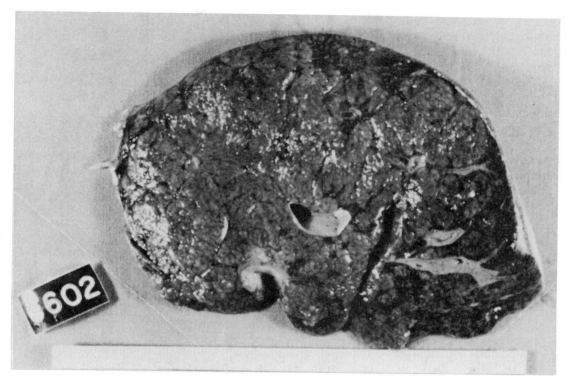

**Figure 14-5.** Massive necrosis of liver from isoniazid ingestion. Also shown in color section, p C-4.

vated; the bilirubin is about equally conjugated and unconjugated. Hepatic encephalopathy with neurologic effects ranging from a minor disturbance of consciousness to a flapping tremor of the extremities may develop. This is attributed to the production of ammonia by urea-splitting bacteria in the intestine; the ammonia is not cleared by the damaged liver and thus escapes into the general circulation. Death may occur within 24 hours or after a few days.

## Inflammations

Hepatitis is caused by three viruses, type A (HAV), type B (HBV), and neither A nor B (NAB). Most of these infections are subclinical, although some cause a mild, transient illness and a few go on to a fulminant, massive necrosis. The most frequent is HAV disease, which is epidemic and was previously known as infectious hepatitis or catarrhal jaundice. It is passed by fecal-oral contamination and thus tends to occur in children and under conditions of crowding and poor hygiene. The incubation period is one to two months. The virus, of the RNA type, appears to proliferate in the cytoplasm of hepatocytes. The symptoms are fever, anorexia, nausea, and vomiting. The liver enlarges, the abdomen is tender, and lymphadenopathy develops. Jaundice appears, bile darkens the urine, and viral particles may be identified in the stool. The illness ordinarily subsides spontaneously six to eight weeks after the onset of jaundice. During this time a serum antibody develops that confers lifelong immunity. An exposed person may be protected from the infection by passive transfer of convalescent serum. The disease is worldwide in distribution and occurs almost entirely in humans. Oysters and clams concentrate the virus, and ingestion of these uncooked mollusks may transmit the disease.[11] Human carriers are rare.

HBV disease, or serum hepatitis, is somewhat different. Inoculation takes place through the skin, the incubation period is longer, two to six months, and the disease affects adults more often than children. The illness is severer than HAV disease. The virus, called a Dane particle after its discoverer, consists of an outer envelope and an inner core. The envelope is composed of a surface antigen ($HB_sAg$) that is abundant and appears in the serum, and the illness can be specifically diagnosed by means of the antigen. The core, composed of DNA, infects the nuclei of hepatocytes. Inflammation of the liver develops and massive necrosis may follow. The illness is transmitted by the sharing of needles among drug abusers and by the pooling of blood components for transfusion. The pathologic stages vary from slight to pronounced and are indistinguishable from those of HAV disease. Asymptomatic human carriers of the virus are common, and progression to a stage of subclinical but chronic disease is often observed. Active immunity is conferred by the inoculation of heated $HB_sAg$. Both chronic active hepatitis and acute fulminant hepatitis may lead to coarse scarring of the liver, i.e., postnecrotic cirrhosis.[12,13] Viral hepatitis was reviewed by Melnick and colleagues.[14]

Cirrhosis is the premier disease of the liver. It is the seventh most common cause of death in the United States.[15] The word comes from the Greek *kirrhos*, meaning "orange-colored," "yellowish," or "tawny." Although Laënnec selected this term because of the unique color of the livers he observed, common morphologic features provide a more practical definition. Cirrhosis is a chronic progressive inflammation of the liver characterized by degeneration of hepatocytes, regeneration of hepatocytes,

and fibrosis. These changes are widespread and often uniform. The degeneration may be accompanied by necrosis, the regeneration tends to be nodular, and the fibrosis ranges from fine, diffuse, interlobular strands to massive scars irregularly spread throughout the organ.

Although this triad of changes is common to all, different kinds of cirrhosis exist. No classification is altogether satisfactory. The reason is that a given cause does not always produce the same kind of cirrhosis, and sometimes the cause is not evident at all (cryptogenic cirrhosis). Moreover, intermediate types obscure any single morphologic pattern. The Fifth Havana Conference nevertheless identified three distinct morphologic types: portal, postnecrotic, and biliary.[16] More recent classifications, relying mainly on etiology, seem not to simplify matters.[17,18] Biliary cirrhosis is divided into a primary type, in which the obstruction is within the small bile ductules, and a secondary type, in which the obstruction is at the hilum or outside the liver within the large bile ducts.

Portal cirrhosis is the most frequent. It is also known as alcoholic nutritional or Laënnec's cirrhosis. The term "micronodular" is sometimes used but is not recommended. Portal cirrhosis is the result of restructuring of injured tissue. The injury is due to undernutrition, alcoholism, or both. Each, however, may injure the hepatic tissue independently of the other. For example, cirrhosis develops after ileal bypass without alcoholism, and it arises in primates given alcohol and a nutritious diet.[18,19] Portal cirrhosis is common because alcohol is popular in American society, and the incidence of cirrhosis is proportional to alcohol consumption.[19] Ten to 30 per cent of alcoholics are said to develop cirrhosis.[20] In some cases, however, the lesion develops without alcoholism or other known cause.

The earliest change is steatosis, which may become pronounced, and on this ac-

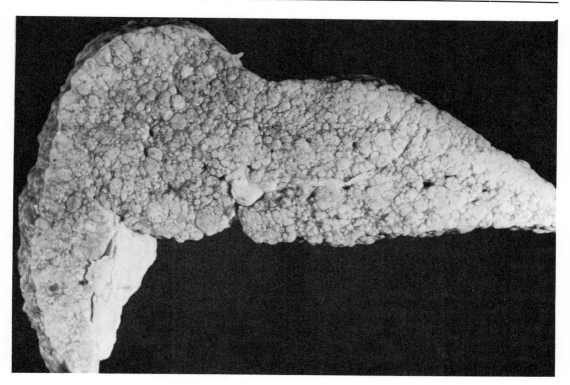

**Figure 14-6.** Cut surface of Laënnec's cirrhosis of liver. Also shown in color section, p C-5.

count the liver is almost always enlarged in the beginning. "Ballooning degeneration" of hepatic cells develops, necrosis follows, and neutrophilic infiltration signals the development of acute alcoholic hepatitis. A protein material of uncertain nature accumulates in the hepatocytes to form the so-called Mallory bodies, which are characteristic but not pathognomonic of alcoholic injury. The clinical manifestations of this stage include fever, leukocytosis, and jaundice with elevation of liver transaminases. The first connective tissue change is pericentral fibrosis.[19] This alters the lobular structure and is followed by portal scarring so that cirrhosis begins. Regeneration of hepatocytes is indicated by nuclear enlargement and binucleate forms. The cells proliferate in small nodules between the fibrous septa. As the connective tissue contracts, the liver gradually shrinks and eventually becomes a small, scarred, micronodular structure. Some of the nodules fuse while others succumb, so that macronodulation does not connote a different type of cirrhosis. At some undefined point in this sequence irreversibility develops, and from that time forward therapy cannot stop the progression of the disease. Cirrhosis is thus the scarred end stage of a chronic inflammation of the liver. The cut surface appearance is shown in Figure 14-6 (see color section, p C-5).

The microcirculation of the lobules is vastly altered by the bands of connective tissue that extend between the lobules and within them. The nodules of regenerating hepatocytes and the periportal scars compress the central veins so that the flow of blood through the liver is obstructed. In

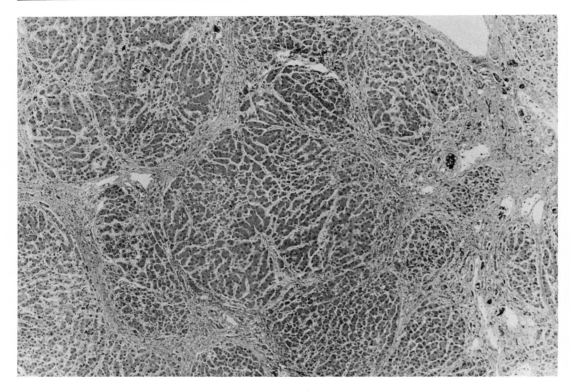

**Figure 14-7.** Scarring and nodular regeneration of cirrhotic liver

addition, the hepatic arteries and portal veins shunt blood into the hepatic veins so that the sinusoids are bypassed and the hepatocytes are increasingly deprived of a blood supply.[21] On this account the liver gradually fails. Indeed, these vascular changes are the key feature of cirrhosis and the main target of therapeutic efforts. Periportal scarring is shown in Figure 14-7.

The consequences of these morphologic alterations may be classified as due to portal obstruction, hypersplenism, or liver failure. Portal obstruction causes the intralobular pressure to rise; the production of lymph increases, and transudation into the peritoneum causes ascites to form.[22] In addition, lymph flow in the thoracic duct increases and the vessel dilates. Blood pressure also rises in the obstructed portal vein, which forces open portasystemic anastomoses especially in the form of

esophageal varices, hemorrhoids, and a caput medusae. The spleen tends to be large and is usually palpable. Hypersplenism is evidenced by anemia, leukopenia, and thrombocytopenia. Thrombocytopenia contributes to a bleeding tendency, as also does failure of the liver to produce clotting factors. Jaundice develops, with a serum bilirubin composed of conjugated and unconjugated pigment. As the intrahepatic circulation is shunted past the hepatocytes, hormonal metabolism falters and estrogens from the adrenal cortex in males are not inactivated in the liver. On this account body hair diminishes, the testes atrophy, and gynecomastia develops. Fetor hepaticus arises as products of the intestine in the portal venous system bypass the liver and gain the systemic circulation. Hepatic encephalopathy, with a wide range of neurologic manifestations, also reflects failure of

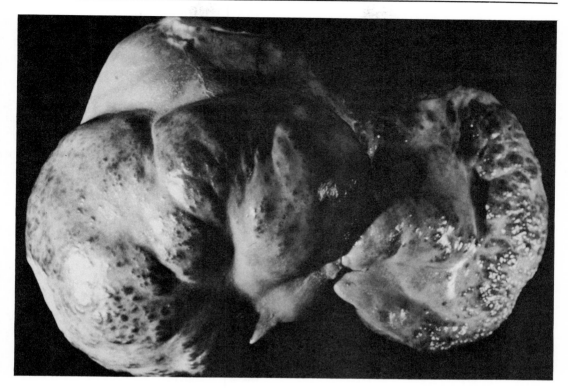

**Figure 14-8.** The coarse, irregular scars of postnecrotic cirrhosis

the liver to metabolize protein. For this reason esophageal hemorrhage, which releases extra protein into the gut, is associated with hepatic coma: Bacteria in the intestine produce nitrogenous substances that are not detoxified in the liver. Unexplained clinical features are vascular "spiders" over the face, chest, and upper arms, and palmar erythema, or "liver palms."

The outlook is, of course, unfavorable as soon as the irreversible stage has been passed. Abstinence from alcohol and surgical shunting of portal blood into the inferior vena cava are helpful therapeutic measures. Nevertheless, approximately 85 per cent of patients die within five years of the time of diagnosis. The three main causes are esophageal hemorrhage, intercurrent infection, and liver failure. Infrequent causes are spontaneous peritonitis and hepatocellular carcinoma.[23],[24]

The second main form of cirrhosis is the postnecrotic type. It is characterized by massive, irregular scarring (Figure 14-8). The regenerating nodules are frequently large, more than 2 cm in diameter, so that postnecrotic cirrhosis is sometimes termed "macronodular." This is inadvisable because the nodules of portal cirrhosis may also become large and the term then fails to distinguish one from the other. The distinctive features of postnecrotic cirrhosis are the width and irregular distribution of the scars. The wide scars represent massive foci of necrosis with disappearance of hepatocytes, collapse of stroma, and gradual conversion of the injury to fibrous connective tissue. Intervening portions of parenchyma may show micronodular scarring. Diagnosis by needle biopsy is somewhat unreliable; precision requires observation of the whole organ.

Clinical manifestations are jaundice, ascites, hematemesis, and abdominal pain. These often are not preceded by an illness suggestive of viral hepatitis. In a series of 221 patients only 24 per cent had had a previous episode of jaundice.[25] Half the patients were alcoholics, half developed esophageal varices, and laboratory tests were not useful in determining the specific kind of cirrhosis. Fourteen per cent, however, developed primary hepatocellular carcinoma. When this happened, the serum alkaline phosphatase tended to rise and the ascitic fluid often became bloody. The outlook after a portacaval shunt is the same as for portal or biliary cirrhosis.[26]

The third main kind of cirrhosis is biliary, which is divided into primary and secondary forms. Both are due to prolonged obstruction to the flow of bile, and both are slow to develop, with months intervening between the onset of the jaundice and the formation of the cirrhosis. In both also the livers are dark green and the cirrhosis is periportal and micronodular. In the primary form the bile ducts are inconspicuous whereas in the secondary form they are large and dilated. The obstruction in the primary form appears to be in the interlobular bile ducts, which display intense, nonsuppurative, chronic inflammation.[27] The condition occurs predominantly in dark-complected, middle-aged women. Patients experience pruritus and a gradually deepening jaundice accompanied by hepatosplenomegaly, xanthomas of the skin, and markedly elevated levels of serum cholesterol and lipids. The most discriminating laboratory value is a positive serum mitochondrial antibody reaction. Microscopically bile retention is evident, the number of bile ductules is decreased, and in about a third of cases nonspecific granulomas occur in the periportal fibrous tissue. Although the cause of the obstructive inflammation is not known, the serum antimitochondrial reaction suggests some kind of immunologic disturbance.

Secondary biliary cirrhosis is due to extrahepatic obstruction of the common bile duct. The usual causes are stricture, gallstones, and neoplasms. A recent history of biliary surgery is suggestive of stricture. Ascending cholangitis tends to develop. On this account the clinical manifestations often include fever, chills, leukocytosis, and pain in the right upper quadrant of the abdomen. Hyperlipidemia is also present, and xanthomas of the skin may develop. The serum antimitochondrial reaction, however, is negative. The liver is remarkable for its dark green cut surface and the pronounced dilation of the bile ducts. Microscopic examination discloses proliferation of bile ductules in the periportal scar tissue and often leukocytes about the dilated biliary channels. Ascites and esophageal varices form less frequently than with portal cirrhosis. Unless the obstruction is relieved, death occurs from liver failure and septicemia.

Hemochromatosis also causes a distinctive cirrhosis. In this disorder, which affects men in the 40- to 60-year age group, excessive amounts of iron are deposited in tissues, especially the liver and pancreas. The total body iron may be 20 to 50 times greater than the normal amount of 3.5 gm. The cause is not clear although some forms are due to an inborn metabolic error.[28] The consequence of the iron deposition is pigmentation and fibrosis. The liver is large with a brownish-red cut surface, and the pattern of fibrosis is like that of portal cirrhosis. The Prussian blue reaction reveals abundant hemosiderin granules in hepatocytes, Kupffer cells, epithelium of bile ducts, and fibrocytes of the periportal scars (Figure 14-9). The pancreas undergoes atrophy and fibrosis, the cut surface is rusty red, and hemosiderin deposition is pronounced in both endocrine and exocrine cells. The skin is discolored slate gray from iron deposition, or brownish-red (bronze) from melanin pigmentation. The characteristic clinical triad is cirrhosis, diabetes mel-

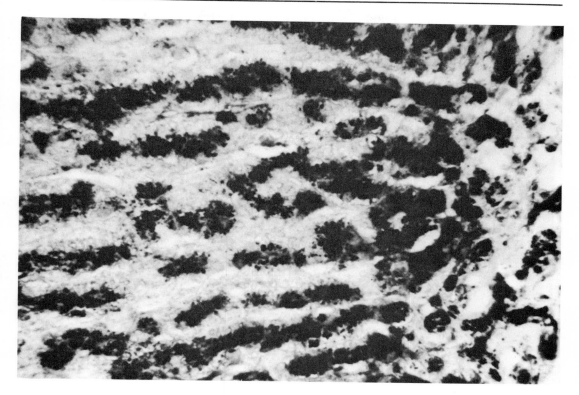

**Figure 14-9.** Prussian blue reaction showing hemosiderin granules in hepatocytes in hemochromatosis

litus, and pigmentation of the skin (bronze diabetes). The course is prolonged, and death eventually results from hepatic failure or esophageal hemorrhage. Primary carcinoma is said to arise in about 15 per cent of patients.[5]

## Tumors

Hemangiomas and adenomas are the benign tumors of the liver. Hemangiomas are frequent, multiple, and of little clinical importance. Adenomas are uncommon and may be related to the ingestion of oral contraceptives, although this point is disputed.[29] They occasionally rupture and cause significant peritoneal hemorrhage.

The common malignant tumors of the liver are carcinomas of hepatocytes and of bile ducts. Three-fourths are hepatocellular, while the remainder are cholangiocarcino-

mas or mixed. Between 3 and 10 per cent of patients with cirrhosis develop cancer of the liver, and of livers with cancer, 60 to 90 per cent are cirrhotic.[30] Portal cirrhosis is the most frequent precursor. The proportion of cancers is higher in both the postnecrotic and pigmentary (hemochromatosis) forms. The cause is unknown, although contamination of food with aflatoxin may account for the high incidence of liver cancer in Africa.[31] Schistosomiasis and liver flukes may have the same effect in Asia.

Characteristic symptoms are abdominal pain, intermittent fever, and weight loss. Signs include hepatomegaly, jaundice, and ascites. Blood-tinged ascitic fluid in a patient with cirrhosis is especially suggestive. The tumors display three gross patterns: a single large mass, usually in the right lobe; a nodular form evenly distribut-

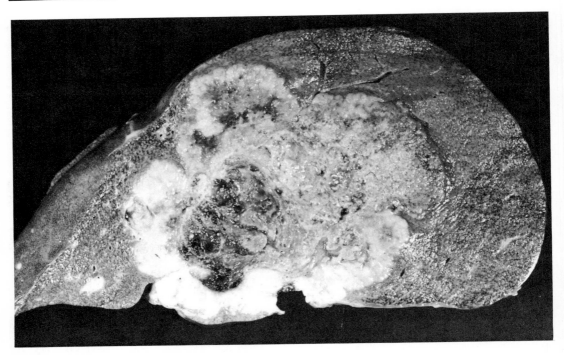

**Figure 14-10.** Primary carcinoma of liver

ed throughout all lobes; and a diffuse pattern in which the gross diagnosis is not evident. The nodular form is most frequent. The cut surface of a primary liver cell cancer is shown in Figure 14-10. The tumor cells are polygonal and resemble hepatocytes. Extension into branches of the portal vein is frequent, and metastases are most common in regional lymph nodes and the lungs. Cholangiocarcinomas are similar clinically and grossly and are composed of cuboidal cells that produce mucin. These cancers arise more often in noncirrhotic livers. Resection has been recommended for localized cancers of either type. The mean survival in one series of 64 cases of widespread tumor was 3.8 months after the diagnosis was established.[31]

## THE EXTRAHEPATIC BILIARY SYSTEM

The extrahepatic biliary system consists of the right and left hepatic ducts, which merge at the porta hepatis to form the main hepatic duct; the cystic duct, which leads to a blind diverticulum; the gallbladder; and the common bile duct, which proceeds from the junction of the cystic duct to the duodenum. The opening into the duodenum is at the ampulla of Vater, 7 to 10 cm distal to the pyloric ring. The function of this system is to collect bile from the liver, concentrate it in the gallbladder, and deliver it into the duodenum. Bile is 97 per cent water and 3 per cent solids. The main solid components are bilirubin, cholesterol, lecithin, mucus, and the sodium salts of taurocholic and glycocholic acids. Bile salts and lecithin tend to keep cholesterol in solution. Gastric contents in the duodenum, especially fatty foods, cause release of a hormone from the duodenal mucosa (cholecystokinin) that stimulates the gallbladder to contract. Bile then flows down the cystic duct into the common duct, and thence into the duodenum. The capacity of the gallbladder is about 50 ml, and it is able to concentrate the bile to 1/10 its original volume by selective absorption of water and bile acids.[32] In over half of persons the pancreatic duct opens into the common bile duct just before it reaches the duodenum; in the remainder it opens separately into the duodenum at the papilla of Vater.

The main pathologic processes of the extrahepatic biliary system are concretions, inflammation, and tumors. It is estimated that 12 million women and 4 million men in the United States have gallstones.[33] The stones form in the gallbladder and most are asymptomatic. They are composed mainly of a mixture of cholesterol, calcium bilirubinate, and calcium carbonate. The stones are small, smooth, and black, and often number in the hundreds. They form because of stagnation, infection, or abnormal bile composition due to faulty bile production by the liver or to excessive absorption of water and bile acids by the gallbladder.[34] Stones of calcium bilirubinate tend to form as a consequence of conditions such as sickle cell anemia, thalassemia major, and congenital spherocytic anemia. When a stone passes into the cystic duct and obstructs it, or into the common duct with the same effect, symptoms arise. This occurs four times more often in women than in men, usually after the age of 40, and especially in women who have borne babies and are overweight. Obstruction of the cystic duct causes intense pain in the right upper quadrant of the abdomen that is often spasmodic (biliary colic) and is associated with fever, leukocytosis, nausea, and vomiting. The abdomen may be tense but jaundice does not develop. The gallbladder becomes distended, the wall is edematous and hyperemic, and the serosa is covered with fibrin. The mucosa ulcerates and the infected wall is infiltrated with neutrophilic leukocytes. The organisms are mainly staphylococci and coliform bacteria. The lumen is filled with blood, bile, and pus, which is known as empyema of the gallbladder. Surgical re-

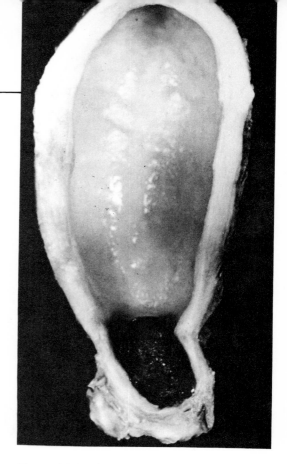

**Figure 14-11.** Cholelithiasis with chronic cholecystitis and fibrosis of gallbladder wall

moval is curative. Without removal the inflammation may subside, chronic cholecystitis may develop, or complications may arise. If the reaction subsides and the obstruction persists, the content of the lumen is absorbed and the re-formed mucosa secretes a colorless mucoprotein that fills and eventually distends the gallbladder to form hydrops of that structure. It can be diagnosed by ultrasound.[35] If the inflammation becomes chronic, fibrosis of the wall develops and distention of the gallbladder is no longer possible (Figure 14-11). The complications include perforation with pericholic abscess, subdiaphragmatic abscess, diffuse peritonitis, septicemia, or cholecystointestinal fistula with passage of concretions into the ileum or colon. If the stone is large and passes into the ileum, impaction at the ileocecal junction may cause intestinal obstruction, or gallstone ileus.

An obstructing stone in the common duct is attended by similar clinical events, although jaundice develops and tends to be intermittent as one stone passes and another takes its place. The serum bilirubin is conjugated, the stool loses its color, and the urine darkens as water-soluble pigment is passed. The complications of common-duct obstruction are also similar, with the additional possibilities of ascending cholangitis, abscess formation in the liver, and biliary cirrhosis if the common-duct obstruction persists. Finally, a concretion at the papilla of Vater may also block the pancreatic duct and thus be associated with acute hemorrhagic pancreatitis.

It is often clinically difficult to distinguish a stone in the common duct from a carcinoma of the head of the pancreas because both cause biliary obstruction. However, stones are frequently associated with chronic cholecystitis, so that the gallbladder will not dilate, whereas carcinoma of the pancreas is not associated with a fibrotic gallbladder and the gallbladder will dilate under the pressure of the obstruction. Therefore obstructive jaundice with a palpable gallbladder is more likely to be the result of cancer of the head of the pancreas than to be due to a stone in the common duct. This rule, known as Courvoisier's law, has many exceptions.

Acute cholecystitis may also occur in the absence of concretions and is due to chemical irritation from overconcentrated bile, infection, or reflux of pancreatic secretions. Chronic cholecystitis may also arise without known cause. It produces a vague illness of long duration that is characterized by abdominal discomfort, intolerance of fatty foods, frequent eructations, and transient biliary colic. Cholecystography reveals the concretions or a nonfunctioning gallbladder.

Cholesterolosis is yellow flecking of the mucosa from the accumulation of lipid-laden macrophages beneath the basement membrane. The condition does not have any clinical significance and is not associated with hypercholesterolemia.

Tumors occur in the gallbladder and bile ducts. The benign lesions are papillomas and adenomas, which are infrequent and clinically silent.[36] The malignant tumors are scirrhous, well-differentiated adenocarcinomas that fungate into the lumen of the gallbladder, massively invade the attached right lobe of the liver, or encircle the common duct and obstruct it. Tumors of these kinds are encountered in something over 1 per cent of biliary operations.[37] The outlook is poor because metastases to the liver and regional lymph nodes often precede the development of clinical signs.

## THE PANCREAS

The pancreas is a retroperitoneal organ of the upper abdomen. Its head nestles into the C loop of the duodenum, the body crosses the spine, and the tail extends to the hilum of the spleen. The organ normally weighs 60 to 120 gm and consists of exocrine and endocrine parts. Exocrine glands are arranged in lobules that secrete digestive enzymes into ductules that merge to form the pancreatic duct of Wirsung, which opens into the duodenum at the ampulla of Vater or joins the common bile duct just before it opens into the duodenum. The enzymes are trypsin, lipase, amylase, elastase, and phospholipase. They are secreted in a precursor form and activated in the duodenum by enterokinase. The endocrine part consists of the islets of Langerhans, which have no ducts and secrete directly into capillaries. Islets are composed of $\alpha$, $\beta$, and $\delta$ cells, which respectively secrete glucagon, insulin, and perhaps gastrin. The main pathologic reactions of the exocrine portion are cystic fibrosis, chronic calcifying inflammation, acute necrotizing inflammation, and carcinoma. The principal pathologic reactions of the endocrine portion are diabetes mellitus and tumors of the islet cells.

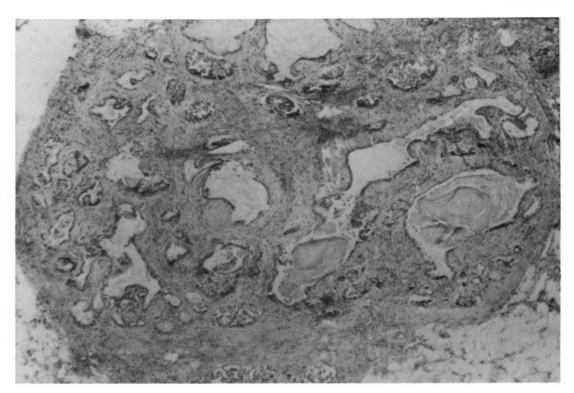

**Figure 14-12.** Cystic fibrosis of pancreas with atrophy, fibrosis, and dilated ducts filled with inspissated secretions

## Exocrine glands

Cystic fibrosis is an inherited disorder of exocrine glands in which the two central changes are a mucous secretion that is abnormally viscous and sweat secretion that is abnormally salty. The sweat glands are structurally normal, but the high concentration of sodium chloride leads to salt depletion, and occasionally to heat prostration. The mucous glands are abnormal; their viscous secretions will not flow through the ductules or other outflow channels, so that obstruction is gradually followed by dilation, atrophy, and fibrosis. Since the condition is hereditary, it is present in utero, and on this account the intestinal mucus forms into a black, solid, ropy cord that will not pass. The consequences are intestinal obstruction in the newborn, known as meconium ileus, and, later, rectal

prolapse from straining at stool to pass the viscous material. From infancy to young adulthood, the main pathologic changes develop in the pancreas, liver, and especially the lungs. The sequence is again obstruction, dilation, atrophy, and fibrosis. Atrophy of the pancreas becomes so pronounced that diabetes mellitus may develop, and failure of pancreatic enzymes to reach the intestine causes malabsorption, diarrhea, and weight loss.[38] The histologic appearance is shown in Figure 14-12. In the liver, bile ducts are obstructed by mucous plugs so that cholestasis arises and biliary cirrhosis may develop. The most conspicuous changes, however, take place in the lungs, where the bronchial mucous glands become blocked, squamous metaplasia follows, and chronic bronchitis often progresses to bronchiectasis. There is also mucous plugging of peripheral airways so that emphysema develops.[39] The pulmonary reaction dominates the clinical events and largely determines the outlook.

Cystic fibrosis is the most common lethal genetic disease of Caucasians. It was recognized as an entity in 1936.[40] At that time the term applied to the pancreas. When it was learned that mucous glands throughout the body are affected, the term mucoviscidosis was proposed. In 1953, however, Sant'Agnese showed that serous and sweat glands are also affected so that the term cystic fibrosis regained favor and now prevails.[41] The condition is inherited as an autosomal recessive mendelian trait. Heterozygotes are unaffected, and no method of identifying them has been found.[39] Carriers number one in 20, or about 5 per cent of the Caucasian population. Only homozygotes develop the disease, and their frequency in the population is between one in 1,500 and one in 2,000.

The condition affects the sexes equally and is virtually limited to Caucasians. The principal clinical manifestations are recurrent pulmonary infections, malnutrition, and growth failure. The diagnosis is easily overlooked, however, because the onset varies from infancy to young adulthood, different anatomic systems may be affected, and the severity of symptoms is markedly variable. Nevertheless, the sweat as collected by pilocarpine stimulation regularly reveals increased sodium and chloride, a finding diagnostic of the condition. Therapy consists of antibiotics, pancreatic enzymes, postural drainage, and aerosols to loosen the mucous plugs in the bronchi. Although the outlook has been improved, the diagnosis is extremely serious: 50 per cent of patients die before reaching the age of 21 years, and 95 per cent of deaths are due to pulmonary complications.[39, 42]

Inflammations of the pancreas range from trivial to calamitous. Two forms stand out: recurrent calcifying pancreatitis and acute necrotizing pancreatitis. Recurrent calcifying pancreatitis tends to be a "hidden disease" because the pancreas is covered on one surface by the posterior body wall and on the other by the stomach and transverse colon. Therefore the organ cannot be palpated and epigastric symptoms are easily ascribed to other structures. Recurring pancreatitis is due to precipitation of protein secretions within the ducts.[43] The cause is not certain, but most cases are associated with alcoholism or liver disease. Alcohol stimulates the pancreas to secrete its enzymes and the sphincter of Oddi to contract. Intraductal stagnation then develops, proteins precipitate, and these inspissated masses gradually calcify so that they may become visible on an abdominal X-ray. The concretions consist of calcium carbonate and are scattered throughout the ducts. Pancreatitis follows ductal obstruction, and recurrences follow repeated bouts of alcoholism. Repair of the foci of inflammation leads to extensive atrophy and fibrosis so that the pancreas is gradually reduced to a firm, fibrous cord one-sixth the normal size. The cut surface appearance is shown in Figure 14-13. The endocrine portions are eventually affected. The characteristic clinical features are thus abdominal pain, diabetes mellitus, steatorrhea, and calcification of the pancreas.[44] Many patients also have cirrhosis, although ascites is uncommon. However, rupture of a dilated duct may release enzymes into the peritoneum with the formation of massive "pancreatic ascites." The diagnosis is indicated by a nontender abdomen and an extremely high amylase content with over 3 gm of protein per deciliter of fluid.[45] Surgical drainage of the ruptured duct is sometimes possible, and cannulation of the thoracic duct has been helpful.[46]

Acute necrotizing pancreatitis is a catastrophic illness of sudden onset characterized by constant, severe pain in the epigastrium that often radiates to the back and is associated with nausea, vomiting, jaundice, shock, and collapse.[47] It affects adults of

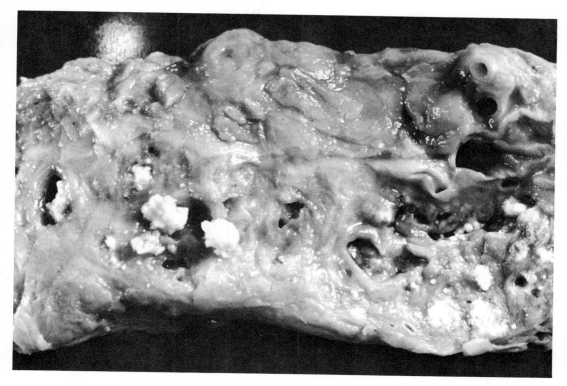

**Figure 14-13.** Calculi in ducts of pancreas of alcoholic patient

either sex, especially the 40- to 70-year age group, and the onset often follows a large meal rich in fats and intemperate use of alcohol. The diagnosis is indicated by a high serum amylase and lipase early in the course of the illness. Grossly the pancreas is edematous, hemorrhagic, and massively necrotic (Figure 14-14). Yellowish-gray foci of fat necrosis affect the peripancreatic adipose tissue and spread throughout the omentum and mesentery. A slightly turbid peritoneal effusion containing abundant free fat droplets forms. Necrosis of arteries with rupture accounts for the hemorrhage, which is occasionally massive. Bacteria reach the peritoneum from blood or necrotic tissue and often cause suppuration, including localized subdiaphragmatic abscess and diffuse acute suppurative peritonitis. The mortality is about 25 per cent.[47] With survival, pseudocyst formation is frequent.

The pseudocysts measure up to 15 cm in diameter, the chambers are lined with granulation tissue that matures to a fibrous margin, and the lumen is filled with exudate and fragments of necrotic debris. Most pseudocysts subside spontaneously, some require surgical drainage, and a few leak into the peritoneum and cause recurrent ascites.[48]

Seventy to 90 per cent of cases are associated with biliary calculi, alcoholism, or trauma.[49] Most of the rest are due to mumps, hypercalcemia, or certain drugs, especially adrenal corticosteroids.[50] By ductal obstruction with reflux of bile, introduction of bacteria, or induced transition of precursor enzymes to active forms (hypercalcemia), proteolytic and lipolytic enzymes are activated and begin the process of pancreatic autodigestion. Elastase digests arteries and causes hemorrhage. Trypsin

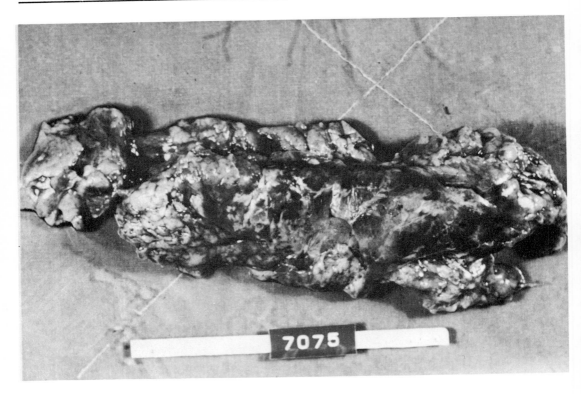

**Figure 14-14.** Acute necrotizing pancreatitis

digests protein. Lipase hydrolyzes triglycerides to fatty acids and glycerol. The glycerol is absorbed, and the fatty acids combine with calcium to form calcium "soaps" (saponification). On this account a low serum calcium is one other characteristic clinical finding. Treatment is symptomatic, although surgical relief of a ductal obstruction may be helpful.

Carcinoma of the exocrine pancreas now ranks as the fourth most common fatal cancer in the United States. It is exceeded in frequency only by tumors of the lung, colon, and breast. The incidence in the whole population is about 10/100,000. The cancer affects men twice as often as women. It is uncommon under 45 years; most cases arise after age 60. Although the cause is not known, the incidence is increased in persons who smoke cigarettes, have diabetes, or eat foods rich in cholesterol and pro-

tein.[51] The cancer is not more frequent, however, in patients with pancreatitis. Methylnitrosourea and other nitroso compounds cause the cancer in experimental animals.

Two-thirds of the tumors arise in the head of the pancreas, with the remainder scattered about the body and tail. All are white, firm, densely fibrous, and poorly demarcated. The gross cut surface is shown in Figure 14-15 (see color section, p C-5). The tumors arise from ductal epithelium, mucin is secreted, and nearly all are adenocarcinomas. An occasional adenoacanthoma (mixed glandular and squamous cells) and a rare squamous-cell carcinoma may occur. The duct of the pancreas is obstructed as it passes through the tumor, and the tissue proximal to the obstruction shows ductal dilation with atrophy and fibrosis of the adjacent parenchyma. Cancers of the head

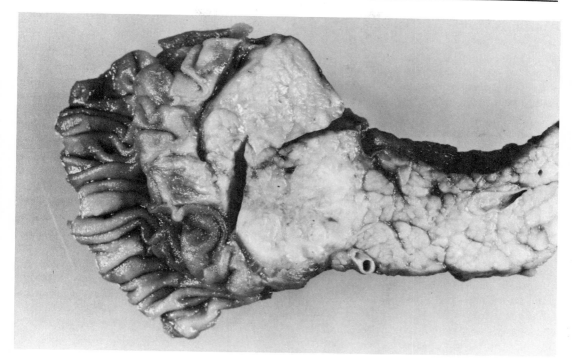

**Figure 14-15.** Duodenal mucosa (left), carcinoma of head of pancreas (center), and normal pancreas with dilated duct of Wirsung cut obliquely (right). Also shown in color section, p C-5.

of the pancreas also obstruct the common bile duct early in the course of the disease. Later the cancer spreads in the perineural lymphatics to the lymph nodes of the porta hepatis and invades the portal vein. The perineural spread may account for the abdominal pain. Death from biliary obstruction and metastatic disease in the liver occurs before wide dissemination takes place. For cancers of the body and tail, biliary obstruction is late but spread throughout the peritoneal cavity is early and extensive. For this reason death is often due to intestinal complications rather than to widespread metastatic disease.

The earliest symptom of pancreatic cancer is vague abdominal discomfort that tends to be neglected until anorexia, weight loss, jaundice, or abdominal pain develops. The abdominal symptom is a constant, progressive, dull ache in the epigastrium that is often referred to the back. Examination reveals jaundice, hepatomegaly, and tenderness of the abdomen. The gallbladder is often enlarged and palpable when the cancer is in the head (Courvoisier's law). In the body and tail, metastases are frequently found at the first examination; the sites include supraclavicular lymph nodes, a rectal shelf (Blumer's shelf), and the peritoneum with ascites formation. The cancer is extremely difficult to cure because spread is early, the initial symptoms are vague, and resection is limited by the importance of adjacent organs. Carcinoembryonic antigen has not proved reliable as a screening procedure, and detection by ultrasonography has not yet proved successful.[52] Improvement of diagnosis by coaxial tomography is under assessment.[53] Nevertheless, the only hope of cure is early detection and total surgical removal. The outlook is accordingly poor because removal of the stomach, pancreas, duodenum, and spleen is a formidable surgical undertaking. In a compilation of results the operative mortality was 21 per cent, only 4 per cent of patients survived five years, and nearly all died within six months of the time of diagnosis. This outlook is so grave that biliary bypass to relieve the cholestasis without any attempt to cure the cancer has been suggested to provide an equally good result.[54]

## Endocrine

Diabetes mellitus is a genetically determined disorder of carbohydrate metabolism. The primary disorder appears to be in the $\beta$ cells of the islets of Langerhans of the pancreas. The disorder causes a lack of insulin resulting in a metabolic derangement that may be controlled by injections of insulin or taking hypoglycemic agents by mouth. Even though the diabetes is controlled, however, tissue changes gradually take place, life tends to be shortened, and complications involve the kidneys, with renal failure; the eyes, with blindness; the nerves, with pain; and the arteries, with disabling or fatal thrombotic disease. The condition affects 2 to 4 per cent of the American public. Diabetes mellitus is therefore a common, serious, and extremely important disease.

The normal pancreas weighs 60 to 120 gm. One to 3 per cent of that weight consists of islets of Langerhans. The islets are composed of 20 to 30 per cent $\alpha$ cells, which secrete glucagon; 60 to 80 per cent $\beta$ cells, which secrete insulin; and 2 to 8 per cent $\delta$ cells, which secrete other hormones, possibly gastrin. In diabetes the $\beta$ cells produce either too little insulin or a normal amount. If they produce a normal amount, diabetes may be caused either by a defective release mechanism, by neutralization of the insulin emerging from the cell, or by an abnormality of the insulin that makes it functionally useless. Whatever the mechanism, diabetes is presumably due to a genetic fault within the $\beta$ cells. The mode of transmission of the heritable defect is not known.

Without insulin glucose metabolism is blocked, hyperglycemia develops, and glucosuria follows as the blood sugar surmounts the renal threshold and spills over into the urine. The hypertonic urine pulls water with it, so that dehydration develops and polydipsia follows. Protein catabolism is undertaken for gluconeogenesis, so that weakness and wasting develop despite a vigorous appetite. But because the glucose cannot be used, the body turns to its fat depots for a source of energy. Fats are stored mainly in the form of triglycerides, and these are hydrolyzed to glycerol and fatty acids. In the metabolism of fatty acids, acetoacetic acid is formed. Derivatives of this are acetone and $\beta$-hydroxybutyric acid. Acetone, diacetic acid, and $\beta$-hydroxybutyric acid are collectively known as ketone bodies. When fatty acid metabolism speeds up, large amounts of these ketone bodies are produced, and their accumulation in the blood causes ketosis. Since two of the ketone bodies are acids, diabetic acidosis also develops. The urine of an untreated diabetic thus reveals glucose and acetone as well as diacetic and $\beta$-hydroxybutyric acids. The clinical manifestations of diabetic ketoacidosis are dehydration with dry mucous membranes, deep, sighing Kussmaul respirations to expel carbon dioxide and lessen the acidosis, and the odor of acetone on the breath. Without treatment the condition progresses to somnolence, coma, and eventually death.

Diabetes takes two main clinical forms. In the juvenile-onset form, or type I, insulin-dependent diabetes, the disease begins during childhood, often abruptly, or before the age of 25 years. It is characterized by failure of the islet cells to produce insulin. This form is often difficult to control, complications tend to develop, and life may be shortened by as much as 20 to 25 years. The second form is maturity-onset or type

II, non-insulin-dependent diabetes, in which the process begins gradually, usually after the age of 40, and the metabolic disorder is easier to control. Usually oral hypoglycemics and diet suffice. Longevity is less limited in this form. The β cells produce sufficient insulin, but either the hormone cannot escape from the cell, it is defective, or it is neutralized on emergence from the cell. About 60 per cent of all diabetes is the maturity-onset form. Both insulin-dependent and non-insulin-dependent forms are hereditarily determined, with no genetic difference between them.

Although the genetic effect is evident, onset in both forms of the disease is also influenced by environmental factors such as trauma, infection, pregnancy, emotional stress, and especially obesity. Moreover, any of these conditions occurring in a diabetic worsens the disease and requires additional insulin for control. The diabetogenic nature of obesity is evidenced by the facts that a majority of maturity-onset diabetics are overweight and loss of weight tends to restore carbohydrate tolerance to normal.[55] Thus heredity and environment both play roles in the onset and progress of the disease.

Diabetes is classified according to six degrees of severity. The least severe is prediabetes, a theoretical form in which no disease is recognizable but the subject is an offspring of two diabetic parents and thus has a potential abnormality of glucose tolerance. The second is latent diabetes, in which a previously abnormal glucose tolerance curve is brought back to normal by weight reduction and/or elimination of stress. The third form is gestational diabetes, which develops or is first recognized in pregnancy. It carries a higher-than-normal risk of perinatal complications but almost always disappears at birth. The fourth is chemical or "borderline" diabetes, in which the glucose tolerance curve is abnormal only after meals. The most pronounced degrees are those of overt diabetes, types I

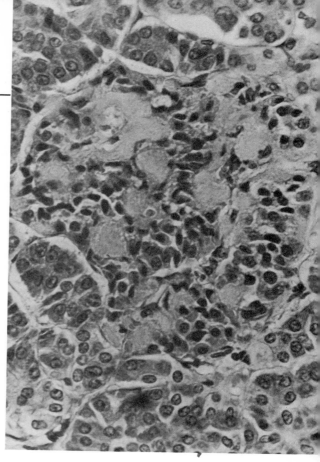

**Figure 14-16.** Amyloid infiltration of islets of Langerhans in diabetic patient

and II, in which hyperglycemia is present in the fasting state as well as after meals. It is in these last two conditions that tissue alterations are especially prominent and complications tend to develop.

In 20 per cent of cases of overt diabetes the pancreas is structurally normal. In the insulin-dependent portion of the other 80 per cent, the number of islets is reduced, the β cells are degranulated, and fibrosis or lymphocytic infiltration affects a part of the remaining islets. In the non-insulin-dependent form, however, the number of islets is normal but infiltration with amyloid replaces some of the β cells. This change is secondary, patchy, and characteristic of but not specific for diabetes mellitus. The islet changes in either clinical form of the disease correlate more with the duration of the condition than with the severity of the process. Amyloid infiltration of an islet is shown in Figure 14-16.

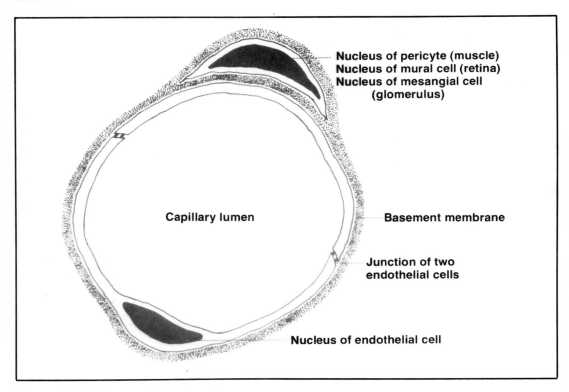

Labels on figure:
Nucleus of pericyte (muscle)
Nucleus of mural cell (retina)
Nucleus of mesangial cell (glomerulus)

Capillary lumen

Basement membrane

Junction of two endothelial cells

Nucleus of endothelial cell

**Figure 14-17.** Diagram of normal capillary

Outside the pancreas tissue changes are especially prominent in the kidneys, eyes, peripheral nerves, and medium-sized arteries. At most sites the underlying change is a "microangiopathy" consisting of thickening of the basement membranes of capillaries. The normal capillary is diagrammed in Figure 14-17. The supporting cell embedded in the basement membrane is called a pericyte in skeletal muscle, a mural cell in the retina of the eye, and a mesangial cell in a glomerulus of the kidney. It is not clear whether this cell or the endothelial cells of the capillary wall form or remove the substance of the basement membrane. In the kidney thickening of this layer results in diffuse or nodular thickening of the intercapillary portion of the glomerular tuft. Diffuse thickening is nonspecific, but nodular change is virtually diagnostic of diabetes (Figure 14-18). The nodular sclerosis gradually obliterates the glomerular capillaries and causes the Kimmelstiel-Wilson syndrome, which is characterized by hypertension, albuminuria, and subcutaneous edema. The second renal lesion characteristic of diabetes is necrosis of the tips of the renal papillae (Figure 14-19). This is a consequence of pyelonephritis and is associated with renal failure of abrupt onset. The presence of glycogen in the epithelial cells of the convoluted tubules is termed the Armanni-Ebstein lesion. It disappears with subsidence of the hyperglycemia.

In the retina focal loss of mural cells changes the pattern of capillary flow with subsequent development of microaneurysms. The reason for the mural cell loss is not clear. In addition to microaneurysms hemorrhages occur within the vitreous, and repair by granulation tissue often causes blindness.[56] Segmental demyelination of peripheral nerves is a cause of pain, especially in the extremities, as well as reflex changes that develop after diabetes has been prolonged.

Atherosclerosis is accelerated throughout the life of the diabetic, and the patient becomes especially prone to coronary thrombosis with myocardial infarction, strokes, and ischemic necrosis of the lower extremities. Myocardial infarction is twice as common, and ischemic necrosis of the feet and toes is considerably more common, in diabetics than in nondiabetics.[57] These effects of accelerated atherosclerosis, in association with such complications as renal failure, ketoacidosis, and a tendency to infections, shorten life. In one tabulation the life expectancy for male and female diabetics was shortened by 9.1 and 6.7 years as compared with nondiabetics.[58] The topic of diabetes has been admirably essayed by Lacy and Kissane.[59]

Tumors of the islet cells are uncommon, and those of $\alpha$ cells, which secrete glucagon, are rare. The two common tumors are those of $\beta$ cells, which secrete insulin, and

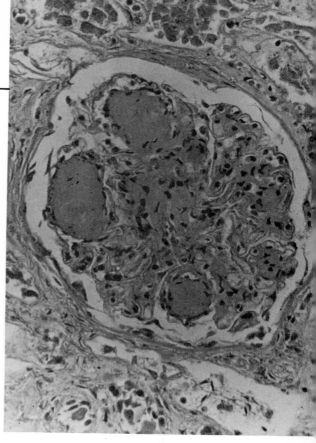

Figure 14-18. Nodular intercapillary glomerulosclerosis characteristic of diabetes mellitus and the lesion associated with the Kimmelstiel-Wilson syndrome

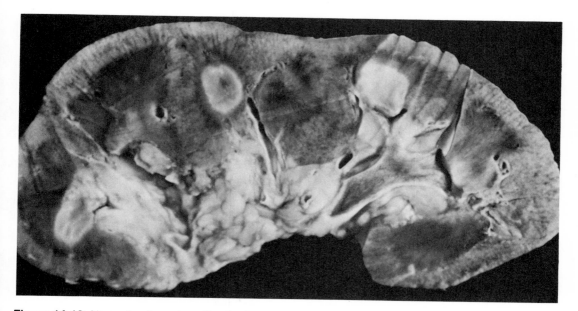

Figure 14-19. Necrosis of renal papillae in diabetic with acute pyelonephritis

those of δ cells, which may secrete gastrin. β-Cell tumors, or insulinomas, cause hypoglycemia, and δ-cell tumors, which increase the secretion of gastrin, cause the Zollinger-Ellison syndrome.

The clinical manifestations of an insulinoma are hypoglycemia that tends to become evident before meals and is manifested by disturbances of consciousness due to neuroglycopenia. The reaction may be brought on by fasting and is abolished by oral or intravenous glucose. The blood glucose is, of course, low. The diagnosis is established by demonstrating hyperinsulinemia by radioimmunoassay at the time of the reaction. The tumors causing this condition are usually single, occur in any part of the pancreas, and often measure less than 1 cm in diameter. The cells are small, cuboidal, and arranged in clusters without noticeable anaplasia even though malignancy is frequent. In fact, metastases are present in 10 to 15 per cent of cases at the time of diagnosis.[60] Although the tumors are often diffi-cult to locate, surgical excision is the favored method of treatment.

In 1955 Zollinger and Ellison described two patients with non-β-cell tumors that were associated with pronounced gastric hyperacidity and intractable peptic ulcerations.[61] The condition became known as the Zollinger-Ellison syndrome. The tumors are small, often multiple, and frequently malignant, although the rate of growth is extremely slow. The gastric acidity may be 20 times normal, and the ulcers are often found in unusual locations such as the second and third parts of the duodenum or beyond the ligament of Treitz. Patients complain of severe ulcer pain and upper gastrointestinal hemorrhage. Diarrhea, perforation, and hyperparathyroidism are frequent accompaniments of the condition. The type of islet cell causing the tumor is uncertain, but gastrin is secreted and hypergastrinemia as determined by radioimmunoassay is diagnostic. Gastrectomy is the treatment of choice.[60]

## REFERENCES

1. Kramer K, Kuller L, Eisher R: The increasing mortality attributed to cirrhosis and fatty liver in Baltimore (1957-1966). *Ann Intern Med* 69:273, 1968

2. Levy M, Polliack A, Lender M, et al: The liver in amyloidosis. *Digestion* 10:40, 1974

3. Seeley TT, Blumenfeld CM, Ikeda R, et al: Hepatic infarction. *Hum Pathol* 3:265, 1972

4. Cerra FB, Nolan JP, Upson JR: Cruveilhier-Baumgarten disease with associated splenic artery aneurysms. *Am J Dig Dis* 22:559, 1977

5. Schiff L: *Diseases of the Liver*, 4th ed, p 1359. Philadelphia: Lippincott, 1975

6. Parker RGF: Occlusion of the hepatic veins in man. *Medicine* 38:369, 1959

7. Wu SM, Spurny OM, Klotz AP: Budd-Chiari syndrome after taking oral contraceptives. A case report and review of 14 reported cases. *Am J Dig Dis* 22:623, 1977

8. Albert LI: Veno-occlusive disease of the liver associated with oral contraceptives: Case report and review of the literature. *Hum Pathol* 7:709, 1976

9. Tandon RK, Tandon BN, Tandon HD, et al: Study of an epidemic of venoocclusive disease in India. *Gut* 17:849, 1976

10. Maddrey WC, Boitnott JK: Isoniazid hepatitis. *Ann Intern Med* 79:1, 1973

11. Dougherty WJ, Altman R: Viral hepatitis in New Jersey 1960-1961. *Am J Med* 32:704, 1962

12. Boyer JL, Klatskin G: Pattern of necrosis in acute viral hepatitis. Prognostic value of bridging (subacute hepatic necrosis). *N Engl J Med* 283:1063, 1970

13. Baggenstoss AH, Soloway RD, Summerskill WHJ, et al: Chronic active liver disease. The range of histologic lesions, their response to treatment, and evolution. *Hum Pathol* 3:183, 1972

14. Melnick JL, Hollinger FB, Dreesman GR: Recent advances in viral hepatitis. *South Med J* 69:468, 634, 1976

15. Silverberg E: Cancer statistics, 1978. *CA—Cancer J Clin* 28:17, 1978

16. Fifth Pan-American Congress of Gastroenterology, La Habana, Cuba, January 20-27, 1956: Report of the Board for Classif ication and Nomenclature of Cirrhosis of the Liver. *Gastroenterology* 31:213, 1956

17. Galambos JT: Classification of cirrhosis. *Am J Gastroenterol* 64:437, 1975

18. Edmondson HA, Peters RL: Liver. In *Pathology

(Anderson WAD, Kissane JM, eds), 7th ed, vol 2, p 1333. St Louis: Mosby, 1977

19. Lieber CS: Pathogenesis and early diagnosis of alcoholic liver injury. *N Engl J Med* 298:888, 1978

20. Popper H: Pathologic aspects of cirrhosis. A review. *Am J Pathol* 87:228, 1977

21. Groszmann WJ, Kravetz D, Parysow O: Intrahepatic arteriovenous shunting in cirrhosis of the liver. *Gastroenterology* 73:201, 1977

22. Gibson J, Smith JC: The origin of ascites in experimental cirrhosis in the rat. *Am J Pathol* 41:535, 1962

23. Weinstein MP, Iannini PB, Stratton CW, et al: Spontaneous bacterial peritonitis. A review of 28 cases with emphasis on improved survival and factors influencing prognosis. *Am J Med* 64:592, 1978

24. Brancaccio M, Smith JC: Spontaneous peritonitis in an adult. Report of a case. *Med Ann DC* 40:753, 1971

25. MacDonald RA, Mallory GK: The natural history of postnecrotic cirrhosis. A study of 221 autopsy cases. *Am J Med* 24:334, 1958

26. Kanel GC, Kaplan MM, Zawacki JK, et al: Survival in patients with postnecrotic cirrhosis and Laennec's cirrhosis undergoing therapeutic portacaval shunt. *Gastroenterology* 73:679, 1977

27. Sherlock S, Scheuer PJ: The presentation and diagnosis of 100 patients with primary biliary cirrhosis. *N Engl J Med* 289:674, 1973

28. Richter GW: The iron-loaded cell—The cytopathology of iron storage. A review. *Am J Pathol* 91:363, 1978

29. Guzman IJ, Gold JH, Rosai J, et al: Benign hepatocellular tumors. *Surgery* 82:495, 1977

30. Edmondson HA: *Tumors of the Liver and Intrahepatic Bile Ducts. Atlas of Tumor Pathology*, fasc 25. Washington, DC: Armed Forces Institute of Pathology, 1958

31. Curutchet HP, Terz JJ, Kay S, et al: Primary liver cancer. *Surgery* 70:467, 1971

32. Wheeler HD: Concentrating function of the gallbladder. *Am J Med* 51:588, 1971

33. Small DM: The etiology and pathogenesis of gallstones. *Adv Surg* 10:63, 1976

34. Carey MD, Small DM: Micelle formation by bile salts. Physical-chemical and thermodynamic considerations. *Arch Intern Med* 130:506, 1972

35. Chandnani PC, Chhabria PB, Perrill CV, et al: Ultrasound as an aid in the diagnosis of hydrops of the gallbladder. *JAMA* 237:996, 1977

36. Christensen AH, Ishak KG: Benign tumors and pseudotumors of the gallbladder. Report of 180 cases. *Arch Pathol* 90:423, 1970

37. Piehler JM, Crichlow RW: Primary carcinoma of the gallbladder. *Arch Surg* 112:26, 1977

38. Lobeck CC: Cystic fibrosis of the pancreas. In *The Metabolic Basis of Inherited Disease* (Stanbury JB, Wyngarden JB, Fredrickson DS, eds), 2nd

ed, pp 1300-1317. New York: McGraw-Hill, 1966

39. di Sant'Agnese PA, David PB: Research in cystic fibrosis. *N Engl J Med* 295:481, 1976

40. Fanconi G, Uehlinger E, Knauer C: Das Coeliaksyndrom bei angeborener zysticher Pankreasfibromatose und Bronchiecktasien. *Wien Med Wochenschr* 86:753, 1936

41. Bowman BH, Mangos JA: Current concepts in genetics. Cystic fibrosis. *N Engl J Med* 294:937, 1976

42. Wood RE, Boat TF, Doershuk CF: Cystic fibrosis. *Am Rev Respir Dis* 113:833, 1976

43. Sarles H, Sahel J: Pathology of chronic calcifying pancreatitis. *Am J Gastroenterol* 66:117, 1976

44. Spiro HM: *Clinical Gastroenterology*, p 837. Toronto: Macmillan, 1970

45. Donowitz M, Kerstein MD, Spiro HM: Pancreatic ascites. *Medicine* 53:183, 1974

46. Chaves FJZ, Amarante M, Lopes C: Pancreatic ascites. Calcification as a clue to diagnosis. *Am J Gastroenterol* 67:253, 1977

47. Read G, Braganza JM, Howat HT: Pancreatitis— A retrospective study. *Gut* 17:945, 1976

48. Winship D: Pancreatitis: Pancreatic pseudocysts and their complications. *Gastroenterology* 73:593, 1977

49. Pellegrini CA, Paloyan D, Acosta JM, et al: Acute pancreatitis of rare causation. *Surg Gynecol Obstet* 114:899, 1977

50. Nakashima Y, Howard JM: Drug-induced pancreatitis. *Surg Gynecol Obstet* 145:105, 1977

51. Morgan RGH, Wormsley KG: Progress report. Cancer of the pancreas. *Gut* 18:580, 1977

52. McCormack LR, Seat SG, Strum WB: Pancreatic carcinoma. Survival following detection by ultrasonic scanning. *JAMA* 238:240, 1977

53. MacDonald JS, Widerlite L, Schein PS: Current diagnosis and management of pancreatic carcinoma. *J Nat Cancer Inst* 56:1093, 1976

54. Shapiro TM: Adenocarcinoma of the pancreas. A statistical analysis of biliary bypass vs Whipple resection in good risk patients. *Ann Surg* 182:715, 1975

55. Yalow RS, Glick SM, Roth J, et al: Plasma insulin and growth hormone levels in obesity and diabetes. *Ann NY Acad Sci* 131:357, 1965

56. Palmberg PF: Diabetic retinopathy. *Diabetes* 26:703, 1977

57. Goldenberg S, Alex M, Blumenthal HT: Sequelae of arteriosclerosis of the aorta and coronary arteries. *Diabetes* 7:98, 1958

58. Bale GS, Entmacher PS: Estimated life expectancy of diabetics. *Diabetes* 26:434, 1977

59. Lacy PE, Kissane JM: Pancreas and diabetes mellitus. In *Pathology* (Anderson WAD, Kissane JM, eds), 7th ed, vol 2, pp 1467-1477. St Louis: Mosby, 1977

60. Zollinger RM, Mazzaferri EL: Tumors of the islets of Langerhans. *Adv Surg* 10:137, 1976

61. Zollinger RM, Ellison EH: Primary peptic ulcerations of the jejunum associated with islet cell tumors of the pancreas. *Ann Surg* 142:709, 1955

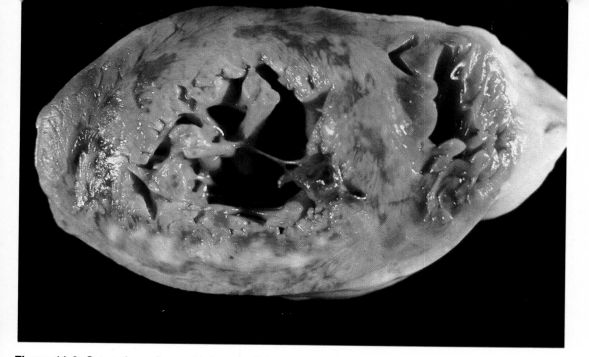

Figure 11-9. Cut surface of recent infarct (pallid zone), seven to 10 days after onset

Figure 11-19. Destruction of aortic cusps by acute bacterial endocarditis

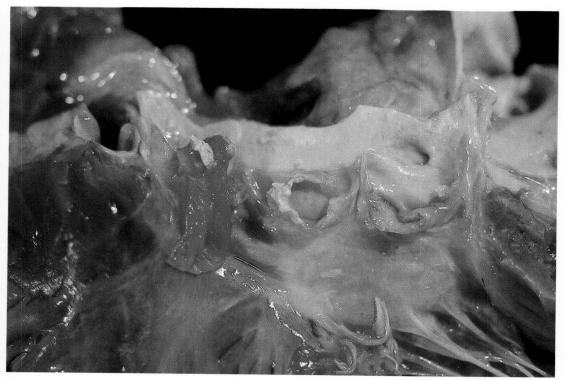

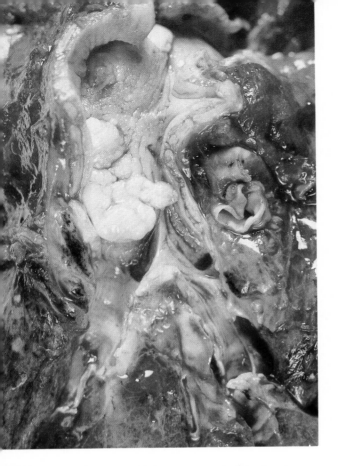

**Figure 12-18.** Bronchogenic carcinoma

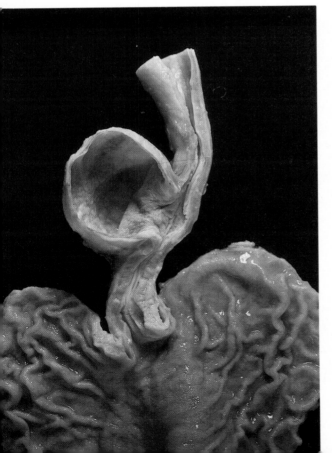

**Figure 13-6.** Large traction diverticulum of esophagus

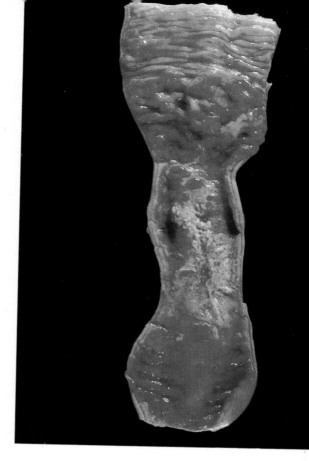

**Figure 13-17.** Affected segment of distal ileum in regional enteritis

**Figure 13-21.** Mucosal surface in chronic ulcerative colitis. Only the dark, hyperemic portion is affected.

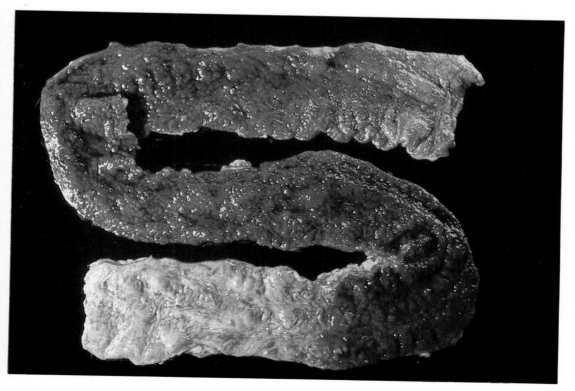

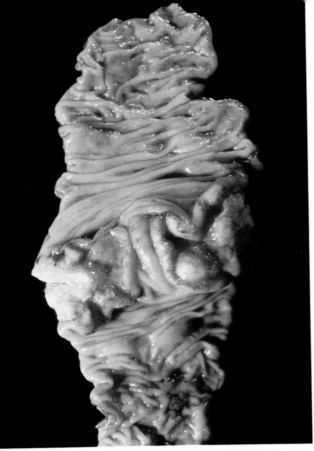

**Figure 13-28.** Encircling or "napkin ring" carcinoma of descending colon

**Figure 14-5.** Massive necrosis of liver from isoniazid ingestion

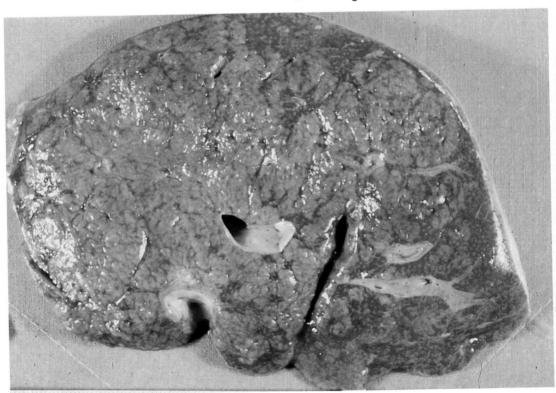

C-4

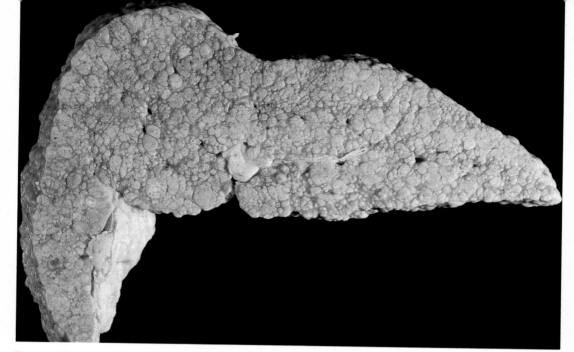

**Figure 14-6.** Cut surface of Laënnec's cirrhosis of liver

**Figure 14-15.** Duodenal mucosa (left), carcinoma of head of pancreas (center), and normal pancreas with dilated duct of Wirsung cut obliquely (right)

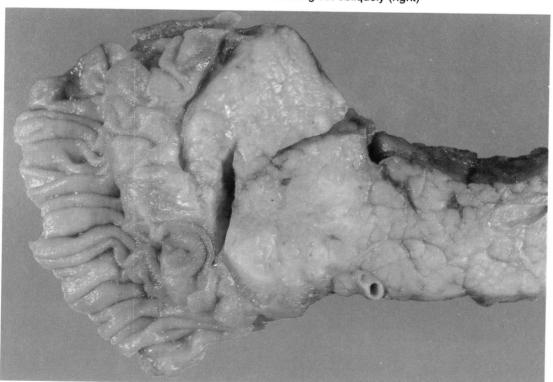

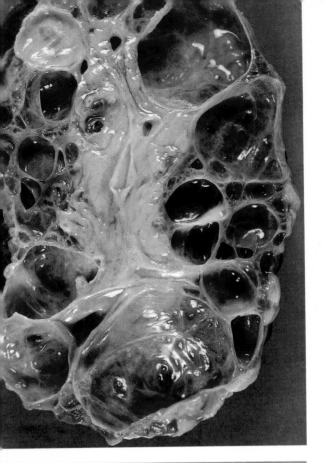

**Figure 15-3.** Cut surface of a polycystic kidney

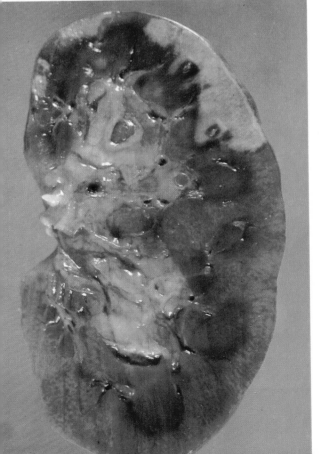

**Figure 15-12.** Recent infarct of kidney

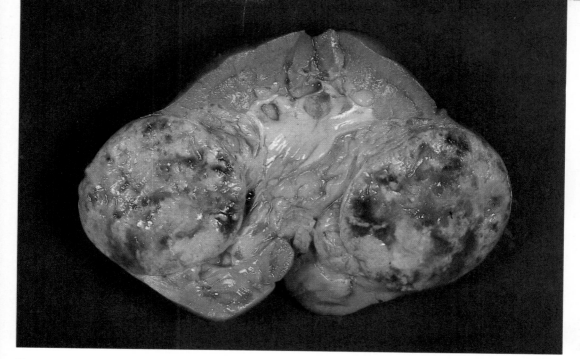

**Figure 15-14.** Carcinoma of kidney

**Figure 16-10.** Cut surface of embryonal carcinoma of testis

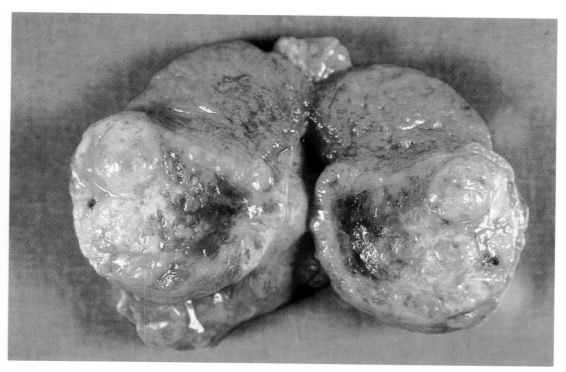

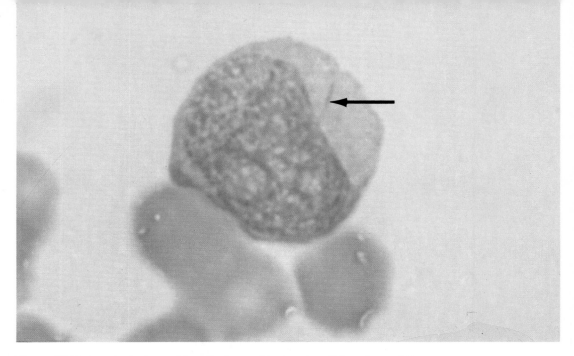

**Figure 19-7.** Auer body (arrow) in cytoplasm of leukemic cell (courtesy of Dr. Carl Johnson, Drew Postgraduate School of Medicine, Los Angeles)

**Figure 20-5.** Cut surface of pheochromocytoma of adrenal medulla

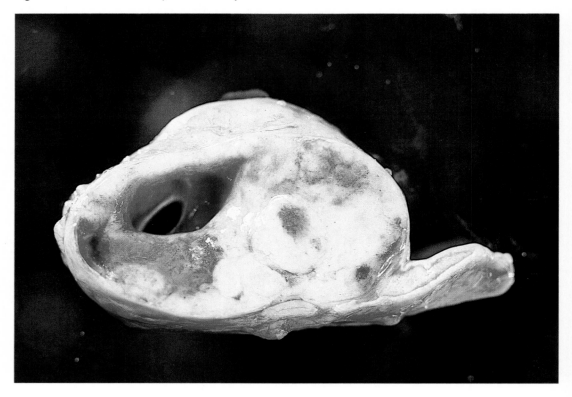

**Figure 21-1.** Pott's disease (tuberculosis) of the spine

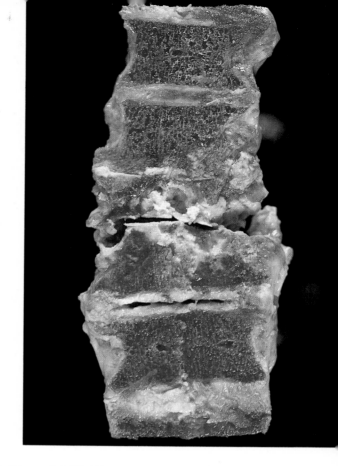

**Figure 21-9.** Fragmented articular surface of head of femur in osteoarthritis

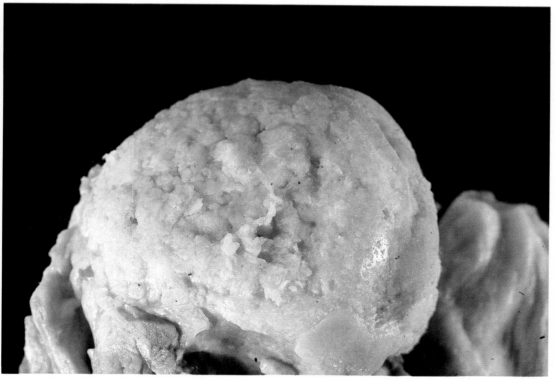

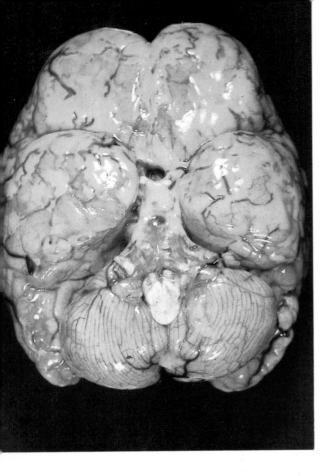

**Figure 22-1.** The pale exudate of acute bacterial meningitis

**Figure 22-4.** Petechiae over cut surface of cerebrum in acute anterior poliomyelitis. The patient was an 8-year-old girl who died after five days in the hospital.

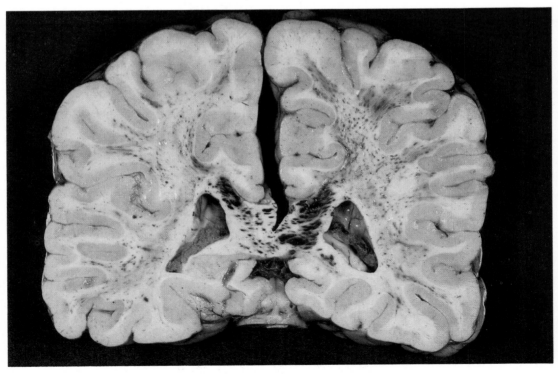

**Figure 22-8.** Saccular (berry) aneurysm of circle of Willis

**Figure 22-6.** Recent hemorrhagic infarct of brain

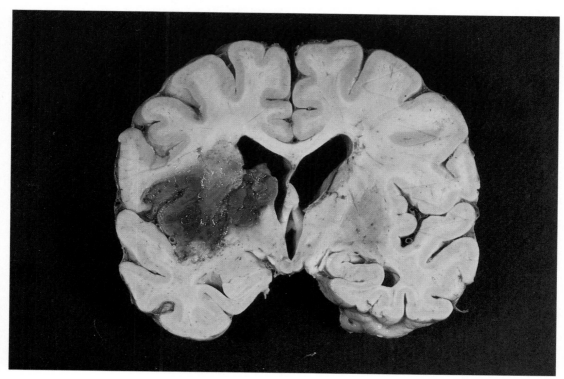

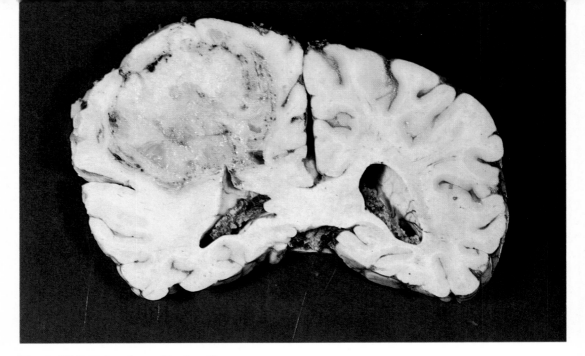

**Figure 22-9.** Cut surface of brain with glioblastoma multiforme

**Figure 22-12.** Large meningioma of dura markedly indenting the subjacent brain

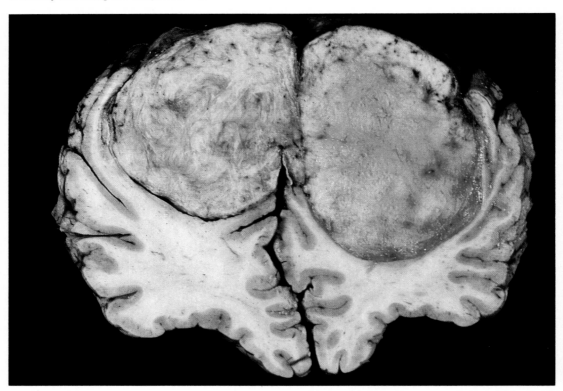

# 15

# RENAL DISEASE

## THE NORMAL KIDNEY

Each kidney weighs 140 to 160 gm and contains 1.3 million nephrons. A nephron consists of a glomerulus, proximal convoluted tubule, loop of Henle, distal convoluted tubule, and a collecting duct that opens at the tip of the renal papilla into the pelvis of the kidney. An afferent arteriole enters each glomerulus and divides into a capillary network, which then fuses to form the efferent arteriole that leaves the glomerulus. One-fourth of the cardiac output passes through the kidneys; the hydrostatic pressure in the glomerular capillaries is three times higher than in capillaries elsewhere in the body. The endothelium of the capillary is separated from the epithelium of the glomerulus by a basement membrane (Figure 15-1). Soluble components of the blood move across the basement membrane to form a nearly protein-free glomerular filtrate. The filtrate moves down the tubules, where the needs of the body are reabsorbed and the remainder is excreted. In 24 hours 180 liters of glomerular filtrate are formed, 178 liters are reabsorbed, and about 2 liters are excreted as urine. Although this transaction is enormous, each glomerulus produces only about 70 $\mu$l of filtrate per day.

The juxtaglomerular apparatus lies just outside the glomerulus, where the muscle cells of the arteriole take on an epithelioid appearance and show granules that contain renin. The cells of the distal convoluted tubule apposed to this site are also specialized

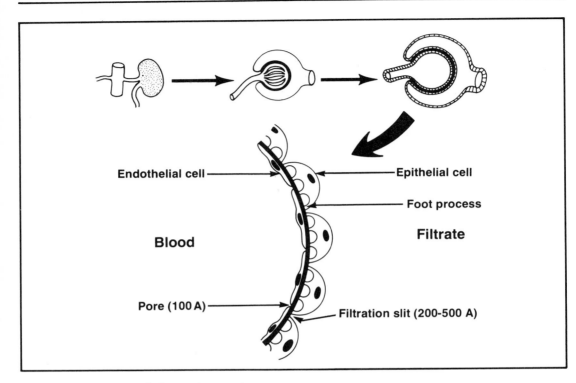

**Figure 15-1.** Diagram of glomerular membrane

and constitute the macula densa. These structures form the juxtaglomerular apparatus, which appears to monitor the pressure in the glomerular arterioles as well as the composition of the urine in the distal tubules. In this way it may control the rate of glomerular filtration and the production of renin, respectively.

Approximately 70 per cent of the glomerular filtrate is reabsorbed in the proximal convoluted tubule, leaving 25 per cent to progress to the loop of Henle. The loop is arranged so as to provide a countercurrent multiplier that concentrates solutes in the fluid passing into the renal pelvis. Little change takes place in the urine once it enters the renal pelvis, moves through the ureter, and collects in the urinary bladder.

The main functions of the kidney are the excretion of waste products, regulation of fluid volume, maintenance of acid-base balance, synthesis of vitamin D and prosta-

glandins, and secretion of renin and erythropoietin. The clinical manifestations of renal disease reflect disturbances of these various functions.

## CONGENITAL ABNORMALITIES

Common anomalies of the urinary system include renal agenesis, hypoplasia, horseshoe kidney, and bifid ureter. These range from lethal (agenesis) to inconsequential (bifid ureter). Horseshoe kidney (Figure 15-2) may be associated with an aneurysm of the abdominal aorta.[1] Of particular interest is polycystic kidney, a familial disorder transmitted as a mendelian recessive characteristic that occurs approximately once in every 250 births.[2] One-third of cases become evident in infancy, causing renal failure, while the rest become clinically manifest in adult life and are characterized by pain, hematuria, and palpable masses in both flanks. The condition is bilateral and is due to multiple developmental failures anywhere along the nephrons.[3] A multicystic kidney (Figure 15-3; see color section, p C-6) is prone to infection so that pyuria is also common. As the cysts slowly enlarge, atrophy of the intervening parenchyma takes place and renal failure gradually develops. The kidneys are huge, and the diagnosis is aided by retrograde pyelography, which reveals pronounced distortion of the caliceal system. Half the patients die within two to four years of symptomatic onset, and life seldom persists for more than 10 years after onset.[2]

## RENAL FAILURE

Aside from congenital and neoplastic disease, there are only four main categories of renal disorder: glomerular, tubular, infectious/obstructive, and vascular. All often progress to acute or chronic renal failure. Acute failure is characterized by oliguria (less than 400 ml/24 hours) and azotemia (elevation of blood urea nitrogen). It is not necessarily due to renal disease, however, and for this reason acute failure also has prerenal and postrenal forms. The cause of prerenal failure is hypotension with reduced perfusion, as occurs with shock, hemorrhage, or congestive heart failure. When the blood pressure in the afferent arteriole is lower than 60 mm Hg, glomerular filtration begins to fail; as this happens, the small molecules of urea take longer to be reabsorbed by the tubular cells while the larger molecules of creatinine tend to pass quickly through the tubules and be excreted in the urine. An indication of prerenal failure is accordingly a ratio of blood urea nitrogen to creatinine that rises substantially above the normal of 15:1. Prerenal failure is corrected by restoring blood pressure to normal if this can be done before ischemic damage becomes pronounced.

Renal disease causing acute failure is due to diminished glomerular filtration or sup-

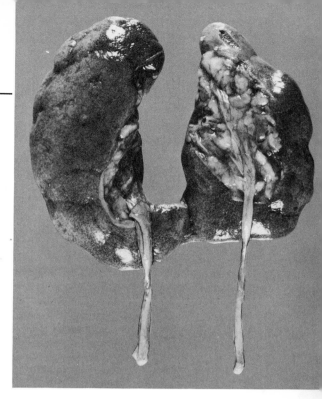

**Figure 15-2.** Horseshoe kidney

pressed tubular function. The former is due to glomerulonephritis and the latter to infection, to nephrotoxins, or to prolonged hypoperfusion from such conditions as trauma, hemorrhage, heart failure, sepsis, and dehydration. After 40 minutes of hypoxia, restoring the blood pressure no longer reverses the tubular impairment. The ischemic injury is reversible, however, and if the patient can be kept alive for 10 days to two weeks, the oliguria gives way to pronounced diuresis and tubular function is gradually restored.

Postrenal failure is associated especially with obstruction. The common cause is nodular hyperplasia of the prostate; others include neurogenic bladder, periureteral fibrosis, calculi of the ureters, and carcinoma of the prostate growing into the trigone or obstructing the prostatic urethra. The history, sequence of events, time intervals, and laboratory findings usually reveal whether the acute failure is due to prerenal hypoperfusion, renal parenchymal disease, or postrenal obstruction of outflow.

Disease of the kidneys may also go on to chronic renal failure. The clinical manifes-

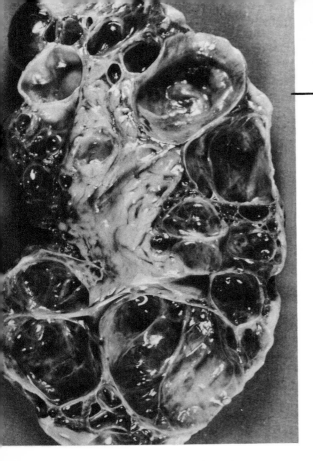

**Figure 15-3.** Cut surface of a polycystic kidney. Also shown in color section, p C-6.

tations include lassitude, weight loss, nausea, anorexia, vomiting, itching, anemia, acidosis, a bleeding tendency, and often hypertension. The blood urea nitrogen is, of course, raised above the normal 15 mg/dl, but this only signals the accumulation of various excretory products, including phenols and organic acids. No one substance is known to be the cause of the uremic syndrome. Associated lesions are found outside the kidneys and include fibrinous pericarditis, uremic pneumonitis and gastroenteritis, hyperparathyroidism secondary to phosphorus retention, and cardiac hypertrophy due to hypertension.

## Glomerulonephritis

The term given to primary glomerular injury is glomerulonephritis. The morphologic changes consist of proliferation of glomerular cells, exudation of neutrophils, and at-

tachment of immune complexes to the basement membrane. These alterations may be focal or diffuse, and may occur singly or in various combinations. About 70 per cent of glomerulonephritis is due to the attachment of antigen-antibody complexes to the basement membrane, 5 per cent is due to antibodies directed against the basement membrane, and the rest is poorly understood.[4] As the acute injury passes into the chronic phase, fibrosis and hyalinization replace the glomerular tufts regardless of the nature of the initial injury.

Acute glomerulonephritis is manifested by the nephritic syndrome or the nephrotic syndrome. The nephritic syndrome consists of hematuria, azotemia, and hypertension. The patient also manifests oliguria, slight proteinuria, and facial edema, especially about the eyes. The nephrotic syndrome is characterized by massive proteinuria, hypoalbuminemia, hypercholesterolemia, and generalized subcutaneous edema. In a patient with acute glomerulonephritis, one of these two syndromes may prevail. It is therefore useful to consider glomerular disease from the standpoint of these two clinical presentations. It should be borne in mind, however, that no classification of glomerulonephritis is entirely satisfactory, and renal biopsy is often necessary to establish an accurate diagnosis.[5]

Poststreptococcal glomerulonephritis is the main cause of the nephritic syndrome. The patients are usually children, but the condition may affect adults. The onset follows a streptococcal infection, usually of the throat, by an interval of one to two weeks. During this time antibodies are forming to the bacteria, which are usually strains 12, 4, and 1 of group A. The laboratory evidence of this formation is elevation of the antistreptolysin titer in the patient's serum. At the end of this interval, when the throat infection has subsided, glomerulonephritis begins. The onset is abrupt and consists of smoky urine (hematuria), proteinuria, oliguria, periorbital edema, and hypertension. The kidneys grossly are swollen and hyperemic but are not otherwise unusual. Microscopically, however, there is proliferation of endothelial, epithelial, and mesangial cells, as well as swelling of endothelial cells. Because of the cellular proliferation the condition is also known as proliferative glomerulonephritis. A light infiltration of neutrophilic leukocytes is present in the glomeruli. These changes encroach on the capillary lumens so that glomerular flow is reduced and filtration is diminished. In addition, "humps" of immune complexes attach to the basement membrane on the epithelial side of this layer, and this establishes the condition as an immune complex disease. In 95 per cent of children it subsides spontaneously; the remainder go on to rapidly progressive renal failure or gradually progressive chronic glomerulonephritis. In adults the condition often fails to resolve completely, and a higher proportion go on to chronic failure.[6]

The nephrotic syndrome is caused by lipoid nephrosis and membranous glomerulonephritis. Lipoid nephrosis has a peak incidence at two to three years of age, and 85 per cent of cases occur before the age of 15. The clinical manifestations begin gradually and consist of massive proteinuria, hypoalbuminemia, and anasarca. There is no hematuria, hypertension, or renal failure. On light microscopy the glomeruli appear normal, and for this reason the condition has also been called nil disease or minimal-change glomerulonephritis. With electron microscopy, however, the foot processes of the epithelial cells are swollen and flattened and appear fused. The basement membrane is normal, no immune complexes are deposited, and there is no proliferation of glomerular cells. How "fusion" of the foot processes causes increased permeability of the glomeruli is not clear. Nevertheless, protein and lipids spill into the tubules, and the term lipoid nephrosis arose because the glomeruli appear normal, lipids are found in the tubular cells, and fat

bodies are present in the urine. Although the pathogenesis remains clouded, patients respond favorably to corticosteroids with disappearance of the proteinuria and recovery of the epithelial foot processes. The outlook is therefore altogether favorable.

Membranous glomerulonephritis causes the nephrotic syndrome in adults. The onset is gradual, and the patient develops massive proteinuria, losing more than 3.5 gm/24 hours. With this occur hypoalbuminemia, widespread edema, hypercholesterolemia, and lipiduria. In the kidneys the basement membranes of the glomeruli appear uniformly thickened because of the presence of dense bodies, presumably consisting of antibody and complement, and destruction of the foot processes of the podocytes. Eventually the deposits, which are on the epithelial side of the membrane, fuse with it. The antigen causing these deposits has not been identified. The course is progressive, the value of corticosteroids is doubtful, and renal failure gradually develops between two and 20 years after the onset of the disease.[7]

The foregoing types of glomerulonephritis are more or less distinct. The proliferative poststreptococcal type causes the nephritic syndrome, affects mainly children, and usually subsides spontaneously; lipoid nephrosis also affects children, is manifested by the nephrotic syndrome, and responds favorably to steroid therapy. In adults the nephrotic syndrome signals membranous glomerulonephritis with an uncertain response to therapy and a generally unfavorable outlook. In addition to these three clinically recognizable types there is a combined type, membranoproliferative glomerulonephritis, which is less distinct from the standpoints of clinical manifestations and anatomic changes. Membranoproliferative glomerulonephritis may present with the nephrotic or the nephritic syndrome, mainly children and young adults are affected, and the course is variable, with most progressing to chronic renal failure. The glomeruli reveal proliferation of mesangial cells and deposits of immune bodies and complement on both sides of the basement membrane as well as within it. The blood complement level is characteristically low; it is not clear whether this is due to insufficient formation in the liver or to increased destruction after the complement is formed. The cause of this type of glomerulonephritis is not known, although it has been suggested that hypocomplementemia may predispose to it.[4] There are probably divers causes, many associated with persistent antigenemia, which may have a role in pathogenesis.[8]

Finally, the nephrotic syndrome is also seen in adults with diseases that secondarily affect the kidneys. Chief among these are amyloidosis, diabetes mellitus, and disseminated lupus erythematosus. The main features of the four types of acute glomerulonephritis are summarized in Table 15-1.

All of the four main types of acute glomerulonephritis may go on to chronic glomerular disease, in which the kidneys are small, the surface is granular, and the cortex is thin (Figure 15-4). The histologic hallmark is uniform sclerosis of all glomeruli, often with hyalinization. Interstitial fibrosis and arterial thickening are also

**Table 15-1.**

## Characteristics of acute glomerulonephritis

| | |
|---|---|
| **Proliferative** | Children and adults affected |
| | Nephritic syndrome |
| | Increased glomerular cells |
| | Treatment symptomatic |
| | Outlook favorable |
| **Lipoid nephrosis** | Children affected |
| | Nephrotic syndrome |
| | Foot process "fusion" |
| | Treated with steroids |
| | Outlook favorable |
| **Membranous** | Adults affected |
| | Nephrotic syndrome |
| | Thickened basement membrane |
| | Treatment controversial |
| | Outlook unfavorable |
| **Membranoproliferative** | Children and adults affected |
| | Nephritic/nephrotic syndrome |
| | Increased glomerular cells, thickened basement membrane |
| | Treatment symptomatic |
| | Outlook unfavorable |

present (Figure 15-5). Chronic glomerulonephritis is the most common cause of chronic renal failure. About one-third of patients give no history of having had a preceding acute glomerular disease. The subject is reviewed by Leaf and Cotran.[4]

### Tubular disease

Nephrosis is the term for tubular disease. It is produced by ischemia, which is usually associated with shock, and by toxins that cause necrosis of the tubular cells. Among the toxins are heavy metals such as gold, arsenic, bismuth, and bichloride of mercury, solvents such as chloroform, carbon tetrachloride, and methyl alcohol, and antibacterial agents such as neomycin, polymyxin, and methicillin. Ethylene glycol (antifreeze), some pesticides, and mushroom poisoning also injure the sensitive tubular epithelium. The clinical onset begins within 24 hours of the injurious event and is manifested by oliguria, proteinuria, and a rising serum creatinine and blood urea nitrogen. Electrolyte imbalance and hydration disturbances also develop. Grossly the kidneys are smooth, pale, and large, often weighing more than 250 gm each. On section the cortex is thick and the cortical striations are indistinct. Microscopically the tubular cells are necrotic and sloughing of them into the lumen causes tubular casts that gradually dissolve. If the patient survives for 10 days to two weeks, the tubular epithelium will regenerate, and after massive diuresis renal function will gradually resume. The outlook therefore is determined by the severity of the event causing the nephrosis rather than by the inability of the kidneys to recover from the injury.

Two special forms are cholemic and myeloma nephrosis. When shock and jaundice occur together, as may happen with biliary operations, renal failure often develops. This is known as cholemic nephrosis. Morphologic changes are minimal. The failure has been attributed to the circulating bilirubin, but recovery on transplantation of

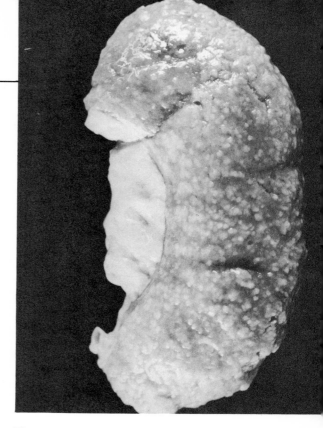

**Figure 15-4.** External surface of kidney in chronic glomerulonephritis

the kidney suggests that an alteration of blood flow may be the cause.[4] In multiple myeloma, γ-globulins are overproduced. Some are so small, i.e., under mol wt 40,000, that they are filtered at the glomerulus with and are reabsorbed into the tubular cells. The tubular cells burst, the tubular lumens become clogged, and extension of the debris into the peritubular parenchyma incites a chronic granulomatous inflammation. This condition is known as myeloma kidney.

### Pyelonephritis

Pyelonephritis is a bacterial infection of the pelvis and parenchyma of the kidney. The organism is usually *Escherichia coli*, and the main route of infection is through the ureter from the lower tract. Evidence for this is the frequency of such infections with indwelling catheters, neurogenic flaccid bladders, and other obstructions such as strictures of the ureter, calculi, tumors of

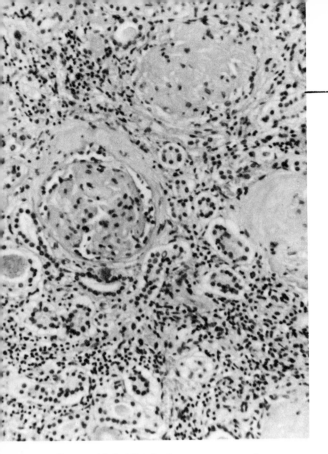

**Figure 15-5.** Histologic appearance of chronic glomerulonephritis

the bladder, and hyperplasia of the prostate. An additional obstruction is pregnancy with compression of the ureters as they cross the pelvic brim. Attention is also given to a dysfunction of the vesicoureteral sphincter that allows urine to gush into the ureter when the bladder contracts. The renal tissue discloses multiple abscesses appearing on the surface as slightly raised, pale gray foci. If the abscesses become large and interconnect, the condition is referred to as a carbuncle of the kidney. Destruction of the parenchyma may convert the kidney to a pus sac, which is termed pyonephrosis (Figure 15-6). Extension through the capsule produces a perinephric abscess. In some instances, with obstruction and overwhelming infection, necrosis of the papillary tips develops even though the patient is not diabetic. This is also a cause of acute renal failure. Otherwise the clinical features are fever, malaise, leuko-

cytosis, urinary frequency, pyuria, and pain over the costovertebral angles. The urine is loaded with bacteria and granular (pus) casts. Death results from sepsis and renal failure.

Ordinarily, however, the reaction subsides and the patient lives. In this event the kidney is scarred but renal function is sufficient to sustain life. In other instances the infection is low-grade from the outset so that chronic pyelonephritis develops from both reactions. Analgesic overuse also leads to chronic pyelonephritis, perhaps through the mechanism of papillary tip necrosis.[9] Grossly the characteristic scar is large, irregular, flat-based, finely granular, and located over the lateral or "saddle" portion of the kidney (Figure 15-7). On histologic examination tubular dilation, colloid casts, interstitial fibrosis, and varying infiltration of leukocytes are the principal findings. Thickening of arterial vessels is also conspicuous. The process may be focal and asymptomatic or it may be widespread and progress to atrophy with contraction and hypertension. If the process is bilateral and advanced, renal failure may develop. If it is unilateral, however, nephrectomy is curative and the hypertension abates.

## Calculi

Closely associated with pyelonephritis is obstruction of the urinary tract. Among the common causes of urinary-tract obstruction are nodular hyperplasia of the prostate and calculi that form in the renal pelvis. Less frequent causes are congenital valves of the urethra, an aberrant renal artery compressing the ureteropelvic junction, neurogenic flaccid bladder, and carcinomas of the urinary bladder or adjacent structures such as the endometrium, cervix, or prostate with extension to the urethra. Stagnant, impassable urine exerts pressure and becomes infected so that hydronephrosis and pyelonephritis result.

Calculi arise in the kidneys, usually in the 20- to 40-year age group. They are unilateral, measure 2 to 3 mm in diameter, and are smooth or spiculate. Over 50 per cent are composed of calcium oxalate with or without calcium phosphate.[10] Less frequent are cystine and uric acid stones. The formation of calculi is attributed to supersaturation of the constituents of the urine.[11] No clinical signs are produced until the mucosa is ulcerated. This tends to occur when the concretion passes into the ureter, the smooth muscle contracts about it, and renal colic develops. The colic consists of extremely severe pain over the costovertebral angle that recurs at regular intervals, is referred to the urethra, and is associated with microscopic hematuria. Calculi under 0.5 cm in diameter tend to pass down the ureter and seldom recur, but those over 1.0 cm remain in the renal pelvis, require operative removal, and recur more frequently.[12] The larger concretions gradually come to fill the renal pelvis and conform to its shape. These are called staghorn calculi; they obstruct the flow of urine, abrade the

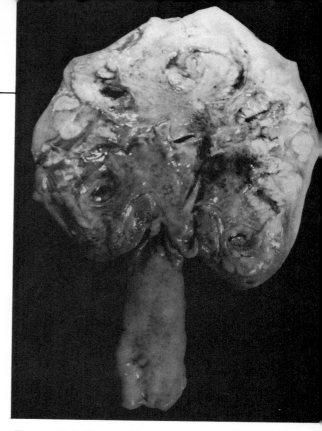

**Figure 15-6.** Opened kidney of pyonephrosis. The pelvis is dilated, abscesses are present, and the kidney has been converted into a "pus sac."

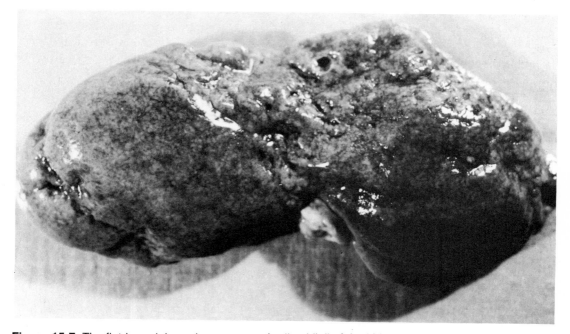

**Figure 15-7.** The flat-based, irregular scar over the "saddle" of the kidney that is characteristic of chronic pyelonephritis

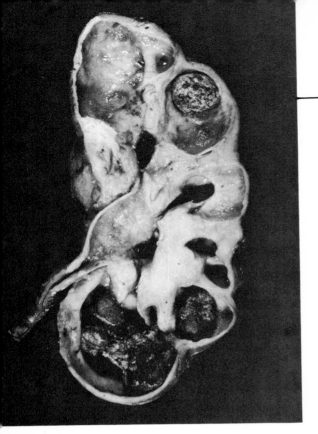

**Figure 15-8.** Calculi in pelvis of hydronephrotic kidney. Atrophy of the renal parenchyma is pronounced.

pelvic mucosa, and lead to both hydronephrosis and pyelonephritis (Figure 15-8).

## Vascular disease

The two main vascular lesions of the kidney are arteriolar nephrosclerosis and thromboembolism. Two other, much less frequent lesions are atherosclerosis of the renal artery and cortical necrosis of the renal parenchyma. The relationship of renal vascular change to hypertension is an especially interesting aspect of renal disease.

Arteriolar nephrosclerosis consists of hyaline thickening of the afferent arterioles (Figure 15-9). The process is uniform and bilateral, ischemic atrophy gradually develops, and the tubular portions of the cortex are affected first. The kidneys are symmetrically reduced in size, and the cortical surfaces are evenly and finely granular (Figure 15-10). Histologic examination reveals, in addition to the vascular thickening, interstitial fibrosis, crowding of glomeruli

from the reduced tubular tissue, and light infiltration with lymphocytes. The condition is extremely common, affecting 70 per cent of autopsy subjects over the age of 60. It is also associated with hypertension. It is not clear whether the vascular narrowing is the cause or effect of high blood pressure. However, the juxtaglomerular apparatus, which forms and stores renin, is hyperplastic, and the mechanism of the hypertension involves this complex renin-angiotensin system. Between 90 and 95 per cent of hypertension is "essential" and associated with this vascular lesion.

In a small proportion of patients, usually after several years of essential hypertension, the blood pressure abruptly rises to a high level and renal failure rapidly develops. Fibrinoid necrosis is then added to the hyaline thickening of the arterioles, the damaged vessels bleed, and the surface of the kidneys develops a characteristic "flea-bitten" appearance (Figure 15-11). The vascular lesion is necrotizing arteriolitis. This syndrome of accelerated (malignant) hypertension progresses, without treatment, to a fatal outcome in six months to a year. The cause of this abrupt clinical and pathologic change is not known, although unusually high levels of renin and aldosterone are found in such patients.[13] With antihypertensive therapy, half of patients live five years.[4]

Renal artery stenosis due to atherosclerosis, most often at the aortic ostium, also causes hypertension. This form constitutes only 2 to 5 per cent of cases of high blood pressure. The condition is often unilateral and is curable by resection of the kidney or bypass of the arterial obstruction by an autologous saphenous vein graft.[14]

Since blood flow to the kidneys is five to 10 times greater than that to the heart, lungs, or liver, the renal tissue is especially vulnerable to embolic obstruction of its arteries. Renal infarcts are thus common. They come mainly from the left atrial appendage in cases of fibrillation, from the

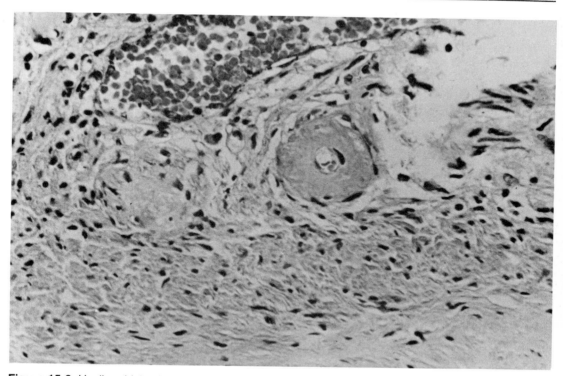

**Figure 15-9.** Hyaline thickening of the arteriolar wall; arteriolar nephrosclerosis

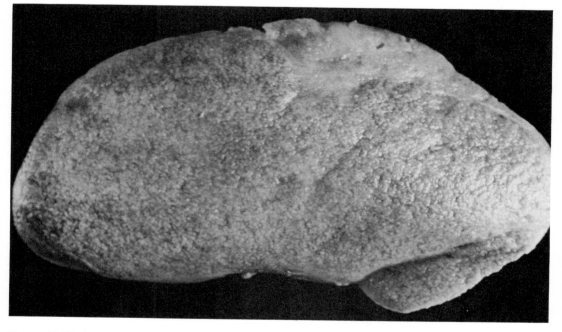

**Figure 15-10.** The finely granular external surface of the kidney in arteriolar disease

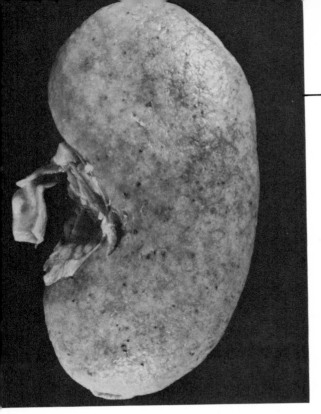

**Figure 15-11.** The "fleabitten" kidney of necrotizing arteriolitis

**Figure 15-12.** Recent infarct of kidney. Also shown in color section, p C-6.

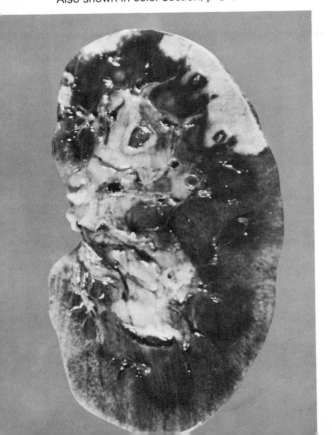

mitral valve in bacterial endocarditis, and from the mural endocardium of the left ventricle in cases of myocardial infarction. A large artery within the kidney is usually obstructed, and the infarct takes a wedge shape with the base extending to the cortical surface. The reaction is a focus of coagulation necrosis that is swollen and hyperemic early, becomes decolorized later, and eventually results in a white, fibrous, sunken scar. Clinical manifestations may be absent or include a slight, steady pain in the flank that is associated with microscopic hematuria or, less often, normal urine. Renal failure is uncommon, but hypertension frequently develops. A recent infarct is shown in Figure 15-12 (see color section, p C-6). Emboli also reach the kidneys from ulcerated atheromas of the aorta. This occurs either spontaneously or after renal aortography or operations on the abdominal aorta.[15] The occluded vessels display the characteristic acicular slits of cholesterol crystals (see Figure 11-31).

The least frequent of the vascular disorders is renal cortical necrosis. The mechanism of the ischemia is not clear, but the condition is associated with gram-negative sepsis, large-area burns, and especially hemorrhagic complications of late pregnancy. The kidneys reveal cortical "ribbons" of pale yellow necrosis, although the process may be patchy (Figure 15-13). The intralobular arteries are only occasionally occluded by fibrin thrombi.[16] The clinical onset is abrupt, with anuria and rapidly progressive renal failure that is often fatal. Bilateral acute renal cortical necrosis is one of the few causes of total absence of urine.

## TUMORS

Benign tumors of the kidney are not clinically significant; fibromas and adenomas of the cortex and medulla are minute and tend to remain localized. Only two malignant tumors of the kidney are common in adults; 90 per cent are carcinomas of the renal pa-

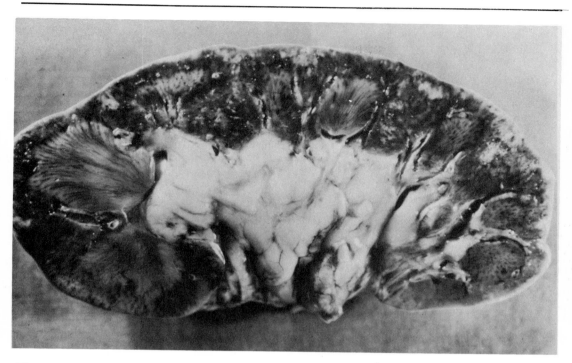

**Figure 15-13.** The cortical pallor of renal cortical necrosis

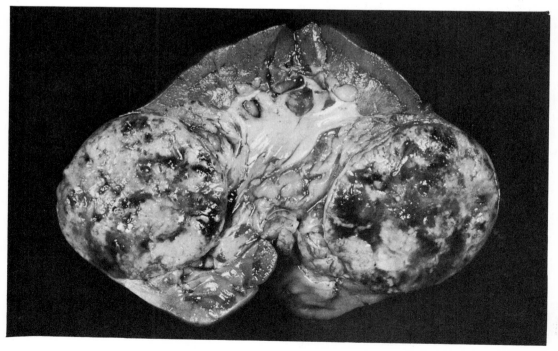

**Figure 15-14.** Carcinoma of kidney. Also shown in color section, p C-7.

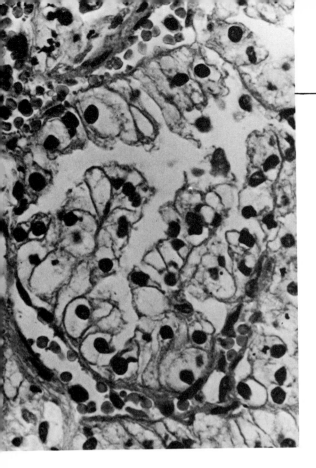

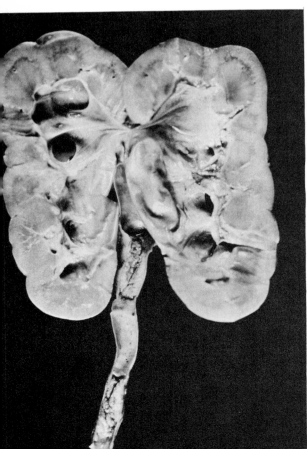

renchyma and 10 per cent are transitional cancers of the pelvic mucosa. Grawitz used the term "hypernephroma" for carcinoma of the renal parenchyma, thinking that the tumor arose from ectopic adrenal cells in the renal cortex. It is now known that the cancer arises in the epithelial cells of the proximal convoluted tubules.[17] The tumors average 5 to 7.5 cm in diameter at the time of removal, and the cut surfaces are red from hemorrhage, gray from fibrous septa, and yellow from necrotic foci or lipids in the tumor cells. A cut surface is shown in Figure 15-14 (see color section, p C-7). Microscopically the cells lie in solid clusters and tubular arrangements with infrequent gland formation. The characteristic cell is "clear" from lipids being dissolved out in the embedding process (Figure 15-15). For this reason the neoplasm has been called a clear-cell tumor. The cancer tends to grow into the renal vein and thence into the inferior vena cava. By the time the tumor has reached 5 cm in diameter, the chances are even that it has already spread outside the kidney.[18] The most frequent sites of metastasis are the liver, lungs, bone, and retroperitoneal lymph nodes.

The cancer appears clinically most often after the age of 50. It affects men twice as often as women and occurs equally on either side of the body. As the tumor enlarges, a characteristic triad develops: pain in the abdomen, a mass in the flank, and blood in the urine. This triad, which indicates advanced disease, is often preceded by fever, weight loss, and fatigue. Polycythemia from tumor cell production of erythropoietin is observed in as many as 6 per cent of cases. Although radiographic procedures are helpful in establishing the diag-

**Figure 15-15** (top). The "clear cells" of renal carcinoma

**Figure 15-16** (bottom). Transitional-cell carcinoma of the first portion of the ureter with an additional tumor in the midureter

nosis, cytologic examination of the urine is not. Treatment consists of nephrectomy, which achieves a 10-year survival rate of about 25 per cent.[18]

Tumors of the renal pelvis and ureters are composed of transitional epithelial cells. Hematuria, dysuria, and frequency are the main clinical signs. The outstanding pathologic feature is that the tumors are often multiple. Such a tumor of the ureter is shown in Figure 15-16. Hydronephrosis and pyelonephritis are common consequences of the obstruction. Excretory urograms identify pelvic cancers whereas retrograde urography is preferred for ureteral tumors. In addition, cytologic examination of urinary sediment is often helpful in making the diagnosis. Invasion of adjacent structures is late, and metastases are first seen in retroperitoneal lymph nodes. Because of the multiple foci of tumors, nephroureterectomy is required for cure.

Wilms's tumor arises in infants and children. It occurs equally in boys and girls, affects either or both kidneys, and is manifested clinically by pain and a sizable mass in the abdomen. The tumor, also known as a nephroblastoma, is composed of a mixture of epithelial, stromal, and undifferentiated tissues. Skeletal muscle and neural elements are often present. Metastatic spread takes place to the liver, lungs, and retroperitoneal lymph nodes. With surgical excision followed by irradiation and chemotherapy, metastases regress and a formerly unfavorable prognosis has been converted in recent years to a five-year survival rate that often exceeds 80 per cent.[18]

## REFERENCES

1. Ezzet F, Dorazio R, Herzberg R: Horseshoe and pelvic kidneys associated with abdominal aortic aneurysms. *Am J Surg* 134:196, 1977

2. Campbell MF, Harrison JH: *Urology*, 3rd ed, vol 2, pp 1416-1486. Philadelphia: Saunders, 1970

3. Osathanondh V, Potter EL: Pathogenesis of polycystic kidneys. Type 3 due to multiple abnormalities of development. *Arch Pathol* 7:485, 1964

4. Leaf A, Cotran R: *Renal Pathophysiology.* New York: Oxford University Press, 1976

5. Kincaid-Smith P: Glomerulonephritis. Med J Aust 2:260, 1976

6. Baldwin DS: Poststreptococcal glomerulonephritis. A progressive disease? *Am J Med* 62:1, 1977

7. Pierides AM, Malasit P, Morley AR, et al: Idiopathic membranous nephropathy. *Q J Med* 46:163, 1977

8. Jones DB: Membranoproliferative glomerulonephritis. One or many diseases? *Arch Pathol Lab Med* 101:457, 1977

9. Kincaid-Smith P: Pathogenesis of the renal lesion associated with the abuse of analgesics. *Lancet* 1:859, 1967

10. Rose GA: The causes and medical treatment of renal calculi. *Practitioner* 218:74, 1977

11. Finlayson B: Renal lithiasis in review. *Urol Clin North Am* 1:181, 1974

12. Blandy JP, Marshall VR: Size of renal calculi, recurrence rate and follow-up. *Br J Urol* 48:525, 1976

13. McAllister RG Jr, VanWay CW III, Dayani K, et al: Malignant hypertension: Effect of therapy on renin and aldosterone. *Circ Res Suppl* 2, 29:160, 1971

14. Foster JH, Oates JA: Recognition and management of renovascular hypertension. *Hosp Pract* 10:61, 1975

15. Gore I, Collins DP: Spontaneous atheromatous embolization. Review of the literature and report of 16 additional cases. *Am J Clin Pathol* 33:416, 1960

16. Kleinknecht D, Grunfeld J, Gomez PC, et al: Diagnostic procedures and long-term prognosis in bilateral renal cortical necrosis. *Kidney Int* 4:390, 1973

17. Oberling C, Riviere M, Haguenau F: Ultrastructure of the clear cells in renal carcinomas and its importance for the demonstration of their renal origin. *Nature* 186:402, 1960

18. Bennington JL, Beckwith JB: *Tumors of the Kidney, Renal Pelvis, and Ureter. Atlas of Tumor Pathology,* 2nd series, fasc 12. Washington, DC: Armed Forces Institute of Pathology, 1975

# 16

## DISORDERS OF MALE GENITALIA

### INFECTIONS

Venus was the ancient Roman goddess of love. Venereal infections are therefore those connected with sexual activity. The five main venereal infections are syphilis, gonorrhea, lymphogranuloma venereum, chancroid, and granuloma inguinale. The first three were discussed in Chapter 5. For syphilis the two genital lesions are the chancre, in the first stage, and the condyloma latum, in the second stage. The chancre usually occurs on the penis in the region of the glans or prepuce, and the flat condyloma occurs on the perianal skin. Both teem with spirochetes, which can be identified by dark-field illumination, and both are, of course, infective lesions. Gonorrhea is a word made up of the Greek words *gonos*, meaning "seed," and *rhoia*, meaning "flow." The gram-negative cocci *Neisseria gonorrhoeae* incite a superficial exudative inflammation that spreads over the genital mucosa from the urethra to the prostate. The reaction is due to an endotoxin liberated on the death of the organisms. The reaction is superficial and especially pronounced in the glands of the urethra, and healing takes place by the formation of granulation tissue that matures to a dense scar. The consequence is stenosis that obstructs the urinary tract and leads to the sequence of stagnation, dilation, and infection. Although the organisms are sensitive to penicillin, immunity does not develop and recurrent infection is always possible.

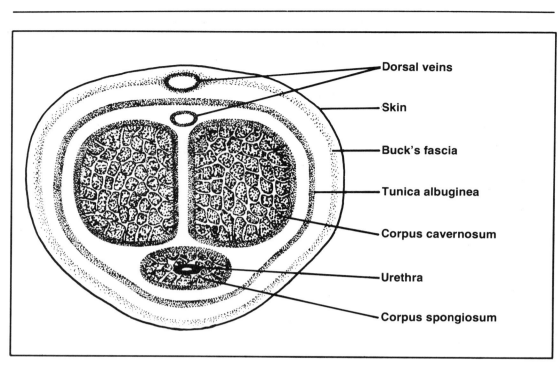

Dorsal veins

Skin

Buck's fascia

Tunica albuginea

Corpus cavernosum

Urethra

Corpus spongiosum

**Figure 16-1.** Diagram of cross section of penis

Chancroid ("soft chancre") and granuloma inguinale are uncommon. The former is caused by *Haemophilus ducreyi*, a small bacillus that invades the penile skin through a minute abrasion during intercourse. A vesicle at the site develops approximately a week later and progresses to a pustule and then a small ulcer, the "soft chancre." The base shows acute, nonspecific exudative inflammation. In about half of cases the organism is carried to the inguinal lymph nodes, where suppuration develops. Fistulae to the skin of the groin occasionally follow.

Granuloma inguinale is even less common and occurs mostly in the tropics. Blacks are most frequently affected. The responsible organism is *Calymmatobacterium (Donovania) granulomatis*, an encapsulated coccobacillus that is phagocytized by macrophages, in which it is known as the Donovan body. The process begins as an inflammatory papule that enlarges, ul-

cerates, and spreads. The entire perineum may become ulcerated. The organism is carried in the lymph stream to the regional lymph nodes, where suppuration, rupture, and drainage develop. Healing takes place by scar formation with notable fibrosis that disfigures the surface and causes lymph obstruction as well.

## PENIS

Anomalies of the penis and urethra are uncommon; hypospadias is the most frequent. *Span* is a Greek word meaning "tear," "pluck off," "pull," or "draw." In hypospadias the urethra opens onto the ventral surface of the penis anywhere from the glans to the perineum. The usual site is at the coronal sulcus, next is the shaft of the organ, and least frequent is a scrotal or perineal opening. Surgical correction is possible.[1] The condition is often associated with chordee, which is a sharp ventroflexion of the shaft due to associated fibrosis of the corpus spongiosum. Epispadias, in which the urethra opens onto the dorsal surface of the penis, is rare. Other anomalies of the urethra include meatal stricture, duplication, and posterior valves, all of which cause obstruction and dilation of the bladder, ureters, and renal pelves.[2]

When the aperture of the prepuce is small, the foreskin cannot be retracted over the glans. This is known as phimosis. It precludes the removal of smegma from the coronal sulcus, and infections of the glans tend to develop. When the prepuce is retracted, however, and then cannot be drawn forward over the glans, paraphimosis exists. This tends to obstruct the venous circulation so that edema of the glans develops.

Priapism is penile erection without prior sexual stimulation. It occurs in conditions associated with venous thrombosis. These include especially leukemia, sickle cell anemia, and, less commonly, trauma. When the dorsal vein of the penis is thrombosed, blood is entrapped in the large vascular sinuses of the corpora cavernosa so that the erection tends to persist. The corpus spongiosum, however, which surrounds the urethra as indicated in Figure 16-1, is less affected so that urination is unimpeded.

François Gigot de la Peyronie was physician to King Louis XIV of France. In 1743 he described several conditions that impede micturition, one of which eventually came to bear his name. Peyronie's disease is fibrous thickening of the shaft of the penis that causes a painful or bent erection. The median age is 52 years, and the fibrosis occurs in plaques measuring up to 3 cm in diameter that lie between the corpus cavernosum and the tunica albuginea on either side over the dorsolateral portion of the penis. The plaques are presumed to begin as foci of inflammation that subsequently undergo fibrosis and later proceed to calcification or ossification.[3] The cause is unknown and the treatment is uncertain, although

cortisone is helpful in the early inflammatory stage. Ten per cent of patients also have Dupuytren's contracture, which suggests a widespread abnormality of connective tissue. Also, Peyronie's disease may be the presenting sign of the carcinoid syndrome.[4] The connection between these two conditions is that carcinoid tumors secrete serotonin (5-hydroxytryptamine) and serotonin alters human collagen. A urinary screen for serotonin indicating a carcinoid tumor is therefore recommended for patients with Peyronie's disease.

Carcinoma of the penis is primarily a disease of societies in which circumcision is not practiced so that filth and smegma accumulate under the prepuce. It is extremely rare in Jews, who are regularly circumcised, and it causes fewer than 1 per cent of malignancies in male gentiles in the United States. It accounts for 12 per cent of cancers of male Hindus of India, however, and is common in China and Africa as well.[5] The tumor arises between the ages of 40 and 70 years, mostly on the glans, prepuce, or coronal sulcus.[6] The presenting indications are a mass or phimosis of recent onset. Examination discloses a small ulcer or a fungating mass. The cancers are squamous and well differentiated. Spread takes place through the profuse penile lymphatics to the inguinal and iliac lymph nodes. About half of patients reveal inguinal node involvement at the time of diagnosis. Treatment consists of amputation of the penis 2 cm proximal to the margin of the tumor, with inguinal node resection in order to prevent recurrence from occult metastatic disease. Irradiation is useful only when the cancer is superficial and the patient is young. Survival is determined by the stage of the disease, and is 95 per cent at three years when the tumor is clinically localized.[5]

Although the cause is unknown, some cases are preceded by erythroplasia of Queyrat, which is a raised, firm, shiny red plaque on the glans or prepuce that usually measures 1 cm in diameter and causes scaliness, itching, and sometimes pain. Microscopically the mucosa is thick (acanthosis) and the cell pattern is in disarray (dysplasia). The condition is similar to but different from Bowen's disease, or intraepithelial carcinoma of the skin. In a series of 100 patients, 10 developed cancer at the site of the lesion.[7]

## SCROTUM

The scrotum is a dependent bag covered by rugose skin and supported by the tunica dartos. It contains the testes and spermatic cords. The testes descend into the scrotum during the seventh to eighth month of intrauterine life, and the descent takes place in the inguinal canal through a peritoneal evagination called the tunica vaginalis. After the descent is completed, the neck of the tunica vaginalis closes off so that the chamber is separated from the peritoneum and consists of a continuous serosal membrane with a visceral and parietal layer entirely within the scrotum. It is a kind of miniature peritoneum. A few drops of fluid normally lubricate the smooth, glistening surfaces.

Enlargement of the scrotum has six causes, four of which are common: hydrocele, hematocele, spermatocele, and varicocele. Hydrocele is an accumulation of transudate often associated with inflammation, especially gonorrhea, and less often with trauma. Heart failure with widespread edema may cause it. Often the cause is unknown. The amount of fluid is usually about 100 ml, and almost always less than 400 ml. The bag of fluid transilluminates in a dark room, which aids in the diagnosis and locates the position of the testis as well. Treatment consists of excision of the sac, plication of it, or aspiration with injection of a sclerosing solution. Aspiration with injection is reported to cause fewer complications, such as hemorrhage or infection, and can be done on an outpatient basis.[8] Hema-

tocele is associated with trauma, does not transilluminate, and may resolve or go on to dense fibrosis and then calcification. Spermatocele is cystic dilation of the ducts of the epididymis that arises at the upper pole of the testis. It subsides with aspiration, which yields a milky fluid containing spermatozoa. Varicocele is dilation of the veins of the spermatic cord. Congestive failure is the usual cause. The vessels do not transilluminate but do collapse on recumbency, which is a diagnostic feature. It is of incidental interest that *pampinus* means "tendril," the veins that ascend the spermatic cord in a tortuous manner resemble tendrils, and on this account the spermatic veins are known as the pampiniform plexus. For this reason a varicocele is also referred to as a pampinocele.

The two uncommon causes of scrotal enlargement are tuberculosis and syphilis. Tuberculous enlargement occurs as a conglomerate tubercle in the epididymis; it is never miliary and is secondary to active pulmonary disease. In tertiary syphilis the epididymis is bypassed so that gummas form in the testis proper. Neither disease is now likely to reach this stage.

## PROSTATE

Prostatitis may be due to tuberculosis from pulmonary disease but is more often caused by *N. gonorrhoeae* from local infection. Infrequently hematogenous spread allows streptococci or staphylococci to reach the gland from boils or tonsillitis. Instrumentation of the urethra may also be a cause. Foci of acute exudative inflammation develop. Abscesses may form, and these tend to rupture into the urethra and drain in this manner rather than by the formation of fistulous tracts that drain into the rectum or onto the perineum. Obstruction of prostatic ducts leads to rupture with spillage of secretions into the stromal tissue, where noncaseating granulomas form. These granulomas should not be mistaken for tubercu-

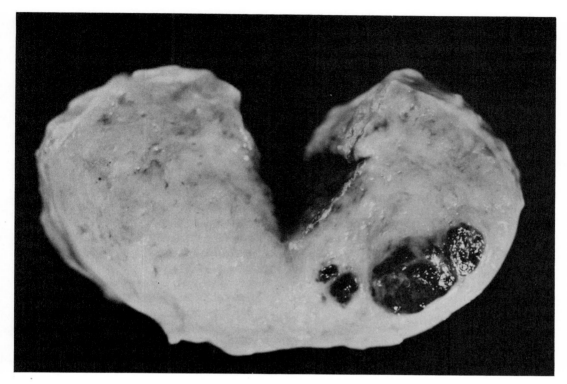

**Figure 16-2.** Hemorrhagic nature of recent infarct of prostate

losis; the absence of both pulmonary disease and caseous necrosis aids in making the distinction.

Vascular lesions of the prostate include thrombi in the periprostatic veins and arterial obstructions from emboli, vascular inflammation as with polyarteritis, or thrombosis from local atherosclerosis. Also in the tissue are small, common, localized, hemorrhagic infarcts (Figure 16-2). As the infarcts resolve, squamous metaplasia of the marginal epithelium becomes pronounced. Periprostatic phlebothrombosis may occasionally give rise to pulmonary emboli, but the consequences are not often clinically significant.

A principal lesion of the prostate is hyperplasia, which is seldom seen before the age of 50 but becomes increasingly common thereafter. It is nearly universal to some degree by the age of 80. It is due to a mid-life diminution of the secretion of androgens by the testes, which leaves a relative abundance of estrogen that continues to be produced in undiminished amount by the adrenal cortex.[9] The inner cell mass of the prostate, which surrounds the urethra, is responsive to estrogen, whereas the outer cell mass is androgen-dependent. On this account the inner cell mass becomes hyperplastic and compresses the urethra (Figure 16-3). The patient experiences dysuria, frequency, dribbling, and difficulty in starting and stopping the urinary stream. Obstruction gradually develops, the bladder dilates and becomes trabeculated from hyperplasia, and eventually hydroureter, hydronephrosis, and pyelonephritis follow.

The gland is two to 10 times normal size, and the cut surfaces reveal discrete, bulging, rubbery nodules measuring 1 to 2 cm in diameter. On histologic section these are

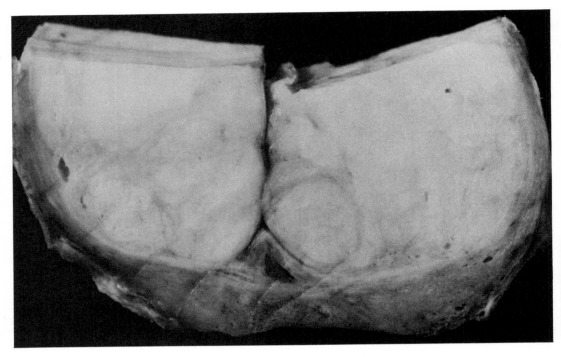

**Figure 16-3.** Nodular hyperplasia of prostate compressing the urethra at the midline

composed of clusters of dilated glands (Figure 16-4). The stimulated unit is the tall columnar epithelial cell; the cuboidal cells are old and degenerating.[10] Infolding of lining cells into the glandular lumens is common. Nodules of solid fibromuscular stroma also form, although these are less frequent and less well demarcated. When both are present, the diagnosis of glandular and stromal hyperplasia is appropriate. The process is evenly bilateral so that a symmetrical rubbery enlargement is felt on rectal examination. The process also affects the middle lobe lying at the point of the trigone, which is at the internal entrance to the prostatic urethra. Middle-lobe hyperplasia is thus especially likely to obstruct the urinary flow. Glandular hyperplasia does not proceed to malignant disease. The obstruction, which only occasionally requires surgical relief, is most often treated by transurethral prostatectomy.

It was said in 1900 that carcinoma of the prostate is rare.[11] That was an error; the cancer was much more common even then, and today it represents 17 per cent of all male malignant disease.[12] It is second only to cancer of the lung. This figure of 17 per cent represents only the clinically evident cases. In 1941 Moore made step sections of whole prostates and found many small cancers that were confined to the gland and were asymptomatic.[13] Subsequent studies have revealed that the tumor is rare before age 50, increases with age thereafter, and is present in as many as 80 per cent of men over the age of 90.[14] The clinically silent cancers are thus much more frequent than those that give rise to symptoms. Taken altogether, carcinoma of the prostate is the most common cancer of men in the United States.

The tumor presents in three ways: as clinically evident disease, as metastatic disease without an apparent primary site (occult cancer), and as small quiescent tumors that are essentially localized to the gland (latent cancer).[15] The tumors arise for the most part from the posterior lobes, which lie against the capsule of the gland and constitute the outer cell mass. The marginal location places the tumor at a distance from the urethra so that symptoms do not arise until metastases have formed outside the gland or the tumor has spread through the inner cell mass to the urethra. Involvement of the urethra is manifested by hematuria, infection, or urinary obstruction. Metastatic disease causes pathologic fractures or bone pain at the sites of the malignant deposits. A hard nodule can be felt through the rectum on either side of the posterior surface of the gland. All clinical manifestations therefore indicate advanced disease that is usually incurable, as early diagnosis is extremely difficult.

Grossly the tumors are hard and pale gray with somewhat poorly defined margins (Figure 16-5). Nearly all are adenocarcinomas although a few, perhaps 10 per cent, are undifferentiated. Anaplasia is often extremely slight so that the existence of the cancer is certified more by the presence of tumor cells in the perineural lymphatics than by cytologic features. Perineural invasion is shown in Figure 16-6. From the capsular lymphatics metastatic spread extends to the pelvic lymph nodes and to bone, especially the sacrum, pelvis, and spine. Eventually spread to the lungs takes place. Cerebral metastases are uncommon and may develop through Batson's plexus of paravertebral veins.[16] Metastases in fatal disease are often widespread, as evidenced by the high frequency with which tumor cells are found in aspirated bone marrow.

The epithelium of the prostate produces acid phosphatase, which normally flows out of the gland through ducts that open into the urethra. With metastatic disease, however, no outflow path is available and the

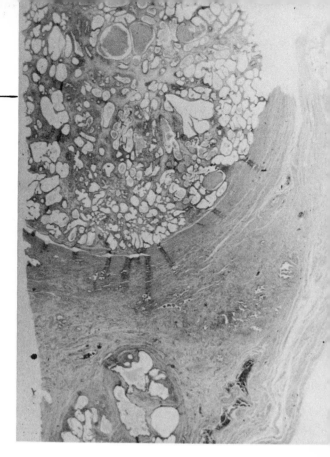

**Figure 16-4.** Dilated glands in discrete nodule of hyperplastic prostate

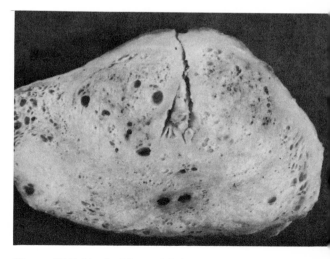

**Figure 16-5.** Hard white nodule in external cell mass at left; carcinoma of prostate

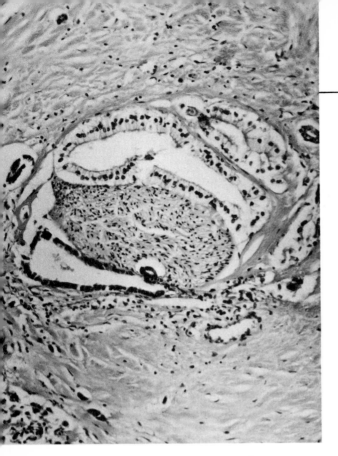

**Figure 16-6.** Perineural invasion of prostatic cancer

enzyme accumulates in the serum. This is especially true with metastatic disease to bone.[17] The metastatic sites, moreover, are osteoblastic, and with new bone formation the serum alkaline phosphatase also rises. These enzyme changes are useful in monitoring the effects of treatment. Cytologic examination of the urine sediment rarely discloses tumor cells when the cancer is not clinically evident; when it is clinically evident, the yield of tumor cells is improved by massage of the gland. However, the advisability of massaging a malignant tumor is doubtful. Diagnosis therefore rests more with needle biopsy than with serum changes or cytologic findings.

A staging system for prostatic cancer is in use but is only an amplification of the clinical presentations cited earlier. Moreover, the system is fraught with several difficulties, as pointed out by Franks.[9] Foremost among these is the unavoidable error of extrapolating clinical findings to an accurate delineation of tumor spread. The goal of treatment, nevertheless, is to eradicate all of the tumor. Local means have seldom succeeded because tumor spread is ordinarily extensive by the time clinical signs arise. This situation changed in 1941, when Huggins discovered the principle of "physiologic surgery," i.e., removal of a normal structure to heal an abnormal part.[18] He found that castration or the use of estrogens would cause not only the tumor to shrink, but the metastatic lesions as well. Antiandrogenic measures are the keystone of current therapy. An estimated 20 per cent of patients, however, fail to respond.[15] Local surgical excision and irradiation are also used. Results of all these treatments are difficult to interpret because of variation in the natural history of the tumors, the use of multiple therapeutic methods, and the frequency of death from other causes at this time of life. Nevertheless, about half of patients with clinically evident cases survive for five years, 20 per cent of latent cancers become aggressive, and the remainder continue to be indolent whether or not treatment is given.[9] The prolonged estrogen therapy that is required may cause gynecomastia.

Clinically evident cancer of the prostate is rare in Orientals, which suggests the influence of a genetic or environmental factor in the United States, where the tumor is common. However, latent cancers of the prostate are common in Japanese men.[15] There is no chemical or physical way to identify those latent cancers that will become aggressive. The prostate is stimulated by androgenic and inhibited by estrogenic hormones, but these are said to play no part in carcinogenesis.[9] Since androgen production diminishes with old age while estrogen continues to be secreted from the adrenal cortex in normal amounts, the cancer is not associated with an abnormality of hormone production. Moreover, no relationship is known between the blood or

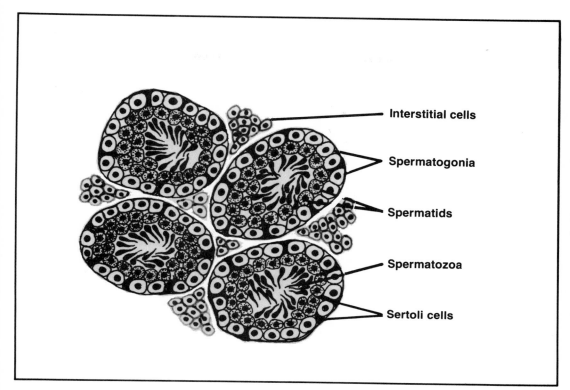

**Figure 16-7.** Diagram of histologic structure of testicular tissue

Labels in figure:
- Interstitial cells
- Spermatogonia
- Spermatids
- Spermatozoa
- Sertoli cells

urine levels of androgens, estrogens, or steroid hormones and the development of the cancers. The tumor appears unrelated to nodular hyperplasia of the inner cell mass and is not prevented by treatment of that condition. Virus-like particles have been identified in the tumor cells in some cases but are also found in nodular hyperplasia, and their relationship to malignant tumor formation is not yet clear.[19] Thus the cause of the second most common clinically evident cancer in men is still unknown.

### TESTIS

The Greek words *orchis* and *kryptos* mean "testis" and "hidden." Cryptorchidism is thus the term for an undescended testis. Actually only 25 per cent are intra-abdominal; 70 per cent are located in the inguinal canal and are therefore not quite hidden. (The remaining 5 per cent are perineal, pubic, or otherwise unusually situated.) The condition occurs in 3 per cent of infants, but spontaneous descent takes place in the first few weeks or months of life so that the incidence drops to 0.5 per cent in men.[20] The cause is unknown, although deformities of the inguinal canal play a role, and inguinal hernia often accompanies the condition. Even though undescended, the malpositioned testis undergoes normal development until the age of 5 years, and surgical treatment (orchiorrhaphy, orchiopexy) allows continued normal development if performed prior to that time.[21]

Without treatment atrophy develops, the texture becomes firm, and dense connective tissue replaces the seminiferous tubules. Spermatogenesis then ceases so that the patient is sterile when the condition is bilateral. The atrophy is due to the higher intra-abdominal temperature compared with that of the scrotum. The condition is

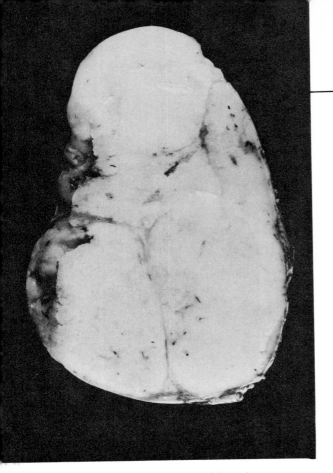

**Figure 16-8.** Fleshy, soft, white cut surface of seminoma. The tumor measures 13 × 9 × 7 cm.

Table 16-1.

## Main tumors of testes

| Type | Proportion |
|------|------------|
| Germinal | |
| Seminoma | 35-70% |
| Embryonal carcinoma | 20% |
| Teratocarcinoma | 9% |
| Choriocarcinoma | Rare |
| | |
| Stromal | |
| Interstitial tumor | Rare |

usually asymptomatic. The incidence of malignant tumors in undescended testes, however, is alarmingly high. Campbell, cited by Grove, found that of 1,422 malignant testicular tumors, 12 per cent arose in undescended testes.[22] Moreover, orchiopexy after the age of 6 does not necessarily reduce the malignant potential; a cancer has arisen as long as 34 years after that procedure.[23]

Klinefelter's syndrome includes gynecomastia, sterility, eunuchoid habitus, absence of libido, and low intelligence. Although the external genitalia are normal, the testes are aspermic and hypoplastic, measuring only 2 cm in greatest dimension. In 80 per cent of patients the body cells contain 47 nuclei with an XXY sex chromosome pattern. For this reason buccal smears reveal Barr bodies, and neutrophils show the drumstick configuration of normal females. In the other 20 per cent the syndrome is unaccompanied by an abnormal number of sex chromosomes.[24]

There are only three main tumors of the testis, and all are malignant. They are uncommon and collectively constitute only 1 per cent of cancers in males. The average age at onset is 32 years, and 80 per cent occur before the age of 40. The cause is not known although roughly 10 per cent arise in undescended testes.[22] The histologic structure of the testis is shown in Figure 16-7. The germinal cells line the seminiferous tubules and progress from spermatogonia along the basement membranes to the intermediate spermatids and then to spermatozoa, which occupy the lumens. The three main tumors of the testis arise from these germinal cells and collectively make up 95 per cent of the total. These are the seminoma, embryonal carcinoma, and teratocarcinoma. A fourth germinal tumor, the choriocarcinoma, is extremely rare. The nongerminal units are the Sertoli cells, which provide support for the spermatogonia, and the interstitial cells of Leydig, which lie between the seminiferous tubules

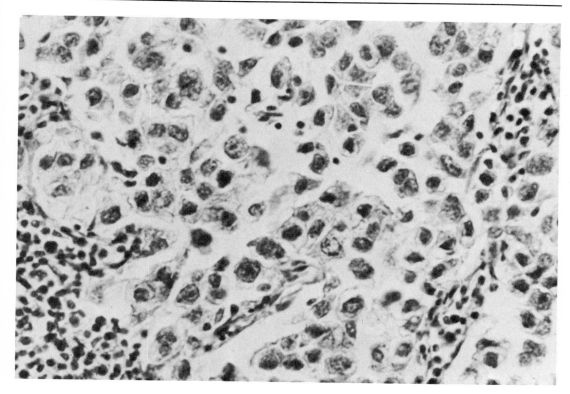

**Figure 16-9.** Histologic structure of seminoma

and secrete androgens. Tumors of Leydig cells are virilizing and rare. Adenomas of Sertoli cells are too rare to be included here. The main tumors and their relative frequencies are shown in Table 16-1.

Although Table 16-1 suggests histologic uniformity, examination reveals that in about 40 per cent of patients more than one tumor type is present in the same lesion. All cause a palpable mass in the scrotum, and usually pain or discomfort as well. Spread tends to occur early, and metastases are frequently present by the time the diagnosis is made. Orchiectomy is the proper diagnostic procedure because biopsy ruptures the tunica albuginea and hastens spread of the tumor.

Seminoma is the most frequent. It occurs in adults. The testis is enlarged, the tunica albuginea is intact, and the cut surface is pale, soft, and fleshy with scant stroma (Figure 16-8). The cells are large and uniform with few mitotic figures or other evidence of anaplasia (Figure 16-9). It is an extremely radiosensitive tumor, and orchiectomy, either with or without irradiation, achieves a five-year survival rate of about 95 per cent.[25] The counterpart of this tumor in the ovary is the dysgerminoma.

Embryonal carcinoma is less frequent and more malignant than seminoma. It occurs in infants and adults. The tumor is small, unencapsulated, soft, and focally hemorrhagic (Figure 16-10; see color section, p C-7). The tumor cells are arranged in acinic or papillary formations, and anaplasia is pronounced. Multinucleated giant cells and mitotic figures are numerous. Spread takes place early up the spermatic cords to the iliac lymph nodes. Metastases to the lungs and liver are frequent. The cancer is not especially radiosensitive. The

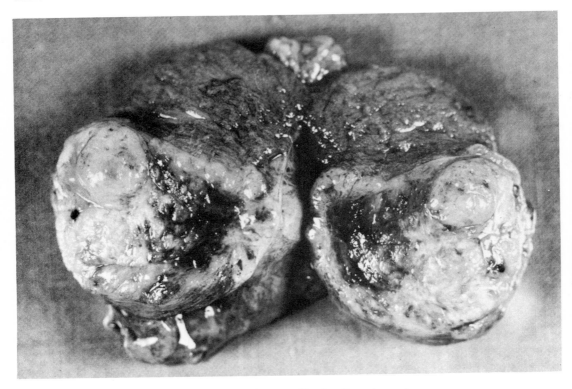

**Figure 16-10.** Cut surface of embryonal carcinoma of testis. Also shown in color section, p C-7.

five-year survival rate is between 60 and 65 per cent.[26]

Teratocarcinomas are characterized by tissue elements from at least two of the three germ layers: endoderm, ectoderm, and mesoderm. They occur in the first three decades of life. The tumors are large and the cut surfaces are soft and multicystic with grossly evident plugs of keratin, accumulations of mucin, islands of cartilage, and spicules of bone. Histologic examination reveals a mix of squamous epithelium, intestinal and bronchial mucosa, neural tissue, skin appendages such as sebaceous glands, and fragments of cartilage. Elements of choriocarcinoma may be present along with the other tissue components. In this case chorionic gonadotrophin

may be present in the blood and urine. Metastases are frequent, although the various tissue components appear well differentiated. The five-year survival rate is about 60 per cent.[26]

Choriocarcinoma rarely arises in the testis. It is clinically silent, spreads early, and is unaffected by any mode of treatment. The primary tumor is soft and markedly hemorrhagic. Metastases are similar in consistency and are widespread. The histologic feature is the combined presence of cytotrophoblasts and syncytiotrophoblasts. The functional feature is the massive production of chorionic gonadotrophin. Identification of this substance in the blood or urine is necessary for the diagnosis of choriocarcinoma.

# REFERENCES

1. Hagerty RF, Taber E: Hypospadias. *Am Surg* 24:244, 1958

2. Mogg RA: Congenital anomalies of the urethra. *Br J Urol* 40:638, 1968

3. Smith BH: Peyronie's disease. *Am J Clin Pathol* 45:670, 1966

4. Bivens CH, Maracek RL, Feldman JM: Peyronie's disease—A presenting complaint of the carcinoid syndrome. *N Engl J Med* 289:844, 1973

5. deKernion JB, Tynberg P, Persky L, et al: Carcinoma of the penis. *Cancer* 32:1256, 1973

6. Staubitz WJ, Lent MH, Oberkircher OJ: Carcinoma of the penis. *Cancer* 8:371, 1955

7. Graham JH, Helwig EB: Erythroplasia of Queyrat. A clinicopathologic and histochemical study. *Cancer* 32:1396, 1973

8. Moloney GE: Comparison of results of treatment of hydrocele and epididymal cysts by surgery and injection. *Br Med J* 3:478, 1975

9. Franks LM: Etiology, epidemiology, and pathology of prostatic cancer. *Cancer* 32:1092, 1973

10. Mao P, Nakao K, Bora R, et al: Human benign prostatic hyperplasia. *Arch Pathol* 79:270, 1965

11. Boyd W: *A Textbook of Pathology*, 8th ed, p 961. Philadelphia: Lea & Febiger, 1970

12. Silverberg BS: Cancer statistics, 1977. *CA—Cancer J Clin* 27:26, 1977

13. Moore RA: Morphology of small prostatic carcinoma. *J Urol* 33:224, 1935

14. Hirst AE Jr, Bergman RT: Carcinoma of the prostate in men 80 or more years old. *Cancer* 7:136, 1954

15. Franks LM: Recent research on prostatic cancer. *Pathol Annu* 2:76, 1967

16. Catane R, Kaufman J, West C, et al: Brain metastases from prostatic carcinoma. *Cancer* 38:2583, 1976

17. Mostofi FK, Price EB Jr: *Tumors of the Male Genital System. Atlas of Tumor Pathology*, fasc 8. Washington, DC: Armed Forces Institute of Pathology, 1973

18. Huggins C, Hodges CV: Studies on prostatic cancer. I. The effect of castration, of estrogen and of androgen injection on serum phosphatases in metastatic carcinoma of the prostate. *Cancer Res* 1:293, 1941

19. Ohtsuki Y, Seman G, Maruyama K, et al: Ultrastructural studies of human prostatic neoplasia. *Cancer* 37:2295, 1976

20. Campbell MF, Harrison JH: *Urology*, 3rd ed, vol 2, pp 1628-1644. Philadelphia: Saunders, 1970

21. Robinson JN, Engle ET: Some observations on the cryptorchid testis. *J Urol* 71:726, 1954

22. Grove JS: The cryptorchid problem. *J Urol* 71:735, 1954

23. Angulo R, Caballerd L, Mejia P: Bilateral seminoma 34 years after orchiopexy. *J Urol* 118:882, 1976

24. Griesemer DA, ed: Klinefelter syndrome and breast cancer. *Bull Johns Hopkins Hosp* 138:102, 1976

25. Mostofi FK: Testicular tumors. Epidemiologic, etiologic, and pathologic features. *Cancer* 32:1186, 1973

26. Newton RA: Malignant tumors of the testis. In *Cancer, A Manual for Practitioners*, 4th ed. Boston: American Cancer Society, Massachusetts Division, 1968

# 17

## DISORDERS OF FEMALE GENITALIA

### INFECTIONS

The female genital tract is subject to venereal infections, including gonorrhea, syphilis, chancroid, granuloma inguinale, and lymphogranuloma venereum. In gonorrhea the gonococci cause an acute exudative inflammation that remains superficial and involves the urethra, paraurethral (Skene's) glands, Bartholin's glands, and, later, the uterine (fallopian) tubes. The vagina and uterine cervix, which are covered by tough squamous mucosa, are unaffected. The endometrium is also bypassed; the reason is not clear. At the sites of disease ulceration occurs, a mucopurulent drip develops, and healing gradually takes place with scar formation. In Bartholin's glands abscesses form, fibrosis follows, duct obstruction develops, and cyst formation is a frequent result. Passage of the newborn through the infected canal leads to ophthalmia neonatorum, which causes acute conjunctivitis with subsequent scarring that eventually leads to blindness. The condition is prevented by instillation of penicillin or a weak solution of silver nitrate into the eyes immediately after birth.

In the uterine tubes pyosalpinx is followed by fibrosis, tortuosity, and eventual blockage of the passage so that ova cannot move through the lumen to the endometrium (Figure 17-1). Sterility results when the process is bilateral, as is frequent. Blockage also results in ectopic (tubal) pregnancy, which sooner or later requires

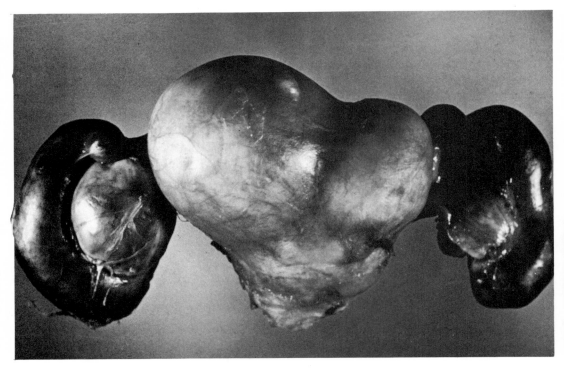

**Figure 17-1.** Pyosalpinx with fibrous tubo-ovarian adhesions

operative attention. Spread of the infection into the peritoneum leads to pelvic inflammatory disease with dense fibrous adhesions that incarcerate all structures—the so-called frozen pelvis. Finally, hematogenous dissemination may lead to suppurative arthritis, vegetative endocarditis, or acute meningitis. None of these, however, is frequent.

A separate consideration is epidemic vulvovaginitis, which affects prepubertal girls beginning any time after infancy. In the prepubertal period the vaginal mucosa is immature and unable to resist infection with *Neisseria*. The infection is transmitted by fomites; it is nonvenereal and has nothing to do with sexual activity.

In female syphilis the chancre usually occurs on the labia, vaginal mucosa, or cervix so that often it is not evident to the patient. It heals spontaneously without a scar. The secondary stage of the disease is character-

ized in the genital tissues by the condyloma latum, which arises on the vulva or perineum. It is a flat, reddish-brown elevation that consists of epithelial hyperplasia, elongation of rete pegs, and infiltration with lymphocytes, macrophages, and plasma cells. The lesion teems with spirochetes, is highly contagious, and responds to treatment with penicillin. It is to be distinguished from the condyloma acuminatum, which arises in the anogenital region and consists of acanthosis with hyperkeratosis. There is little inflammation, and the lesion is not affected by penicillin therapy. Condyloma acuminatum is probably caused by a virus.

Chancroid is similar to the male disease. A vesicle forms on the labia and becomes a pustule, and the organism (*Haemophilus ducreyi*) is carried in the lymph stream to the inguinal nodes, where suppuration develops in about half of patients. The en-

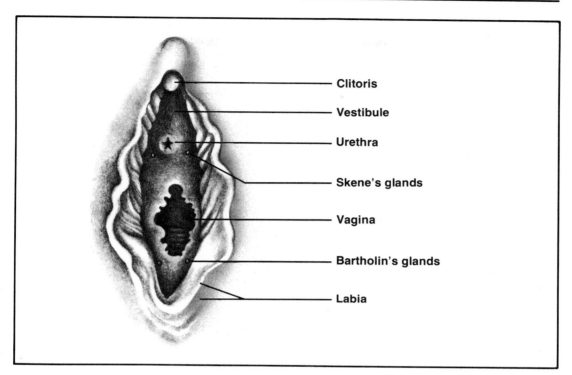

**Figure 17-2.** The structures of the vulva

larged, tender, violaceous nodes constitute a "bubo." The infection does not extend outside the genital tissues and heals spontaneously without scar formation.

Granuloma inguinale in the female also causes a large, irregular, flat ulcer over the groins and perineum that is serpiginous and indolent. The base is richly infiltrated with plasma cells and macrophages in which Donovan bodies are evident. Buboes may form in the inguinal nodes. The ulcer heals with granulation tissue that progresses to scar formation or keloids so that the surface may become disfigured.

To the established causes of venereal infections must now be added nongonococcal urethritis due to *Chlamydia trachomatis*. The organism is an obligate intracellular parasite previously regarded as a large virus but distinguishable from a virus by the presence of two nucleic acids. *C. trachomatis* causes acute exudative urethritis

that may spread in the male to the epididymis or rectum, and in the female to the cervix, uterine tubes, or rectal mucosa. The organism may coexist with the gonococcus, it does not respond to penicillin, and it is a frequent cause of postgonorrheal urethritis. It is also the cause of inclusion conjunctivitis in the neonate who has passed through the birth canal during maternal infection. The disease is transmitted by sexual intercourse, and it is amenable to treatment with tetracycline.[1]

## VULVA

The vulva consists of the mons pubis, both labia, the clitoris, vestibule, and vestibular glands (Figure 17-2).

In addition to the venereal infections that affect the vulva, the two principal lesions are urethral caruncle and epidermoid carcinoma. The caruncle is a discrete, fri-

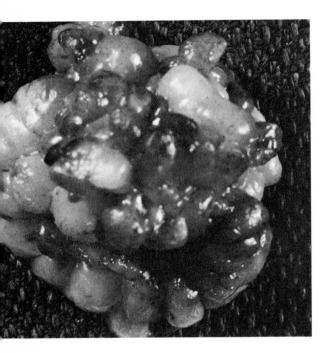

**Figure 17-3.** Multicystic botryoid sarcoma

able tissue mass measuring 0.5 to 1.0 cm in diameter that lies within the distal urethra or at its opening onto the vestibule. The mass is composed of highly vascularized granulation tissue covered by transitional epithelium or squamous mucosa. Ulceration may occur, leukocytes infiltrate the stroma, and bleeding may follow. The cause is unknown. The lesion occurs mainly during adulthood, excruciating pain is the clinical characteristic, and cure is achieved by surgical excision.

Carcinoma of the vulva occurs during adulthood, represents about 4 per cent of female genital cancers, and presents as a "lump," white patch, or focus of itching on the surface. The most frequent site is on either labium on either side. The site is often preceded by a focus of leukoplakia or carcinoma in situ.[2] The cancer ulcerates the surface, invades the subjacent tissue, and is almost always squamous. Extensive lymphatics carry the tumor cells to the lymph nodes on both sides of the pelvis so that surgical treatment requires bilateral dissection of lymph nodes. Results vary with the stage of the disease. When the tumor measures less than 3 cm in diameter, 65 per cent of patients survive for five years.[3] When the cancer measures 3 to 7 cm, however, survival is reduced to 21 per cent.

## VAGINA

The vagina is a collapsed cylinder lying between the bladder in front and the rectum in back. It extends from the vestibule of the vulva to the uterine cervix. After puberty the mucosa is keratinized so that gonococci may no longer invade and inflame the tissue. Two other inflammatory conditions occur, however. The flagellated protozoan *Trichomonas vaginalis* causes a chronic superficial exudative inflammation that is reflected clinically by thin, persistent leukorrhea. The second is a fungus, *Candida albicans (Monilia)*, that is evident grossly in the form of white patches over the rugose mucosa and is also expressed clinically by watery leukorrhea. Both *Trichomonas* and *Candida* are localized to the surface, and neither causes a constitutional reaction.

Carcinoma of the vagina is a vanishingly rare disease. It has shown up recently, however, in a clear-cell variety often associated with endocervical glands in the squamous surface (vaginal adenosis) in the daughters of women who took diethylstilbestrol during pregnancy. The drug is a synthetic estrogenic hormone formerly thought to protect the fetus against hemorrhagic complications during pregnancy. The tumors have also occurred on the cervix. Bleeding is the clinical manifestation. The ages of the daughters range from 7 to 28 years. Irradiation and surgical extirpation are the methods of treatment. No tumors have occurred in the male offspring of exposed mothers. The use of diethylstilbestrol in pregnancy has been discontinued.[4]

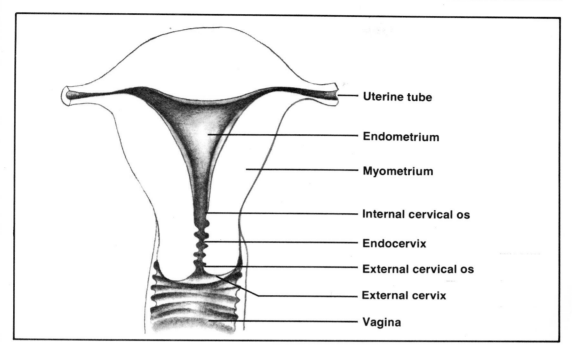

Figure 17-4. Cervix and endocervical canal in relation to uterus above and vagina below

Embryonal rhabdomyosarcoma also arises in the bladder or vagina of infant girls. The mean age is 3 years. The tumor is polypoid and may project through the vagina as a mass that appears multicystic (Figure 17-3). For this reason it is known as a botryoid (grapelike) sarcoma. Normal mucosa covers the "cysts," myxoid tissue makes up most of the mass, and malignant striated muscle fibers are scattered throughout the stroma. Radical surgery is indicated, but it succeeds only in those infrequent instances in which the tumor is localized at the time of treatment.

## CERVIX

From Figure 17-4 it is evident that the cervix is composed of an internal canal and an external portion. The canal begins at the internal cervical os, measures 2 cm in length, and ends at the external cervical os.

It is lined by a single layer of tall columnar cells that extend into clefts, which give the appearance of a superficial layer of glands. The external cervix, or portio vaginalis, begins at the external os and extends to the upper margin of the vagina. It is covered by a smooth layer of squamous epithelium. The squamocolumnar junction divides the two portions of cervix at the external cervical os.

Three minor conditions often affect the cervix: inflammation, erosion, and polyp formation. Gonorrhea causes endocervicitis with sequestration of bacteria in the endocervical glands. Pyogens also affect the tissue, especially from lacerations incurred with abortion. Both produce a superficial exudate and chronic leukorrhea. As the reaction subsides, stenosis of the gland clefts may develop so that small cysts come to occupy the distal part of the endocervical canal. These fill with the mucous secretions of the epithelial cells. Termed nabothian cysts, they are of little clinical import. With chronic inflammation that extends into these glands, squamous metaplasia of the lining cells frequently develops. This change is not to be mistaken for epithelial neoplasia. When fibrosis from the reparative reaction is pronounced, the endocervical canal may become stenosed or closed. If it closes, atrophy of the endometrium with or without accumulation of exudate in the chamber (pyometrium) follows.

The second minor condition is erosion, in which the endocervical mucosa slips out of the canal and extends for a variable distance over the portio vaginalis. The surface grossly reveals a pink, velvety discoloration around the external os that is accompanied by persistent leukorrhea. The cause is not known. Microscopically the portio is covered with endocervical mucosa that is chronically inflamed. Antibiotic therapy prevents reinfection. It is important that the red granular surface not be mistaken for a tumor.

Polyps of the endocervix project into the canal and may extend through the external os into the vaginal portion. The globular mass is covered with endocervical mucosa, the stroma consists of highly vascularized loose connective tissue, and the centers disclose irregularly dilated endocervical glands. Polyps tend to be clinically silent unless ulceration develops; leukorrhea or vaginal bleeding is then the clinical manifestation. Severance through the stalk is curative. Polyps are neither neoplastic nor premalignant.

The major lesion of the uterine cervix is carcinoma. It occurs mainly in women over the age of 45 years, it is the second most frequent cancer in women, and it arises at the squamocolumnar junction. Moreover, it evidently arises through a series of cytologic changes that take place over several years. Normally the squamous portion of the cervical mucosa is layered with cuboidal basal cells, large intermediate cells, and huge, flat superficial cells. Mitotic figures are present in the basal cells, which lie against the basement membrane, and their normal proliferation is balanced by equal desquamation of the superficial cells.

Dysplasia is a disturbance of the normal maturation sequence so that the number of mitotic figures increases and they extend into the intermediate cell layer. The superficial cells are spared, however, so that the alteration is not transmural. The condition regresses spontaneously but may recur. According to some, about 10 per cent of cases progress to carcinoma in situ.[5] This condition is transmural and thus involves all layers of the mucosa. The basement membrane, however, remains intact. There is no clinical or gross evidence of the condition, and it is identified by biopsy after the discovery of abnormal cells in the Papanicolaou smear. The lesion is illustrated in Figure 17-5. Carcinoma in situ is irregularly distributed over the cervical surface so that without a special marking the correct site for biopsy cannot be discerned. The superficial cells of the normal mucosa contain glycogen, however, and covering the surface with a weak solution of iodine discolors the normal mucosa brown while leaving the abnormal sites pallid and unstained. This Schiller test is thus useful in identifying the abnormal mucosa that is suitable for biopsy.

The frequencies with which dysplasia progresses to carcinoma in situ, and with which the latter advances to invasive cancer, are somewhat uncertain. It is nevertheless presumed to be a sequence. Part of the reason is that the average age for dysplasia (35 years) precedes that of carcinoma in situ (38 years), which precedes that for invasive cancer (48 years).[6] Uncertainty about the transformations stems largely from the unreliability of the diagnoses. Independent observers, examining the same slides, have difficulty in finding agreement over the diagnoses.[7] There is also question about the propriety of regarding carcinoma

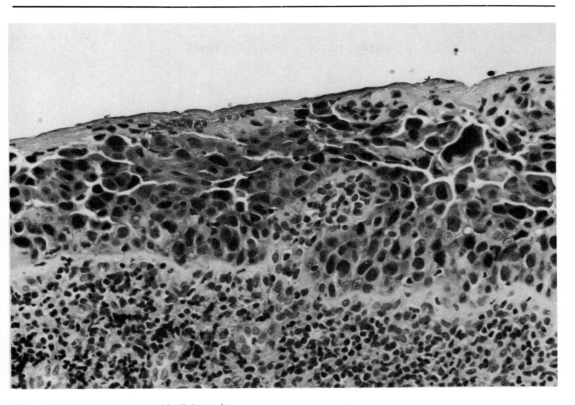

**Figure 17-5.** Transmural epithelial atypia

in situ as malignant when the majority of such lesions do not progress to invasive tumors.[8] There is even question about the use of the term. If carcinoma in situ means cancer, there is little explanation for the majority of cases that do not invade. On the other hand, if the term means that the lesion will become cancerous later, there is doubt about using such a term for a condition that is not now malignant and probably will not become so. Consult reference 9 for a criticism of this nomenclature.

It is estimated that 2 per cent of American women will develop carcinoma of the cervix by the age of 80. Nevertheless, the frequency has been decreasing; in 1930 it was 20/100,000, and in 1970 it regressed to 8/100,000. This decline is attributable to diagnostic techniques, particularly cytologic examination, that detect premalignant disease before an invasive tumor devel-

ops.[6] The importance of pelvic examinations with direct visualization of the cervix and cytologic studies is obvious. The patient with this cancer is usually 45 to 55 years old, married, parous, and aware of a vaginal discharge or intermittent spotting that progresses to recurrent hemorrhage.

Examination of the cervix reveals a raised white plaque or shallow red ulcer in the region of the squamocolumnar junction. The growth extends outward to produce a pendulous mass (exophytic), or inward to form an invasive lesion (endophytic) (Figure 17-6). Whatever the direction, 95 per cent are squamous and the remainder are adenocarcinomas that presumably arise from the endocervical glands. Grading is not of great importance because it is the spread of the cancer rather than its degree of differentiation that determines the prospect for cure. Since spread takes time, the

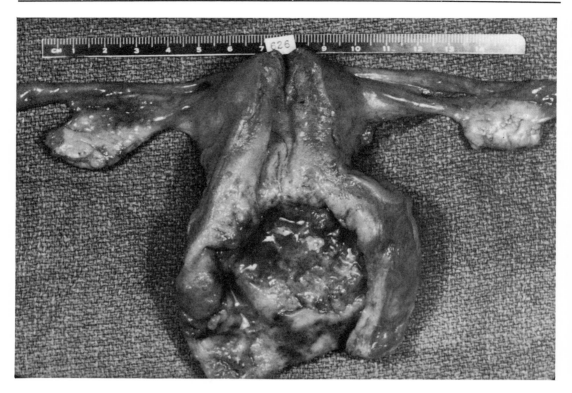

**Figure 17-6.** Endophytic carcinoma of uterine cervix

earlier the treatment begins, the better the outlook.

The cervical cancer spreads upward to the endometrium, downward to the vagina, anteriorly to the bladder, posteriorly to the rectum, laterally to the round ligaments, outward to the pelvic nodes, and, seldom, outside the pelvis to the liver and lungs. An important feature of the tumor is therefore a tendency to remain in the pelvis, killing the patient not by distant metastases but by urinary obstruction as a result of invasion of the urethra, bladder, and/or ureters, producing hydronephrosis and suppurative pyelonephritis.

The method of treatment and the prospect for cure are determined by the spread of the tumor. This is estimated by examination with X-rays, pyelography, and lymphangiography. Unfortunately, these data are not very accurate.[10,11] Nevertheless, they allow the disease to be assigned a stage—an arbitrary classification of tumor spread utilized within different institutions by common consent. The main aspects of the classification of cervical cancer are shown in Table 17-1.

Treatment consists of irradiation or radical hysterectomy. The latter includes salpingectomy, oophorectomy, and bilateral pelvic lymphadenectomy. Results are about the same regardless of the method.[12] This is not surprising, since it is the stage of the disease rather than the individuality of the method that determines the result of treatment. Prognosis is not worsened by pregnancy. Chemotherapy is ineffective. Five-year survival is equated with cure. The five-year survival rate for stage I is 85 to 90 per cent; for stage II, 70 to 75 per cent; for stage III, 30 to 35 per cent; and for stage IV, 10 per cent.[12]

The cause of the disease is unknown, but several features are of much interest. It is a condition of parous women, especially those of low socioeconomic status and those whose husbands are not circumcised. It is also a condition of women who have had early coitus and continued exposure to different sexual partners. It is therefore rare in women whose husbands are circumcised, nonexistent in those who are celibate, and comparatively common in those who are promiscuous. This suggests that smegma or a virus affecting genital tissue may be carcinogenic. Attention has turned away from smegma and toward a viral cause. Herpes type 2 virus affects genital tissues, and antibodies to this virus are much more frequent in women with cancer of the cervix than in others.[6] This finding raises the possibility that cervical cancer is a "venereal disease." Cervical cancer is not an estrogen-dependent tumor.

## UTERUS

The adult parous uterus weighs 100 to 140 gm and measures 8 to 9 cm in length; the lower third projects into the vagina as the cervix. The serosa is part of the peritoneum, the wall is composed of smooth muscle, and the lining surface, or endometrium, sheds monthly with menstrual periods during reproductive life.

Acute endometritis is due to pyogenic organisms that reach the tissue after abortion, especially when nonsterile devices have been used. After birth, retained placental fragments, which are necrotic, become foci for bacterial growth and suppurative inflammation. The process tends to be transient because of the recurrent shedding of the lining surface. If the endocervical canal is blocked, however, pyometrium with or without pyosalpinx often develops. Chronic endometritis is nonspecific and of little clinical importance unless it is tuberculous. The granulomas are identified in curettings, and the condition is secondary to active pulmonary disease. Caseation does not develop because menstrual periods extrude the infected tissue.

The endometrium may also undergo hyperplasia so that a soft, fleshy tissue mass fills the cavity. The condition occurs near the menopause and may be due to failure of follicles to rupture so that estrogen stimulation is prolonged. The process also occurs in women taking estrogen therapy for menopausal symptoms. The condition is manifested by bleeding that tends to be continuous throughout the menstrual cycle. Curettings reveal large tissue fragments with compact stroma and abundant glands that are irregularly dilated. An earlier tendency was to relate this to the pattern of holes in Swiss cheese. The epithelial cells lining the glands are present in a single layer without anaplasia. Although it is widely accepted that the condition precedes the development of carcinoma of the endometrium, the precise relationship between the two conditions is uncertain.

Polyps of the endometrium are common. They occur around the menopause, i.e., 45 to 55 years, and cause intermittent bleed-

Table 17-1.

## Staging of cervical cancer

| Stage | Disease process |
|-------|-----------------|
| 0 | Carcinoma in situ |
| I | Localized to cervix |
| II | Spread to lower fundus or upper two-thirds of vagina |
| III | Spread to pelvic wall or lower one-third of vagina |
| IV | Spread to bladder, rectum, or extrapelvic site |

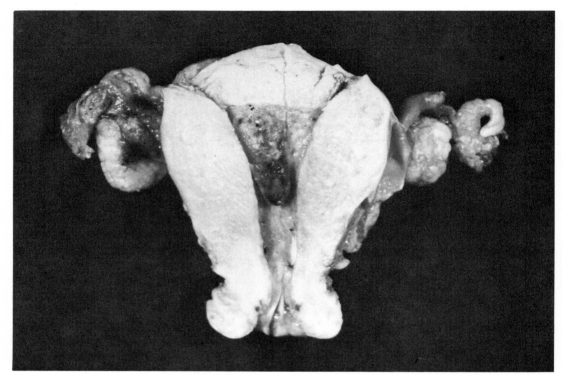

**Figure 17-7.** Polyp of endometrium

ing between the menstrual periods or after the menopause. The polyps are oval, fleshy, dark red, and sessile or pedunculated. They distort the shape of the endometrium and are neither neoplastic nor preneoplastic. About 20 per cent are multiple. The cause is unknown, although they may represent a focal response of the endometrium to estrogen stimulation. Polyps are the most common cause of postmenopausal bleeding. Curettage establishes the diagnosis and cures the condition at the same time. The gross appearance is shown in Figure 17-7.

Adenomyosis, or endometriosis interna, is the presence of ectopic foci of endometrium throughout the uterine wall. The favored site is the posterior wall, where the fascicles of muscle undergo hypertrophy. The uterus is therefore enlarged and sagit-

tal section reveals asymmetrical thickening of the posterior wall. If the ectopic foci are localized to one area, thickening of the myometrium produces a poorly defined muscle mass known as an adenomyoma. Since ectopic endometrium also occurs outside the uterus, the terms endometriosis interna and externa are in use. Romney and colleagues regard the two conditions as different.[6] The cut surface of the myometrium reveals coarse trabeculation and a scattering of minute colorless cysts or discrete foci of dark red discoloration that measure 1 to 4 mm in diameter. These discolorations are islands of ectopic endometrium in which menstrual hemorrhage has taken place. The histologic change has three features: ectopic glands, a narrow collar of ectopic stroma, and a light infiltration of macrophages that are brown from

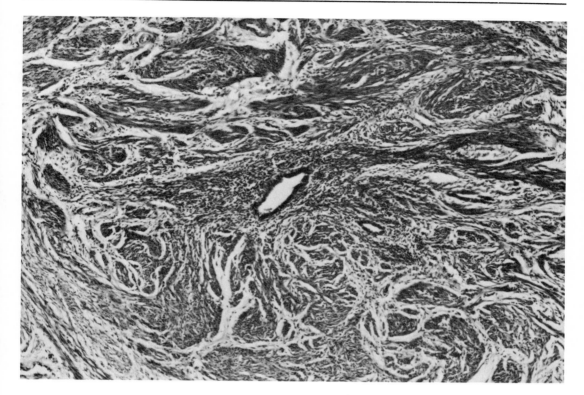

**Figure 17-8.** Ectopic endometrial gland with surrounding stroma deep in myometrium

the phagocytosis of hemosiderin (Figure 17-8). The cause of the condition is not known, although the ectopic foci are connected by tortuous routes to the endometrial cavity.[13] Endometriosis interna is thus displacement rather than neoplastic invasion. The patients are usually parous and 40 to 50 years old, and they complain of premenstrual pain, colicky dysmenorrhea that may be severe, and excessive menstrual bleeding. Hysterectomy is a suitable treatment for many patients.

Foci of endometrium spread throughout the pelvic tissues are also called endometriosis, or endometriosis externa. This differs from adenomyosis in several particulars. Patients are usually single, nulliparous, and 20 to 40 years old. The ectopic tissue is more responsive to the hormonal tides of the menstrual cycle so that bleeding is regular, symptoms are more pronounced, and the reparative reaction evokes granulation tissue and scar formation. The hemorrhagic debris discolors the tissue so that blue nodules are evident at the ectopic sites.

The characteristic clinical feature is sacral pain associated with menstrual periods. Additional symptoms depend on the site of involvement. In the uterine tubes fibrosis, distortion, and sterility develop. Severe dysmenorrhea is the feature of ovarian involvement; "chocolate cysts" measuring up to 10 cm in diameter may form. In the uterine ligaments pelvic or sacral pain is prominent, and extension to the peritoneum with attendant fibrosis fixes the tissue ("frozen pelvis") and also causes sacral pain. In the rectal wall tenesmus or obstruction may develop, and in the urinary bladder dysuria is the clinical aspect.

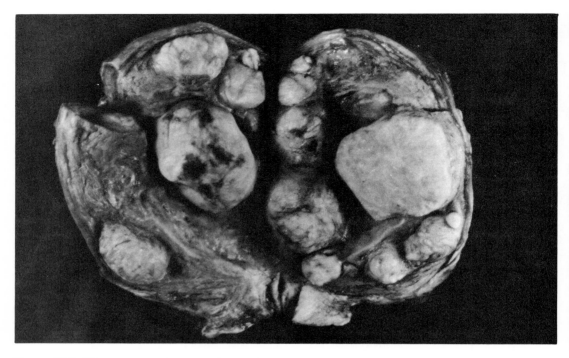

**Figure 17-9.** Fibromyomas of myometrium: submucosal, intramural, and subserosal

Occasionally the ectopic tissue is found in the umbilicus or a laparotomy scar, and at both sites recurring pain is the main complaint. Rarely, the appendix, ileum, or pleural surface is affected. How the deposits of endometrium reach these extrauterine sites is not known, although suggestions include abnormal differentiation of the celomic epithelium and regurgitation of endometrial fragments through the ends of the uterine tubes with implantation at the various sites. The condition is neither premalignant nor caused by hyperestrinism.

The most common benign tumor of the female genitalia is leiomyoma of the myometrium. It is present in one of every four women. The tumor is also known as a fibroid, fibroma, or fibromyoma. It consists of coarse interlacing fascicles of smooth muscle and fibrous connective tissue. The tumors may be small or large, usually measuring 1 to 10 cm in diameter, with sharply demarcated and nonencapsulated margins

(Figure 17-9). The tumors are often multiple. Those projecting into the endometrial cavity are submucosal, those within the wall are intramural, and those projecting beneath the serosa, which are sometimes pedunculated, are subserosal. Giant fibromyomas weighing several pounds are occasionally encountered. Large tumors may undergo central infarction with cyst formation; this is especially common during pregnancy when edema develops and the tissue swells. After the menopause the fibroids shrink, become dense, and frequently calcify. Rarely, transition to leiomyosarcoma takes place. Most fibromyomas are small and asymptomatic. Larger tumors cause heaviness and discomfort in the pelvis with occasional menorrhagia from compression of pelvic veins. Large fibromyomas may interfere with pregnancy, and pedunculated subserosal tumors may undergo torsion and infarction with the development of pelvic pain. The cause of the tumors is not

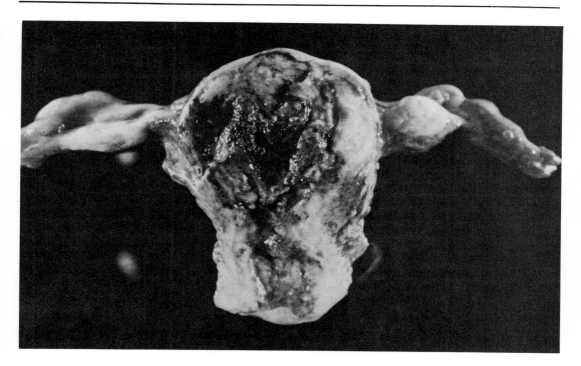

**Figure 17-10.** Carcinoma of endometrium invading myometrium

known, but their appearance during reproductive life, enlargement with pregnancy, and regression after the menopause indicate that they are estrogen-dependent.

Carcinoma of the endometrium is the most common cancer of the female genital tract. It was estimated that 38,000 new cases would be detected and 3,200 deaths would occur from this tumor in 1980.[14] Moreover, the incidence is increasing. Although the cause is not known, hyperestrinism appears to be important. Nulliparity with uninterrupted menstrual pulses of estrogenic stimulation, late menopause (over 52), obesity, estrogen-secreting ovarian tumors, and polycystic ovarian disease are all associated with the cancer. Estrogen stimulation is prolonged with nonrupture of ovarian follicles, and serum levels of estrone are high in overweight women. In addition, concern is directed to the wide use of estrogenic substances in the treatment of menopausal symptoms, with a si-

multaneous increase in the incidence of the cancer.[15] No strong family history is noted.

Cancer of the endometrium arises mainly in postmenopausal women; 80 per cent occur after the age of 50. It is especially likely to occur in women who are obese, hypertensive, and diabetic. The earliest clinical manifestation is leukorrhea, spotting (blood), or vaginal bleeding. Although more frequently caused by polyps, vaginal bleeding more than one year after cessation of the menses should never fail to bring to mind the possibility of endometrial cancer. Biopsy by curettage establishes the diagnosis. The tumor appears to be preceded by a sequence of proliferative changes of increasing atypia that include cystic hyperplasia, focal dysplasia, and carcinoma in situ.[16] The histologic distinction among these, however, is imprecise.

Grossly the endometrium reveals a friable polypoid nodule that may display necrosis or hemorrhage. With extension the cavity fills with tumor and invasion of the muscle wall begins. The gross appearance is shown in Figure 17-10. The histologic diagnosis requires apposed glands of irregular size without intervening stroma (back to back), and lining cells that display anaplasia. Necrosis, hemorrhage, and leukocytic infiltration are frequent. Almost all are adenocarcinomas that tend to be well differentiated. When foci of squamous metaplasia are conspicuous, the term adenoacanthoma is used. This occurs in about 10 per cent of cases and is of no prognostic import.[6]

The cancer grows slowly and gradually spreads outside the uterus. It invades the myometrium and extends downward into the cervix, upward to the uterine tubes, and outward to the pelvic lymph nodes. All these precede late spread to the liver and lungs. A staging classification for equating therapeutic results at different institutions has been provided by the International Federation of Gynecology and Obstetrics. The main features are listed in Table 17-2. Over two-thirds of cases are at stage I in most series.[17] Unfortunately, clinical staging is not very accurate.[18] The keystone of therapy is surgical removal of the uterus. The extent of the procedure, however, and the use of irradiation are arguable.[19, 20] When the cancer is at stage I and appears limited to the endometrium, the survival rate at five years is over 90 per cent.[6] With successive stages, each indicating deeper spread, survival rates decline, and stage IV patients rarely survive. The usual cause of death is urinary obstruction with uremia, or ileal obstruction from peritoneal metastasis.

## UTERINE TUBES

Acute salpingitis is due especially to gonorrhea but is also a consequence of contraceptive devices and nonsterile abortifacient instrumentation. Organisms in addition to the gonococcus include staphylococci, streptococci, and *Escherichia coli*. The tubes are swollen, hyperemic, and roughened with fibrin over the serosa. The patient experiences fever, abdominal pain, and tenderness over the lower abdomen. Leukocytosis with neutrophilia is constant. The complication is extension of infected exudate out of the fimbriated ends of the tubes to cause peritonitis or pelvic abscesses, especially in the rectouterine fossa. Tubo-ovarian abscess formation is also common. As the acute reaction subsides granulation tissue appears, the plicae of the mucosa fuse, and the subsequent scar formation distorts or blocks the lumen. Proximal to the obstruction pus collects if the lumen is infected (pyosalpinx), or clear fluid if it is not (hydrosalpinx). After these changes the patient may be sterile or vulnerable to ectopic pregnancy.

With ectopic pregnancy the chorionic villi burrow into the tubal wall, vascular sinuses form and rupture, hematosalpinx develops, and eventually the tube perforates. The patient experiences severe pain in the lower abdomen, urine tests reveal that she is pregnant, and surgical excision

Table 17-2.

## Staging of endometrial cancer*

| Stage | Disease process |
|---|---|
| I | Confined to corpus |
| II | Corpus and cervix |
| III | Extrauterine but confined to pelvis |
| IV | Spread to bladder, rectum, or outside pelvis |

*International Federation of Gynecology and Obstetrics.

of the tube is necessary for control of the bleeding.

Ectopic endometrium in the tubal wall (endometriosis externa) is also a cause of discomfort and dysfunction. With repeated hemorrhagic sloughing of the displaced mucosa, macrophages abound, granulation tissue converts to scar tissue, and the lumen is distorted. Other lesions of the uterine tubes, especially primary tumors or metastatic disease, are uncommon.

## OVARIES

The normal ovary measures 2.5 cm in diameter and is firm and pale gray with coarse creases indenting the surface. Section reveals small cysts around the cortex. Each represents a graafian follicle where an ovum may be extruded by rupture of the overlying cortex. After rupture, the cyst fills with fibrin and blood. Later the lining cells enlarge and lipids accumulate so that the margin turns yellowish-orange and a corpus luteum is formed. This gradually hyalinizes and converts to a white corpus albicans. After reproductive life the ovaries atrophy.

Abnormalities of the ovary are inflammation, endometriosis, polycystic disease, and tumor formation. Oophoritis occurs as an extension of acute salpingitis; the reaction may subside or progress to fibrous adhesions with tubo-ovarian abscess. Endometriosis converts the ovary to a "chocolate cyst" that measures up to 10 cm in diameter. The blood has no route of escape. Its breakdown produces the chocolate color and recurrence of the hemorrhage causes the gradual enlargement.

In 1935 Stein and Leventhal described seven patients with hirsutism, oligomenorrhea, and infertility associated with large ovaries that on section revealed 20 to 100 cortical cysts covered by a thick fibrous capsule.[21] They regarded the condition as a hormonal disturbance in which the follicles were unable to rupture through the tough surface layer. The nature of the hormonal disturbance is not clear, although the clinical features suggest an increase in androgen production. Wedge resection of the ovaries restored menstruation in all seven patients, and two became pregnant. Since then a similar syndrome due to adrenal overactivity has been identified. In this condition the ovaries also contain cortical cysts. Both conditions are now grouped under the term polycystic ovary syndrome, with type I the condition described by Stein and Leventhal, and type II the condition due to adrenal disturbance. In type I polycystic ovary, ovulation-stimulating drugs often eliminate the need for wedge resection; adrenal suppressive therapy is suitable in the type II syndrome.[22] Peripheral conversion of androgens to estrogens, with prolonged estrogenic stimulation, is thought to account for the increased incidence of endometrial cancer that is seen with polycystic ovarian disease.[23]

Tumors of the ovary arise from surface cells (celomic epithelium), germ cells that line the follicles, and stromal cells. Surface-cell tumors are much the most frequent, constituting about 65 per cent of all ovarian tumors; germ-cell tumors make up about 15 per cent of the total, and stromal tumors are the least common. Table 17-3 classifies

Table 17-3.

## Origins of ovarian tumors

| Site | Tumor type |
| --- | --- |
| Surface cells | Cystadenoma<br>Brenner tumor |
| Germ cells | Teratoma<br>Dysgerminoma |
| Stromal cells | Granulosa cell tumor |

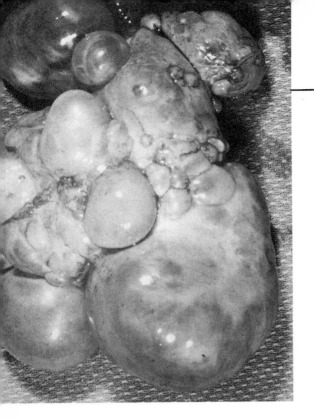

**Figure 17-11.** Multiloculated serous cystadenoma

the main ovarian tumors according to these three sites of origin.

Cystadenomas occur in the 20- to 50-year age group. They are multilocular and large, often measuring 15 to 30 cm in diameter. The walls are thin, and the lining cells, which are present in a single layer, distinguish between the serous type and the mucinous type. In the serous type the cells are cuboidal or flat, some are ciliated, and calcified psammoma bodies are often present in the subepithelial stroma. Papillary or cystic excrescences in the form of small granular clusters roughen the otherwise smooth gray lining surfaces. The lumens are distended with a clear, watery fluid. The cysts enlarge slowly, and slightly more than half become malignant with excrescences that extend through the wall to appear on the serosal surface (Figure 17-11). The tumor is then a serous cystadenocarcinoma. Care must be taken during operative removal

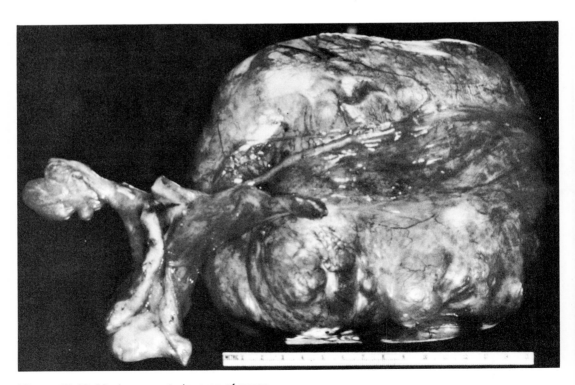

**Figure 17-12.** Mucinous cystadenoma of ovary

not to rupture the tumor and seed the peritoneum with neoplastic cells. Without rupture, the outlook for cure is good.

Mucinous cystadenomas are also large and multilocular, but the lumens contain a clear, viscid fluid and excrescences are not present over the lining surface (Figure 17-12). The epithelial cells are columnar, nonciliated, and present in a single layer with basal nuclei and cytoplasm that fills with mucin (Figure 17-13). Only about 5 per cent of these tumors become malignant, i.e., mucinous cystadenocarcinoma.[24]

The Brenner tumor is white, tough, and small, usually measuring less than 6 cm in diameter (Figure 17-14). It is solid and sharply demarcated with uroepithelial cells scattered in clusters over a dense ovarian stroma that is mainly fibrous. The epithelial component arises from the Walthard cell rests, which are invaginations of metaplastic celomic epithelium.[25] The tumor is benign and has no hormonal or secretory effect; it is of little clinical significance.

The tumors that arise from germ cells are the teratoma and dysgerminoma. The teratoma, also called a dermoid, is a cystic tumor that contains mature remnants of all three germ layers: ectoderm, endoderm, and mesoderm. Teratomas arise during early adulthood, are occasionally bilateral, and usually measure 6 to 12 cm in diameter. The texture is doughy, and sections reveal a thin wall with a large lumen containing pale yellow sebum that has the consistency of soft butter (Figure 17-15). The lumen may also contain particles of bone, portions of teeth, and strands of black hair. Histologic sections disclose mature epidermis, hair follicles, sebaceous glands, bronchial mucosa, intestinal mucosa, and neural tissue in various mixtures. Cartilage may also be present. Surgical excision is curative. The tumor is thought to arise from a single

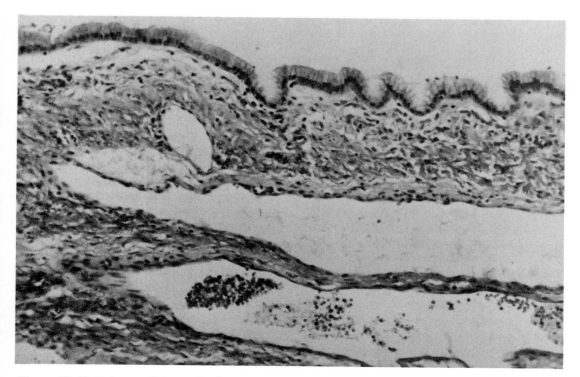

**Figure 17-13.** Columnar lining cells of pseudomucinous cystadenoma

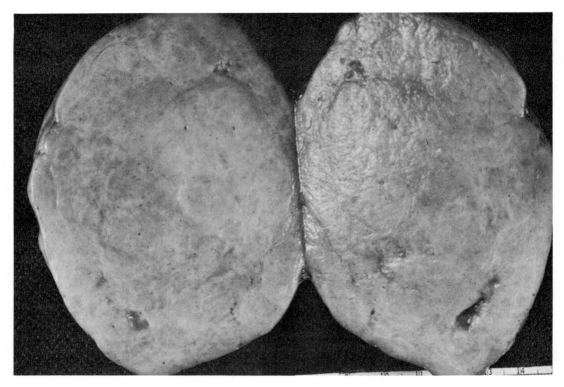

**Figure 17-14.** Cut surfaces of Brenner's tumor of ovary

germ cell that is fertilized by parthenogenesis.[26] Malignant transformation, especially of squamous cells, occurs but is extremely uncommon.

Dysgerminomas are solid epithelial ovarian tumors of girls or young women that cause an abdominal mass with pelvic discomfort and occasional menstrual disturbance. The average age is 22 years, and the symptomatic period to the time of diagnosis is about six months. The tumor measures up to 50 cm in diameter and presents a soft, pale pink, fleshy cut surface mottled with foci of hemorrhage and necrosis. Microsections reveal solid masses of large epithelial cells of uniform appearance supported by a scant stroma and infiltrated sparsely with lymphocytes. The dysgerminoma is the female counterpart of the testicular seminoma, and it is thought to arise from a pri-

mordial germ cell of the ovary. Treatment consists of surgical removal and irradiation. The rate of survival at five years is about 90 per cent.[27]

The principal neoplasm arising from the stroma of the ovary is the granulosa-cell tumor. It secretes estrogen, and the mean age of occurrence is 53 years.[28] The age spread, however, is wide so that if it occurs in childhood puberty is precocious, during reproductive life no clinical changes are conspicuous, and after the menopause both endometrial hyperplasia and endometrial cancer tend to occur. Otherwise abdominal pain and an adnexal mass are the main clinical features. The tumor measures 13 cm in mean diameter, and the cut surface is pale yellow and solid or partially cystic. The neoplastic cells are small and basophilic with rosette formations known as Call-

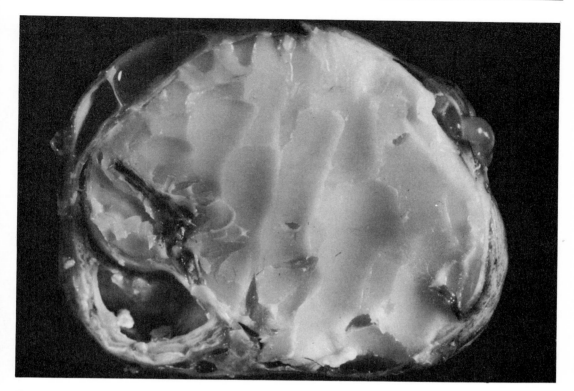

**Figure 17-15.** Hair, calcifications, and sebum on the cut surface of an ovarian teratoma

Exner bodies. The tumor grows slowly and is seldom malignant. Surgical excision is the only treatment that achieves cure. The outlook is favorable unless lymphatic or capsular invasion indicates metastatic spread.

Not listed in Table 17-3 is the arrheno-blastoma, which also arises from stromal cells but is extremely rare. The tumor contains Leydig cells, secretes testosterone, and causes masculinization. The clinical evidence of this is hirsutism, deepening of the voice, and enlargement of the larynx and clitoris.

## REFERENCES

1. Schachter J: Chlamydial infections. *N Engl J Med* 298:428, 490, 540, 1978

2. Japaze H, Garcia-Bunuel R, Woodruff JD: Primary vulvar neoplasm. A review of in situ and invasive carcinoma, 1935-1972. *Obstet Gynecol* 49:404, 1977

3. Merrill JA, Ross NL: Cancer of the vulva. *Cancer* 14:13, 1961

4. Ulfelder H: The stilbestrol-adenosis-carcinoma syndrome. *Cancer* 38:426, 1976

5. Kraus FT: *Gynecologic Pathology*, p 173. St Louis: Mosby, 1967

6. Romney SL, Gray MJ, Little AB, et al: *Gynecology and Obstetrics: The Health Care of Women.* New York: McGraw-Hill, 1975

7. Klionsky B: Editorial statement of the Ad Hoc Committee on Reproducibility of Histopathologic Diagnoses of Uterine Cervical Lesions. *Am J Clin Pathol* 52:358, 1969

8. Kolstad P, Klem V: Long-term followup of 1121 cases of carcinoma in situ. *Obstet Gynecol* 48:125, 1976

9. Smith JC: Carcinoma in situ. *Hum Pathol* 9:373, 1978

10. van Nagell JR Jr, Roddick JW Jr, Lowin DM: The staging of cervical cancer: Inevitable discrepancies between clinical staging and pathologic findings. *Am J Obstet Gynecol* 110:973, 1971

11. van Nagell JR Jr, Harralson JD, Roddick JW Jr: The effect of examination under anesthesia on staging accuracy in cervical cancer. *Am J Obstet Gynecol* 113:938, 1972

12. Marchant DJ: Cancer of the cervix. *N Engl J Med* 281:602, 1969

13. Novak ER, Woodruff JD: *Gynecologic and Obstetric Pathology with Clinical and Endocrine Relations*, 6th ed, p 232. Philadelphia: Saunders, 1967

14. Silverberg E: Cancer statistics, 1980. *CA—Cancer J Clin* 30:23, 1980

15. Weiss NS, Szekely DR, Austin DF: Increasing incidence of endometrial cancer in the United States. *N Engl J Med* 294:1259, 1976

16. Vellios F: Endometrial hyperplasia and carcinoma in-situ. *Gynecol Oncol* 2:152, 1974

17. Rutledge F: The role of radical hysterectomy in adenocarcinoma of the endometrium. *Gynecol Oncol* 2:331, 1974

18. Goodman R, Hellman S: The role of postoperative irradiation in carcinoma of the endometrium. *Gynecol Oncol* 2:354, 1974

19. Smith JC: The superiority of surgical treatment of endometrial carcinoma. *JAMA* 160:1460, 1956

20. Brady LW, Lewis GC Jr, Antoniades J, et al: Evolution of radiotherapeutic techniques. *Gynecol Oncol* 2:314, 1974

21. Stein IF, Leventhal ML: Amenorrhea associated with bilateral polycystic ovaries. *Am J Obstet Gynecol* 29:181, 1935

22. Raj SG, Thompson IE, Berger MJ, et al: Clinical aspects of the polycystic ovary syndrome. *Obstet Gynecol* 49:552, 1977

23. McDonald TW, Malkasian GD, Gaffey TA: Endometrial cancer associated with ovarian tumor and polycystic ovarian disease. *Obstet Gynecol* 49:654, 1977

24. Hart WR, Norris HJ: Borderline and malignant mucinous tumors of the ovary. Histologic criteria and clinical behavior. *Cancer* 31:1031, 1975

25. Roth LM: The Brenner tumor and the Walthard cell rest. An electron microscopic study. *Lab Invest* 31:15, 1974

26. Linder D, McCaw BK, Hecht F: Parthenogenetic origin of benign ovarian teratomas. *N Engl J Med* 292:63, 1975

27. Asadourian LA, Taylor HB: Dysgerminoma. An analysis of 105 cases. *Obstet Gynecol* 33:370, 1969

28. Fox H, Agrawal K, Langley FA: A clinicopathologic study of 92 cases of granulosa cell tumor of the ovary with special reference to the factors influencing prognosis. *Cancer* 35:231, 1975

# 18

## DISEASES OF THE BREAST

### THE NORMAL BREAST

Glands are classified according to whether part of the cytoplasm becomes the secretion (apocrine), all of the cytoplasm becomes the secretion (holocrine), or none of the cytoplasm is given up for this purpose (merocrine). Sweat glands are apocrine, and the breast is a clump of modified sweat glands. It consists of 10 to 18 separate glands that open onto the nipple through five to nine individual ducts.[1] Before puberty the breast consists of branching ducts in myxomatous connective tissue with only saccular gland buds. At the beginning of the menses (menarche) estrogen is secreted by the ovaries, and this causes growth of both the glands and the ducts. With the appearance of progesterone in the latter half of the menstrual cycle, stromal growth also takes place and edema is associated with this. When menstruation commences the edema subsides, the lobular (gland) cells desquamate, the ducts shrink, and a degree of atrophy affects the connective tissue stroma. Throughout reproductive life, therefore, the female breast is subject to alternating cycles of stimulation and regression.

With pregnancy and a prolonged estrogenic effect, the proliferation of glands outpaces the stroma, and over the nine-month period the breast comes to consist almost entirely of glands. Secretory activity begins in the third trimester, and the milklike substance appearing at the nipple before

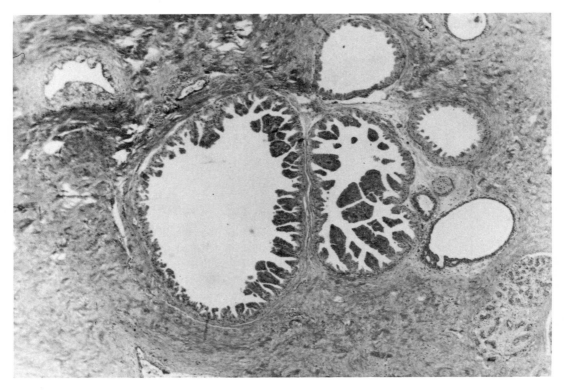

**Figure 18-1.** Large eosinophilic epithelial cells (apocrine gland change) in fibrocystic disease

and just after birth is called colostrum. At the end of reproductive life (menopause) the breast undergoes atrophy, the glands largely disappear, and the structure comes to resemble the male breast, which consists of only small ducts lying in a scant stroma. Sufficient estrogen from the adrenals, however, causes some of the glandular elements to persist.

## ABNORMALITIES OF THE BREAST

Abnormalities of the breast include supernumerary (extra) nipples, which usually are single and are located at any point on a curved line extending from the axilla to the breast and over the abdomen to the groin. This is the so-called milk line. Supernumerary nipples, which may be accompanied by small amounts of breast tissue, are mainly a cosmetic disturbance and are corrected by excision.

Mastitis is due to bacterial infections of the breast, especially by staphylococci and streptococci. It occurs mainly during lactation, when fissures of the nipple allow entry of bacteria into the tissue. Abscess and cellulitis are the common forms. Incision and drainage of an abscess may be required. Chronic granulomatous mastitis is tuberculous, rare, and secondary to active pulmonary disease. A chancre may occur on the nipple; it is highly contagious.

Fat necrosis is a focal reaction that occurs in middle-aged women with large, pendulous breasts. It is due to bruising of the tissue or to a surgical procedure but may also arise spontaneously, presumably from ductal perforation with spillage of debris into the adjacent adipose tissue.[2] The site is small, well circumscribed, and indurated. The reaction gradually subsides but may undergo calcification or cyst formation. The resemblance to cancer by palpation or mammography may necessitate surgical excision to make certain.[3]

## FIBROCYSTIC DISEASE

The most common disease of the breast is chronic cystic mastitis. The condition has many synonyms, including fibrocystic disease, fibrocystic mastopathy, cystic disease, chronic mastitis, and Schimmelbusch's disease. It occurs during adult life, especially near the menopause, and is characterized by symptoms that are often slight and more noticeable before menstrual periods than after. The complaints include pain, tenderness, a burning sensation, and palpable nodularity of the tissue. Examination reveals coarse or fine nodularity that may be localized but is ordinarily widespread throughout both breasts. The contour of the breasts is not grossly altered. The pathologic features are chronic inflammation, focal fibrosis, and the development of cysts lined with a single layer of epithelial cells. The cysts are usually small, measuring 0.2 to 0.5 cm in diameter, and often contain a turbid fluid that gives a "blue-domed" appearance. The lining epithelial cells are large and columnar with deeply eosinophilic cytoplasm. This aspect of the lining cells constitutes the characteristic apocrine gland change (Figure 18-1). The pericystic connective tissue is lightly infiltrated with lymphocytes. There is no specific treatment, although surgical attention is necessary when the disease is present in the form of a single cyst that is large and may be clinically indistinguishable from cancer. The cause may be an uneven response of the tissue to the alternating tides of hormonal stimulation and regression that take place during the long period of reproductive life. It is difficult to be certain of the relationship between cystic disease

and carcinoma, although several authors find a four- to five-times greater risk of malignant disease in patients with the inflammatory condition.[4,5] Although that relationship may exist, it is important to emphasize that multiplicity of nodules, bilateral involvement, and pain and tenderness are the three clinical features that distinguish the condition from cancer.

A lesion much more closely resembling cancer is sclerosing adenosis. It is uncommon and occurs after the menopause. It tends to be asymptomatic and presents as a discrete, nontender focus of induration in one breast. Although it is freely movable and unattached to the overlying skin, the possibility of cancer requires surgical exploration. The lesion measures 1 to 2 cm in diameter, the margin is poorly delineated, and the consistency is hard. The cut surface fails to reveal the "chalk lines" characteristic of malignant tumors. Microsections disclose interlacing bundles of fibrous stroma and irregular proliferations of epithelial cells. However, anaplasia is not seen and marginal invasion of the adjacent normal tissue is not evident. The condition is neither malignant nor premalignant, and it is cured by surgical excision.

## BENIGN TUMORS

The most common benign tumor of the breast is the fibroadenoma. It occurs after puberty, especially throughout young adult life, and dwindles in frequency toward the menopause. When a fibroadenoma persists into the postmenopausal period, it often undergoes calcification. The tumor is mainly asymptomatic and is detected by self-examination, which reveals a painless, movable, unattached mass in one breast. The tumor grows extremely slowly. Excision reveals a bulging, round, white, firmly resilient tumor mass that is sharply circumscribed but unencapsulated and usually measures less than 3 cm in diameter. Microsections disclose ducts of markedly dis-

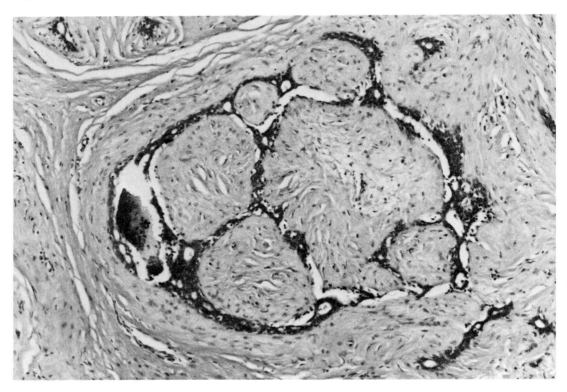

**Figure 18-2.** Distorted ductal lumen stretched over nodular masses of connective tissue in fibroadenoma

torted outline caused by stretching over nodular masses of connective tissue (Figure 18-2). The histologic distinction between periductal and intraductal types has no clinical usefulness. The cause is unknown but may be a localized overreaction to estrogenic stimulation. In about 15 per cent of patients more than one tumor is present in the same or opposite breast.[2]

Rarely, an indolent fibroadenoma suddenly begins to grow so that a giant tumor rapidly develops. The skin becomes stretched and discolored, and the tumor becomes heavy and painful. Such a giant fibroadenoma is known as a cystosarcoma phyllodes. The term was coined by Johannes Müller in 1838; *phyllodes* means "leaf-like," an appearance perhaps suggested to him by the cut surface. The "cystosarcoma" is inexplicable since Müller regarded the tumor as benign.[6] The lesion occurs any time after puberty and becomes evident as a palpable, disfiguring breast mass. It may exceed 15 cm in diameter, with a sharply delimited margin and a cut surface that is pale gray and slightly firm (Figure 18-3). Microsections reveal the same tissue components as a fibroadenoma. Wide local excision ordinarily suffices. About 15 per cent of cases, however, show malignant change, and it is the stromal part that undergoes this transformation. In such cases radical mastectomy may be required.[7] Metastases spread by hematogenous dissemination to the lungs and bone, often bypassing the axillary lymph nodes.

The second most common benign tumor of the breast is the intraductal papilloma. It is a discrete lesion that is often accompanied by epithelial proliferations in other

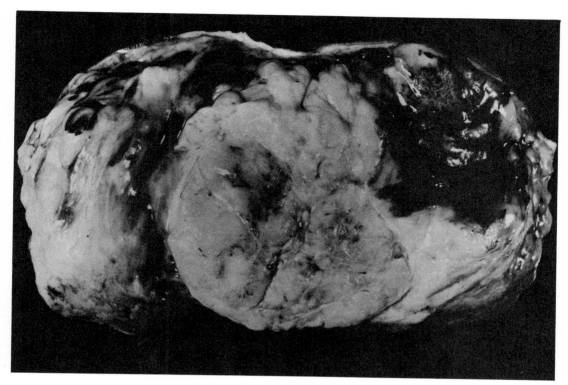

**Figure 18-3.** Cut surface of cystosarcoma phyllodes. The tumor measured 33×11×7 cm.

parts of the duct, i.e., papillomatosis. The lesion is most common in early adult life, decreasing in frequency thereafter. It is asymptomatic except for a serous or bloody discharge from the nipple. Often no mass is palpable. The tumor is small, pink, villous, and composed of delicate fibrovascular fronds covered by a single layer of cuboidal epithelial cells. Local excision is curative. Transition to carcinoma is rare.[6]

## MALIGNANT TUMORS

Cancer of the breast is the most common malignant tumor of women in the United States. The approximate but sobering figures are that 90,000 new cases will be diagnosed each year, 33,000 deaths will occur, and one of every 15 women will develop the cancer. Moreover, one patient will die of this disease and two to three new cases will be discovered every 17 minutes of every day.[8] In addition, over half of the patients treated will develop recurrent disease and most will die of disseminated tumor.[9]

**Cause**
The cause of the cancer is unknown, although attention is focused especially on racial, hormonal, familial, and viral factors. Although the incidence of breast cancer is about five times greater in the United States than in Asia, especially Japan, that difference may be related more to affluence than to geography. The incidence in Japanese women rises as they move to the Western Hemisphere and become affluent.[10] It is perhaps the greater caloric intake and increased animal fat in the diet that associate affluence with the tumor.[11]

Hormonal factors also operate: Estrogens are cocarcinogenic in rodents, women have 100 times more breast cancer than men, the tumor arises only after puberty, and cancer does not occur in patients with ovarian dysgenesis or frequently in patients after castration. Moreover, early pregnancy protects against the lesion so that the cancer is more frequent in nulliparous than in parous women. That the protection is due to the low carcinogenic activity of estriol, which is secreted in large amounts during pregnancy, is now disputed.[12] It has been pointed out that estrogens used for contraception or menopausal symptoms may increase the risk of breast cancer. According to Kirschner, however, the evidence for this is not yet convincing.[13] Although hormonal factors are certainly important, therefore, no clinical abnormality of the hormonal milieu has so far been identified in women with increased risk of the tumor.

Familial aggregation, on the other hand, is irrefutable. The risk in daughters of a patient with breast cancer is three times greater than in others, provided the tumor was premenopausal, and this risk increases markedly if a mother and sister are both affected or if the disease was bilateral.[12] It may be pointed out, however, that over 90 per cent of patients with breast cancer have no history of the disease in their female relatives.

Since the report of Bittner regarding a "milk factor" in mice, the possibility of a viral cause of breast cancer has been of interest.[14] However, little validation of this prospect has been forthcoming; an RNA-virus is present in the milk of women with and without a family history of breast cancer, and both parents seem to be involved in transmitting the susceptibility to their offspring so that the transmission of a cancer factor in mice does not appear applicable to humans. Despite laboratory findings, therefore, little epidemiologic evidence that a virus causes breast cancer in humans

is available.[10] It is evidently the interaction of two or more of the foregoing factors that ultimately leads to the development of the tumor. Whatever the cause or combination of factors, however, the women at highest risk are those who are nulliparous and affluent with previous breast disease and a family history of breast cancer.

**Morphology**

The cancer arises mainly after the age of 45, occurs slightly more often in the left breast than in the right (110:100), and appears clinically as a painless lump or, less often, as a nipple discharge. Most are discovered by self-examination and measure less than 4 cm in diameter at the time of detection. The tumor is firm and attached to the adjacent adipose tissue with frequent extension to the overlying skin, which causes dimpling that has been likened to the skin of an orange (peau d'orange). About 50 per cent arise in the upper outer quadrant, 20 per cent are pericentral, and the remainder are distributed evenly throughout the other quadrants. Multicentric sites of origin are claimed by Qualheim and Gall[15] and by Gallager and Martin.[16] Spread takes place through the lymphatics to the axillary lymph nodes from the upper outer tumors, and to the retrosternal nodes from the tumors of the inner quadrants. At least half of patients have nodal disease at the time of diagnosis.[5] The third most frequent regional site is the supraclavicular nodes on the side of the tumor. Distant spread, which may bypass any of the nodes, goes mainly to the lungs, bone, liver, adrenals, and brain.

Most of the cancers are hard and pale gray with serrated margins and central pale yellow "chalk lines" due to necrotic tumor cells that accumulate within dilated duct lumens. A characteristic cut surface is shown in Figure 18-4. Less frequently the cut surface is mucoid and gelatinous or fleshy and soft. These features lead to a descriptive classification that is also based on the presumed site of origin. In 1946 Foote and Stewart proposed that breast cancers arise from ducts or lobules, and that either may be infiltrative or localized (in situ).[17] The difference between a ductal and a lobular origin is not objective, however, and others have proposed that most cancers arise in intralobular terminal ducts rather than in medium-sized ducts.[18] Nevertheless, the classification of Foote and Stewart prevails, and this is shown in Table 18-1 in abbreviated and simplified form. Only carcinomas are included; they constitute over 99 per cent of breast cancers.

It is evident from Table 18-1 that the great majority of breast cancers are infiltrating ductal carcinomas. A few are identified while still in situ, and the rest are scarce to rare. Of the infiltrating ductal tumors, 75 per cent are scirrhous, with medullary and colloid cancers making up 5 to 10 per cent each. Medullary carcinomas are soft, pale pink, and fleshy on gross inspection; histologic sections reveal solid masses of epithelial tumor cells supported by a scant, delicate stroma. Colloid carcinomas, in contrast, present a gray, mucoid, glairy

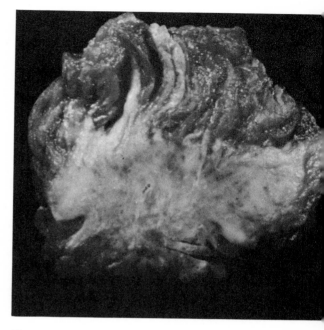

**Figure 18-4.** Cut surface of scirrhous carcinoma. The margins are irregular, "chalk lines" extend through the center, and the tissue is hard.

cut surface that on microsection discloses large lakes of mucin with small numbers of marginal and central (floating) tumor cells. Both medullary and colloid cancers grow slowly and provide a better outlook than the more common scirrhous cancers.[6] In all, however, the tumor cells are infrequently arranged in a glandular pattern so that the term carcinoma is appropriate more often than adenocarcinoma.

Inflammatory carcinoma is a rare and special type. It begins with pain and tenderness in the breast, with moderate enlargement and the rapid development of induration. The breast is firm, warm, and red with dilation of superficial veins. These changes suggest an acute diffuse mastitis. There is no fever, however, or leukocytosis. Moreover, metastatic disease in the axillary nodes is frequent. Biopsy reveals undifferentiated epithelial tumor cells spread widely throughout the tissue with con-

Table 18-1. _____

## Carcinoma of the breast

| Type | Incidence |
| --- | --- |
| Infiltrating ductal | 90% |
| Scirrhous | |
| Medullary | |
| Colloid | |
| Inflammatory | |
| Paget's disease | |
| | |
| In situ ductal | 5% |
| | |
| Infiltrating lobular | |
| | |
| In situ lobular | |

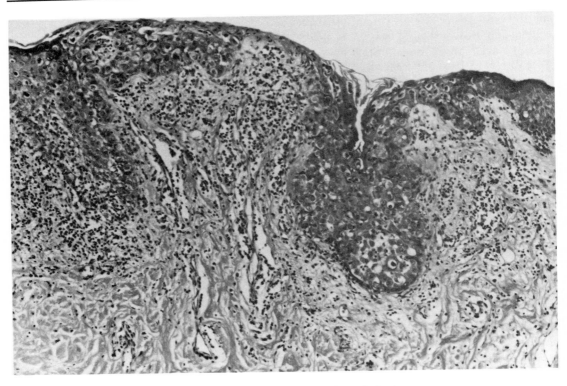

**Figure 18-5.** Paget's disease with huge tumor cells in epithelium of nipple

spicuous extension to lymphatic vessels of the skin. The cancer spreads so rapidly that, regardless of treatment, five-year survival is rare. Radiation alone is the favored method of therapy; neither surgical resection nor ablative endocrine measures have shown promise. It is postulated that the rapid spread of the disease is due to a lack of host resistance to the tumor cells. The cancer is not associated with pregnancy or lactation.[19]

In 1874 Paget called attention to the association of an eczematoid change in the nipple and a cancer of the underlying breast. The present consensus is that the nipple lesion is an intraepithelial extension of a subjacent ductal carcinoma.[20] The disease is uncommon, occurs before or after the menopause, and is characterized by itching, scaliness, erosion, and crusting of the nipple and areola. Because these fea-

tures suggest eczema, the possibility of cancer may be overlooked. An underlying mass may or may not be palpable. Histologic examination reveals large epithelial tumor (Paget) cells in the deep layer of the epidermis (Figure 18-5). Mastectomy is the treatment of choice. When no underlying tumor is palpable, the frequency of metastatic axillary disease is lower and the survival rate is higher than when the subjacent tumor can be felt.[20]

Ductal carcinoma in situ precedes infiltrating ductal cancer. It arises by intraluminal proliferation of malignant tumor cells that line and distend medium-sized ducts without perforation of the basement membrane. The central cells, deprived of their blood supply, undergo necrosis so that on gross section the ducts are filled with a pale yellowish-gray material of caseous consistency that is easily expressed. On this account the tumor is also referred to as a comedocarcinoma. The affected ducts are usually localized to one quadrant of the breast. With time, however, extension through the basement membrane converts the lesion to an infiltrating duct cancer.

In 1941 Foote and Stewart described the lobular carcinoma in situ.[21] It consists of a solid mass of epithelial cells within one or more adjacent lobules. The cells may be larger than normal, but atypia is not conspicuous.[22] The lesion is hard to distinguish microscopically from lobular hyperplasia. Moreover, it is neither clinically evident nor grossly discernible. It is found in premenstrual females on histologic examination of random sections of breast tissue usually removed because of fibrocystic disease. No causal association is implied. The lesion is often multicentric in one breast, and is bilateral in about 15 per cent of cases.[22] The progression of the lesion to invasive tumor, however, is uncertain. In one series of 122 cases only 22 became invasive over a period of 15 years.[5] Toker and Goldberg estimated the risk of invasive carcinoma at about 19 per cent for the ipsilateral breast and an almost equivalent risk for the contralateral breast.[23] They suggested the term "in situ small cell lesion," deleting the word "carcinoma" with its

greater risk of overreaction on the part of the patient or the physician. Indeed, the propriety of using a term meaning "cancer" for a condition that is neither invasive nor likely to become invasive over a period of several years is in some doubt.[24]

### Staging

Cancer of the breast is regarded as clinically curable when there is no evidence of metastatic disease beyond the axilla. Local methods of treatment include partial mastectomy, simple mastectomy, or modified radical mastectomy with or without radiation, which may be given before or after any of the surgical procedures. The result of treatment is expressed as the rate of survival. In order to compare results, different treatments have to be used in patients with approximately the same distribution of tumor. The practice of staging came into being for this purpose; it is a clinical estimate of the extent of the tumor spread. It is based on tumor size, axillary node involvement, and distant metastatic disease. Although various systems are extant, in a general way the patient is classified as summarized in Table 18-2. With this grouping it is possible to apply different methods of treatment to patients with presumably the same extent of tumor spread so that comparison of the subsequent rates of survival will reveal which method is superior.

The practice has not worked, for two main reasons. First, clinical staging is extremely inaccurate. With respect to axillary node involvement, for example, the frequency of false-negatives is as great as 40 per cent, and false-positives vary from 28 to 46 per cent.[25] The second reason is that the difference in treatment methods has only a slight effect on the rate of survival. When the cancer is localized to the breast, radical and conservative methods equally succeed, and when metastases have formed in the lungs or liver, both methods equally fail. The radical method is superior to the conservative method only when the tumor

Table 18-2.

## Staging of breast cancer

| Stage | Disease process |
|---|---|
| I | Localized to breast; <2 cm in diameter |
| II | 2-5 cm in diameter; axillary nodes movable |
| III | Axillary nodes involved |
| IV | Disseminated metastatic disease |

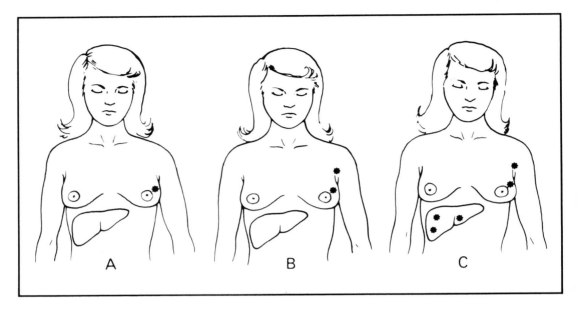

**Figure 18-6.** When the tumor is localized to the breast (A), both conservative and radical methods equally succeed. When the tumor is spread beyond the axilla (C), both methods equally fail. Only when the tumor is spread to the axilla but not beyond (B) is one method superior to the other.

has spread to the axilla but not beyond. These relationships are illustrated in Figure 18-6. Since cases with this precise distribution of tumor are scarce, the rates of survival are affected more by the inaccuracy of staging than by the efficacy of the various methods of treatment. Perhaps for these reasons a comparison of survival rates has not settled the question of which method is superior. Thus Forrest stated that different forms of local therapy have little influence in determining the duration of survival,[26] and Bloom and Field previously pointed out that the variation within each stage is so great that this grouping of cases appears inadequate for determining the relative merits of the different methods of treatment.[27]

Comparative survival rates are useful, however, when the treatment is systemic rather than local. Under the premise that micrometastases are often disseminated by the time the breast lesion becomes clinically evident, Fisher and colleagues recommended the use of adjunctive chemothera-

py.[28] In this event the rate of survival must be depended on because the cancerocidal agent diffuses through the entire circulation and the result is not due to the local procedure alone. The practice of staging is less important because disseminated spread is already presumed. The usefulness of clinical staging in the evaluation of treatment under either circumstance is therefore modest.[24]

**Treatment**

The tumor will enlarge with the passage of time. It has been found that the doubling time—the period required for the tumor to increase its diameter by twice (an eightfold increase in mass)—is highly variable. The median period, however, as found by Gullino, is 100 days.[29] At this rate a tumor grows for years before it becomes palpable so that the clinical phase of the disease is perhaps only one-third of the total duration of the tumor. During the preclinical period tumor cells are discharged into blood and lymphatic vessels although most of these cells are destroyed. Therefore, the longer the duration and the larger the tumor, the greater the exfoliation and the higher the risk of metastatic disease.[30] For this reason treatment should be applied at the earliest possible time. The validity of this principle is corroborated by the report of Gilbertsen: Immediate treatment of 54 patients with cancers detected by annual physical examinations produced a five-year survival rate of 98 per cent.[9] The principles of curative breast cancer therapy have been outlined elsewhere.[31, 32]

Without treatment the rate of survival at five years is approximately 20 per cent.[29] Such patients are not cured, but simply harbor indolent tumors of low biologic aggressiveness. With local treatment, however, survival depends on the stage of the disease. For stage I over 95 per cent of patients are alive five years after therapy. At stage II the survival drops to 65 per cent, and at stage III, to 25 per cent.[33] These figures are only approximations. Moreover, almost one-third of patients who are alive five years after treatment will succumb to metastatic disease that develops in the following five-year period.[8] The success of treatment therefore appears to depend on whether the cancer is localized and can be totally ablated.

In recent years attention has swung away from radical surgical treatment to more conservative local measures combined with postoperative chemotherapy and radiation. The reasons are that cosmesis is important to patients, the probability of disseminated disease at the time of diagnosis is high, and the rates of survival are only slightly affected by whether the method is conservative or radical. Trials of postoperative chemotherapy are now in progress, and only preliminary results, albeit promising, were available at this writing.[28]

Since so many patients develop metastatic disease, palliative measures are commonly needed. In addition to chemotherapy, these include irradiation and endocrine manipulations, including ovariectomy, adrenalectomy, and hypophysectomy. The purpose of these procedures is to remove the source of hormones that sustain or stimulate the growth of the tumor cells. Only about one-third of unselected patients will benefit, however, and they are those in whom the malignant cells have retained specific receptor proteins to which the hormones attach. Receptor assays are thus useful in limiting strenuous endocrine treatments to patients who are likely to benefit from them. Approximately 50 to 70 per cent of estrogen receptor-positive tumors and 5 to 10 per cent of estrogen receptor-negative tumors respond to endocrine treatment.[34] The response includes both palliation and prolongation of survival. The assays apply to both the primary tumors and the metastatic deposits.

## THE MALE BREAST

Enlargement of the male breast is due to hyperplasia and is called gynecomastia. It occurs commonly in boys at the time of puberty, when a transient hormonal imbalance may exist. The enlargement consists of a firm, discrete, discoid subareolar mass that is unilateral and asymptomatic and disappears spontaneously.[35] Biopsy is not necessary. In adulthood the enlargement is bilateral and diffuse. Although some cases are idiopathic, others are associated with estrogen or diethylstilbestrol therapy, estrogen-secreting tumors, cirrhosis with failure of the liver to detoxify estrogen, and Klinefelter's syndrome with its extra female (X) chromosome. In addition, gynecomastia is often seen with hyperthyroidism; the mechanism is unknown and the enlargement disappears with restoration of the euthyroid state.[36] In all these cases the tissue shows ductal elongation and tortuosity, a wide collar of edematous periductal connective tissue, and a light infiltration of lymphocytes about the duct (Figure 18-7). Gynecomastia is not premalignant.

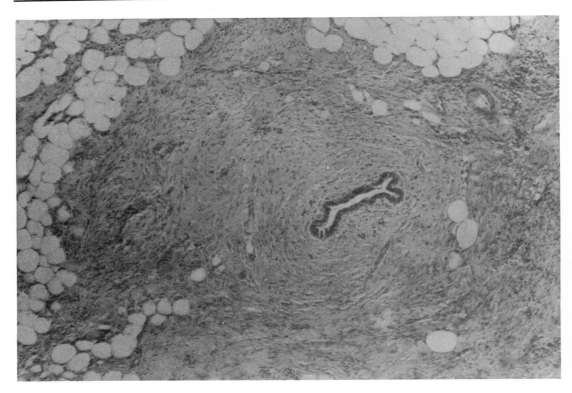

**Figure 18-7.** Histologic appearance of gynecomastia

Carcinoma of the breast also occurs in men although it is 100 times less frequent than in women. The median age is 60, the tumor begins as a subareolar mass, and a nipple discharge may be produced as well as eventual ulceration of the skin. The histologic types, patterns of spread, and epidemiologic features are much the same as for breast cancer in women. The principle of surgical treatment is also the same although for the incurable patient needing palliation, castration is more effective in men than in women.[37] Overall, the outlook is somewhat worse for men, possibly because they tend to seek medical attention later than women.

## REFERENCES

1. Hartmann WH: Pathologic anatomy and classification of cancer of the breast. *Am J Clin Pathol* 64:718, 1975

2. Farrow JH: Common benign lesions of the adult breast. *Clin Obstet Gynecol* 9:170, 1966

3. Coren GS, Patchefsky AS: Fat necrosis of the breast: Mammographic and thermographic findings. *Br J Radiol* 47:758, 1974

4. Kodlin D, Winger EE, Morgenstern NL, et al: Chronic mastopathy and breast cancer. A follow-up study. *Cancer* 39:2603, 1977

5. Ackerman LV, Katzenstein AL: The concept of minimal breast cancer and the pathologist's role in the diagnosis of "early carcinoma." *Cancer* 39:2755, 1977

6. McDivitt RW, Stewart FW, Berg JW: *Tumors of the Breast. Atlas of Tumor Pathology*, fasc 2, p 117. Washington, DC: Armed Forces Institute of Pathology, 1967

7. Oberman HA: Cystosarcoma phyllodes. *Cancer* 18:697, 1975

8. Kennedy BJ: Breast cancer. Introduction. *Semin Oncol* 1:85, 1974

9. Gilbertsen VA: The early detection of breast cancer. *Semin Oncol* 1:87, 1974

10. Correa P: The epidemiology of cancer of the breast. *Am J Clin Pathol* 64:720, 1975

11. Miller AB: Role of nutrition in the etiology of breast cancer. *Cancer* 39:2704, 1977

12. Petrakis NL: Genetic factors in the etiology of breast cancer. *Cancer* 39:2709, 1977

13. Kirschner MA: The role of hormones in the etiology of human breast cancer. *Cancer* 39:2716, 1977

14. Bittner JJ: Some possible effects of nursing on the mammary gland tumor incidence in mice. *Science* 84:162, 1936

15. Qualheim RE, Gall EA: Breast carcinoma with multiple sites of origin. *Cancer* 10:460, 1957

16. Gallager HS, Martin JE: The study of mammary carcinoma by mammography and whole organ sectioning. Early observations. *Cancer* 23:855, 1969

17. Foote FW Jr, Stewart FW: A histologic classification of carcinoma of the breast. *Surgery* 19:74, 1946

18. Wellings SR, Jensen HM: On the origin and progression of ductal carcinoma in the human breast. *J Nat Cancer Inst* 50:1111, 1973

19. Stocks LH, Patterson FMS: Inflammatory carcinoma of the breast. *Surg Gynecol Obstet* 143:885, 1976

20. Freund H, Maydovnik M, Laufer N, et al: Paget's disease of the breast. *J Surg Oncol* 9:93, 1977

21. Foote FW Jr, Stewart FW: Lobular carcinoma in situ: A rare form of mammary cancer. *Am J Pathol* 17:491, 1941

22. Fisher ER, Fisher B: Lobular carcinoma of the breast: An overview. *Ann Surg* 185:377, 1977

23. Toker C, Goldberg JD: The small cell lesion of mammary ducts and lobules. *Pathol Annu* 1:217, 1977

24. Smith JC: The questionable practice of clinical staging. *Perspect Biol Med* 19:273, 1976

25. Silverberg SG: Staging in the therapy of cancer of the breast. *Am J Clin Pathol* 64:756, 1975

26. Forrest APM: Conservative local treatment of breast cancer. *Cancer* 39:2813, 1977

27. Bloom HJG, Field JR: Impact of tumor grade and host resistance on survival of women with breast cancer. *Cancer* 28:1580, 1971

28. Fisher B, Glass A, Redmond C, et al: L-Phenylalanine mustard (L-PAM) in the management of primary breast cancer. An update of earlier findings and a comparison with those utilizing L-PAM plus 5-fluorouracil (5-FU). *Cancer* 39:2883, 1977

29. Gullino PM: Natural history of breast cancer. Progression from hyperplasia to neoplasia as predicted by angiogenesis. *Cancer* 39:2697, 1977

30. Fisher B, Slack NH, Bross IDJ, et al: Cancer of the breast: Size of neoplasm and prognosis. *Cancer* 24:1071, 1969

31. Smith JC: The treatment of breast cancer. *Hum Pathol* 5:625, 1974

32. Smith JC: Interpreting the rate of survival in carcinoma. *Can J Surg* 18:129, 1975

33. Levene MB, Harris JR, Hellman S: Treatment of carcinoma of the breast by radiation therapy. *Cancer* 39:2840, 1977

34. Lippman ME, Allegra JC: Receptors in breast cancer. *N Engl J Med* 299:930, 1978

35. Bannayan GA, Hajdu SI: Gynecomastia. Study of 351 cases. *Am J Clin Pathol* 57:431, 1972

36. Becker KL, Matthews MJ, Higgins GA, et al: Histologic evidence of gynecomastia in hyperthyroidism. *Arch Pathol* 98:257, 1974

37. Crichlow RW: Breast cancer in men. *Semin Oncol* 1:145, 1974

# 19

# HEMOLYMPHATIC DISEASE

## BLOOD AND BONE MARROW

### Normal

Blood is formed in utero in all bone marrow, the liver, and the spleen. In the liver and spleen this is known as extramedullary hemopoiesis. The liver and spleen activities subside at birth, but the marrow activity persists until puberty; thereafter red marrow is found only in the skull, sternum, ribs, spine, innominate bones, and upper thirds of the humerus and femur. Elsewhere hemopoietic tissue disappears, fatty replacement occurs, and the tissue is referred to as yellow marrow. In time of need, however, hemopoiesis expands and all of the marrow again turns red with erythrocytic production.

Blood is formed through a series of chemical and cellular changes. Glycine from the protein pool joins with succinate from the carbohydrate pool to form adipic acid.[1] From this aminolevulinic acid develops, porphobilinogen follows, and four molecules of porphobilinogen plus iron constitute heme. The attachment of globin produces the final molecule of hemoglobin. In the red marrow this assembly begins in the earliest cell, which is undifferentiated, and proceeds through recognizable stages that include the megaloblast, proerythrocyte, normoblast, reticulocyte, and erythrocyte. The transition over this sequence takes about four days. The main changes include a nucleus that gradually disappears and a cytoplasm that gradually fills with hem-globin. Once formed, the cells leave the bone marrow, circulate for 120 days, and then are disposed of in the reticuloendothelial system. A normal adult synthesizes and disposes of about 8 gm of hemoglobin daily. The function of hemoglobin, which is packaged in erythrocytes, is to transport oxygen, which attaches reversibly to the iron in the heme portion of the molecule. Hemoglobin production is stimulated by erythropoietin, which is elaborated by the kidneys.

## Abnormalities: Anemias

The abnormalities of this nicely balanced renewal-depletion system are too much blood (polycythemia) or too little hemoglobin (anemia). Polycythemia is infrequent and is described later. Anemia is perhaps the most common illness of the human species. It is defined as a significant reduction in the normal concentration of hemoglobin, which is 14 gm/dl for women and 16 gm/dl for men. With less than these amounts, tissue is underoxygenated; that is the mechanism of the illness. At 9 to 11 gm/dl pallor is evident and tachycardia develops. At 7 to 7.5 gm/dl exertional dyspnea begins, at 6 gm/dl weakness is evident, at 3 gm/dl dyspnea exists at rest, and at 2 gm/dl cardiac failure develops. Other signs and symptoms, depending on the degree of the anemia, include fatigability, dizziness, anorexia, atrophic skin, concave fingernails, and precordial murmurs. Other pathologic changes include fatty degeneration of the heart, liver, and proximal tubules of the kidneys as well as degeneration of the cortical cells of the cerebrum. Also, when the anemia involves blood destruction, hemosiderin is deposited in the tissues, especially those of the reticuloendothelial system. Although specific features are characteristic of the main anemias, the general clinical and pathologic findings are independent of the cause of the process and reflect only the degree of the deficiency.

Various mechanisms compensate for the scant hemoglobin. Capillaries open up so that oxygen is brought deeper into the tissues. Shunts redirect blood from the skin and kidneys to vital structures, including the heart and brain. Tachycardia increases output and causes hypertrophy but maintains oxygen pressure for more tissue. Hyperpnea also develops although it is an inappropriate response because the hemoglobin is already fully saturated with oxygen. Erythropoietin secretion increases as much as 10 times so that the bone marrow is stimulated to a maximum rate of hemoglobin production. Although these adjustments are temporarily helpful, high output failure gradually develops and is evidenced by an increasing shortness of breath. The compensatory mechanisms were described by Linman.[2]

The anemia of hemorrhage is rather set apart because it is not associated with a failure of the bone marrow or intravascular destruction of the blood. Moreover, it is quickly corrected because of the large functional reserve of the hemopoietic tissue. With acute hemorrhage blood loss is substantial, but the concentration of hemoglobin is unchanged even though the total amount of hemoglobin is reduced. Thus the hemoglobin and hematocrit are normal immediately after the event. However, the patient suffers from hypovolemia, which may induce shock, and treatment should consist of transfusions of whole blood. Unless the volume is made up, fluid moves from the extravascular compartment into the vessels, and this restores the circulating volume within 12 to 36 hours after the bleeding has stopped. The influx of fluid, however, dilutes the formed elements so that anemia exists and the hemoglobin and hematocrit are both low. At this stage treatment should consist of packed red cells. Recovery is rapid since marrow production of red cells may increase four to five times over the basal value without expansion of the red marrow within the bones.[3] If the requirements for erythropoiesis are met and the hemorrhage does not recur, the red cell mass is restored to normal within four to eight weeks.[2]

The anemias may be classified according to their mechanisms of pathogenesis. Aside from acute hemorrhage, the main anemias are due to impaired production or excessive destruction of red cells. Anemias due to impaired production are much more common than the latter.[3] The principal anemias are listed in Table 19-1.

**Iron-deficiency anemia.** In normal adults the daily intake of iron in the diet is 10 to 20 mg, although only 1 mg of this is absorbed each day. This is sufficient to balance the daily loss in tissues from necrobiosis, e.g., sloughing of squamous cells from the skin and columnar cells from the intestinal mucosa. The absorbed iron is carried in the serum attached to a protein, transferrin. The normal level of transferrin is 300 $\mu$g/dl, and one-third of this is used for the transport of iron. Transferrin is therefore about one-third saturated. This arrangement gives rise to the terms serum iron (the amount bound to transferrin, or 100 $\mu$g), latent iron-binding capacity (the transferrin unattached to iron, or 200 $\mu$g), and total

Table 19-1. _____

## Pathogenesis
## of anemia

Impaired production
    Iron deficiency
    Pernicious anemia
    Folate deficiency
    Aplastic anemia
    Secondary anemias

Excessive destruction
    Congenital spherocytosis
    Sickle cell anemia
    Thalassemia
    G6PD anemia
    Autoimmune anemia

iron-binding capacity (the sum of the bound and unbound transferrin, or 300 $\mu$g). The transported iron is deposited in the marrow.

Hemoglobin production is determined both by the stimulation of erythropoietin and by the availability of iron. The availability of iron thus limits the production of hemoglobin. An inadequate supply of iron is due to a faulty diet, as in an infant restricted to intake of milk; malabsorption from intestinal inflammations, such as regional enteritis; or chronic bleeding in which the daily loss of iron is more than can be absorbed from the diet. The causes of such bleeding include varices, hemorrhoids, carcinoma of the colon, especially of the cecum, and extensive hookworm disease. Whatever the mechanism, when iron is unavailable, the red cells become increasingly poor in hemoglobin and small in size (Figure 19-1). The consequence of iron deficiency is therefore hypochromic microcytic anemia. Other features are low serum iron (i.e., under 50 $\mu$g/dl), increased latent iron-binding capacity, and depletion of iron from the bone marrow as shown by the Prussian blue staining reaction. Iron-deficiency anemia affects both sexes and all ages, and exists worldwide. It is the most common of all the anemias.

**Pernicious anemia.** For reasons not yet known, some persons develop antibodies against the epithelial cells of their own gastric mucosa.[4] Evidently as a result of this, the mucosa undergoes atrophy, the rugal pattern is effaced, and the gastric wall is so thin that the pattern of veins could be seen if the stomach were held up to the light. The atrophy is thus pronounced and diffuse; it affects both the parietal and chief cells. As a result the volume of gastric secretion is reduced and there is no acid, no pepsin, and no factor necessary for the absorption of vitamin $B_{12}$. Normally vitamin $B_{12}$ (cyanocobalamin) is ingested in the diet and combines with a secretion of the parietal cells of the stomach; this complex is

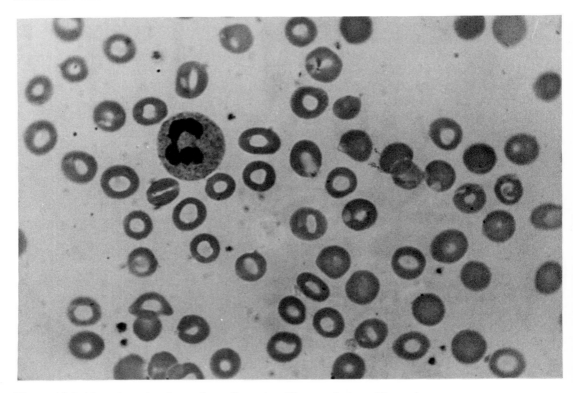

**Figure 19-1.** Hypochromic microcytic erythrocytes. The small size of the red cells can be seen by comparison with the neutrophilic leukocyte.

carried to the distal ileum, where the vitamin enters the mucosa and is absorbed into the body. Of course, without parietal cells there is no intrinsic factor so that the vitamin cannot be carried to the terminal ileum for absorption.

All cells of the body need vitamin $B_{12}$ for the synthesis of thymidine, which is needed for the production of deoxyribonucleic acid. Therefore, without $B_{12}$, DNA production is impaired and cell maturation is delayed. These functional effects are most evident in those cells that divide rapidly or are present on visible surfaces. These include the tongue, the buccal epithelium, the mucosa of the ileum, the vaginal mucosa, and the hemopoietic cells of the bone marrow. Therefore, in a person without vitamin $B_{12}$, the tongue becomes sore, diarrhea may develop, and anemia gradually arises. In its

struggle to function normally, the red marrow expands throughout the long bones, the proportion of immature cells increases, and the erythrocytes turned out into the circulation are large, dark, and few. These features define "hyperchromic" macrocytic anemia. Although the cells are dark and appear to be rich in hemoglobin, in fact the mean corpuscular hemoglobin concentration is normal. The anemia may become pronounced with only 1 million red cells per cubic millimeter and only 2 to 3 gm of hemoglobin per deciliter. In addition, leukopenia is often present and the neutrophils have five to six nuclear segments rather than the normal three to four. They are thus hypersegmented (Figure 19-2). The bone marrow is overactive with many immature cells, including 10 to 25 per cent megaloblasts.

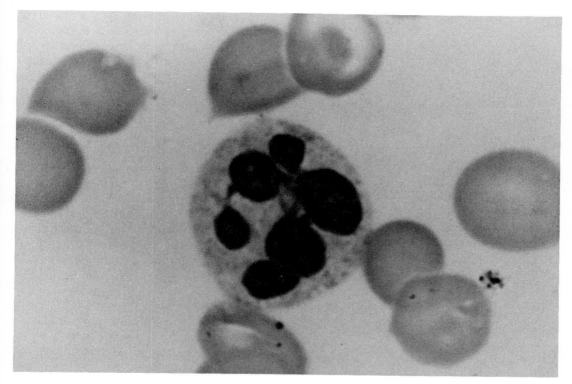

**Figure 19-2.** Hypersegmented neutrophil and macrocytic erythrocytes in pernicious anemia

Vitamin $B_{12}$ is also needed for the function of peripheral nerves and the dorsal and lateral tracts of the spinal cord. The mechanism of this need is not known. Nevertheless, without $B_{12}$, both the peripheral nerves and spinal cord undergo myelin degeneration. The cord changes, which are most pronounced in the thoracic segment, are referred to as subacute combined degeneration. On account of these neural aspects, the onset of pernicious anemia is characterized not only by pallor, weakness, and soreness of the tongue, which becomes smooth and red, but also by numbness and tingling of the extremities. Intramedullary hemolysis also causes a slight degree of jaundice so that the skin takes on a pale lemon-yellow tinge. Thus the patient tends to present with glossitis, jaundice, and neural symptoms. Without treatment the clini-

cal aspects worsen through a series of remissions and exacerbations, and finally the anemia becomes pronounced and ataxia with loss of position sense develops. Weakness becomes extreme, resistance to disease declines, and terminal infection finally claims its victim.

Pernicious anemia begins in middle or old age and affects Caucasians, especially those of Scandinavian descent with blue eyes, blond hair, and fair complexions. A familial factor is present, as relatives of the patient have a higher incidence of the disease than others do. The sexes are equally affected. Vitamin $B_{12}$, given parenterally, corrects the metabolic need; the megaloblastosis subsides, the red cells resume their normal size, and showers of reticulocytes herald the resumption of normal hemopoiesis. All the abnormalities are cor-

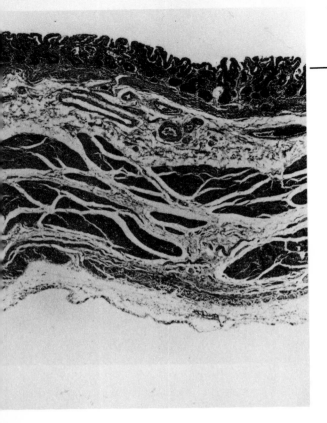

**Figure 19-3.** Atrophy of gastric mucosa in pernicious anemia

rected except the atrophic gastritis and achlorhydria, which are permanent (Figure 19-3). Pernicious anemia is therefore a life-long state. It is not a deficient-intake disease, but a blocked-absorption disease.

From the standpoint of the laboratory, the diagnostic features of pernicious anemia are "hypochromic" macrocytic anemia, hypersegmented neutrophils, gastric achlorhydria, megaloblastosis of bone marrow, low serum cyanocobalamin, and abrupt hematologic improvement with parenteral vitamin $B_{12}$. Atrophic glossitis, pallor of the skin, and numbness and tingling of the extremities with eventual loss of vibration sense fill out the clinical aspects of the disorder.

Understanding the pathogenesis of pernicious anemia did not come easily. The condition was originally described by Addison in 1855, but the term "pernicious," meaning "deadly," was not applied until 1872. Advances were then meager until

1926, when Minot and Murphy discovered that the feeding of liver had a therapeutic effect. From that time forward pernicious anemia was no longer a hopelessly incurable disease. In 1929 Castle identified the need for a gastric substance that he called "intrinsic factor." It was then understood that an "extrinsic factor" from the diet and an "intrinsic factor" from the stomach were required in order to prevent the development of the disease. In 1948 vitamin $B_{12}$ was crystallized, so that the extrinsic factor became cyanocobalamin and the intrinsic factor was found to be a glycoprotein secreted by the gastric mucosa. The availability of crystalline cyanocobalamin completed the therapeutic triumph; it takes only 1 mg given by intramuscular injections at monthly intervals to prevent recurrence of the disease.[5]

Understanding pernicious anemia led to the recognition that megaloblastosis with hyperchromic macrocytic anemia could also be caused by absence of the stomach (gastrectomy), absence or dysfunction of the ileum (ileal resection, regional enteritis), and malabsorption syndromes (pancreatitis, sprue, Whipple's disease). In addition, intestinal stasis from diverticula or blind loops permits overgrowth of bacteria that render dietary $B_{12}$ unavailable for absorption. Thus different mechanisms cause the same hemopoietic disturbance; pernicious anemia is merely the form of the disease that is due to atrophic gastritis.

**Folate-deficiency anemia.** Folic acid (pteroylglutamic acid) is also a dietary substance needed for thymidine synthesis and hence DNA production. As would therefore be expected, a shortage of this substance also causes macrocytic anemia with megaloblastosis of the bone marrow. The cellular changes are indistinguishable from those of pernicious anemia; the diagnosis is made on the basis of acid in the gastric juice, absence of subacute combined degeneration of the spinal cord, and the presence of a low serum folate level as determined by radioimmunoassay. Also, the serum cyanocobalamin is normal and the anemia is unresponsive to parenteral $B_{12}$. The cause of this anemia is either an inadequate supply of folate, an increased need for it, or failure to absorb it. It is therefore seen in conditions of abject poverty, in alcoholism, in malnourished populations, in malabsorption syndromes, and in conditions of increased need, especially pregnancy. All such folate-deficiency anemias are corrected with folic acid therapy. Even the hematologic findings of pernicious anemia subside with folic acid; the neurologic aspects, however, are unaffected or made worse.[6]

**Aplastic anemia.** In some individuals an idiopathic failure of the bone marrow develops and the red cells begin to disappear from the blood. The resulting anemia, which is termed aplastic, is normochromic and normocytic. Biopsy of bone marrow discloses absence of hemopoietic elements and replacement with fatty tissue. In other persons all the formed elements of the blood (red cells, white cells, platelets) disappear so that pancytopenia results. Both conditions are often relentlessly progressive and fatal. In about half of cases the reason for this devastating illness is entirely unknown; it is altogether idiopathic. In the rest, exposure to a bone marrow toxin (benzene compounds, radiation) is identified or special sensitivity to a drug (chloramphenicol, phenylbutazone, nitrogen mustards) is presumed.

**Secondary anemias.** Hemopoietic failure is also a secondary aspect of other diseases, especially those of the liver and kidney. With cirrhosis, for example, anemia is common and in some instances may be macrocytic. The explanation for this is not known although it is tempting to suppose that folate intake is inadequate or that vitamin $B_{12}$, which is normally stored in the liver, is either depleted or altered so that it is not available to the bone marrow. Normochromic normocytic anemia is also a constant feature of chronic renal disease regardless of the type. It is attributed to failure of the kidneys to produce erythropoietin.[2] Marrow failure is also occasioned by the infiltrations of metastatic disease. The most common cancers are those of the breast, lung, and prostate. Leukemic infiltrations of bone marrow also force out the normal hemopoietic elements so that normochromic normocytic anemia results. Multiple myeloma has the same effect; plasma cell proliferations replace the hemopoietic tissue. The term for anemias due to bone marrow replacement by malignant tumor is myelophthisic.

### Excessive destruction

The globin part of hemoglobin consists of four chains of amino acids, each in a particular sequence. During intrauterine life most of the hemoglobin is fetal in type (Hb F) and consists of two $\alpha$ chains and two $\gamma$ chains. In adult life almost all the hemoglobin is of the adult type (Hb $A_1$) and consists of two $\alpha$ chains and two $\beta$ chains. The transition from Hb F to Hb $A_1$ takes place in about the first six months after birth. A third kind of hemoglobin, Hb $A_2$, is present in trace amounts in adults; it consists of two $\alpha$ chains and two $\delta$ chains. The differences among the various chains are found in the specific sequences of the amino acids. A normal person inherits a gene for one $\alpha$ chain and one $\beta$ chain from each parent. Genetic faults may, of course, cause alterations in any of these chains. When that happens, a hemoglobinopathy develops.

**Sickle cell anemia.** In Hb $A_1$ each $\alpha$ chain has 141 amino acids and each $\beta$ chain 146 amino acids, so that normal adult hemoglobin is composed of a total of 574 amino acids. On one end of each chain is an amino group ($NH_2$), and on the other end a carboxyl group (COOH). The sixth amino acid from the $NH_2$ terminus in the $\beta$ chain is

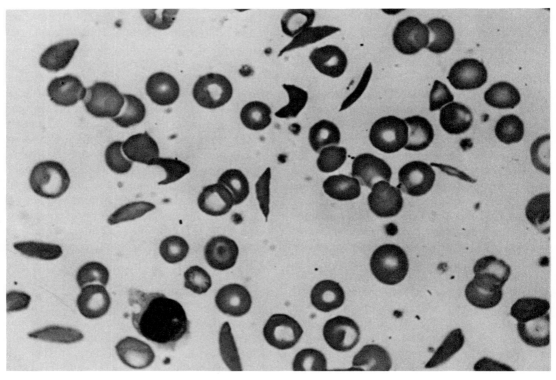

**Figure 19-4.** Sickle cells with pointed ends in sickle cell anemia

normally glutamic acid. When that is re-placed with valine, sickle cell hemoglobin (Hb S) results. The reason for this substitu-tion is a fault in the gene that directs the construction of the $\beta$ chain. When the sub-stitution is present in only one of the two $\beta$ chains, the individual is heterozygous and asymptomatic although as much as 40 per cent of his or her hemoglobin may be in the Hb S form. Such persons have the sickle cell trait. When both $\beta$ chains carry the va-line substitution, however, the person is homozygous and has sickle cell anemia with over 70 per cent of the hemoglobin in the Hb S form. Whether the patient is hetero-zygous or homozygous depends on whether the genetic fault was inherited from one or both parents.

The amino acid substitution in the $\beta$ chain causes the hemoglobin to react to low oxy-gen tension by forming rigid structures,

called tactoids, within the cell. These de-form the cell so that it takes on the configu-ration of the blade of a sickle (Figure 19-4). This occurs spontaneously in the red cells of homozygotes and can be induced by low oxygen tension in the cells of heterozy-gotes. Adding sodium metabisulfite, a re-ducing agent, to the blood smear in the lab-oratory thus induces tactoid formation and reveals the presence of the sickle cell trait.

The significance of the sickle deformity is that the stiff, elongated cells cannot pass through capillaries easily, and as the lu-mens are blocked, hypoxia develops, the red cells hemolyze, and microinfarcts form. The hemolysis causes anemia, and on this account the bone marrow undergoes hyper-plasia, filling up the long bones and project-ing trabeculae outside the tables of the skull to form additional hemopoietic tissue. This gives a characteristic radiographic ap-

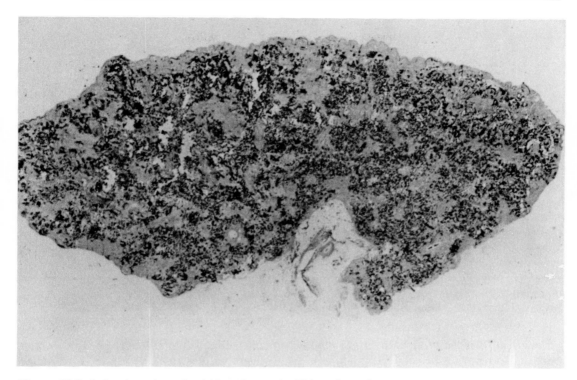

**Figure 19-5.** Autosplenectomy in sickle cell anemia. This entire spleen weighed only 10 gm.

pearance, the "hair-on-end" skull. The hemolysis also causes jaundice with unconjugated hyperbilirubinemia. In the beginning splenomegaly is common, but after a few years and the formation of hundreds of microinfarcts, the spleen is reduced to a minute, fibrotic, calcified structure (Figure 19-5). The virtual disappearance of the spleen by this process is called autosplenectomy. The liver may be large from extramedullary hemopoiesis, the heart may be hypertrophic from compensatory tachycardia, and the tips of the renal pyramids may show necrosis from ischemia.

The clinical signs of sickle cell disease are mainly pallor and weakness with joint pains, leg ulcers, and hemolytic crises. The ulcers occur about the ankles and persist as long as the hemoglobin is low. The hemolytic crises consist of excruciating pain in the bones, joints, and abdomen. They last four to six days, gradually subside, and may not be associated with pronounced hemolysis. Laboratory examination of the blood reveals evidence of hemolysis and hyperactivity of the bone marrow: sickle cells, normocytes, reticulocytes, and an anemia of 2 million to 3.5 million red cells per cubic millimeter. There are also unconjugated bilirubin in the serum and increased urobilinogen in the stool, and electrophoresis shows an abundance of sickle hemoglobin (Hb S) as well as a compensatory increase of fetal hemoglobin (Hb F). Without treatment homozygotes may die in infancy or live into early adulthood. With treatment consisting of exchange transfusions and measures to counteract dehydration and acidosis, the outlook is improved. Most hope attaches to the prospect of finding an antisickling agent or a mechanism for correcting the single gene mutation.[7]

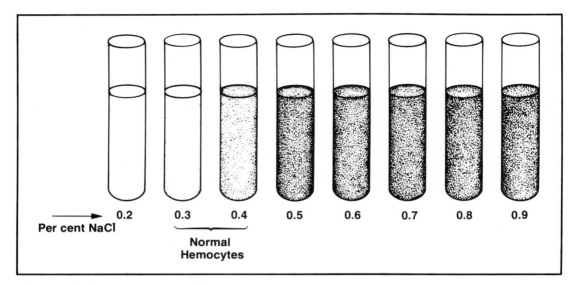

Figure 19-6. The mechanism for identifying increased osmotic fragility in congenital hemolytic anemia. Each tube contains the same amount of blood.

Sickle cell disease is virtually restricted to blacks and is widespread in Africa and in other malaria-infested parts of the world. In the United States the sickle cell trait is present in 8 per cent of blacks (heterozygotes) while the disease occurs in 1 per cent (homozygotes). Why does such a devastating disturbance have such a wide distribution? It has been discovered that sickle hemoglobin in some way interferes with the proliferation of the malarial parasite, *Plasmodium falciparum*, in red cells. An interesting situation thus arises: The sickle homozygote dies of anemia, the normal child dies of *P. falciparum* malaria, and the heterozygote is protected from both conditions. The heterozygote thus has an advantage that favors proliferation and spread. This perhaps explains the unusually wide distribution of the disease. The pattern of inheritance is autosomal codominant.[8]

**Congenital hemolytic anemia.** An inherited trait transmitted as a mendelian dominant causes red cells to have an abnormal membrane. The molecular nature of the disturbance is not known, but the abnor-

mality diminishes the surface area of the cell so that it is small and spheroidal rather than biconcave. The cell is known as a spherocyte. It has a dark center because of the thickness of the central region. This change of shape prevents the erythrocyte from squeezing through the capillary filters of the spleen so that stasis and destruction occur in that organ. Hemolytic anemia thus results. It is termed congenital hemolytic or congenital spherocytic anemia. The deficiency of hemoglobin is only slight, however, because the bone marrow undergoes hyperplasia of six to 10 times normal and the red cell production is nearly able to keep up with the rate of hemolysis. The condition begins in infancy or childhood and affects the sexes equally. It is manifested by pallor, jaundice, and splenomegaly. Four laboratory features are characteristic: a mean corpuscular hemoglobin above normal (spherocytosis), a reticulocytosis of 5 to 20 per cent, a bilirubinemia of 2 to 3 mg/dl, and an increase in the osmotic fragility of the red cells.

Erythrocytes absorb water as they are immersed in decreasing concentrations of saline. Normal cells burst (hemolyze) at 0.45 to 0.32 per cent salt solution, while spherocytes hemolyze at 0.68 to 0.55 per cent (Figure 19-6).

If treatment is not given the hemolysis continues, the bone marrow responds, and the jaundice persists. The spleen enlarges to 500 to 2,000 gm as a result of both hemolysis and extramedullary hemopoiesis. The complication of this ongoing disturbance is the formation of bilirubin gallstones, which may be present even in childhood.[8] Fortunately, removal of the spleen, which is the sole site of the hemolyzing process, cures the anemia. The spherocytes remain, of course, but the hemolysis stops and normal hemopoiesis is restored. It is of incidental interest that normal red cells transfused into a patient with this condition and an intact spleen do not hemolyze.

**Thalassemia.** *Thalassa* means "sea." The word is adapted to a disease affecting inhabitants of the Mediterranean littoral, i.e., persons of Greek and Italian ancestry. It is an inherited condition in which a genetic fault causes failure of an amino acid chain in the globin molecule to form. Thalassemia is therefore not due to an abnormal structure of a globin chain, but to absence of one or more of the chains. Three consequences result: Compensatory globin chains develop, the red cells become poor in hemoglobin, and they are sequestered and destroyed, especially in the spleen. Thalassemia is therefore an inherited hypochromic microcytic anemia of the hemolytic type. The genetic fault is inherited as an incomplete autosomal dominant. The condition is sometimes referred to as Cooley's anemia, after its discoverer.

The fault may affect either the $\alpha$ or the $\beta$ chains and the disturbance may be either heterozygous or homozygous. $\alpha$-Chain deficiency that is heterozygous tends to be asymptomatic. The homozygous state, however, is fatal in utero or early in life. Heterozygous $\beta$-chain deficiency, with only one chain affected, causes thalassemia minor, in which Hb $A_1$ is suppressed and compensation comes from the production of hemoglobins not requiring $\beta$ chains, i.e., Hb F and Hb $A_2$. The anemia is slight and the patient is asymptomatic, although the spleen may be enlarged. Homozygous $\beta$-chain deficiency, with both chains affected, causes thalassemia major; $\gamma$-chain production is compensatory so that the hemoglobin is almost entirely fetal in type (Hb F). Thalassemia major is usually fatal in utero, or in childhood or adolescence.

Thalassemia major becomes noticeable early in life, always within the first decade. The clinical signs include pallor, weakness, and protuberance of the abdomen from marked hepatosplenomegaly due to extramedullary hemopoiesis. The bone marrow is overactive, and a skull X-ray reveals the "hair-on-end" appearance. A blood smear shows nucleated red cells, reticulocytes, and a pronounced hypochromic microcytic anemia. In addition, inclusion bodies form within the red cells from precipitation of excess $\alpha$ chains.[9,10] The key diagnostic observation is the presence of more than 50 per cent fetal hemoglobin (Hb F) in the electrophoretic pattern. The evidence of increased blood destruction includes unconjugated hyperbilirubinemia and an increased excretion of urobilinogen in the stool. A high serum iron level, perhaps indicating deficient utilization, distinguishes the hypochromic microcytic anemia from that due to iron deficiency. Life may be sustained by transfusions, but otherwise the child rarely progresses to adult life.

**Enzyme-deficiency anemia.** Normal red cells contain an enzyme, glucose 6-phosphate dehydrogenase (G6PD), that is necessary for protection against certain chemicals. The chemicals include antimalarial agents, especially primaquine, and less often others such as aspirin, acetanilide, and nitrofurantoin. These drugs, given to a G6PD-deficient individual, denature protein within the cell, Heinz bodies form, and the spleen destroys the cells with such inclusions. A hemolytic anemia thus develops. It begins within two to four days and subsides within 72 hours after the drug is discontinued. The anemia is present only after exposure to the drug. The bone marrow reacts by hyperplasia with reticulocytosis, and the signs of hemolysis develop: unconjugated bilirubinemia and increased excretion of urobilinogen in the stool.

The condition is inherited; the gene for G6PD is carried on the X chromosome. The clinical disturbance is therefore more frequent in males (XY), in whom the affected chromosome is unopposed, than in females (XX), who are usually heterozygous and protected, at least partially, by one normal chromosome. The condition is common in blacks, in whom the anemia is only moderate, and is uncommon in men of Italian or Greek ancestry, in whom the anemia is often pronounced when it does occur. About 11 per cent of black males in the United States are affected.[6]

**Autoimmune hemolysis.** Antibodies generated by an individual against his own erythrocytes are the cause of "autoimmune hemolytic anemia." The condition may be idiopathic or secondary to a known disease, such as leukemia, lymphoma, Hodgkin's disease, lupus erythematosus, viral infections, advanced cirrhosis, and carcinomatosis. The antibodies may be evident in vitro at body temperature (warm) or at room temperature (cold). Warm antibodies are more frequent and the anemias are more pronounced. The characteristic laboratory feature of both warm and cold autoimmune hemolysis is a positive Coombs test, in which serum containing antihuman globulin developed in a rabbit is added to washed human red cells coated with self-generated antibody. Such antibodies are composed of human globulin. Clumping of the cells reveals the presence of antibody on the patient's erythrocytes. Otherwise the anemia

is hemolytic, of varying degree, and nonspecific.

Although the foregoing descriptions account for the principal anemias, several conditions have been omitted from this brief review. For example, lead poisoning interferes with hemoglobin production so that normochromic normocytic anemia develops. The process is gradual, and clinical features that distinguish the condition include encephalopathy, abdominal pain, and paresthesias of the extremities. In the laboratory, basophilic stippling of the young erythrocytes is especially characteristic. Malaria causes hemolytic anemia as the parasites multiply within the red cells and cause them to burst. The spleen is usually enlarged and a recent visit to an endemic area may be discovered from the history. *Clostridium perfringens (welchii)* infection may also cause pronounced hemolytic anemia. Hypersplenism, often associated with cirrhosis, also causes a sharp reduction in one or more of the formed elements circulating in the blood. Sequestration of erythrocytes in the spleen is presumed. The topic is mentioned in Chapter 14.

## RETICULOENDOTHELIAL TISSUE

The reticuloendothelial tissues are found in the bone marrow, spleen, lymph nodes, liver, and lymphoid deposits of the walls of the bronchi and the mucosa of the intestine. At these sites two main kinds of tissue are present. One is the hemopoietic component, which occupies the bone marrow and consists of the formative and mature cells of the erythrocytic, myelocytic, and megakaryocytic series. Each of these is in constant renewal-depletion balance so that in any unit of time some cells succumb and are disposed of while an equal number are generated to replace them. The other component is the lymphopoietic tissue, which occupies the remainder of the anatomic sites mentioned above and is also spread lightly throughout the bone marrow. Both components undergo regressive and progressive changes. The regressive changes of the hemopoietic component are anemia, leukopenia, and thrombocytopenia, while those of the lymphopoietic component consist of the immunodeficient disorders.

This section reviews the progressive disorders of both components of the system. The classification is shown in Table 19-2. Burkitt's tumor and Hodgkin's disease are usually classified as subtypes of the lymphomas. They are set apart in Table 19-2 because of unique clinical or morphologic features that distinguish them from the "ordinary" lymphomas.

Leukemia is a malignant disease characterized by an increased number of circulating leukocytes, an increased proportion of immature leukocytes, and leukemic infiltration (leukosis) of a wide variety of tissues. Craigie described the condition in

Table 19-2. _____

## Progressive disorders of the reticuloendothelial system

Hemopoietic
    Acute myeloid leukemia
    Chronic myeloid leukemia
    Erythroleukemia (Di Guglielmo)
    Myeloproliferative disorders
        Primary polycythemia
        Myeloid metaplasia
        Megakaryocytic myelosis
        Idiopathic thrombocythemia

Lymphopoietic
    Acute lymphoid leukemia
    Chronic lymphoid leukemia
    Hairy-cell leukemia
    Lymphoma
        Nodular
        Diffuse
    Hodgkin's disease
    Burkitt's lymphoma
    Multiple myeloma

1839, although he attributed his findings to suppuration of the blood. In 1845 Virchow distinguished the process from suppuration, and two years later he coined the term leukemia. In 1877 Ehrlich developed the stains that specify the granules in the various types of leukocytes, and by 1930 all the kinds of leukemia were known. Chemotherapeutic agents were discovered about 100 years after the condition was first recognized. These historical events have been reviewed by Williams and his colleagues.[8]

The incidence of leukemia, with all types included, is six per 100,000 population, and when these are combined with the lymphomas, they cause approximately 10 per cent of all cancer deaths.[11] The leukemias are classified by cell type, cell number, and disease duration. Classification by duration, which consists of acute, subacute, and chronic categories, is not altogether favored because it is retrospective and may also be affected by treatment. Classification by cell number consists of leukemic and aleukemic categories, but aleukemic disease, in which the leukocyte count is normal or low, is so infrequent that this scheme is seldom useful. The prevailing classification is thus by cell type, modified by the valid expectation that the process will be rapid when the leukocytes are immature, and gradual when they are not. The main varieties are thus lymphoblastic, in which most of the cells are undifferentiated; chronic lymphoid, in which most of the cells are mature; and acute and chronic myeloid leukemia. These four make up about 85 per cent of the total. Lymphoblastic and chronic lymphoid leukemias are diseases of the lymphoreticular tissue, while acute and chronic myeloid leukemias are disorders of the hemopoietic tissue.

The cause of leukemia is not precisely known, although a role is given to chemicals, radiation, viral infection, and genetic predisposition. Prolonged exposure to benzene, as with the use of glue in shoemaking, is a cause of leukemia although benzene is

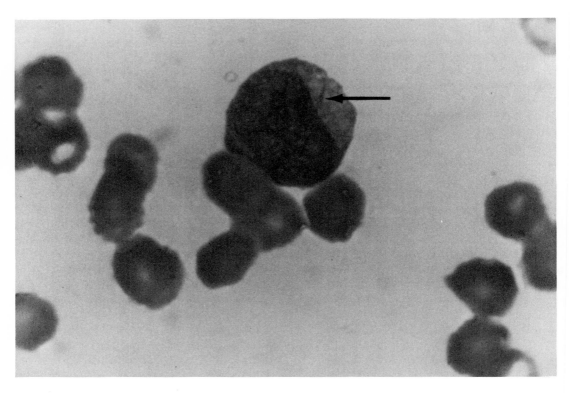

**Figure 19-7.** Auer body (arrow) in cytoplasm of leukemic cell (courtesy of Dr. Carl Johnson, Drew Postgraduate School of Medicine, Los Angeles). Also shown in color section, p C-8.

the least important of the etiologic agents.[12,13] Radiation is unquestionably a cause, with increases occurring after treatment for ankylosing spondylitis and after the whole-body exposures of the atomic bombing in Japan. The occurrence is dose-related and the type is almost invariably chronic myeloid. The first cases in Japan occurred two years after the exposure, the peak incidence was at five to seven years, and the frequency declined gradually thereafter but remained slightly elevated 20 years later.[14]

A viral cause was identified by Gross, who produced the disease in animals by transfer of a cell-free filtrate to mice within 48 hours of birth.[15] Later it was learned that type C RNA tumor viruses occur in leukemic animals, and a type C RNA virus

has been identified in a case of human disease.[16] The viral particles are also found in controls, however, so that proof of causation is still wanting. Although a viral cause suggests the possibility of contagion, leukemia is not excessive in the marital partners of patients with the disease, or in the children of women with leukemia whether or not they are breast-fed by their mothers.[8]

The best evidence of a genetic predisposition is the increased frequency of the disease in identical twins as compared with dizygotic (fraternal) twins or sibs.[17] That the leukemia does not always occur in the identical twin, however, may indicate that an environmental factor is also needed. A genetic fault is further suggested by the increased incidence of leukemia in patients with Down's syndrome, who have a trisomy of chromosome 21, and by an abnormally small chromosome 22—i.e., the Philadelphia chromosome—in 85 per cent of patients with chronic myeloid leukemia.[18] The possibility that the cause of leukemia is multifactorial, cannot, of course, be discounted.

The pathogenesis of leukemia is also not clear. In the past the disease was attributed to uncontrolled proliferation of cells, but more recently it was found that cell division is not more rapid in the leukemic population; rather, the cell cycle may be prolonged.[19] Thus the mechanism may be more one of accumulation than of proliferation. Although that issue is unsettled, it is clear that the main varieties are those that arise from the myeloid tissue (hemopoietic) and the lymphoid tissue (lymphoreticular).

## Hemopoietic disorders

**Acute myeloid leukemia.** Acute myeloid leukemia occurs more often in adults than in children. The onset is usually abrupt but is occasionally gradual, and males are affected slightly more often than females. The initial symptoms are anorexia, malaise, and weakness. Weight loss may be noticed. The liver and spleen are only moderately enlarged, and the subcutaneous lymph nodes may not be palpable. The leukocyte count is often only slightly raised, although many of the cells are immature. A diagnostic feature seen in the blood smear is the Auer body. This inclusion (Figure 19-7; see color section, p C-8) occurs in myeloid cells and is a cytoplasmic rod composed of abnormal neutrophilic granules. Hemorrhage and anemia develop as the normal elements of the bone marrow are crowded out by the leukemic cells. Leukemic cell infiltrations (leukosis) occur in many organs, especially the liver, spleen, lymph nodes, and kidneys. The bone marrow turns pale on account of the masses of myeloid cells. Chemotherapeutic agents that are effective against the leukemic cells

are also myelosuppressive so that marrow atrophy tends to be produced in the course of treatment. Without treatment the average survival time is three months; few patients live more than six months. With treatment about 50 per cent of patients achieve complete remission, and their median survival is one year.[8]

**Chronic myeloid leukemia.** Chronic myeloid (granulomatous) leukemia constitutes about 15 per cent of all adult leukemias. It occurs in either sex and affects all ages but is rare in children. The clinical features include a gradual onset of fatigue, weight loss, occasional night sweats, and low-grade fever. The main physical finding is splenomegaly. Laboratory investigation reveals slight anemia, normal or increased platelets, and a leukocyte count of 20,000 to 50,000 with a generous proportion of myelocytes and metamyelocytes in the differential count. All the tumor cells belong to the same clone. Of special importance are low or absent alkaline phosphatase activity in the myeloid cells, and a Philadelphia chromosome in 85 per cent of cases.[20] The Philadelphia chromosome is diagnostic: An arm of chromosome 22 is translocated elsewhere, usually to chromosome 9. The spleen tends to become enormous, often weighing over 5,000 gm and extending into the pelvis. In no other leukemia, and in virtually no other disease, does it become so large. Histologic examination reveals leukosis of many tissues in addition to the spleen and bone marrow. Solid masses of leukemic cells in bone or soft tissues, especially about the head, occasionally form discrete tumors known as chloromas. These give a green cut surface because of the enzyme myeloperoxidase. They are of no special significance and their presence does not affect the prognosis.[8] Therapy consists of alkylating agents and the use of radioactive phosphorus.[21] The median survival is about three years, although 20 per cent of patients will have remissions lasting 10 to 15 years.[21] The terminal event is often a "blast crisis" in which the blood suddenly becomes inundated with extremely immature cells. As responsiveness to therapy declines, secondary bacterial and fungal infections herald the end.

Other progressive conditions affect the hemopoietic tissue of the reticuloendothelial system. Erythroleukemia, described by Di Guglielmo, is a rare malignant process in which the cells in the blood and tissues are mainly erythroblasts. The condition affects adults, tends to be acute, and is associated with anemia due to massive replacement of the bone marrow with erythroblasts. Leukocytosis is not pronounced, but leukosis of the liver and spleen, with enlargement, is characteristic. Immature myeloid cells are also numerous, and the distinction from acute myeloid leukemia is not always possible. The cause is not known although cases have been reported after prolonged exposure to thorium oxide, chlorambucil, and cyclophosphamide.[22-24] The outlook is poor, with few surviving more than two years after the onset of the disease. Monocytic (Schilling) and myelomonocytic (Naegeli) leukemias are clinically like the myeloid leukemias and are classified with them.[25]

**Myeloproliferative disorders.** There are also separate proliferations of red cells, myeloid cells, megakaryocytes, and platelets. These are benign, are uncommon or rare, and are known collectively as the myeloproliferative disorders. The individual conditions are graced respectively with the formal names of primary polycythemia (polycythemia rubra vera), myeloid metaplasia, megakaryocytic myelosis, and idiopathic thrombocythemia. Primary polycythemia occurs in adults and is characterized by a florid complexion, an increased blood volume, and a red cell count of 7 million to 10 million. Increases of platelets (300,000 to 600,000) and leukocytes (12,000 to 20,000) signify a panmyelosis affecting all elements. The central lesion is a diffuse myelofibrosis; its cause is not known. Splenomegaly arises from extramedullary hemopoiesis and is characteristic of polycythemia. The circulating myeloid cells show an increased leukocyte alkaline phosphatase, which distinguishes the condition from leukemia. The course lasts 10 to 20 years and ends with thrombotic complications or, less frequently, the transition to acute myeloid leukemia. The condition must be distinguished from secondary polycythemia due to insufficient oxygenation, as seen with congestive heart failure, congenital heart disease, or pulmonary emphysema. In the secondary form the spleen is not enlarged, the leukocyte alkaline phosphatase is normal, and only the erythroid cells show hyperactivity in the bone marrow. Pure erythrocytosis from excretion of erythropoietin by hepatomas and carcinomas of the kidney also occurs.[26,27]

Myeloid metaplasia is a non-neoplastic primary disorder of unknown cause. The clinical features are anemia, extramedullary hemopoiesis, and moderate leukocytosis with immature myeloid cells in the blood. The bone marrow is hypocellular and often fibrotic. The marrow function is taken up by the spleen, which becomes enormously enlarged because of extramedullary hemopoiesis. The course is prolonged. A normal leukocyte alkaline phosphatase and absence of the Philadelphia chromosome distinguish the condition from chronic myeloid leukemia. Therapy is often unsatisfactory, and the condition may transform into acute myeloid leukemia.

Both myeloid metaplasia and myeloid leukemia need to be distinguished from the leukemoid reaction, in which the leukocyte count may rise to 50,000 and immature myeloid cells may appear in the differential count. The usual cause of the leukemoid reaction is widespread infection, miliary tuberculosis, or metastatic carcinoma that stimulates the bone marrow. The absence of a Philadelphia chromosome and the presence of alkaline phosphatase in the leukocytes distinguish the condition from more serious disorders.

Megakaryocytic myelosis and primary thrombocythemia are both myeloproliferative disorders in which the megakaryocyte or platelet count is above normal. In primary thrombocythemia the platelet count often persists above 1 million. The cause is unknown. The clinical features are bleeding and thrombosis. Although splenomegaly occurs, splenectomy worsens the condition. Life may not be shortened, but the possibility of hemorrhage, thrombosis, or thromboembolism persists.

## Lymphoreticular tissue

Although lymphocytes cohabit the bone marrow with myeloid cells, they are found mainly in extramedullary aggregates, including lymph nodes, spleen, tonsils, thymus, and mucosa of the bronchi and intestinal tract. Lymphocytes probably arise in the bone marrow, after which some differentiate in the thymus (T cells) and others remain unprocessed (B cells).[28] T lymphocytes are involved in cellular immunity, as in graft rejection and delayed hypersensitivity, while B lymphocytes are involved in the production of antibodies. The two cell types may be distinguished by specific surface markers. Small lymphocytes, as seen in the differential leukocyte count, will transform under stimulation to become large cells that appear immature and are capable of proliferative activity.[29] Phagocytes, including circulating monocytes, tissue macrophages, and histiocytes, also populate lymphoid tissue as well as other structures such as the liver, lungs, and serosal surfaces. These cells are involved in processing antigens and they also have surface markers that permit identification. Leukemias and extravascular tumors arise from all these identifiable components of the lymphoreticular tissue.

**Acute lymphoid leukemia.** Acute lymphoblastic leukemia is principally a disease of children. The onset is abrupt with fever, fatigue, hemorrhages into skin, and pain over the bones, especially ribs and sternum. Lymph node enlargement is widespread, and distention of the abdomen results from leukosis of the spleen and liver. In the laboratory, circulating leukocytes number 30,000 to 100,000 and most are extremely immature. When the leukocytes are uniformly undifferentiated, surface markers may be helpful in identifying the cell type. When prolymphocytes or mature lymphocytes are present, these serve to indicate the cell type. In all cases the cells are monoclonal and derive from T lymphocytes, B lymphocytes, or "null" cells without surface markers. The null cell group makes up about 70 per cent of the total.[30] As the lymphoid cells infiltrate the bone marrow and crowd out the normal hemopoietic elements, anemia and thrombocytopenia develop. Anemia contributes to weakness, and thrombocytopenia causes hemorrhages into the skin, gingivae, serosal surfaces, and viscera. In lymph nodes the capsule is invaded and the normal follicular pattern of the tissue is effaced. Infarcts form in the spleen, the capsule may rupture, and on both accounts pain may develop in the left upper quadrant of the abdomen. Leukosis also affects such diverse tissues as tonsils, lungs, heart, kidneys, intestine, testes, and orbits.

Infiltration of the meninges with leukemic cells occurs in about 60 per cent of patients with acute lymphoid leukemia and forms the so-called leukemic meningitis. It tends to be a late complication and is associated with increased intracranial pressure. The clinical manifestations are headache, vomiting, papilledema, and stiff neck. In the meninges the leukemic cells are protected from therapeutic drugs by the blood-brain barrier. The cells thus rest in a "pharmacologic sanctuary," and emergence from this protected environment may be the cause of post-therapeutic exacerbation.[31] Treatment consists of external radiation of the head and intrathecal administration of drugs. These prophylactic measures reduce the incidence to about 10 per cent. The complication is rare in adults.

Without treatment 90 per cent of patients die within six months. In 1947 Farber and associates discovered the therapeutic usefulness of the folic acid antagonists, and effective therapy of leukemia was then begun.[32] Currently vincristine and prednisone are favored, and with these agents 65 to 70 per cent of children become disease-free for three years. Moreover, 50 per cent will remain disease-free at five years and the rate of relapse after this will be low.[31] For those in whom the disease progresses, however, infections tend to develop. The usual organism is *Pseudomonas*, and a gram-negative septicemia may arise. Candidiasis, aspergillosis, and *Pneumocystis carinii* also contribute to the terminal condition.[33]

**Chronic lymphoid leukemia.** Chronic lymphoid (lymphocytic) leukemia is the most common form of the disease in adults. It arises in later life, with 90 per cent of patients over 50 and two-thirds over 60 years of age. It is twice as common in men as in women. It is due to a progressive increase in lymphoid cells, which are occasionally large with prominent nucleoli but are more often small and resemble mature lymphocytes. The cause is unknown, but no cases have been attributable to ionizing radiation. The lymphocytes arise from a single clone of B cells, and they are characterized by a long life with little proliferative capacity.[34] Moreover, the cells are immunologically deficient so that hypogammaglobulinemia tends to develop. The deficient cells fail to respond to antigenic stimuli and appear to accumulate passively in the tissues of the reticuloendothelial system, where they lie dormant for long periods. Lymphocytic leukosis thus becomes widespread in the lymph nodes, spleen, liver, bone marrow, and lymphoid deposits in the bronchi and small intestine. The spleen seldom weighs over 2,500 gm. Replacement of bone marrow with lymphoid cells crowds out the hemopoietic tissue, and anemia develops. In addition, the inability to produce immunoglobulins increases susceptibility to secondary infections.

The onset is so gradual that many cases are identified in the course of routine examinations. Fatigue and weakness are the main complaints. Examination reveals enlargement of lymph nodes and splenomegaly, although both may be slight. The leukocyte count is usually between 10,000 and 150,000. Lymphocytosis is evident on the differential smear, prolymphocytes suggest the nature of the disease, and the bone marrow discloses replacement with lymphoid cells, which establishes the diagnosis. The chromosomes of the tumor cells show no characteristic changes. Hemolysis develops through autoimmunity and this adds to the anemia; the Coombs test is positive. Blast crises are infrequent. Therapy with chlorambucil and triethylenemelamine provides a median survival of five years, with 30 per cent alive at 10 years.[34] There is no cure. Death is preceded by unresponsiveness to treatment and the complications of infection.

Less certain is the classification of the infrequent leukemias, i.e., the pure monocytic leukemia of Schilling and the monomyelocytic leukemia of Naegeli. Whether these are distinct and different is still not clear, but in both the tumor cells produce muramidase, which rises to a high level in the serum. Both behave like acute leukemias of other types, with the possible exception of greater leukosis of the gums and soft tissues. They are distinguished from acute lymphoblastic leukemia by the myeloperoxidase and Sudan black stains, which are positive in all the myeloid leukemias.[25] Hairy-cell leukemia is a rare lymphoproliferative disorder characterized by splenomegaly, pancytopenia, and circulating lymphoid cells over which filamentous processes give a unique (hairy) appearance. The filaments are seen by phase contrast microscopy.[29] As many as 50 per cent of the circulating leukocytes may be of this kind. The hairy cells may be derivatives of B lymphocytes.[35] The progress of the disease is slow, and splenectomy is the most helpful therapeutic measure.

**Lymphomas.** The lymphomas are malignant solid tumors of lymphoid tissue that usually arise in one group of lymph nodes. They are diseases of older age, usually begin gradually, and affect men more often than women. The clinical features are painless enlargement of lymph nodes associated later with lassitude, weight loss, and occasionally fever. Splenomegaly develops, hepatomegaly follows, and infiltration of bone marrow gradually replaces the hemopoietic elements so that anemia, leukopenia, and thrombocytopenia tend to develop. An autoimmune hemolytic process may worsen the anemia.

Classification of the lymphomas is based on cell type and tissue pattern. The cells are small lymphocytes, large histiocytes, or a mixture of the two. If the follicular tissue pattern is discernible, the tumor is regarded as nodular. If the follicular pattern is effaced, the tumor is diffuse. Either nodular or diffuse tumors may be composed of the cells noted above. The follicular (nodular) lymphomas constitute only 10 per cent of the total and are much less aggressive than the diffuse lymphomas, which constitute 90 per cent.[28] All of the nodular tumors and most of the diffuse tumors are derived from a single clone of B lymphocytes.[36] The nodular lymphomas may progress to the diffuse tissue pattern, and the diffuse lymphomas may progress to acute or chronic lymphoid leukemia. Change within the group is therefore always in the direction of increasing malignancy.

Grossly the nodes are enlarged, firm, and matted together. The cut surfaces are fleshy and uniformly pale gray, and have

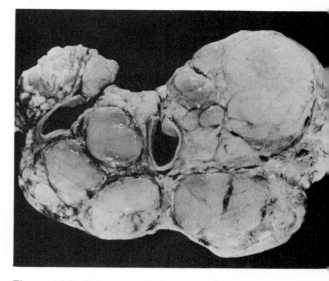

**Figure 19-8.** Enlargement of para-aortic lymph nodes in lymphoma

been likened to the appearance of fish flesh (Figure 19-8). The histologic features include partial or total effacement of the follicular pattern, extension of the tumor cells into and beyond the capsule, and a liberal sprinkling of mitotic figures throughout the microscopic fields (Figure 19-9). Without treatment the tumor cells continue to spread in the nodes, spleen, liver, and bone marrow. Inanition follows and secondary infection develops. With treatment 50 per cent of patients with nodular lymphoma survive five years. Only about half this proportion with diffuse lymphoma live as long.[28] Treatment consists of focal irradiation, total-body irradiation, and various combinations of chemotherapy.[36, 37]

The Sézary syndrome and mycosis fungoides are also malignant diseases of the lymphopoietic tissue. Neither is common, both occur in adults, and the primary involvement is in skin. In both there appear lymphoid cells in the upper dermis, distinguished by cerebriform convolutions of the nuclei. These are of T-lymphocyte origin. Diffuse erythroderma and early blood involvement that progresses to leukemia are

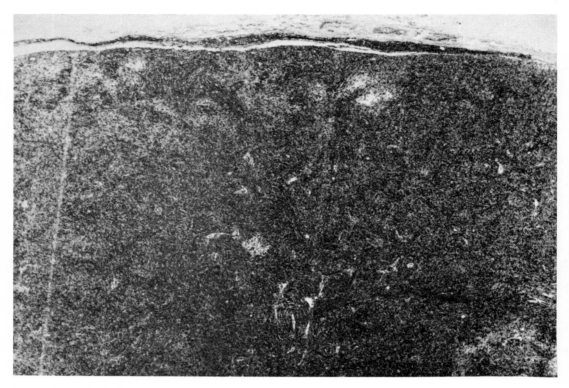

**Figure 19-9.** Follicular effacement and capsular spread in diffuse lymphocytic lymphoma

the features of the Sézary syndrome. Mycosis fungoides is characterized by dermal infiltrations that progress to localized tumors, but leukemia does not develop. Eventually visceral involvement is common in both. Neither is sufficiently frequent to be listed in Table 19-2.

**Hodgkin's disease.** In 1832 Thomas Hodgkin described seven cases of a disease that appeared to arise in lymph nodes. His report aroused no interest for the following 24 years. At that time Sir Samuel Wilks discovered Hodgkin's paper in the course of another investigation and subsequently wrote a more comprehensive account of the condition. Had it not been for Wilks's "chivalrous honesty" in giving credit to the original author, the disease might now have a different name.[8]

Greenfield described the histologic changes in 1878, and 20 years later Sternberg established the cell bearing his name as a characteristic feature of the disease. Four years later Reed embellished that account. Because of this sequence, the multinucleated cell should perhaps be referred to as the Sternberg-Reed cell rather than the other way around. In 1944 Parker and Jackson subordered cases into the paragranuloma, granuloma, and sarcoma categories. Because 90 per cent of patients fell into the granuloma group, however, the prognostic utility of that category was modest. In 1966 Lukes, Butler, and Hicks recommended a new classification consisting of four subgroups: lymphocytic predominance, nodular sclerosis, mixed cellularity, and lymphocytic depletion. The first two categories, constituting about half of cases, have a favorable prognosis; the other two do not. Finally, in 1971, the Ann Arbor Conference specified the staging system that is now widely used. These historical developments have been reviewed by Carr and colleagues.[38]

Hodgkin's disease is the most common of the malignant lymphomas. It has no absolute definition because the histologic features are variable, objective criteria are lacking, and the cause is not known. It arises in lymph nodes, spreads predictably, gradually invades extranodal tissues, and, unless treated, progresses to inanition, intercurrent infection, and death. It affects either sex, occurring twice as often in males as in females, and shows a bimodal peak of incidence, the first between 15 and 30 years and the second after the age of 50. The usual presenting sign is painless enlargement of the lymph nodes on one side of the neck. Subsequently fever, malaise, anorexia, and weight loss gradually develop. Pruritus is likely to occur, and drenching night sweats are common. As the disease progresses anemia, leukocytosis with eosinophilia, and thrombocytosis appear. An undulating febrile reaction, called Pel-Ebstein fever, is characteristic. Peculiar features are the development of anergy with nonreactivity to the tuberculin skin test, and severe pain, especially in bone lesions, after the ingestion of alcohol. The lack of tuberculin reactivity suggests a T-lymphocyte defect; the bone pain phenomenon is unexplained.

The fever, anemia, and night sweats of Hodgkin's disease suggest an infection, but no agent has been identified. The malignant nature of the condition is evidenced by its progressive course and widespread involvement of extranodal tissues. A genetic effect is possible, with a slightly increased risk of the disease in the sibs, parents, and progeny of patients.[39] Also, clusters of cases have suggested an infectious agent, although epidemiologic authorities regard this as "hardly more than suggestive."[28] It

has also been proposed that a viral infection of T lymphocytes causes a change of surface antigens, an interaction with nontransformed cells takes place, and from this a clone of malignant cells emerges.[29] Although the evidence for this mechanism is indirect, it at least combines the processes of infection and neoplasia.

Grossly the lymph nodes are large, firm, and pale gray. The cut surfaces are flecked with pale yellow foci of necrosis. Initially discrete, the nodes later become joined and matted. Adjacent structures become invaded and compressed. Three microscopic features are required for the diagnosis. The first is effacement of the nodal tissue pattern by proliferation of malignant reticulum cells. A variant of these elements is the multinucleated Sternberg-Reed cell (Figure 19-10). The cell is necessary for the diagnosis but nonspecific otherwise. The cell often displays a mirror-image nucleus. The second feature is an overlay of normal cells of different kinds that include lymphocytes, eosinophils, plasma cells, neutrophils, and macrophages. The third feature is fibrosis that ranges from a slight, diffuse change to coarse bands that encircle nodules of tumor. No single change is pathognomonic, and all are required in some degree for the diagnosis.

When the diagnosis is established, individual histologic features allow subclassification into the categories shown in Table 19-3. The frequency of the different subgroups in one series of 345 patients is also given in Table 19-3.[38]

Mainly by the use of lymphangiography it has become evident that Hodgkin's disease spreads to contiguous nodal structures first with later dissemination through the bloodstream.[28] Hematogenous spread accounts for the involvement of extranodal tissues such as the lungs, kidneys, stomach, adrenals, dura, meninges, thyroid, breasts, gonads, and lower urinary tract (Figure 19-11). In addition to histologic subgroups, the spread of the tumor also af-

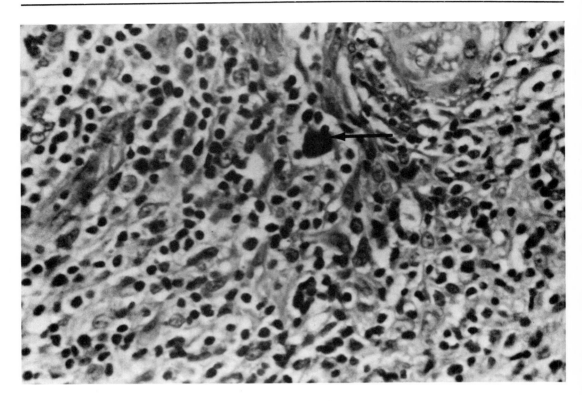

**Figure 19-10.** Multinucleated Sternberg-Reed cell (arrow) in Hodgkin's disease

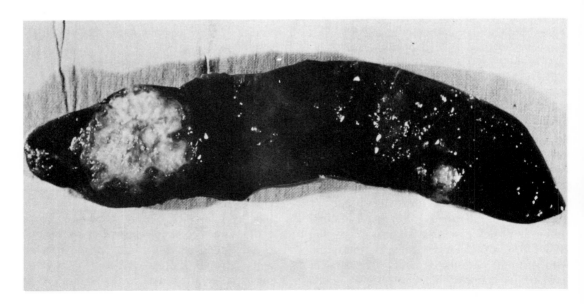

**Figure 19-11.** Nodules of Hodgkin's disease in spleen

fects the outlook for the patient. In order to standardize tumor spread in different series, a staging system has been devised. All the stages are clinical estimates of the spread of the tumor. In stage I the tumor appears localized to one group of lymph nodes. In stage II the involvement includes two groups of nodes, both on the same side of the diaphragm. In stage III nodal groups are affected on both sides of the diaphragm, and in stage IV extranodal tissues are affected with or without nodal involvement. The extent of spread at the time the patient is first seen is, of course, determined by the attitude and alertness of the patient. In 340 cases, stages I and II made up 60 per cent of the total at the time of presentation.[39] Outlook is also affected by the absence or presence of systemic symptoms: fever, pruritus, and night sweats. On this account the stages of the disease are qualified by the letters A, to signify no systemic symptoms, and B, to indicate their presence. The patient with the best outlook has stage I disease of type A with the histologic pattern of lymphocytic dominance.

Treatment of localized disease consists of high-dose, supervoltage radiation therapy. For disseminated tumors radiation or combinations of drugs are used. Among the most popular combinations is MOPP: mechlorethamine (nitrogen mustard), Oncovin (vincristine), procarbazine, and prednisone. Each therapeutic method for the two-thirds of patients with disseminated disease has its own proponents. With these methods the overall five-year survival rate is 73 per cent, with the range extending from 90 per cent for stages I and II to 35 per cent for stage IV.[39]

**Burkitt's lymphoma.** Burkitt's lymphoma was first clearly described in 1958.[40] It accounts for more than half of the childhood neoplasms in East Africa, it is the least differentiated of the lymphomas, and it occurs in children of either sex, mainly in the age group of 3 to 14 years. The illness is short,

the tumors grow rapidly, and the most frequent presentation is a nearly painless enlargement of the jaw that progresses, without treatment, to grotesque distortion of the face (Figure 19-12). The tumor tissue is soft and uniformly pale gray. Abdominal viscera are also primarily affected, and the central nervous system is involved in nearly one-third of cases. Paraplegia and ocular palsies result. Peripheral lymph nodes tend not to be affected.

The tumor is composed of monomorphic cells that resemble lymphoblasts with a scattering of macrophages containing cellular debris that gives a "starry sky" appearance. The cytoplasm is uniquely rich in ribonuclease, as disclosed by the methyl green-Pyronine Y stain.[41] Mitotic figures are abundant. With cyclophosphamide the tumors "melt away" with restoration of normal features (Figure 19-13). Therapy of localized disease achieves long remission and probably cure. The outlook is much less favorable when the disease is widespread. Without treatment the tumor is rapidly fatal and life seldom lasts more than six months after the clinical onset.

Burkitt's lymphoma occurs worldwide but is endemic in equatorial Africa and eastern New Guinea. At these sites the rainfall is abundant and the weather is warm. These conditions correspond to the

Table 19-3.

## Classification and incidence of Hodgkin's disease

| Subgroup | Incidence |
|---|---|
| Lymphocyte dominance | 17% |
| Nodular sclerosis | 37% |
| Mixed cellularity | 30% |
| Lymphocyte depletion | 12% |

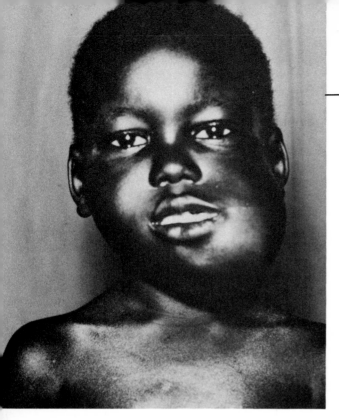

**Figure 19-12.** Burkitt's lymphoma of mandible in 7-year-old boy

**Figure 19-13.** The same patient as in Figure 19-12, 21 days later, after treatment with cyclophosphamide

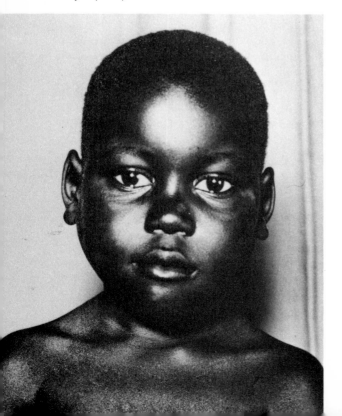

distribution of mosquitoes that could act as vectors. The tumor cells contain a virus of the herpes group (Epstein-Barr). Although the relationship among these factors is not clear, it has been suggested that the virus, which is lymphoproliferative, acts as an initiating factor, and malaria, which is localized to vector-borne regions, acts as a cofactor in the development of the malignant process.[41]

**Myelomatosis.** Multiple myeloma is a malignant proliferation of plasma cells that occurs after the age of 50 and is more common in men than in women. The cause is unknown. Pathogenesis devolves on two mechanisms: the production of excess tissue and the elaboration of excess immunoglobulin. The tumor cells are scattered throughout the bone marrow, where nodular proliferations cause "punched-out" foci of radiolucency, especially in the spine, skull, ribs, and pelvic bones. The marrow discloses pale red, soft, gelatinous tumor nodules that cause bone pain, osteoporosis, and pathologic fractures (Figure 19-14). Marrow aspiration reveals 30 per cent or more plasma cells. As the bone is eroded, calcium is liberated and the serum calcium rises. Normal erythroid precursors are gradually replaced by the advancing tumor cells so that anemia develops. The tumor cells may also spread to the periosteum or other soft tissues to form solid tumor masses. Occasionally the bloodstream in the terminal phase is invaded with the development of a plasma-cell leukemia.

The second mechanism is the production of immunoglobulin. The tumor cells are monoclonal derivatives of B lymphocytes, and the immunoglobulins are complete or incomplete, usually IgG but occasionally IgA, and are ordinarily the same for any given patient throughout the course of the disease. The globulin lacks receptor sites, so that it is useless as an antibody for the protection of the host. Since all tumor cells produce the same protein, serum electrophoresis reveals a characteristic monoclonal spike in the γ-globulin region. The useless protein combines with clotting factors and causes bleeding, forms rouleaux structures that induce thrombosis, and replaces normal immunoglobulins so that protection against infection gradually diminishes. Amyloidosis in the primary distribution, affecting the tongue, heart, and gut, is common although the relationship to the plasma-cell tumors is obscure.

The immunoglobulin produced by each patient is usually complete, with light and heavy chains held together by disulfide bonds. In some cases, however, additional light chains are produced, and these, which have a molecular weight of about 22,000, pass easily into the urine. Their presence in urine was discovered by Henry Bence Jones, who noticed that this protein coagulates at 45° to 55°C and dissolves at higher temperatures. Normal proteins do not dissolve after coagulating. Bence Jones proteinuria is thus characteristic of multiple myeloma and occurs in 50 to 60 per cent of cases. In the kidneys the Bence Jones protein, with or without albumin, forms hyaline casts in the distal tubules and collecting ducts. The tubules dilate and syncytial epithelioid cells form about the margins of the casts. Together with interstitial inflammation, these changes constitute the "my-

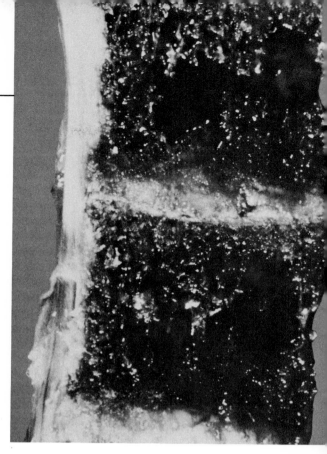

**Figure 19-14.** Tumor erosion of vertebral trabeculae in multiple myeloma

eloma kidney."[42] The progress of the disease is slow; bone destruction forces the patient to become bedridden, and anemia precedes terminal infection. Remissions are induced with alkylating agents, especially melphalan, and prednisone.

## REFERENCES

1. Smith JC: Heme pigment metabolism: A clinicopathologic spectrum. *Med Ann DC* 37:353, 1968

2. Linman JW: Physiologic and pathophysiologic effects of anemia. *N Engl J Med* 279:812, 1968

3. Hillman RS, Finch CA: Erythropoiesis. *N Engl J Med* 285:99, 1971

4. Castle WB: Current concepts of pernicious anemia. *Am J Med* 48:541, 1970

5. Sullivan LW: Differential diagnosis and management of the patient with megaloblastic anemia. *Am J Med* 48:609, 1970

6. Ravel R: *Clinical Laboratory Medicine: Clinical Application of Laboratory Data*, 3rd ed. Chicago: Year Book Medical Publishers, 1978

7. Trubowitz S: The management of sickle cell anemia. *Med Clin North Am* 60:933, 1976

8. Williams WJ, Beutler E, Erslev AJ, et al: *Hematology*, pp 385, 717. New York: McGraw-Hill, 1972

9. Marks PA, Bank A: Molecular pathology of thalassemia syndromes. *Fed Proc* 30:977, 1971

10. Weatherall DJ: Molecular pathology of the thalassemia disorders. *West J Med* 124:388, 1976

11. Silverberg E: Cancer statistics, 1977. *CA—Cancer J Clin* 27:26, 1977

12. Aksoy M, Erdem S, Dincol G: Types of leukemia in chronic benzene poisoning. A study of thirty-four patients. *Acta Haematol* 55:65, 1976

13. Vigliani EC, Saita G: Benzene and leukemia. *N Engl J Med* 271:872, 1964

14. Cronkite EP: Evidence for radiation and chemicals as leukemogenic agents. *Arch Environ Health* 3:297, 1961

15. Gross L: The role of viruses in the etiology of cancer and leukemia. *JAMA* 230:1029, 1974

16. Gallagher RE, Gallo RC: Type C RNA virus isolated from cultured human acute myelogenous leukemia cells. *Science* 187:350, 1975

17. McMahon B, Levy MA: Prenatal origin of childhood leukemia. *N Engl J Med* 270:1082, 1964

18. Trujillo JM, Ahearn MJ, Cork A: General implications of chromosomal alterations in human leukemia. *Hum Pathol* 5:675, 1974

19. Mauer AM: Cell kinetics and practical consequences for therapy of acute leukemia. *N Engl J Med* 293:389, 1975

20. Jackson L: Chromosomes and cancer: Current aspects. *Semin Oncol* 5:3, 1978

21. Moloney WC: Chronic myelogenous leukemia. *Cancer* 42:865, 1978

22. West WO: Acute erythroid leukemia after cyclophosphamide therapy for multiple myeloma: Report of two cases. *South Med J* 69:1331, 1976

23. Waddell CC, Brown JA, Rueb DL: Erythroleukemia (Di Guglielmo's disease). Occurrence 28 years after thorium administration. *JAMA* 238:423, 1977

24. Khandekar JD, Kurtides ES, Stalzer RC: Acute erythroleukemia complicating prolonged chemotherapy for ovarian carcinoma. *Arch Intern Med* 137:355, 1977

25. Bennett JM, Catovsky D, Daniel MT, et al: Proposals for the classification of the acute leukemias. *Br J Haematol* 33:451, 1976

26. Gallagher NI, Donati RM: Inappropriate erythropoietin elaboration. *Ann NY Acad Sci* 149:528, 1968

27. Brownstein MH, Ballard HS: Hepatoma associated with erythrocytosis. Report of eleven new cases. *Am J Med* 40:204, 1966

28. Aisenberg AC: Malignant lymphoma. *N Engl J Med* 288:833, 935, 1973

29. Braylan RC, Jaffe ES, Berard CW: Malignant lymphomas: Current classification and new observations. *Pathol Annu* 10:213, 1975

30. Brouet JC, Seligmann M: The immunological classification of acute lymphoblastic leukemias. *Cancer* 42:817, 1978

31. Frei E III, Salan SE: Acute lymphoblastic leukemia: Treatment. *Cancer* 42:828, 1978

32. Farber S, Cutler EC, Hawkins JW, et al: The action of pteroylglutamic acid conjugates in man. *Science* 100:619, 1947

33. Hersh EM, Bodey GP, Nies BA, et al: Causes of death in acute leukemia. *JAMA* 193:105, 1965

34. Rundles RW, Moore JO: Chronic lymphocytic leukemia. *Cancer* 42:941, 1978

35. Golomb HM: Hairy cell leukemia: An unusual lymphoproliferative disease. A study of 24 patients. *Cancer* 42:946, 1978

36. Berard CW, Jaffe ES, Braylan RC, et al: Immunologic aspects and pathology of the malignant lymphomas. *Cancer* 42:911, 1978

37. Canellos GP, Lister XA, Skarin AT: Chemotherapy of the non-Hodgkin's lymphomas. *Cancer* 42:932, 1978

38. Carr I, Hancock BW, Henry L, et al: *Lymphoreticular Disease*, p 64. Philadelphia: Lippincott, 1977

39. Kaplan HS: On the natural history, treatment, and prognosis of Hodgkin's disease. *Harvey Lect* 64:215, 1968-1969

40. Burkitt D: A sarcoma involving the jaws in African children. *Br J Surg* 46:218, 1958

41. Burkitt DP, Wright DH: *Burkitt's Lymphoma*. Edinburgh: Livingstone, 1970

42. Zlotnick A, Rosenmann E: Renal pathologic findings associated with monoclonal gammopathies. *Arch Intern Med* 135:40, 1975

# 20

# ENDOCRINE DISORDERS

The main components of the endocrine system are the pituitary, adrenals, thyroid, parathyroids, and islets of Langerhans. The islets are discussed in Chapter 14. The endocrine organs secrete hormones that regulate physiologic processes. Because the hormones enter vascular sinuses directly from the secreting cells, no ductal systems are involved. Since only some of these structures have an acinic pattern, the word "gland" need not be attached to each.

## PITUITARY

The pituitary is a solid ovoid structure weighing 0.5 to 1.0 gm that is cradled in the sella turcica and is connected to the hypothalamus by a slender stalk. It consists of an anterior lobe (adenohypophysis), which makes up two-thirds of the volume, and a posterior lobe (neurohypophysis), which makes up the rest. The anterior lobe arises from an upgrowing bud of the foregut (Rathke's pouch), and the posterior lobe from a downgrowing bud of the forebrain. The adenohypophysis is composed of epithelial cells; 50 per cent are chromophobic and do not take the hematoxylin-eosin stain, while the remainder are chromophilic with 40 per cent taking eosin (red) and 10 per cent taking hematoxylin (blue).[1] Venous blood from the capillaries of the hypothalamus flows down the stalk in the portal veins to reach the sinusoids of the anterior lobe. These channels then converge to form another vein that leaves the pituitary and

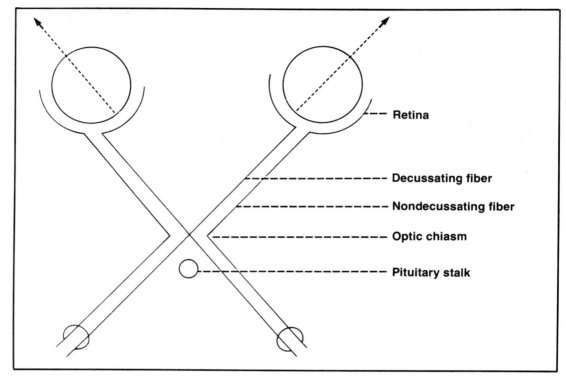

**Figure 20-1.** Relationship of pituitary stalk to optic chiasm

opens into the systemic circulation. Releasing factors of the hypothalamus flow in the portal veins to the anterior lobe, where hormones are discharged into the vascular sinusoids and thence into the venous blood. These hormones include prolactin as well as growth, thyroid-stimulating, melanocyte-stimulating, adrenocorticotrophic, luteinizing, and follicle-stimulating hormones. The last two are also known as the pituitary gonadotrophins.

## Hypopituitarism

Most diseases of the anterior lobe cause pituitary insufficiency. The conditions include primary tumors, infarcts, expanding cysts, metastatic cancers, and granulomatous diseases such as sarcoidosis, which is uncommon, and tuberculosis, which is rare. The clinical manifestations depend on the time of onset. In children failure to grow is

the main manifestation of lesions that destroy the pituitary. The most common is the craniopharyngioma, which is a primary tumor. The somatic hypoplasia is symmetrical so that no disproportion develops. Pituitary dwarfism thus differs sharply from achondroplastic dwarfism, in which the extremities are short but the head and trunk are of normal size. Both ablative lesions of the pituitary and functional disturbances of the hypothalamus are associated with Fröhlich's syndrome, in which marked obesity is associated with gonadal underdevelopment. The condition is rare and affects children.

Adenomas that cause hormonal insufficiency are most often chromophobic, occur in middle life, and become large enough to expand the sella and compress the adjacent fibers of the optic chiasm. Sellar enlargement is noticeable on lateral X-rays of the head, and pressure on the optic chiasm obscures the lateral fields of vision so that bitemporal hemianopsia develops. The relationship of the pituitary stalk to the fibers of the optic chiasm is shown in Figure 20-1. Headache and visual disturbance characterize the early phase of the condition; later hormonal insufficiency becomes evident. The tumors are nodular, encapsulated, and composed of solid sheets of nonstaining (chromophobic) cells that lack anaplasia. Malignant transformation is rare. Basophilic adenomas are small and ordinarily do not deform the sella. Eosinophilic adenomas are reviewed in the next section.

A less frequent primary tumor is the craniopharyngioma. It arises in children, usually before the age of 15, from remnants of Rathke's pouch. It is benign, multicystic, and lies below, within, or above the sella. Both squamous and columnar cells line the cysts, which contain a dark, oily fluid in which cholesterol crystals may be found. Foci of stromal calcification are often so pronounced as to be visible on X-rays of the head. The tumor distorts the sella, compresses the optic tracts, and eventually causes hypopituitarism, manifested by retarded growth, amenorrhea in girls, polyuria from posterior lobe pressure, and obesity from extension to the hypothalamus. The tumor remains localized and is cured by surgical excision.

Because the arterial supply is not sufficient to sustain the pituitary tissue,[2] its lifeline is the portal venous system, which delivers blood from the hypothalamus to the anterior lobe. Interruption of the portal flow thus causes ischemic necrosis of the anterior pituitary. The posterior lobe (neurohypophysis) is less dependent on the portal flow and is only rarely affected. The ensuing hormonal deficiency may be acute or chronic. The former is manifested by pallor and lethargy progressing to coma and death within two weeks after the onset of symptoms. If the patient survives, chronic insufficiency develops slowly over

several years. The clinical aspects are weakness, amenorrhea, loss of pubic and axillary hair, and trophic disturbances of the skin that cause it to become sallow, smooth, and shiny. Both the acute and chronic forms of insufficiency are often due to postpartum hemorrhage with its attendant shock. The pituitary is especially vulnerable at this time because it swells during gestation, the sinusoids are compressed in the bony cage, and the underperfusion associated with shock completes the circulatory impairment. The clinical features are known as Sheehan's syndrome when associated with pregnancy, and otherwise are called Simmonds's disease. The common causes are prolonged shock with underperfusion and chromophobe adenoma with gradual compression. Necrosis of the pituitary from shock is shown in Figure 20-2. Other causes include a wide variety of uncommon lesions such as intrasellar cysts, healed inflammations, gliomas of the hypothalamus, suprasellar meningiomas, and angiomas of the pituitary stalk. The anterior lobe becomes atrophic and scarred with occasional calcification. Hypothyroidism may develop, and atrophy affects the somatic, endocrine, and gonadal organs. Emaciation, however, is not prominent.[3] Pituitary insufficiency is thus associated with symmetrical dwarfism, Fröhlich's syndrome, Sheehan's postpartum necrosis, Simmonds's disease, the common chromophobe adenoma, which affects adults, and the uncommon craniopharyngioma, which affects children.

## Hyperpituitarism

Adenomas of the pituitary are chromophobic, eosinophilic, or basophilic. Their frequency is about 60, 33, and 5 per cent, respectively. Hyperfunction is caused by the eosinophilic adenoma, which secretes growth hormone. When the tumor arises in children before the epiphyses of the long bones have fused, gigantism results. The patients may grow to a height of eight feet,

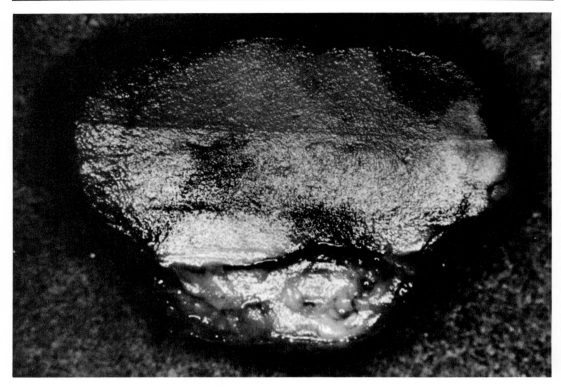

**Figure 20-2.** Widespread necrosis of the pituitary associated with shock and vascular underperfusion

and a corresponding organomegaly develops. When the tumor arises after epiphysial closure, acromegaly arises. In this condition the distal (acral) parts enlarge: nose, mandible, supraorbital ridges, hands, and feet. In addition, a characteristic coarsening of facial features develops over several years. Visceral enlargement also takes place but is not clinically conspicuous. The adenomas form nodular tumors that displace the other cellular elements, distort the sella, and extend out of it to compress the optic chiasm with the gradual development of blindness. The eosinophilic cells are arranged in solid masses without anaplasia or conspicuous stroma. As the tumors become large, hemorrhage, necrosis, and cyst formation tend to develop. The tumors remain localized, however, and may be treated by irradiation or surgical exci-

sion. Occasionally eosinophilic adenomas secrete prolactin, which causes galactorrhea in association with amenorrhea.[4] Electron microscopy has also shown that some adenomas classified as chromophobic by light microscopy are in fact secretory so that hyperpituitarism is occasionally caused by noneosinophilic adenomas.[5]

**The posterior lobe**

The posterior lobe, or neurohypophysis, secretes two hormones: oxytocin and vasopressin. Oxytocin causes the uterus to contract, and vasopressin causes the renal tubular cells to absorb the glomerular filtrate. Vasopressin is therefore also known as antidiuretic hormone. Destruction of the hypothalamus, which initiates the secretion of vasopressin, causes diabetes insipidus, as does destruction of the posterior lobe itself. This condition is rare and is characterized by enormous thirst (polydipsia) and excessive excretion of urine (polyuria). Excretion of 5 to 10 liters of urine per day is not unusual. The specific gravity stays close to 1.002. Patients are not otherwise ill and in most cases suffer only this excretory disturbance. The primary form of the disease is due to idiopathic degeneration of the hypothalamus that initiates the hormone secretion. About half the cases studied by Blotner were due to this cause.[6] The secondary form, caused by actual destruction of the posterior lobe, was due to such lesions as trauma, infection, and metastatic carcinoma in the series of cases studied by Blotner. Vasopressin distinguishes between the pituitary lack and renal disease, which may also be a cause of polyuria; exogenous vasopressin causes the polyuria to cease when the kidneys are normal.

## ADRENALS

The adrenals, which are located at the upper pole of each kidney, are composed of a cortex and a medulla. Each weighs 3 to 5 gm in the adult. The cortex consists of an outer zona glomerulosa, a middle zona fasciculata, and an inner zona reticularis. These zones secrete mineralocorticoids, glucocorticoids, and sex hormones, respectively. Mineralocorticoids (aldosterone) cause the renal tubular cells to conserve sodium and secrete potassium; glucocorticoids (cortisone) suppress the inflammatory and immune responses; and the sex hormones (androgens, estrogens) stimulate development of the secondary sex characteristics. The medulla of each adrenal consists of pheochromocytes, which secrete epinephrine and norepinephrine. Epinephrine causes vasoconstriction and increased cardiac output, while norepinephrine causes vasoconstriction and elevation of blood pressure. Lesions of the adrenals cause too much or too little of these substances to be secreted.

### Hypoadrenalism

Acute cortical insufficiency is extremely uncommon, affects children and young adults, and is due to overwhelming bacteremia, most often with meningococci. Less often the organisms are pneumococci or streptococci. The onset is abrupt with widespread purpura, shock, and circulatory collapse. The clinical course is fulminant, with death occurring six to 24 hours after the onset of symptoms. The condition is known as the Waterhouse-Friderichsen syndrome and should be thought of whenever shock suddenly develops in a patient with septicemia. Bacteria may be seen in smears of the skin hemorrhages and can be cultured from them. Autopsy examination reveals hemorrhagic necrosis of both adrenals, especially the cortical tissue, and petechiae throughout the serosal surfaces elsewhere. Recent thrombi in the capsular and central veins of the adrenals are often seen.[7,8] It is not clear whether the circulatory collapse is due to acute hormonal insufficiency or to overwhelming bacterial toxicity.[9] Recovery is possible if antibiotics and cortical steroids are given in large amounts in the earliest part of the illness.

Chronic cortical insufficiency was described by Addison in 1855. The disease, which bears his name, is uncommon, affects either sex, mostly in middle age, and is manifested by hypotension, weight loss, and intestinal disturbances, including vomiting, diarrhea, and abdominal pain. The patient is languid, indisposed to exertion, and displays a melanotic pigmentation of the skin that is most noticeable over scars, creases, and exposed surfaces. This is due to lack of feedback inhibition so that the pituitary continues to secrete melanocyte-stimulating hormone. The blood sugar is low, as are the serum sodium and chloride, and the urinary excretion of 17-ketosteroids is markedly decreased. The adrenals are reduced to vestiges weighing as little as 1 gm each, and the cortices are largely replaced with fibrous connective tissue.

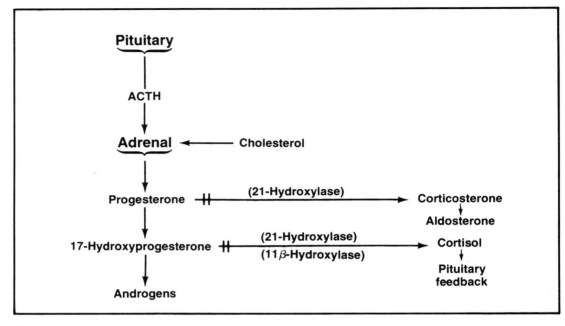

**Figure 20-3.** Metabolic pathways of adrenal steroid production

The cortical destruction was formerly due to caseating tuberculosis but is now more often the result of idiopathic atrophy or, less frequently, due to bilateral histoplasmosis. The atrophy may be an autoimmune reaction, because antibodies to cortical cells are present in over half of patients. Rarely, amyloidosis, hemochromatosis, or metastatic carcinoma is the cause. Health is preserved by corticosteroid replacement therapy. Without treatment, or with inadequate treatment, patients are given to sudden attacks of prostration, circulatory collapse, cyanosis, and pulmonary edema that may be fatal. Such "addisonian crises" are precipitated by minor infections or surgical procedures. Immediate hormonal replacement is required.

### Hyperadrenalism
Three clinical conditions are due to overproduction of adrenocortical hormones: congenital cortical hyperplasia, Conn's syndrome, and Cushing's disease. Congenital cortical hyperplasia is extremely uncommon and is characterized by virilism in children and young adults. It was formerly known as the adrenogenital syndrome. Girls develop hirsutism and a large clitoris. Later there are amenorrhea, small breasts, baldness, and male musculature. In boys the penis is enlarged and pubic hair appears early, but later the normal changes of puberty tend to mask the virilism. The cause is an insufficiency of 21-hydroxylase, which is due to an autosomal recessive mutation. Without enough of this enzyme, normal steroid synthesis is impaired and the raw material of cortisol formation is routed to the overproduction of androgens. These relationships are shown in Figure 20-3. The insufficiency of cortisol prevents feedback to the pituitary so that it overproduces ACTH. There is accordingly an excess of ACTH in the blood and increased excretion of androgens (17-ketosteroids) in the urine. The adrenals may be normal or show cortical thickening. Rarely, cortical carcinoma is the cause of ACTH overproduction. Other enzyme faults of steroid production (11β-hydroxylase, 17-hydroxylase) are less common.

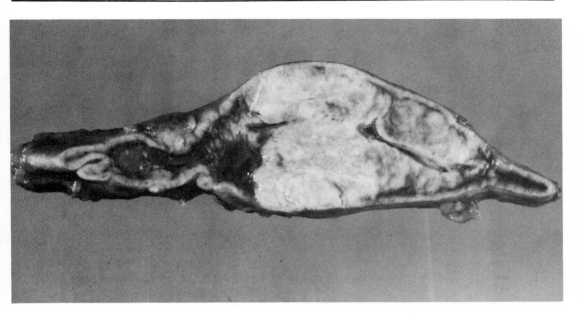

**Figure 20-4.** Adenoma of adrenal cortex

Conn's syndrome is due to overproduction of aldosterone. Over 90 per cent of cases show an adenoma of the cortex (Figure 20-4). The consequences of too much aldosterone are hypertension, tetany, periodic muscle weakness, and excessive thirst and urine formation. The blood contains increased sodium, decreased potassium, and a high level of aldosterone. Removal of the adenoma is curative.

Cushing's disease is due to excess circulating glucocorticoids. It affects middle-aged adults, women three times more often than men, and is characterized by diabetes, central-body obesity, plethora, hypertension, weakness, osteoporosis, and cutaneous striae. Cortisol stimulates the appetite and promotes obesity. It is also diabetogenic so that protein catabolism fuels hyperglycemia through gluconeogenesis. The glucose is converted to fat and deposited in the cheeks and trunk to give the characteristic "moon face," dorsal hump, and central-body obesity. The protein breakdown causes weakness, muscle wasting, osteoporosis, and atrophy of the skin with fra-

gility and purple stria formation. Cortisol also stimulates hemopoiesis and is immunosuppressive so that neutrophilia and polycythemia develop along with lymphopenia, impaired reaction to infections, and delayed healing of wounds. The hypertension may represent an increased sensitivity to catecholamines.[10] A small increase in androgen production is the cause of acne and hirsutism, which complete the syndrome. Diagnosis depends on finding an excess of cortisol in the blood and urine.

The common cause of this syndrome is prolonged use of commercially available glucocorticoids, such as prednisone. The spontaneous syndrome is relatively rare and is due to production of excess cortisol. In 60 per cent of cases the cause is unknown and increased secretion of pituitary ACTH is presumed. In these patients the adrenals show cortical hyperplasia and the pituitary is normal or contains a basophilic microadenoma. In another 25 per cent of cases an adenoma or carcinoma of the adrenal cortex is the cause. In the remaining cases ectopic cortisol is produced by nonpi-

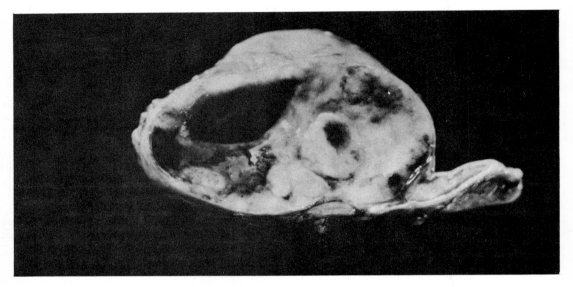

**Figure 20-5.** Cut surface of pheochromocytoma of adrenal medulla. Also shown in color section, p C-8.

**Figure 20-6.** Pheochromocytes above, normal cortical cells below

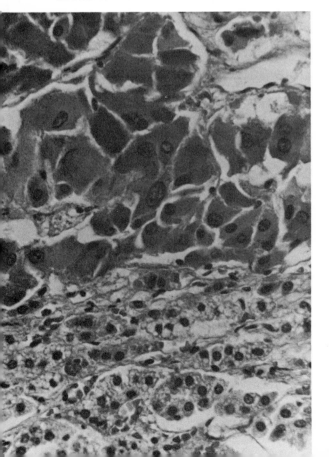

tuitary tumors, especially oat-cell carcinomas of the lung, thymomas, and carcinomas of the pancreas. Therapeutic methods include bilateral adrenalectomy, irradiation of the pituitary, and transsphenoidal microsurgery to remove a basophilic adenoma from the pituitary.[11]

## Medulla

The adrenal medulla originates in cells from the neural crest that differentiate into chromaffin and nonchromaffin tissues.[12] The chromaffin derivative consists of pheochromocytes, meaning cells that stain darkly with chrome salts. Pheochromocytes secrete the catecholamines epinephrine and norepinephrine in regulated amounts and in the approximate ratio of 9:1. Virtually all of the normal adult medulla consists of mature chromaffin tissue. The nonchromaffin derivative consists of neuroblasts, which differentiate into ganglion cells of the autonomic nervous system. Ganglion cells are seen only occasionally in histologic sections. All primary lesions of the medulla are extremely uncommon. In terms of relative frequency, however, the neuroblastoma is common, the pheochromocytoma is uncommon, and the ganglioneuroma is rare.

Pheochromocytomas are soft, brownish-pink, sharply delimited tumors that average 90 gm and show central hemorrhage with frequent cyst formation.[13] A cut surface is shown in Figure 20-5 (see color section, p C-8). Thin slices of tumor immersed in potassium dichromate turn brown in the presence of catecholamines. On microsection the cells are large and polygonal with abundant granular cytoplasm and bizarre nuclei in which there is much variation in size, shape, and density of basophilic staining (Figure 20-6). Mitotic figures, however, are scarce. Although 80 to 90 per cent are benign, metastases may develop, and the presence of tumor in such tissues as lymph nodes, liver, lungs, or bone is the surest distinction between benign and malignant disease; histologic features are not reliable in this regard.[14]

Pheochromocytomas occur in children but more often in adults, especially during the 30- to 50-year age span. The tumor cells relentlessly synthesize, store, and secrete epinephrine and norepinephrine in varying proportions. Hypertension results, but the tumor is so uncommon that less than 0.1 per cent of all high blood pressure can be attributed to this cause.[15] In nearly half of patients the hypertension is sustained. In the rest it is paroxysmal so that the patients experience intermittent attacks of excruciating headache and profuse sweating together with palpitations, trembling, and weakness. Diagnosis rests on the detection of catecholamines or of a derivative, 4-hydroxy-3-methoxymandelic acid (vanillyl-mandelic acid), in the urine. Adrenalectomy is curative.

The neuroblastoma is the most common solid tumor of infancy and childhood. The median age is 2 years, and most occur before the age of 5. The tumors are extremely malignant. They arise from neural crest

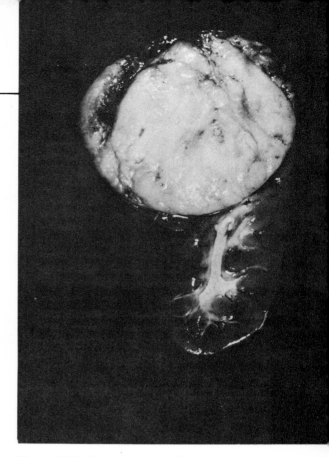

**Figure 20-7.** Neuroblastoma of adrenal medulla impinging on subjacent kidney

remnants in the abdomen (75 per cent), thorax (15 per cent), or pelvis (4 per cent).[16] Half of those in the abdomen are located in the adrenal medulla. The tumors weigh 100 to 200 gm, and the cut surfaces are soft and pale (Figure 20-7). Microsections reveal uniform sheets of small cells in which the nuclei are round, deeply basophilic, and enclosed within a thin rim of barely noticeable cytoplasm. Rosettes often form and neurofibrils may be demonstrated by special stains. Foci of calcification are sometimes visible on X-rays of the abdomen. Seventy-five per cent of patients excrete metabolites of catecholamines in their urine.[17] Rarely, neuroblasts mature into ganglion cells. Metastases are early and widespread. The liver is massively involved so that the abdomen is protuberant, the bone marrow is extensively infiltrated so that myelophthisic anemia develops, and proptosis may occur from extension of the tumor to the orbit. Adrenalectomy is the treatment for localized disease; chemotherapy and radiation, for metastatic spread. The outlook is poor because 70 per cent of tumors have disseminated at the time of diagnosis.[16] The overall survival rate is about 30 per cent two years after diagnosis.

Ganglioneuromas of the adrenal medulla are rare. They arise in young adults and are bulky, firm, and pale gray. Microsections reveal interlacing bands of collagen with interspersed Schwann cells and a scattering of ganglia. The tumors are benign and grow slowly. Excision is curative.

## THYROID

The thyroid consists of two lateral lobes connected by an isthmus. The lobes are symmetrical and the gland normally weighs 25 to 40 gm. The cut surfaces are fleshy and light brownish-red. The individual glands, also known as follicles, are round, uniform in size, and lined by a single layer of cuboidal cells. The lumens are filled with clear, pink colloid. The gland preferentially absorbs iodine from the blood, concentrates it at least 40 times, and incorporates it into thyroxine ($T_4$) and triiodothyronine ($T_3$). The hypothalamus elaborates a releasing factor that causes the pituitary to secrete a thyroid-stimulating hormone, which induces the thyroid to produce its two hormones. These, in turn, monitor pituitary activity through a feedback mechanism. Parafollicular or C cells, which require special stains for identification, are also found in the thyroid; they secrete calcitonin, which lowers the blood calcium and counteracts the effect of parathyroid hormone.

The thyroid originates from a downgrowth of the root of the tongue at a point called the foramen cecum. After it reaches its destination in the neck, no remnants of the downward migration normally remain. When they do persist, such remnants form the thyroglossal duct or cyst, which lies an-

terior to the trachea, measures 1 to 2 cm in diameter, and contains a sticky, pale yellow fluid. Fistulae to the skin may develop. Failure of the thyroid to form at all, which is rare, causes athyrotic cretinism, in which growth is retarded, the head is abnormally large, the eyes are wideset (hypertelorism), and the tongue is large and protruding. Mental development is also impaired.

Acquired diseases of the thyroid may be classified on the basis of function or structure. Functional diseases include the consequences of secreting either too much hormone (hyperthyroidism) or too little hormone (hypothyroidism). Hyperthyroidism is most often due to Graves's disease. It is characterized by increased sensitivity to heat, a tendency to perspire, a ravenous appetite, loss of weight, and easy fatigability. Examination reveals tachycardia, warm, moist skin, and, in slightly more than half of patients, protrusion of the eyes (exophthalmos). The onset of this syndrome is usually gradual but may be abrupt. It occurs four times more often in women than in men, and ordinarily begins in the second to fourth decade. Laboratory confirmation includes an increased metabolic rate, an increased uptake of radioactive iodine, and an elevation of thyroxine and protein-bound iodine in the serum. Without treatment the condition gradually worsens. Physical or emotional stress may induce a sudden excess of hormone so that delirium, hypertension, tachycardia, and high fever suddenly develop. This is the so-called thyroid storm, which, unless controlled, may be fatal. Therapy for hyperthyroidism includes drugs and ablative measures, i.e., thyroidectomy or irradiation.

The gland is symmetrically and only moderately enlarged. The cut surfaces are fleshy and bulging, and microsections reveal columnar enlargement of the lining cells, papillary infolding of the epithelium, reduction of colloid, and vacuolization about the margins of the glands (Figure 20-8). If death occurs, there are also foci of

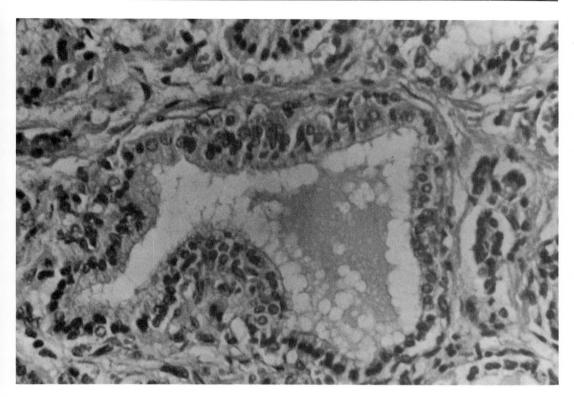

**Figure 20-8.** Thyroid follicle in hyperthyroidism

necrosis in the heart and liver. Such a reaction in myocardium is shown in Figure 20-9. The ocular protrusion is due to edema and slight inflammation of the retro-orbital tissues that push the eyes forward. The exophthalmos may persist even though the hyperthyroidism is well controlled. The cause of the syndrome is attributed to an immunologic disturbance that stimulates the gland to hyperactivity.[18]

Hypothyroidism is due to a deficiency of thyroid hormone. Cretinism is the congenital form, myxedema the acquired form. The causes are insufficiency of dietary iodine for the production of thyroxine, increased need for iodine as encountered in puberty and pregnancy, and goitrogenic drugs (propylthiouracil) or foods (cabbage, turnips). Additional causes include thyroiditis with fibrous replacement, atrophy from old age, replacement with amyloid, abla-

tion by radiation, and removal by surgery. The clinical features are lethargy, malaise, increased fatigability, sensitivity to cold, muscle weakness, and slow mentation. Examination also discloses puffiness of the face, a thick, dry skin, and sparse, coarse hair. Thyroid hormone levels in the blood are low. Cholesterol tends to rise. The tissues reveal interstitial edema in which proteins and mucopolysaccharides are abundant. The heart is dilated and flabby with mucoproteins in the interstitium. Death may be due to ventricular failure.

Structural alterations of the thyroid include enlargement (goiter), inflammations, and tumors. Goiter is usually defined as a thyroid weight that exceeds 40 gm. It often develops in females during puberty or pregnancy. It is not clear whether the enlargement at these times is due to increased metabolic need for thyroid hor-

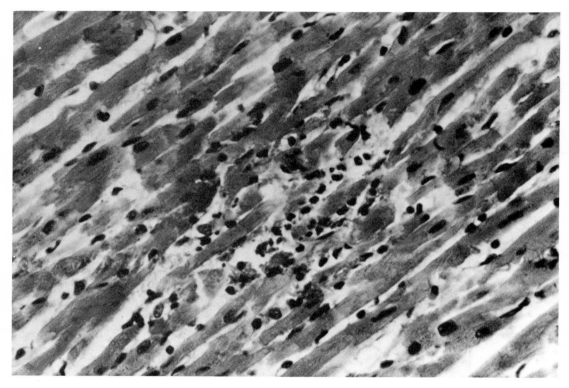

**Figure 20-9.** Focal necrosis of myocardium in hyperthyroidism

mone or to increased production of thyroid-binding globulins. Both reduce thyroxine, decrease feedback notice, and result in oversecretion of thyroid-stimulating hormone by the pituitary. By whichever mechanism, the gland is symmetrically and slightly enlarged so that fullness in the neck is the main manifestation. The follicles are dilated, the lumens are filled with colloid, and the epithelial cells are cuboidal to flat. The condition is self-limited. More important is the nodular colloid goiter, which is large, distorts the neck, and is attributed to cycles of stimulation and involution that affect the tissue unevenly. Goitrogenic foods and drugs block hormone production so that feedback is diminished and too much thyroid-stimulating hormone is secreted. Coarse bands of connective tissue contribute to the nodularity. Pressure symptoms on the trachea, esophagus, and

large vessels are frequent and necessitate surgical removal. A nodule may become "toxic" so that hyperthyroidism develops and, less often, malignant transformation takes place.

The most frequent inflammation of the thyroid is Hashimoto's disease. It is an autoimmune disorder in which antibodies to thyroglobulin as well as to microsomal particles of the epithelial cells are present. The gland is enlarged two to four times, rubbery in consistency, and extensively replaced with lymphocytes that form numerous follicles with large germinal centers. Fibrosis gradually develops so that the cut surface becomes firm and pale yellowish-gray (Figure 20-10). The connective tissue does not bridge the capsule, however, and the gland is not abnormally attached to adjacent structures. Almost all patients are women, the lesion appears at the time of menopause, and the symptoms are those of either hypothyroidism or pressure against adjacent structures.

A second form of thyroiditis is de Quervain's disease, presumably viral in cause, in which the gland reveals granulomatous inflammation. Multinucleated giant cells are numerous and suggest a foreign-body reaction to the colloid of the follicles. Riedel's struma (cast-iron struma) is a rare inflammation characterized by massive fibrosis that replaces the thyroid tissue, extends through the capsule, and binds the gland to adjacent structures in the neck. On this account interference with swallowing and breathing is the main clinical feature. The condition is not an end stage of Hashimoto's disease because it occurs at an earlier time in life and affects the sexes equally. Bacterial thyroiditis with staphylococci and streptococci also occurs; the gland is swollen and tender. Fluctuation indicates abscess formation, and incision and drainage may be required.

The common tumors of the thyroid are adenomas. These are 10 times more frequent in women than in men.[19] They are distinguished from colloid nodules by a uniform internal structure, an intact fibrous capsule, and a different histologic pattern in the tissue outside the capsule. Most are follicular, with colloid-containing small or large glands of approximately uniform size. The descriptive terminology of microfollicular and macrofollicular adenomas has thus arisen. The tumors are single, round, and discrete, and measure 2 to 4 cm in diameter (Figure 20-11). Hemorrhage, fibrosis, and calcification occur. Aside from a cosmetic disturbance, adenomas are significant because they may become "toxic" with the development of hyperthyroidism, or malignant with spreading disease. "Toxic" adenomas are uncommon, and malignancy is rare.[20] Nevertheless, the clinical distinction is aided by the uptake of radioactive iodine: The functional tumor becomes "hot" from uptake of the radioactivity

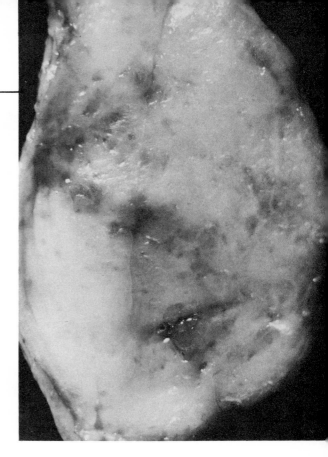

**Figure 20-10.** Widespread fibrosis of thyroid in Hashimoto's disease

whereas the malignant lesion remains "cold" from lack of it. The likelihood that a single thyroid nodule is malignant has been reported to be about 10 per cent.[21] For this reason surgical removal is standard.

Carcinoma of the thyroid is uncommon, causing only six deaths per million per year.[20] Known causes include thyroid-stimulating hormone (TSH) and irradiation. TSH takes a long exposure period, and radiation a long latent period. For example, nodular thyroid disease, not infrequently malignant, was found in 27 per cent of patients given nasopharyngeal irradiation 18 to 25 years previously.[22] The naturally occurring cancers are found in women four times more often than in men, and are often discovered as an incidental lump in the neck. The tumor is pale gray and firm (Figure 20-12). About 40 per cent are papillary, 25 per cent follicular, 25 per cent mixed, and 10 per cent undifferentiated. In one se-

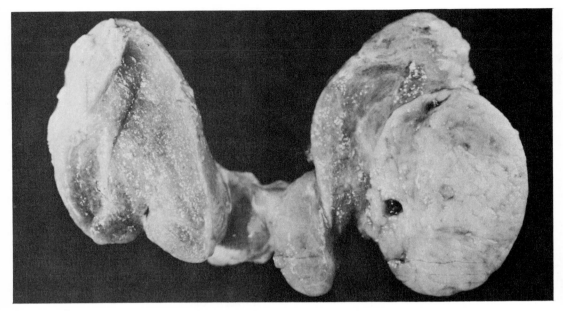

**Figure 20-11.** Cut surface of thyroid showing unilateral discrete adenoma

**Figure 20-12.** Cut surface of carcinoma of thyroid

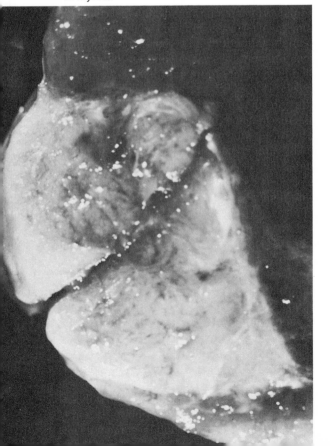

ries of 156 cases, only one medullary carcinoma was found.[23] The papillary cancers grow slowly and are indolent. They arise in the third and fourth decades, remain in the thyroid for a long time, and eventually spread to the nodes of the neck. Total thyroidectomy is often curative, especially in young patients, and the five-year survival rate exceeds 90 per cent.[24] Follicular cancers arise in the fifth decade and, although they grow slowly, tend to metastasize, especially to bone, so that the rate of survival is only about 50 per cent over 10 to 15 years.[20] Undifferentiated carcinomas metastasize early and carry a bleak prognosis.

The medullary cancer is the least frequent and most interesting. It arises from parafollicular (C) cells, secretes calcitonin, and stimulates hyperplasia of the parathyroids from reduction of the blood calcium.[25] It is an undifferentiated tumor with "rivers" of amyloid streaming through the solid masses of tumor cells. It occurs in the third and fourth decades, twice as often in women as in men, and causes a lump in the neck with frequent palpable extension to regional lymph nodes. The cancer is of intermediate malignancy. It occurs sporadically in association with neuromas, especially about the lips and tongue, and less frequently in a familial form in association with parathyroid hyperplasia and pheochromocytomas of the adrenals. The latter combination is known as Sipple's syndrome. The cancer is often present in both lobes of the gland so that total thyroidectomy is recommended. Metastatic carcinoma of the thyroid is seen in about 5 per cent of autopsy series.[20]

## PARATHYROIDS

The four parathyroids are located on the posterior surface of the thyroid, one at each upper and lower pole. They are oval, light yellowish-brown, and less than 0.5 cm in greatest dimension. The main structural unit is the chief cell, which synthesizes and secretes parathyroid hormone. Water-clear and oxyphil cells are derived from chief cells and are present in small numbers. Parathyroid hormone is a polypeptide that regulates serum calcium. When the normal serum calcium value of 9 to 11 mg/dl is exceeded the parathyroids become inactive, and when the serum level is low hyperplasia takes place, the secretion of parathyroid hormone increases, and the blood calcium rises.

Hyperparathyroidism causes an elevated serum calcium, a low serum phosphorus, and an increased excretion of calcium in the urine. The calcium comes from the skeleton by the process of osteoclastic resorption. Osteoporosis gradually develops, and when this becomes advanced, cysts form and the patient is said to have osteitis fibrosa cystica. As the term indicates, the cysts fill with fibrous connective tissue. The condition is also known as von Recklinghausen's disease of bone. The process is symmetrical, bone pain is common, and pathologic fractures may occur, especially in the long bones. In addition, calcium is deposited in

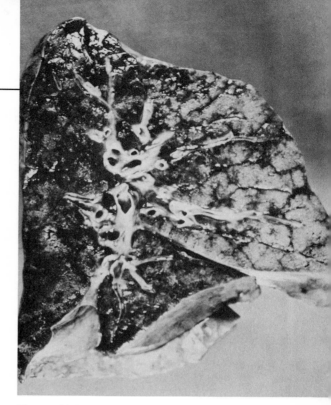

**Figure 20-13.** Extensive metastatic calcification of lung in patient with a parathyroid adenoma

normal tissues (metastatic calcification) whenever the product of the serum calcium and phosphorus in milligrams exceeds the number 75.[26] The tissues affected are the lungs, stomach, and kidneys. In the pulmonary tissue the process may be massive (Figure 20-13). Only minute deposits occur in the gastric mucosa. In the kidneys, however, deposits form in the tubules (nephrocalcinosis) and on the pelvic mucosa (nephrolithiasis). In fact, a stone in the kidney, ureter, or bladder may be the first clinical evidence of hyperparathyroidism.

Primary hyperparathyroidism is autonomous excessive secretion of parathyroid hormone. About 75 per cent of cases are due to a single adenoma of one gland, and 20 per cent to uniform hyperplasia of all four glands.[27] The adenoma is a discrete, encapsulated tumor that compresses the adjoining normal tissue. Adenomas ordinarily measure up to 5 cm in diameter and usually consist of chief cells, although the population may be mixed. Women are af-

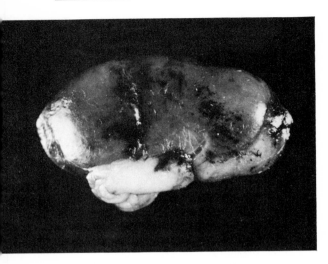

**Figure 20-14.** External surface of parathyroid adenoma. The tumor measures 3.5 × 3.0 × 1.2 cm.

fected more often than men, and the lower glands are affected more than the upper. The lesion is shown in Figure 20-14. The adenoma is not premalignant.

Chief-cell hyperplasia of all four glands is the second main cause of the primary condition. Each gland weighs more than 60 mg, the disturbance is often asymptomatic, and the diagnosis is suggested by a high-calcium, low-phosphorus finding on routine examination of the blood. The cause is not known, although a deficiency of calcitonin has been suggested.[25,28] The distinction between hyperplasia and adenoma may be extremely difficult, especially on frozen section, so that all four glands should be surgically exposed. If only one is enlarged, adenoma is likely, whereas if all four are enlarged, hyperplasia is virtually certain.

Rarely, carcinoma of a parathyroid causes the secretion of too much hormone. Mitoses, vascular invasion, and extension through the capsule distinguish the condition from adenoma.[29] The average weight of the affected gland is 12 gm, and the mean largest diameter is 3 cm. The tumor is not very malignant and is amenable to en-bloc resection.

Secondary hyperparathyroidism is due to low blood calcium regardless of the cause. The most frequent is chronic renal failure, in which phosphorus is retained, the serum calcium falls because of its reciprocal relationship with phosphorus, and the parathyroids respond by hyperplasia with the secretion of increased parathyroid hormone. Infrequently lack of vitamin D, with inability to absorb calcium from the intestine, and, rarely, medullary carcinoma of the thyroid, with increased secretion of calcitonin, are causative. The effects are indistinguishable from those of the primary disturbance. Secondary hyperparathyroidism, however, is more common than the primary process because of the frequency of chronic renal failure.[26]

Hypoparathyroidism causes a low serum calcium, a high serum phosphorus, and tetanic convulsions that resemble epilepsy but do not respond to antiepileptic medications. The condition may be idiopathic but most often is iatrogenic and follows total thyroidectomy.

## REFERENCES

1. Kernohan JW, Sayre GP: *Tumors of the Pituitary Gland and Infundibulum. Atlas of Tumor Pathology*, fasc 36. Washington, DC: Armed Forces Institute of Pathology, 1956

2. Russell DS: Effects of dividing the pituitary stalk in man. *Lancet* 1:466, 1956

3. Sheehan HL: The incidence of postpartum hypopituitarism. *Am J Obstet Gynecol* 68:202, 1954

4. Forbes AP, Henneman PH, Griswold GC, et al: Syndrome characterized by galactorrhea, amenorrhea and low urinary FSH: Comparison with acromegaly and normal lactation. *J Clin Endocrinol Metab* 14:265, 1954

5. Warner NE: Pituitary gland. In *Pathology* (Anderson WAD, Kissane JM, eds), 7th ed, ch 36. St Louis: Mosby, 1977

6. Blotner H: Primary or idiopathic diabetes insipidus: A systemic disease. *Metab (Clin Exp)* 7:191, 1958

7. Fox B: Venous infarction of the adrenal glands. *J Pathol* 119:65, 1976

8. Kaufman G: Adrenal cortical necrosis. An autopsy study. *Arch Pathol* 97:395, 1974

9. Kissane JM: Bacterial diseases. In *Pathology* (Anderson WAD, Kissane JM, eds), 7th ed, ch 9. St Louis: Mosby, 1977

10. McPherson HT: Cushing's syndrome. *Urol Clin North Am* 4:211, 1977

11. Daughaday WH: Cushing's disease and microadenomas of the pituitary. *N Engl J Med* 298:793, 1978

12. Anderson EE: Nonfunctioning tumors of the adrenal gland. *Urol Clin North Am* 4:263, 1977

13. Sherwin RP: Histopathology of pheochromocytoma. *Cancer* 12:861, 1959

14. Gittes RF, Mahoney EM: Pheochromocytoma. *Urol Clin North Am* 4:239, 1977

15. Shoback D: Pheochromocytoma. Clinical conferences at the Johns Hopkins Hospital. *Johns Hopkins Med J* 139:131, 1976

16. Duckett JW, Koop CE: Neuroblastoma. *Urol Clin North Am* 4:285, 1977

17. Maurer HM: Current concepts in cancer. Solid tumors in children. *N Engl J Med* 299:1345, 1978

18. Green WL: Humoral and genetic factors in thyrotoxic Graves disease and neonatal thyrotoxicosis. *JAMA* 235:1449, 1976

19. Wright HK, Burrow GN, Spaulding S, et al: Current therapy of thyroid nodules. *Surg Clin North Am* 54:277, 1974

20. DeGroot LJ: Thyroid carcinoma. *Med Clin North Am* 59:1253, 1975

21. Psarras A, Papadopoulos SN, Livadas D, et al: The single thyroid nodule. *Br J Surg* 59:545, 1972

22. Favus MJ, Schneider AB, Stachura ME, et al: Thyroid cancer occurring as a late consequence of head-and-neck irradiation. Evaluation of 1056 patients. *N Engl J Med* 294:1019, 1976

23. Shields JA, Farringer JL Jr: Thyroid cancer. Twenty-three years' experience at Baptist and St. Thomas hospitals. *Am J Surg* 133:211, 1977

24. Tollefsen HR, DeCosse JJ, Hutter VP: Papillary carcinoma of the thyroid. A clinical and pathological study of 70 fatal cases. *Cancer* 17:1035, 1964

25. Raynor AC, Sowden D: Medullary thyroid carcinoma. *J Surg Oncol* 7:435, 1975

26. Smith JC, Stanton LW, Kramer NC, et al: Nodular pulmonary calcification in renal failure. Report of a case. *Am Rev Respir Dis* 100:723, 1969

27. Kay S: The abnormal parathyroid. *Hum Pathol* 7:127, 1976

28. Haff RC, Black WC, Ballinger WF II: Primary hyperparathyroidism: Changing clinical, surgical and pathological aspects. *Ann Surg* 171:85, 1970

29. Schantz A, Castleman C: Parathyroid carcinoma. A study of 70 cases. *Cancer* 31:600, 1973

# 21

# MUSCULOSKELETAL DISORDERS

The main components of the musculoskeletal system are the bones, joints, muscles, and tendons, and their principal pathologic changes are taken up in that order. The marrow spaces of the bones enclose the erythroid and myeloid tissues, disorders of which are discussed in Chapter 19.

## BONES

All bones arise from connective tissue. In some, such as the head and spine, the transition is direct and is called membranous bone formation. In others, especially the long bones and bridge of the nose, the connective tissue first transforms into cartilage, and it is the cartilage from which the bones then arise. This is known as endochondral bone formation. In both, osteoid is the pale pink protein matrix that is mineralized to produce the mature bone. The long bones consist of an epiphysis, metaphysis, and diaphysis. The epiphysis is covered with cartilage to form the articular surface. The metaphysis is the growth band between the epiphysis and diaphysis. The shaft, or diaphysis, is made up of a solid cortex and a porous center in which bony trabeculae serve as bone struts. Hemopoietic tissue lies between the trabeculae. Osteoclasts, which are multinucleated, resorb or break down bone so that it can be remodeled by osteoblasts, which are mononuclear and form new bone. In this way bones elongate and bodies grow. Throughout life, in response to various stresses, bone is constantly undergoing resorption by osteoclasts and remodeling by osteoblasts. The net balance between these addition-subtraction effects is an increase in the amount of bone during the first five decades of life. After that the amount is reduced at the rate of 5 to 10 per cent per decade.[1]

Skeletal abnormalities include congenital anomalies, inflammations, acquired deficiencies of bone, acquired excesses of bone, and tumors. The main skeletal abnormalities, which are congenital and therefore evident at birth, are achondroplasia, Marfan's syndrome, osteogenesis imperfecta, and osteopetrosis.

## Anomalies

Achondroplasia results from a fault of endochondral ossification. Accordingly, bones that develop through the ossification of cartilage, such as the limbs and bridge of the nose, are selectively stunted. Thus the achondroplastic dwarf is characterized by a head and trunk of normal size attached to limbs that are uniformly short. In addition, the bridge of the nose has a scooped-out appearance. Loose-jointedness is also present so that lumbar lordosis is often pronounced and the buttocks are prominent. The legs bow, and the gait is ducklike. Muscles, however, are well developed, and the men often are employed as midget wrestlers. The genetic fault is transmitted as an autosomal dominant characteristic. Proliferation of the trait is restrained, however, by the difficulty in finding a marital mate and the difficulty of childbirth. Most cases therefore arise as spontaneous mutations in which the parents are normal. Intelligence is within the normal range and the life span has the usual duration.

Marfan's syndrome, described in 1896, is an uncommon condition that is also inherited in an autosomal dominant manner.[2] It is due to a defect of elastic tissue that is manifested mainly by skeletal, ocular, and cardiovascular effects. The skeleton is elongated so that patients are tall and slim, and the extremities, including the fingers, are slender and spider-like (arachnodactyly). Moreover, the tendons are lax and on this account kyphoscoliosis is frequent. In the eyes the suspensory ligament is elongated or broken, and bilateral dislocation of the lenses is the ocular feature. The media of the aorta, composed mainly of elastica, is also weak; dilation with dissecting aneurysm is the main complication. Elastic fibers in the alveoli are also abnormal and emphysema is frequent.[3] Life is moderately shortened and cardiovascular changes are the usual cause of death.

Osteogenesis imperfecta (brittle bones) is a generalized disorder of the connective tissue that prevents the maturation of collagen and formation of bone. It is transmitted as an autosomal dominant characteristic. The bones are thin and extremely fragile, and fractures occur from such trivial motions as turning over in bed. Healing takes place at a normal rate although the callus is often large. The bones of the middle ear are defective and deafness is frequent. The teeth are yellowish-brown from abnormal dentine. The immature connective tissue accounts for the thin, "Wedgwood blue" sclerae, translucent skin, and loose articular support of the back with kyphoscoliosis, weakness of the knees, and bowed legs. The calvaria bulges from poor ossification so that craniofacial disproportion develops: The ears turn outward and downward, and the head continues to enlarge. Patients soon find it difficult to get hats large enough to fit. The triangular face, outward-pointing ears, blue sclerae, deafness, thin skin, kyphosis, and short, bowed legs with a scissor gait give an unmistakable appearance that is diagnostic. Transmission of the trait is limited because these individuals frequently die from collapse of the skull during the process of birth. Patients who reach adulthood face a lifetime of deformity and severely restricted activity.

In 1904 Heinrich Ernst Albers-Schön-berg described a condition that bears his name and is also known as marble bone disease.[4] It has also been called osteopetrosis, although osteosclerosis is said to be the correct term.[2] It is due to excessive bone formation that obliterates the marrow cavities, causing anemia, and squeezes the nerve foramina of the skull, causing visual and hearing disorders. Although the bones are thick, they are structurally weak and fractures are frequent. In the autosomal recessive form the condition is severe, infants are affected, and death occurs in early life from anemia and infection. In the autosomal dominant form the condition is mild, adults are affected, and longevity is normal. The basic defect appears to be an abnormality of osteoclasts that causes faulty resorption of forming bone.[5]

## Infection

An important acquired disease of bone is infection or osteomyelitis. Bacteria reach the bone through puncture wounds, extension from adjacent soft tissues, or hematogenous spread from a distant site. The usual organism is the hemolytic *Staphylococcus aureus*, less often pneumococci or streptococci. Gram-negative bacteria have been common in cases caused by drug injections with unsterile equipment.[6] The most frequent sites in children are the tibia, femur, and phalanges.[7] Patients experience fever and pain of sudden onset that is aggravated by motion. Physical signs include redness, swelling, and tenderness. A suppurative exudate forms in the metaphysis, erodes the trabecular bone, and leaves necrotic fragments (sequestra) that cause the reaction to persist. Erosion also extends through cartilage into joint spaces, and through cortical bone to form sinuses that spread along fascial planes and drain onto the skin. In children bone growth is retarded by destruction of the metaphysial cartilage so that the extremities tend to form asymmetrically. The most disabling compli-

cation is dislocation of the femoral head after it has been destroyed by the inflammatory process. Surgical evacuation of the exudate and the use of antibiotics are methods of treatment. Brodie's abscess is a circumscribed focus of osteomyelitis in a single bone, usually the tibia or femur, that is frequently not attended by a history of trauma or infection. The exudate is often sterile, the lesion tends to be clinically silent, and it is often discovered on routine X-ray examination.[8]

Much less frequent is tuberculosis, which arises from pulmonary disease, often affects the spine, and tends to form fistulae that open onto the skin of the groin after following the fascial sheath of the psoas muscle. Thus the fluctuant mass on the upper inner thigh that perforates the skin to form a draining sinus is known as a psoas abscess. An example of vertebral tuberculosis, or Pott's disease, is illustrated in Figure 21-1 (see color section, p C-9). The centrum may collapse with sharp angulation of the spine so that a gibbus (hump) forms, the spinal cord is crushed, and paralysis or paraplegia results. Syphilis of bone usually takes the form of periostitis but is now a rare condition in any form. However, a case of osteomyelitis of the clavicle due to syphilis in the secondary stage was reported as recently as 1976.[9]

## Bone deficiency

Primary bone deficiency includes osteoporosis, osteomalacia, hyperparathyroidism, renal rickets, aseptic necrosis, and fibrous dysplasia. Secondary bone deficiency is due to metastatic tumor, hyperactive myeloid marrow, as in leukemia, hyperactive erythroid marrow, as in congenital anemia, infiltrations, as in myeloma, and storage disorders, such as Gaucher's disease, in which the marrow becomes clogged with macrophages. Only the primary deficiencies are considered here.

Osteoporosis is atrophy of bone with a normal ratio of mineralized portion to un-

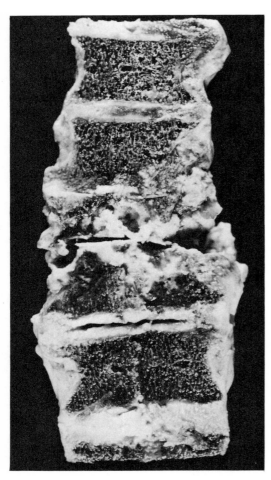

**Figure 21-1.** Pott's disease (tuberculosis) of the spine. Also shown in color section, p C-9.

phosphatase are normal. The cause is unknown although disuse, an endocrine disturbance, or a dietary lack of calcium may play a role.[1] The importance of disuse is exemplified by the astronauts, who develop osteoporosis in the weightlessness of space unless they perform exercises to counteract the effect. The condition is also seen locally when disuse is occasioned by paralysis of a body part or immobilization of a limb in a cast. Endocrine disorders that increase bone resorption and hence cause osteoporosis include hyperparathyroidism, thyrotoxicosis, Cushing's disease, and the complications of long-term glucocorticoid therapy.[11] Treatment is aimed at suppressing bone resorption by use of such agents as calcitonin, anabolic steroids, estrogens, and sodium fluoride.[12]

Osteomalacia, or bone softening, is impaired mineralization of the skeleton with accumulation of unmineralized matrix (osteoid) that covers the bone surfaces. It is due to the unavailability of calcium and phosphorus. As a result the bones soften and bend into deformities rather than turn brittle and separate into fractures. The causes include lack of calcium in the diet, lack of vitamin D, which controls calcium absorption (juvenile rickets), failure to absorb calcium because of intestinal disease (cystic fibrosis, sprue, biliary cirrhosis, regional enteritis), and renal disease with a phosphate leak that lowers serum phosphorus and causes secondary hyperparathyroidism (renal rickets). Phosphate-binding antacids also depress the serum phosphorus level and stimulate parathyroid activity.[13] Regardless of the cause of osteomalacia, patients develop weakness, pain, and disability. The spine and femoral neck are mainly affected. The serum calcium and phosphorus are usually low, but their levels vary with the cause of depletion. Although it is radiographically difficult to distinguish osteomalacia from osteoporosis, biopsy reveals thick mantles of osteoid that surround the sparse trabeculae. Treatment

mineralized matrix (osteoid). The mechanism appears to be an excess of bone resorption over bone formation.[10] The condition is almost universal in the elderly and frequent in postmenopausal women. It develops slowly and eventually causes chronic pain or sudden fracture. The bones become thin, brittle, and porous (Figure 21-2). The spine and femoral neck are most often affected so that a dorsal hump gradually develops, height diminishes, and fractures, especially of the hip, become frequent. The serum calcium, phosphorus, and alkaline

depends on the cause, but hinges mainly on dietary supplements of vitamin D.

Primary hyperparathyroidism is usually due to a single adenoma of one gland that secretes excess parathyroid hormone.[14] The hormone activates osteoclasts in the bone and increases the excretion of phosphates in the urine.[1] The osteoclasts erode bone, and after a long period of osteoporosis local cystic lesions develop. These fill with connective tissue that is brown from old hemorrhage ("brown tumors"). The cystlike rarefactions arise mainly in the mandible, spine, and femoral neck. As the bone is eroded, hypercalcemia develops and calcium spills into the urine. The renal effect causes urinary excretion of phosphates. In this way cystic lesions appear in the bone and calcium phosphate stones form in the kidneys. The high serum calcium also causes lethargy, weakness, and weight loss as well as metastatic calcification, especially in the lungs (Figure 21-3). This combination of symptomatic and structural changes is known as osteitis fibrosa cystica. It is also named von Recklinghausen's disease of bone. The chemical features are a high serum calcium, low serum phosphorus, and an increase of both radicals in the urine. The circulating parathyroid hormone is measurable by radioimmunoassay. Surgical removal of the adenoma gradually restores the bone to normal.

Aseptic necrosis, or infarct, of bone affects mainly the spine and femoral heads in adults. The blood supply, especially to the head of the femur, is interrupted by fracture or dislocation that severs the ligamentum teres, in which the nutrient artery runs. Less easily explained is the process following hyperbarism[15] or corticosteroid therapy.[16] In children the process is idiopathic and causes pain, limping, and limitation of movement. Terminology varies with the site affected: Osgood-Schlatter disease for the tibial tubercle, Legg-Calvé-Perthes disease for the head of the femur, and Köhler's disease for the navicular bone of

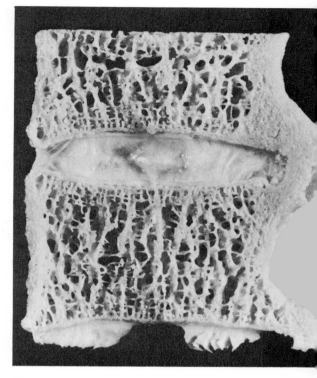

**Figure 21-2.** Osteoporosis of spine. Notice that the anterior spinal ligament is calcified across the intervertebral gap.

the foot. In both adults and children the condition may heal or progress to chronic osteoarthritis.[1]

Aneurysmal bone cysts occur in children and young adults as solitary lesions in any part of the skeleton. They cause pain and swelling. They measure 5 to 8 cm in diameter and give a characteristic multilocular X-ray appearance from delicate septa that divide the chamber. The lumen is filled with liquid blood, and although the cause is not known, an arteriovenous fistula with pressure erosion of bone has been suggested.[17] Therapy consists of curettage. The rate of recurrence is 20 to 40 per cent.

**Bone excess**

Two conditions stand out as examples of primary bone excess: Paget's disease and

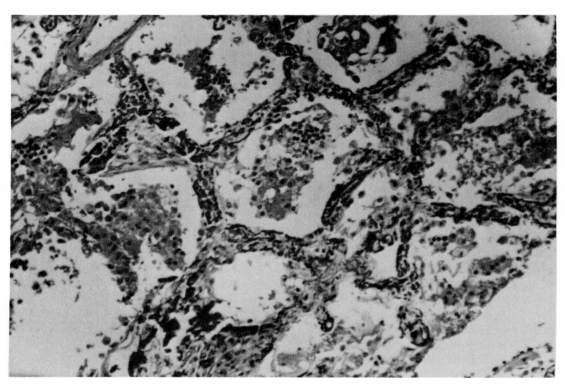

**Figure 21-3.** Metastatic calcification of the lung. The black streaks in the alveolar walls are calcium.

hypertrophic pulmonary osteoarthropathy. In 1877 Paget described osteitis deformans. It is an uncommon condition that arises after the age of 40, twice as often in men as in women, and usually affects the skull, spine, pelvis, or long bones. The process consists of an increased rate of resorption as well as excessive new bone formation, chiefly periosteal, so that over a long period the bone becomes thick, soft, and deformed. Dull pains and gradual enlargement of the affected parts are the clinical aspects. Microscopically the cortical bone reveals an irregular mosaic pattern of cement lines, and the marrow cavities fill with fibrous tissue that is highly vascular. Vascularization of the marrow cavities has the effect of an arteriovenous fistula so that high-output failure of the right ventricle may develop. The serum calcium and phos-

phorus are normal but the alkaline phosphatase is extremely high. The cause of Paget's disease of bone is not known, although viral particles have been described in the osteoclasts of the affected parts.[18] There is no specific treatment for this condition. About 3 per cent of patients subsequently develop osteosarcoma.

Hypertrophic pulmonary osteoarthropathy is the syndrome of clubbed fingers, arthralgias, and periostitis of the long bones that is associated with pulmonary disease. Eighty per cent are due to pulmonary infections or bronchogenic carcinomas, and 10 per cent are associated with sarcomas of the pleura. In children the common cause is cyanotic congenital heart disease. The pathogenesis is unknown, but a neural reflex may stimulate peripheral hypervascularity, which causes the clubbing; transection of the vagus is followed by disappearance of the condition.[19]

## Tumors of bone and cartilage

Tumors of the skeleton arise from bone, cartilage, and marrow. The types and approximate proportions as reported in the large series of Dahlin[20] are shown in Table 21-1. All but a few of the marrow tumors were myelomas, reviewed in Chapter 19.

Tumors of cartilage are benign (chondromas) or malignant (chondrosarcomas). The ratio is approximately 8:5. The most common benign tumor of the skeleton is the bony exostosis or osteochondroma. These result from growth of aberrant foci of cartilage on the surface of the bone.[20] Over 90 per cent are solitary, they tend to occur at the ends of long bones, where tendons insert, and they arise for the most part between 10 and 30 years of age. A slowly enlarging, palpable tumor is produced. Local excision is curative. Chondrosarcomas arise de novo, mainly in middle life, especially from the spine, ribs, and long bones. Pain and swelling are the clinical manifestations, evolution is slow, metastases are late, and wide excision is ordinarily curative. Histologic distinction from the benign chondroma may be difficult.

The benign tumor of bone is the osteoid osteoma, and the malignant tumor is the osteosarcoma. The ratio of incidence of these is about 1:6. Osteoid osteomas occur before the age of 25, three times more often in men than in women, and predominantly in the long bones. The tumors are single and rarely over 2 cm in diameter. The distinctive feature is a central nidus of osteoid surrounded by a peripheral rim of sclerotic bone. The osteoid is radiolucent on X-ray examination, and this is a material aid to the diagnosis. En-bloc surgical excision achieves cure.

The most common primary malignant tumor of bone, next to myeloma, is the osteosarcoma, formerly known as osteogenic sarcoma.[20] The tumor contains osteoid as the central element with varying proportions of other components so that osteoblastic, chondroblastic, and fibroblastic types exist. The tumor infrequently arises in Paget's disease and occasionally occurs after irradiation of bone. The peak incidence is in the second decade, the metaphysial part of the long bones is the site of predilection, and 60 per cent occur in the region of the knee. Pain, swelling, and a palpable mass are the clinical manifestations. X-rays reveal a mixture of lytic and sclerotic changes with destruction of cortex and extension into the adjacent soft tissues. Grossly the tumors are soft with irregular foci of calcification (Figure 21-4). Microsections reveal pronounced anaplasia. Metastases are early, especially in the lungs. The lymph nodes are seldom involved. The tumor is radioresistant and amputation is ordinarily required.[21] Other modalities, including irradiation, chemotherapy, and immunologic manipulations, are still under study. The five-year survival rate for patients who have undergone treatment is about 20 per cent.[20]

The main neoplasms of unknown origin are the giant-cell tumor, which is benign, and Ewing's sarcoma, which is explosively malignant. Giant-cell tumors have a peak incidence in the third decade, most are found in the epiphyses of the long bones,

### Table 21-1.

## Primary tumors of the skeleton

| Site | Incidence |
|------|-----------|
| Marrow (myelomas) | 40% |
| Cartilage | 21% |
| Bone | 19% |
| Fibrous tissue | 4% |
| Notochord | 3% |
| Unknown | 10% |

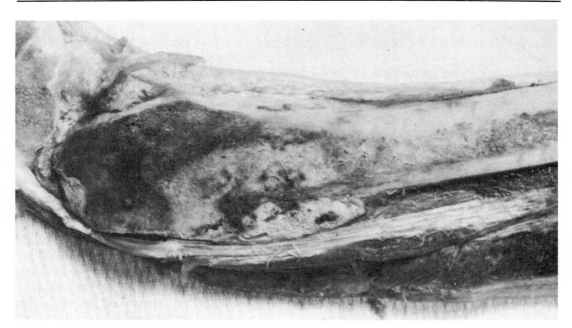

**Figure 21-4.** Osteosarcoma of upper portion of tibia

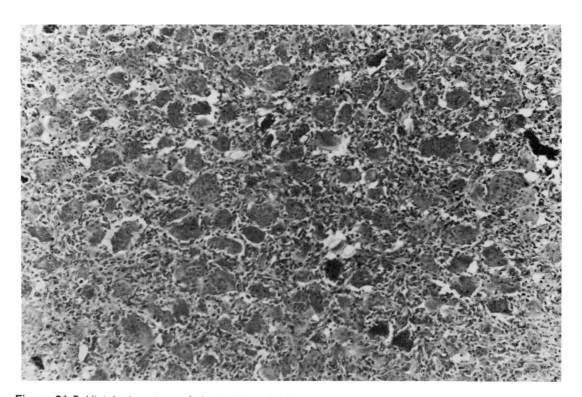

**Figure 21-5.** Histologic pattern of giant-cell tumor of bone

and more than half occur about the knee. Pain, swelling, and a palpable mass are the clinical features. X-rays reveal a focus of radiolucence without a sclerotic margin. Grossly the tumor is soft and red with invariable extension to the articular surface. The presence of giant cells (Figure 21-5) is necessary for the diagnosis but is not unique to the tumor. Removal by curettage is often followed by recurrence so that total resection is preferred. Malignant transformation is uncommon, e.g., 20/264 cases in the series of Dahlin.[20]

Ewing's tumor is a small round-cell sarcoma of uncertain origin that arises in the medullary cavity, mainly in the second decade, and affects any part of the skeleton, with two-thirds being found in the pelvic bones and lower extremities. Pain, swelling, and a tender mass with dilated veins in the overlying skin are the clinical manifestations. Lytic destruction of cortical bone with a laminated elevation of the overlying periosteum is the characteristic radiographic finding. Grossly the tumor is soft, pale gray, and succulent. The histologic nature is shown in Figure 21-6. Widespread metastasis to lungs and other bones is frequent. Amputation and irradiation are both used in therapy. The outlook, however, is guarded; the five-year survival rate in Dahlin's experience was only 16.2 per cent.[20]

Infrequent tumors of bone include the fibroma and chordoma. Fibromas occur almost exclusively in children or adolescents, mainly in the metaphyses and especially in the long bones of the legs. The lesion is usually asymptomatic and comes to attention as an incidental finding. The X-ray characteristic is multilocular radiolucence due to bony trabeculae that extend across the lesion. Microsections reveal connective tissue traversed by calcified trabeculae. Therapy is not necessary as long as the di-

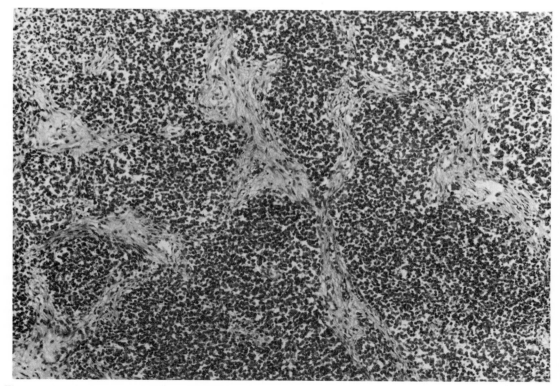

**Figure 21-6.** Histologic structure of Ewing's tumor of bone

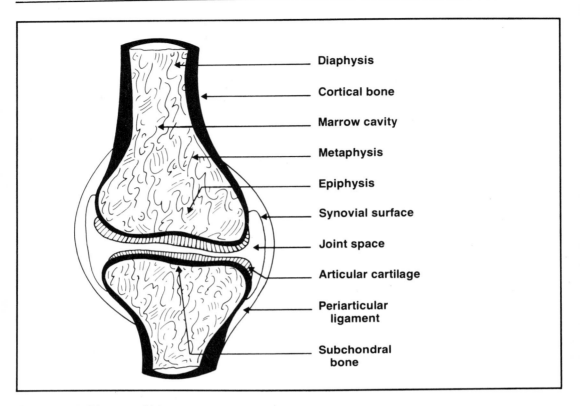

**Figure 21-7.** Diagram of joint structure

agnosis is certain and the function of the bone is not impaired.

Chordomas arise from remnants of the notochord and occur mainly at the base of the brain (spheno-occipital) or spine (sacro-coccygeal). The tumor arises after the age of 30 and causes chronic pain. Tumors of the sacrum and coccyx may be felt by rectal examination. Destruction of bone is seen on X-ray, the tumor is soft and translucent, and microsections reveal solid masses of large, pale cells containing "bubbles" of mucoid droplets. Although the tumor invades slowly and metastasizes late, radical excision is required for cure.

### JOINTS

The joints are three in kind: fibrous (skull), cartilaginous (spine), and synovial (knee).

Only synovial joints are freely movable (Figure 21-7). Arthritis is inflammation of these structures. The main kinds are bacterial, rheumatoid, and degenerative.

Bacterial arthritis usually follows septicemia. The organisms lodge in the synovial tissue, an exudate forms in the synovial fluid, and the joint becomes swollen, red, warm, and painful. The usual bacteria are staphylococci, streptococci, pneumococci, and gonococci. Although septic arthritis occurs uncommonly in pneumococcal septicemia, it occurs in 80 per cent of patients with gonococcal septicemia. Moreover, gonococcal arthritis usually involves more than one joint. A special predisposition of the organism for synovial tissue is thus suggested.[22] In the joint space granulation tissue forms, abscesses develop in the synovium, and lysis of cartilage takes place with erosion of subchondral bone. The bacteria may be cultured from the joint fluid. Early diagnosis, prompt arthrocentesis, and appropriate antibiotics constitute proper treatment. About 1 per cent of patients with tuberculosis have tuberculous arthritis; in half of these the spine is affected, in one-third the hips or knees, and in the remainder the disease is scattered. The condition begins as a subchondral abscess that erodes into the joint space. Culture of the joint fluid reveals the organism, and cure is possible with chemotherapy alone.[22] Mycotic infections of joints are rare.

More common is rheumatoid arthritis, which affects 1 to 5 per cent of the American public, depending on the criteria of diagnosis.[1] It is a disease of adults, twice as frequent in women as in men, that begins gradually with fatigue, anemia, and slight fever followed by morning stiffness of the proximal interphalangeal joints. Polyarticular involvement of large joints then develops and tends to be symmetrical. The joints are swollen and painful. The course is intermittent. In a few cases remission is permanent, and in about 10 per cent of patients the disease progresses to an incapacitating stage. At the onset the synovium is infiltrated with lymphocytes and plasma cells, granulation tissue then forms, and a thick pannus (fibrous covering) develops. The pannus burrows into the subchondral bone, and fibrous adhesions limit joint motion. Fragments of necrotic synovium float in the joint fluid to form the so-called rice bodies. The inflammation spreads to the capsular ligaments, which become weak and allow subluxation. This occurs especially in the metacarpophalangeal joints, with a characteristic ulnar deviation of the fingers. With time adhesions seal the joint space and calcification of the fibrous tissue produces bony ankylosis.

The disease process is not limited to joints; granulomas arise in the skin, lungs, and heart, and pericarditis develops but tends to be clinically silent. The granulo-

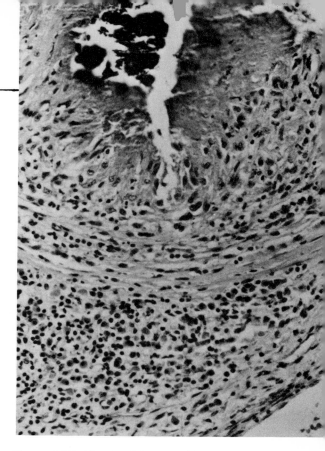

**Figure 21-8.** Margin of rheumatoid granuloma

mas consist of central necrosis with marginal palisading of fibroblasts that are lightly infiltrated with lymphocytes. Such a lesion in the myocardium is shown in Figure 21-8. In the subcutaneous tissue the granulomas often form over the extensor surfaces of the forearms, measure 0.5 to 2.0 cm in diameter, and frequently persist indefinitely. They are painless and are found in about 25 per cent of patients.[22]

The serum in rheumatoid arthritis may contain an abnormal globulin that acts as an antigen and reacts with normal IgG. The abnormal globulin is known as the rheumatoid factor and is present in 70 per cent of patients. It is nonspecific, however, being absent in 30 per cent and also occurring in nonarthritic diseases. The diagnosis of rheumatoid arthritis is thus imprecise; it is based on the characteristic joint changes, subcutaneous nodules, and rheumatoid factor. Although the cause of this common dis-

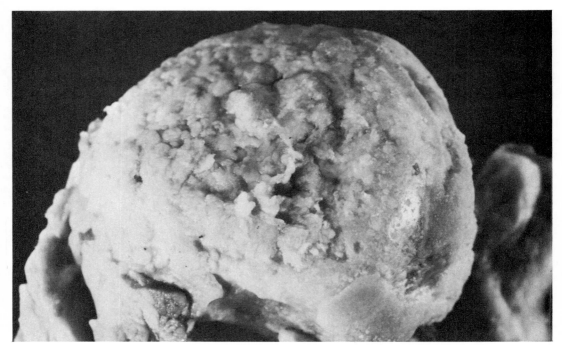

**Figure 21-9.** Fragmented articular surface of head of femur in osteoarthritis. Also shown in color section, p C-9.

ease is unknown, prominent possibilities include an immune disorder of unknown kind that causes a joint component to become antigenic, or an infectious process with an agent such as *Mycoplasma* that is difficult to culture.[1]

When rheumatoid arthritis occurs in children, usually in the 9- to 12-year age group, it is known as Still's disease. Fewer joints are affected, and tests for the rheumatoid factor are negative. Otherwise it resembles the adult condition. The joint disease of rheumatic fever bears no relationship to rheumatoid arthritis.

The most common disorder of joints is osteoarthritis. Although the term indicates inflammation, it is degenerative in nature and leukocytes play no part in the reaction. It affects 40 million American adults, most of whom are asymptomatic. It is a slowly progressive disorder that occurs late in life, affects the weight-bearing joints, and

causes pain on motion, stiffness at rest, and—it is claimed—aching during inclement weather. Later, limitation of motion develops and deformity follows. It is especially common in the spine, hips, and knees. In the knees the smooth articular surfaces become frayed and fragmented, portions break off to become "joint mice," and spurs of new bone (osteophytes) form at the margins of joints and the attachments of tendons. A fragmented articular surface is shown in Figure 21-9 (see color section, p C-9). When bared by this process, the subchondral bone becomes dense and smooth (eburnated). In the spine, new bone formation causes "lipping" around the rims of the vertebral bodies, fusion may take place, and motion is further limited. It is most common in the lumbar portion. An attendant deformity is Heberden's nodes—thickening of the distal interphalangeal joints that is more frequent in women than in men and tends to occur in families. The cause of osteoarthritis is unknown although preceding trauma is frequent, as in the knees of football players, the wrists of jackhammer operators, and the shoulders of baseball pitchers. Joints previously affected by aseptic necrosis are also vulnerable. Beyond this, speculations include an enzyme released by trauma that may digest the cartilage, chondrocytes that are abnormal and cannot maintain the cartilage matrix, and inadequate nutrition of the joint space.[23] The course is slowly progressive. There is no specific treatment.

The intervertebral discs are the shock absorbers of the spine. They are composed of a soft central nucleus pulposus and a peripheral band of dense connective tissue known as the anulus fibrosus. Degenerative changes cause the intervertebral discs to collapse, and this is one of the main causes of short stature in old age. Under pressure the degenerated disc may also herniate through a defect in the anulus fibrosus (Figure 21-10). The extrusion impinges on a spinal nerve root, indents the dura of the spinal cord, and can be located by injecting a contrast medium into the spinal fluid (myelography). The leg pain or sciatica caused by this herniation may be relieved by surgical removal of the extruded portion of the disc. Herniation of the nucleus into the body of the adjacent centrum produces a defect visible by radiographs that is known as a Schmorl nodule. It is usually asymptomatic.

Less often the anterior spinal ligament calcifies to cause ankylosing spondylitis or "poker spine" (Figure 21-2). The condition, also known as Marie-Strümpell disease, affects young men, progresses gradually, and causes a pronounced flexion deformity (kyphosis) so that the patient cannot stand upright. The cause is unknown. Serologic tests for rheumatoid factor are negative, subcutaneous nodules do not form, and the condition is said to be unrelated to rheumatoid arthritis.[1]

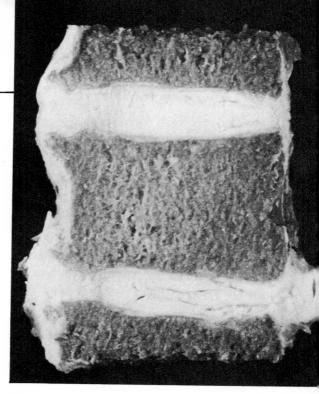

**Figure 21-10.** Cut surface of spine showing herniated intervertebral disc

## Gout

Gout is a hereditary disorder of uncertain genetic transmission that affects chiefly men, begins after the age of 30, and pursues an intermittent course of long duration. It is characterized by hyperuricemia, arthritis, and deposition of urate crystals in joints and connective tissue. The accumulated uric acid precipitates in synovial tissue as monosodium urate crystals, which break into the joint fluid. The crystals are avidly phagocytized, the phagocytes succumb to their own lysosomal enzymes, and the liberated enzymes, chiefly hydrolases, incite an acute exudative synovitis.[24] Ordinarily only one joint is affected—usually the first metatarsophalangeal articulation of either foot. Occasionally the ankle, knee, wrist, or elbow is first affected. The joint fluid contains exudate and yellow, needle-shaped urate crystals, which establish the diagnosis.[25] The joint becomes hot, red, swollen, and so exquisitely tender that the weight of a bed sheet causes excruciating pain. Colchicine relieves the pain of the acute attack but does not change the serum level of uric acid. Without treatment the acute reaction subsides over days to weeks and leaves no residual change. Recurrence after some months is the usual course.

Gradually the acute reaction gives way to chronic tophaceous gout, in which sheaves of urate crystals accumulate in the skin of the ears, periarticular tissue of the fingers and toes, and bones, where punched-out defects adjacent to involved joints are characteristic. In the periarticular tissues the tophi slowly become large and disfiguring. A chronic granulomatous reaction develops, and the overlying skin occasionally ulcerates to discharge the gray, pasty, chalklike crystals. Tophi also form in the kidneys, and involvement of the tubules causes obstruction followed by infection, loss of function, and hypertension. Between 10 and 20 per cent of patients with chronic tophaceous gout develop uric acid calculi in the urinary tract.

Uric acid is derived from purines in the nuclei of cells in the diet and cells of the body, the latter through the normal process of necrobiosis. In gout an inborn error of metabolism causes uric acid to accumulate, either by excessive biosynthesis or by reduced excretion after normal synthesis. The former patients, who constitute 30 per cent of the total, are known as overproducers, while the rest are known as normoproducers. Either way, hyperuricemia is constant. The excretion of uric acid in the urine is normally 420 mg/day. The rest is excreted in the stool (about 330 mg), where it is degraded by bacteria.[26] Urinary excretion of more than 600 mg/day distinguishes overproducers from normoproducers. This distinction is important because agents that suppress uric acid production (allopurinol) are effective for overproducers and agents that increase urinary excretion by blocking tubular reabsorption (probenecid) are effective for normoproducers.[27] The life span of patients is not especially shortened, although the joint disfiguration is an enduring handicap.

Persons with normal metabolism may develop secondary gout from diseases of high cell turnover with the release of nucleotides from which uric acid is formed (for example, tumors, psoriasis, hemolytic anemia, myeloproliferative disorders) and from treatment with cytotoxic drugs, which have the same effect.

### Synovioma

Synoviomas are uncommon malignant tumors of mesenchymal origin that arise in periarticular connective tissue, usually of the lower extremities and most often about the knee. The mean age of patients is 33 years, pain is the most frequent complaint, and the tumors are single and measure 7 to 10 cm in greatest dimension.[28] The cut surfaces are soft and pale gray with occasional grittiness from microdeposits of calcium. The histologic appearance is distinctive (Figure 21-11). The tissue pattern is not constant, however, and varies from a spindle-cell sarcoma resemblance to an adenocarcinomatous appearance. The tumor invades the joint space, extends into adjacent bone, and metastasizes to the lungs and regional lymph nodes. Amputation is the treatment of choice. In the series of Cadman and colleagues 25 per cent survived for five years.[28]

### MUSCLE

Diseases of muscle may be primary or secondary. The main primary diseases are myositis ossificans, the muscle dystrophies, the glycogen storage diseases, polymyositis, and myasthenia gravis. Other primary diseases are too uncommon for the scope of this work. Reference to them may be found in the text of Adams.[29]

The secondary diseases of skeletal muscle are much more common than primary diseases and include denervation atrophy, in which the neural impulse is obstructed by disease of the brain, spinal cord, or peripheral nerves. Cerebral infarction, polio-

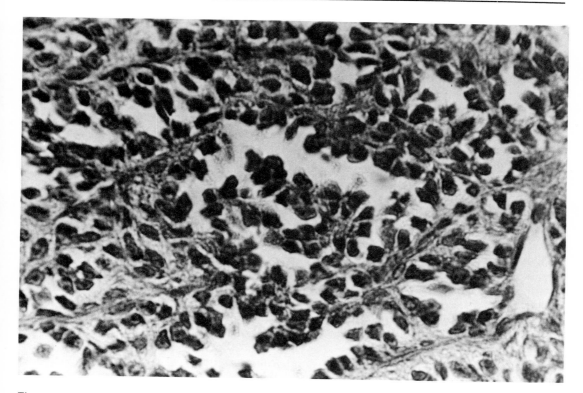

**Figure 21-11.** Histologic pattern of synovioma

myelitis, and traumatic transection of the spinal cord are examples. Systemic conditions affecting skeletal muscle also cause secondary disorders of this tissue. For example, in sarcoidosis noncaseating granulomas form in the myofibrils and biopsy may be diagnostic. In febrile diseases associated with dehydration, especially typhoid fever, Zenker's hyaline degeneration occurs in skeletal muscle, most often the rectus abdominis. In trichinosis, caused by the ingestion of undercooked meat, the nematode *Trichinella spiralis* encysts in skeletal muscle. The condition is now infrequent in the United States because of effective meat inspection. In soiled wounds clostridial organisms cause gas gangrene with the production of crepitant gas and an acute necrotizing myositis. In polyarteritis skeletal muscle is often affected, and biopsy may establish the diagnosis. Both metastatic

disease and primary tumors in skeletal muscle are rare.

## Myositis ossificans

Myositis ossificans is a hereditary disorder that affects children and is characterized by two developmental faults: microdactyly and ossification of connective tissues related to skeletal muscles, i.e., tendons, ligaments, fasciae, and aponeuroses. The term "interstitial ossifying myositis" has been recommended because the primary involvement is of connective tissue.[2] The condition is due to a rare, sporadic dominant mutation with an irregular penetrance. The affected tissues swell, become firm, and gradually turn into hard, bony lumps. Any muscles except those of the tongue, heart, larynx, and diaphragm may be affected and, as the disease progresses, widespread involvement develops. The joint capsules and spine are also involved so that motion gradually becomes limited. Histologic sections reveal inflammation followed by fibrosis, osteoid formation, and finally ossification. The osteoid may be so cellular as to resemble osteosarcoma.[30] Involvement of the intercostal muscles affects breathing, and respiratory failure is the usual cause of death.

### Muscular dystrophy

The muscle dystrophies are degenerative conditions characterized by familial occurrence and symmetrical involvement.[29] Five main kinds are distinguished by incidence and muscle groups involved. The most common is the pseudohypertrophic muscular dystrophy of Duchenne, which begins before the age of 6 years and affects primarily the pelvic and shoulder girdle muscles. The initial clinical feature is a disinclination to walk or run. The condition is due to a sex-linked recessive mutation so that it is carried by females and expressed by males. The muscles become infiltrated with lipid, which causes them to enlarge, and then go on to atrophy. The myocardium may also be affected. The limbs become flaccid and loose, the course is slowly progressive, and death ordinarily occurs before the age of 20. Other clinical types are uncommon or rare and are expressed as autosomal traits that may be recessive or dominant. They include the facioscapulohumeral dystrophy of Landouzy and Déjerine, progressive dystrophic ophthalmoplegia, dystrophia myotonica, and late muscular dystrophy, in which the muscles of the hands and forearms are mainly affected. In all, the muscles are grossly soft and pale, and fibrosis with fragmentation is the histologic aspect of the final stage. Although these disturbances are known to be hereditary, the pathogenesis remains obscure.

### Glycogen storage disease

Glycogen storage disease is a heritable disorder of glycogen metabolism in which this substance accumulates in a variety of tissues. Over 10 types are known, and skeletal muscle is especially affected in type II (Pompe's disease), type III (Cori's disease), and type V (McArdle's disease). The mechanism in each is an inherited enzyme deficiency. Without the enzyme glycogen metabolism is impaired, accumulation develops, and muscle weakness follows. Cardiac muscle is also involved, and heart failure is an occasional complication. All three begin in infancy and often cause death in early childhood. The histologic feature is the presence of large periodic acid-Schiff (PAS)-positive vacuoles of glycogen beneath sarcolemma sheaths of the muscle fibers. Types III and V are due to autosomal recessive genes; the mode of inheritance for type III is not yet established. The remaining types of glycogen storage disease are rare.

### Polymyositis

Polymyositis is a primary degenerative disease of skeletal muscle that is characterized clinically by progressive weakness and anatomically by atrophy and chronic inflammation of muscle fibers. Women are affected twice as often as men, the patients are middle-aged, and the onset is gradual. Weakness begins in the muscles of the shoulder and pelvic girdles. With progression the gait becomes clumsy, inability to stand without assistance develops, and eventually even turning over in bed becomes difficult. In addition to weakness, the affected muscles are tender and sore. In nearly half of patients a violaceous skin rash appears on the face, usually with a butterfly distribution. A dusky lilac suffusion of the upper eyelids is especially characteristic of polymyositis. Such cases were formerly labeled dermatomyositis. In about 20 per cent a malignant tumor of some internal organ is present. In a small proportion of patients skin changes suggest scleroderma; in others joint involvement resembles rheumatoid arthritis. Serum antibodies to stri-

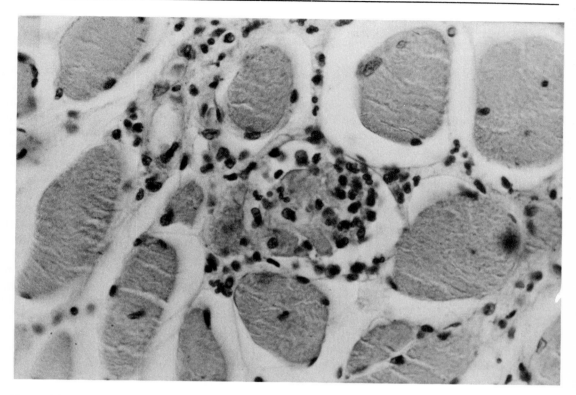

**Figure 21-12.** Focal lymphocytic infiltration of skeletal muscle in polymyositis

ated muscle are generally absent but the serum aldolase, creatine phosphokinase, and glutamate-oxaloacetate transaminase are elevated. Biopsy of muscle reveals degeneration and patchy infiltration with lymphocytes and histiocytes (Figure 21-12). The condition is thought to be a hypersensitivity reaction, but the mechanism is not clear.[31] As the disease progresses the posterior pharyngeal musculature is affected and dysphagia with dysphonia develops. The outlook is determined by the visceral tumor in patients with this associated disease. Otherwise the mortality has been reported to range from 15 to 40 per cent in different series. Death is due to muscular weakness and terminal sepsis.

## Myasthenia gravis

Nerves stimulate muscles. Normally the impulse of a nerve travels down the axis cylinder to the synaptic gap of the neuromuscular junction. The impulse releases acetylcholine into the gap, and the acetylcholine transmits the impulse to the myofibril. Cholinesterase then damps the impulse. If acetylcholine is not produced, or if it is neutralized or blocked in the synaptic gap, the impulse cannot reach the muscle and the muscle will not contract. This is the pathogenesis of myasthenia gravis. The finding of immune complexes at the neuromuscular junctions suggests immune destruction of the postsynaptic membrane.[32] On the other hand, the thymus produces a hormone (thymin) that inhibits neuromuscular transmission, and in most patients with myasthenia gravis the thymus is hyperplastic or neoplastic. Moreover, thymectomy causes clinical improvement or total remission in three-quarters of patients with myasthenia gravis. The disturbance therefore is localized at the neuro-muscular junction, although its precise nature is not understood.

The disease is slightly more frequent in women (3:2), begins after the age of 40, and is manifested by weakness that is especially noticeable after exercise. Often the ocular muscles are first affected, with prominent lid lag. Remissions occur but become less frequent as the disease progresses. Antinuclear antibodies and antibodies to skeletal muscle are often present. The pathologic finding is a widespread distribution of lymphocytes in focal collections ("lymphorrhages") within skeletal muscle. Eventually the respiratory muscles fail and death occurs on this account.

## TENDONS

Included with tendons are the synovial sheaths that enclose them and the bursae of joints. Inflammation of the synovial sheaths constitutes tenosynovitis. It is often due to minor trauma, frequently affects the fingers, and may cause fibrous adhesions that limit the motion of the part. Suppurative tenosynovitis results from a soiled wound or hematogenous dissemination of bacteria from a distant infection. Contracture of the palmar aponeurosis connecting to the fourth and fifth fingers causes the hand to assume the configuration of "papal benediction." It is known as Dupuytren's contracture, is more frequent in men than in women, and is bilateral in about half of cases. Plantar surfaces may also be affected. Although the cause is unknown, metaplasia of fibrocytes to contractile myofibroblasts has been suggested.[33] Bursal sacs are occasionally inflamed, especially about the shoulder and often with calcium deposits, as a result of repeated minor trauma. The inflammation is low-grade and the condition is chronic. Herniation of a bursal sac also occurs over the back of the hand, where it is known as a ganglion, and in back of the knee, where it is known as a Baker cyst. Neither is painful or inflamed, and both are cured by excision.

## REFERENCES

1. Sokoloff L, Bland JH: *The Musculoskeletal System.* Baltimore: Williams & Wilkins, 1975

2. McKusick VA: *Heritable Disorders of Connective Tissue,* 4th ed. St Louis: Mosby, 1972

3. Keye DK, Bale PM: Elastic tissue in pulmonary emphysema in Marfan syndrome. *Arch Pathol* 96:427, 1973

4. Albers-Schonberg disease. *South Med J* 69:788, 1976

5. Schmidt CJ, Marks SC Jr, Jordon CA, et al: A radiographic and histologic study of fracture healing in osteopetrotic rats. *Radiology* 122:517, 1977

6. Fishbach RS, Rosenblatt JE, Dahlgren JG: Pyogenic vertebral osteomyelitis in heroin addicts. *Calif Med* 119:104, 1973

7. Morse TS, Pryles CV: Infections of the bones and joints of children. *N Engl J Med* 262:846, 1960

8. Miller WB, Murphy WA, Gilula LA, et al: Brodie's abscess of the patella. *JAMA* 238:1179, 1977

9. Dismukes WE, Delgado DG, Mallernee SV, et al: Destructive bone disease in early syphilis. *JAMA* 236:2646, 1976

10. Wheeler M: Osteoporosis. *Med Clin North Am* 60:1213, 1976

11. Thomson DL, Frame B: Involutional osteopenia: Current concepts. *Ann Intern Med* 85:789, 1976

12. Wallach S: Management of osteoporosis. *Hosp Pract* 13:91, 1978

13. Cooke N, Teitelbaum S, Avioli LV: Antacid-induced osteomalacia and nephrolithiasis. *Arch Intern Med* 138:1007, 1978

14. Mallette mary hyperparathyroidism: Clinical and biochemical features. *Medicine* 53:127, 1974

15. Nellen JR, Kindwall EP: Aseptic necrosis of bone secondary to occupational exposure to compressed air: Roentgenographic findings in 59 cases. *Am J Roentgenol* 115:512, 1972

16. Fisher DE, Bickel WH: Corticosteroid-induced avascular necrosis. *J Bone Joint Surg* 53A:859, 1971

17. Ruiter Aneurysmal bone cysts. A clinicopathological study of 105 cases. *Cancer* 39:2231, 1977

18. Miller BG, Singer FR: Nuclear inclusions in Paget's disease of bone. *Science* 194:201, 1976

19. Firoozonia pertrophic pulmonary osteoarthropathy in pulmonary metastases. *Radiology* 115:269, 1975

20. Dahlin DC: *Bone Tumors: General Aspects and*

*Data on 6,221 Cases*, 3rd ed. Springfield, Ill: Thomas, 1978

21. Sweetnam R: Primary malignant tumors of bone. *Br Med J* 2:1367, 1976

22. Rodnan on rheumatic diseases, 7th ed. *JAMA* 224:662, 1973

23. Mankin injury and osteoarthritis. *N Engl J Med* 291:1285, 1335, 1974

24. Shirahama T, Cohen AS: Ultrastructural evidence for leakage of lysosomal contents after phagocytosis of monosodium urate crystals. A mechanism of gouty inflammation. *Am J Pathol* 76:501, 1974

25. Agudelo CA, Schumacher HR: The synovitis of acute gouty arthritis. *Hum Pathol* 4:265, 1973

26. Gutman AB, Yu TF: Uric acid metabolism in normal man and in primary gout. *N Engl J Med* 273:252, 313, 1965

27. Gordon GV, Schumacher HR: Management of gout. *Fam Physician* 19:91, 1979

28. Cadman NL, Soule EH, Kelly PJ: Synovial sarcoma. An analysis of 134 tumors. *Cancer* 18:613, 1965

29. Adams RD: *Diseases of Muscle: A Study in Pathology*, 3rd ed. New York: Harper & Row, 1975

30. Lagier R, Cox JN: Pseudomalignant myositis ossificans. A pathological study of eight cases. *Hum Pathol* 6:653, 1975

31. Pearson CM, Bohan A: The spectrum of polymyositis and dermatomyositis. *Med Clin North Am* 61:439, 1977

32. Engel complexes (IgG and C₃) at the motor endplate in myasthenia gravis. Ultrastructural and light microscopic localization and electrophysiologic correlations. *Mayo Clin Proc* 52:267, 1977

33. Gabbiani G, Majno G: Dupuytren's contracture: Fibroblast contraction? An ultrastructural study. *Am J Pathol* 66:131, 1972

# 22

# DISORDERS OF THE CENTRAL NERVOUS SYSTEM

### THE NORMAL CRANIOSPINAL SYSTEM

The normal adult brain weighs 1,250 gm in women and 1,400 gm in men. It consists of two cerebral hemispheres, a connecting corpus callosum, basal ganglia, cerebral peduncles, and a pons, medulla, and cerebellum. The cerebral hemispheres are each divided into frontal, parietal, temporal, and occipital lobes. The brain is enclosed by the skull. The inner surface of the skull is covered by a smooth, fibrous, firmly attached membrane, the dura mater. The surface of the brain is covered by a delicate, transparent membrane, the pia-arachnoid. The pia is attached to the cerebral surface. The arachnoid membrane lies above the pia and is connected to it by delicate, widely spaced filaments of connective tissue. Potential or natural spaces are formed by these structures: the epidural space between the skull and dura, which is unnatural; the subdural space between the dura and arachnoid, which is natural; and the subarachnoid space between the arachnoid and the surface of the brain, which is also natural. The term "leptomeninges" refers to the pia-arachnoid; "pachymeninges" refers to the dura mater alone.

A system of connecting spaces lies within the brain. These include the lateral ventricles, which open through the foramina of Monro into the vertical, slitlike third ventricle. The third ventricle opens through the minute, tubelike aqueduct of Sylvius into the fourth ventricle, which opens onto

**Table 22-1.**

## Comparison of cerebrospinal fluid and blood

| Characteristic | Cerebrospinal fluid | Blood |
|---|---|---|
| Pressure | 100-200 mm H$_2$O | 80-120 mm Hg |
| Protein | 45-55 mg/dl | 4-6 gm/dl |
| Sugar | 45-75 mg/dl | 80-120 mg/dl |
| Chloride | 120-130 mEq/liter | 135-145 mEq/dl |
| Cells | 3-5/cu mm | 5,000-10,000/cu mm |

the subarachnoid space through the medial foramen of Magendie and the lateral foramina of Luschka. These chambers contain the cerebrospinal fluid, which is clear, colorless, and watery and has a volume of about 150 ml. The cerebrospinal fluid cushions the brain and is formed mainly by the choroid plexus in the lateral ventricles. The anterior choroidal artery arises from the internal carotid artery near the posterior communicating branch of the circle of Willis. This vessel pumps blood into the capillaries of the choroid plexus. The fluid that emerges from these capillaries is "conditioned" by the epithelial cells covering the choroid plexus. For this reason ventricular fluid, which becomes the cerebrospinal fluid, differs from a simple filtrate of the blood (Table 22-1).

After the fluid emerges from the foramina of the fourth ventricle, it circulates in the subarachnoid and subdural spaces, passing downward over the spinal cord and also flowing upward over the convexity of the brain. The great sagittal venous sinus runs in the upper part of the dural extension, or falx cerebri, that separates the cerebral hemispheres. Evaginations of the arachnoid extend through the dura into this large venous sinus. It is through these arachnoidal villi (pacchionian granulations) that the cerebrospinal fluid returns to the blood.

## CONGENITAL ABNORMALITIES

Abnormalities of the brain may be taken up in five main categories: congenital, infectious, degenerative, vascular, and neoplastic. Obstruction of the aqueduct of Sylvius causes internal hydrocephalus. The chambers proximal to the obstruction dilate and the cerebral tissue undergoes atrophy to accommodate this change. When this occurs in infancy, before the sutures of the skull are fused, the head enlarges. When a similar process takes place in other individuals later in life, the bones cannot separate and the skull retains its normal size. The internal hydrocephalus is noncommunicating; a dye injected through the skull into a lateral ventricle of the brain will not diffuse into the spinal fluid. When the obstruction is due to disease of the arachnoidal villi, however, the dye does pass into the spinal fluid and the hydrocephalus is "communicating." The frequent cause of hydrocephalus is meningitis with scarring of the cerebral tissue in the healing process. Less frequent is maternal infection with *Toxoplasma* organisms, which pass the placental barrier and reach the fetal cerebral tissue. Least frequent is the Arnold-Chiari malformation, in which an elongated medulla herniates into the foramen magnum and compresses the foramina of the fourth ventricle.

In Down's syndrome the cerebral cortex reveals a reduced number of neurons, and the brain, including the cerebellum, is small. Individuals with cerebral palsy have spastic extremities and sometimes are mentally retarded as well. The brain shows focal agenesis or dysgenesis, either of unknown cause or associated with a condition such as necrosis from hypoxia, hemorrhage from prematurity, kernicterus from erythroblastosis, mechanical injury from the trauma of delivery, or head injury occurring after birth. Epilepsy is not necessarily congenital although most cases develop before the age of 20 years. The disturbance is a paroxysmal burst of motor impulses that causes convulsions (grand mal) or temporary loss of consciousness (petit mal). In most there is no cerebral lesion, although in some a focus of cortical gliosis from previous injury or arachnoidal scarring from previous infection is found.

## INFECTIONS

Infections of the central nervous system are mainly bacterial or viral. Bacteria tend to affect the coverings of the brain (meningitis), whereas viruses tend to spread into the cerebral tissue (encephalitis). The principal bacterial lesion is meningitis, although cerebral abscess and dural sinus thrombosis are also infective.

Meningitis is sporadic in infancy and in old age, and it is epidemic in young adults during conditions of crowding and poor hygiene. The organism in infancy is usually *Haemophilus influenzae*, in old age *Streptococcus pneumoniae*, and in the epidemic form *Neisseria meningitidis*. *N. meningitidis* is carried in the nasopharynges of asymptomatic persons.

The bacteria reach the brain through hematogenous dissemination, through traumatic fractures of the skull, or by extension from an adjacent infection such as otitis media or paranasal sinusitis. In the bloodborne route, two barriers must be surmounted. The first is the blood-cerebral fluid barrier, which is located at the surface of the choroid plexus. The second is the blood-brain barrier. Astrocytes throughout the brain attach foot processes to the surfaces of capillaries. All are covered in this manner. What is in the blood is therefore not necessarily free to diffuse into the cerebral tissue. Water and electrolytes are allowed this passage, but colloid molecules are not. For this reason a colloid dye injected into a systemic artery will not stain the cerebral tissue. Bacteria must cross one or the other of these barriers in order to infect the coverings of the brain.

Clinical aspects, which develop after an incubation period of seven to 10 days, include fever, headache, vomiting, stiffness of the neck, a preference to hold the head tilted backward (opisthotonos), diplopia, photophobia, leukocytosis, and a positive Kernig sign—pain elicited by extension of the knee with the hip flexed. Convulsions may develop. The diagnosis is established by examination of the spinal fluid, which is turbid and under increased pressure. In addition, the level of protein is increased, sugar is decreased, and neutrophilic leukocytes abound. Bacteria are found free in the fluid and within the cytoplasm of white cells. The organisms are ordinarily identified by gram staining of a centrifuged sediment of the spinal fluid.

The exudate forms within the pia-arachnoid on the upper and undersurfaces of the cerebrum so that it becomes covered by a thick, opaque, pale gray layer of neutrophils (Figure 22-1; see color section, p C-10). Microsections reveal that the exudate is confined to this layer (Figure 22-2). It is critically important to identify the organism at the earliest possible time so that an effective antibiotic may be given. When that is done, the outlook is favorable. In the series of Ellsworth and colleagues, the mortality in children was 5 per cent.[1] Although most of the remainder were cured, some developed complications such as optic

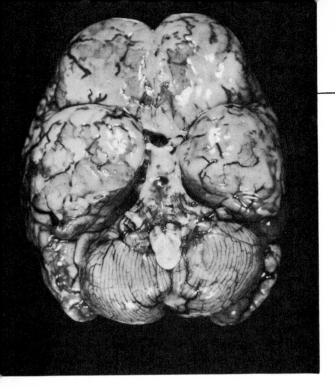

**Figure 22-1.** The pale exudate of acute bacterial meningitis. Also shown in color section, p C-10.

**Figure 22-2.** Confinement of the exudate to the subarachnoid space

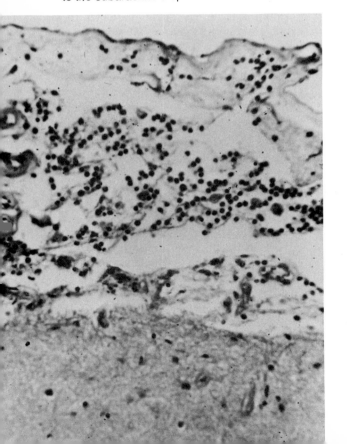

atrophy, facial palsy, or ptosis of the eyelids. Hydrocephalus may be the consequence of postinflammatory fibrosis of the arachnoidal granulations, the foramina of the fourth ventricle, or occasionally the aqueduct of Sylvius.

Tuberculous meningitis is now uncommon but may occur in infants in conjunction with miliary disease. Less often it arises from tuberculosis of the spine, i.e., Pott's disease, which extends through the dura mater. In contrast to pyogenic meningitis, the exudate is pearly gray and translucent, and tends to be localized on the undersurface in the region of the pons (Figure 22-3). In the spinal fluid the cells are mainly lymphocytes, the cell count is relatively low (100 to 500), and the chloride tends to be reduced. In addition, tubercle bacilli are present, and the protein is so high that a pellicle forms as the fluid stands. The condition was formerly fatal, but the effectiveness of chemotherapy, especially isoniazid, streptomycin, and aminosalicylic acid, now allows many patients to recover. The survival rate is on the order of 85 per cent.[2] These agents are also used prophylactically for children who have been exposed to tuberculous patients.[3]

Chronic meningitis is also uncommon. It occurs mainly in the aged, debilitated, and immunosuppressed. The causes are tuberculosis and, more often, fungal infections, including *Cryptococcus neoformans*, *Coccidioides immitis*, *Histoplasma capsulatum*, *Candida albicans*, and *Blastomyces dermatitidis*, as well as *Actinomyces israelii*. The clinical syndrome consists of fever, headache, lethargy, confusion, and a stiff neck. The spinal fluid protein is raised, the cells are mostly lymphocytes, and the glucose is often low. When these aspects persist beyond four weeks, the meningitis is chronic. The inflammatory reaction is often granulomatous rather than exudative. Diagnosis is established by identifying the organism in the spinal fluid. The morbidity and mortality are high.[4]

Abscesses of the brain arise from extension of an adjacent suppurative process, usually producing a single lesion, or by septic embolism from a distant inflammatory site, which tends to cause multiple abscesses. Fracture of the skull or extension of otitis or paranasal sinusitis leads to an epidural abscess that lies between the raised dura and the inner surface of the overlying skull. Fibrin and neomembrane formation then fasten the dura to the brain; the dura later ruptures and the suppurative process extends into the cerebral tissue. Cerebral abscesses caused by septic emboli arise from such conditions as bacterial endocarditis, acute pyelonephritis, and especially suppurative disease of the lungs, including bronchiectasis, pulmonary abscess, and empyema. These abscesses may occur throughout the cerebral hemispheres and cerebellar lobes. Clinical events depend on the size and location of the lesions, although fever, headache, and vomiting are common. The abscess consists of a cavity filled with thick, yellowish-gray, purulent exudate and a shaggy lining. Rupture outward leads to disseminated meningitis, and extension inward spills infected exudate into the ventricular system. The common organisms are staphylococci, streptococci, and *Escherichia coli*. Surgical drainage may allow the inflammation to subside.

The least frequent suppurative process is the dural sinus thrombosis. The veins of the face, including the eyes, drain backward into the head, where they coalesce to form the cavernous sinuses that lie on either side of the hypophysial fossa. Infections of the face may thus pass in the venous current to form septic thrombi in the cavernous sinuses. The thrombotic obstructions cause increased pressure in the facial and periorbital veins so that the face and eyes become markedly edematous and purple from stagnant blood. The thrombi may fragment to form septic emboli that float in the jugular current to lodge in the lungs, producing abscesses there. The

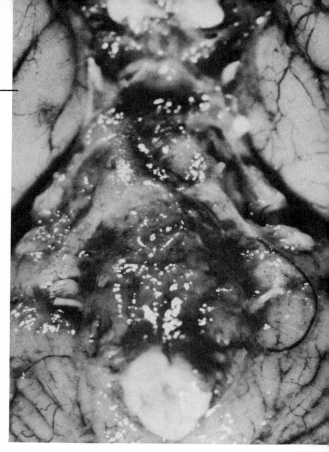

**Figure 22-3.** Gray translucent exudate of tuberculous meningitis with characteristic localization over the base of the brain

same process may also occur in the lateral dural sinuses from extension of infection in the mastoid air cells. Both these infections are inaccessible and therefore are difficult to treat.

Syphilis is also infectious. The central nervous system is involved in the tertiary stage, which takes 10 to 30 years to develop. The tissues mainly affected are the coverings of the brain (meningovascular), the brain itself (paresis), and the spinal cord (tabes dorsalis). All these developments are now extremely uncommon because of the effectiveness of treatment in the primary and secondary stages of the disease.

In meningovascular syphilis the meninges become thick and opaque from fibrosis while the arteries become inflamed and may undergo thrombosis. Thrombosis causes paralysis, and fibrosis gives the clinical manifestations of chronic meningitis. Paresis is characterized by memory loss, mood swings, and muscle weakness. The brain is atrophic with disappearance of cortical ganglion cells, pronounced gliosis develops, and chronic inflammation is reflected by lymphocytes in the perivascular Virchow-Robin spaces. In tabes dorsalis the posterior columns of the spinal cord show demyelination and the axon cylinders undergo degeneration. Both of these tissue components disappear. The patient loses position sense and, less often, the sensation of pain, and on these accounts may develop a painless flail knee (Charcot joint) or penetrating ulcers of the feet. Tendon reflexes and vibration sense are also lost. In these lesions of tertiary syphilis the cerebrospinal fluid discloses a slight lymphocytosis, elevated protein, and antibodies to the spirochete, *Treponema pallidum*. Gummas of the central nervous system are rare.

Viral infections of the brain fall naturally into three categories: those that are secondary to systemic viral diseases, the primary acute infections, and the slow viral diseases. Secondary reactions develop infrequently during convalescence from such common conditions as measles, rubella, and chickenpox. Encephalitis may also follow vaccination for smallpox (an increasingly uncommon practice) by a period of about 10 days. Fever, headache, nuchal rigidity, and ataxia are common clinical features. The spinal fluid discloses lymphocytosis and an increase in protein and pressure. Gross cerebral changes are scant, but microsections reveal perivascular lymphocytosis and focal demyelination of neural tissue. Spontaneous recovery is usual.

Acute primary infections are due to neurotropic viruses that cause inflammation of the brain and spinal cord. The outstanding example of spinal cord inflammation is poliomyelitis. The neurotropic virus enters the gut, passes into the blood, and localizes in the gray matter of the cord (*polio* means gray) with occasional extension to the medulla and brain. Acute inflamma-

tion ensues and the ganglion cells of the anterior horns are especially affected. The cut surfaces of the cord reveal edema grossly, and the cerebral hemispheres may disclose petechiae as well (Figure 22-4; see color section, p C-10. Ganglion degeneration, leukocytic infiltration, and gliosis are the main histologic changes. Paralysis often results when the patient survives. Death occurs when the process ascends to the medulla. In recent years immunization has virtually eliminated the disease.

The brain is also primarily affected by viral infections, i.e., encephalitis. The reaction includes neuronal degeneration, transformation of glial cells to macrophages (neuronophagia), mononuclear cells in the Virchow-Robin spaces (perivascular cuffing), focal necrosis of cerebral tissue, and inclusion bodies within the nuclei of the affected cells. The viruses causing this reaction reside in animal reservoirs, especially birds and small mammals, and are transmitted to humans by the common "rain barrel" mosquito, genus *Culex*. The horse is not a reservoir, as was previously believed, but only a susceptible host.[5] After an incubation period, during which a viremia precedes the cerebral involvement, the patient becomes febrile and experiences headache, nausea, vomiting, and mental aberrations such as disorientation with stupor that may progress to coma. The diagnosis is established by the clinical nature of the disorder plus the findings on examination of the spinal fluid. These include a normal glucose level with elevated protein and cell count, mainly lymphocytes, and a rise in the titer of antibodies to the virus. Recovery tends to be complete although neurologic impairment, such as tremor or dysarthria, may persist.[6] The names of these conditions are derived from the geographic location or presumed animal reservoir. Those of the Western Hemisphere include St. Louis encephalitis, equine encephalitis (eastern and western), and Venezuelan encephalitis. Eastern

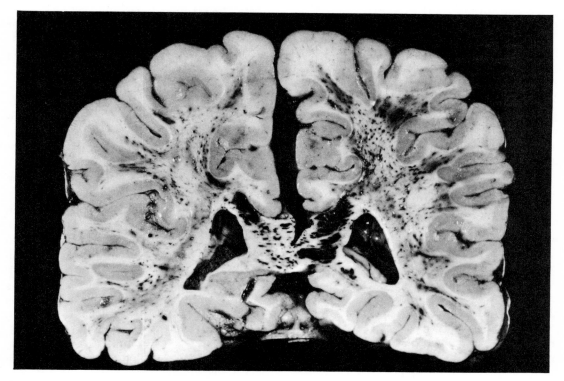

**Figure 22-4.** Petechiae over cut surface of cerebrum in acute anterior poliomyelitis. The patient was an 8-year-old girl who died after five days in the hospital. Also shown in color section, p C-10.

equine encephalitis has an especially high mortality, about 70 per cent.[5]

Variations of these main viral infections also occur. For example, the virus of rubella passes the placenta, infects the fetus, and causes birth defects, including microcephaly and mental retardation. The virus of cytomegalic disease also crosses the placental barrier and causes intracranial calcifications as well as hydrocephalus and microcephaly.[7] Aseptic meningitis is due to the spread of ECHO and Coxsackie enteroviruses from the intestine to the brain, and a necrotizing encephalitis affecting especially the temporal lobes is caused by the herpes simplex virus, whose reservoir is human.

Dogs, skunks, and bats are the usual reservoirs for the rabies virus, which is transferred to humans by the bite of a sick animal whose saliva is infective. The virus then spreads from the site of inoculation to the brain by passing through the Schwann cells of the nerve fibers.[8] On this account the incubation period is extremely variable and tends to be long when the distance from the bite to the brain is great. The medulla and brainstem are primarily affected; the lesions include perivascular cuffing, neural degeneration, neuronophagia, and microglial hyperplasia. The pathognomonic Negri body is found in the cytoplasm of ganglion cells of the hippocampus and in the Purkinje cells of the cerebellum. The patient experiences a prodrome of malaise, fever, and headache followed by fear of water (hydrophobia) and pharyngeal spasms (in 80 per cent) or a symmetrical, flaccid paralysis (in 20 per cent).[9] Serum antibodies to the rabies virus appear within four days of the clinical onset. The condition is nearly always fatal. The autopsy diagnosis is made by fluorescent antibody staining of the virus in the hippocampus. Persons at special risk are hunters, dogcatchers, veterinarians, and cave explorers (spelunkers), as bats abound in caves. Prophylactic immunization is effective.

The concept of slow viral disease arose from an investigation of kuru, a disease that occurred only among the Fore and neighboring inhabitants of the highlands of New Guinea.[10] In that region cannibalism was practiced as a ritual ceremony of mourning, mainly by women and children, who ate poorly cooked cerebral tissue of the deceased. After a latent period that might last as long as 20 years the victims developed a degenerative disease of the cerebrum that was relentlessly progressive and caused death within a year. Kuru was the first degenerative disease of the central nervous system proved to be due to a virus. This discovery opened the possibility that other degenerative diseases of the brain may be of the same nature. It has also discouraged the practice of cannibalism among the Fore.

So far three other slow viral diseases of the brain have been established: subacute sclerosing panencephalitis, progressive multifocal leukodystrophy, and Creutzfeldt-Jakob disease. All affect humans, all are degenerative, and all are transmissible to animals. Moreover, all are preceded by a long latent period and followed by a progressive illness of short duration that is uniformly fatal. Subacute sclerosing panencephalitis is rare, affects children and young adults, and is caused by the rubeola virus.[11] It is therefore also referred to as "slow measles encephalitis." Progressive multifocal leukodystrophy is due to a latent papovavirus that is activated in the course of immunosuppression either from therapeutic intervention or from disease of the

reticuloendothelial tissue such as lymphoma, leukemia, miliary tuberculosis, or widespread metastatic carcinomatosis.[12] Death is due to the cerebral dysfunction rather than to the primary disease process.[8] Creutzfeldt-Jakob disease is similar to kuru, affects adults, and is fatal within one year.[13] These three disorders are manifested by dementia, motor disturbance, and personality changes that worsen relentlessly and progress to coma. Although the brains tend to be grossly normal, the histologic changes are widespread and consist mainly of astrocytic hyperplasia, pronounced gliosis, and swelling and vacuolation of nerve cells. It is noteworthy that no leukocytic infiltration is conspicuous. The cerebrum, cerebellum, brainstem, and spinal cord may be affected. The pathogenesis of these disorders is not yet clear, but it has been suggested that more common degenerative diseases of the brain, such as multiple sclerosis and parkinsonism, may also be due to a slow virus infection.[14]

## DEGENERATIVE DISEASE

Although the main diseases of the central nervous system may be classified as congenital, infectious, vascular, or neoplastic, there remains a diverse group of conditions that have customarily been segregated as either demyelinating or degenerative. This distinction is questionable because demyelination is an aspect of degeneration and because no allowance is made for those conditions in which the pathogenesis is established. Therefore it is more useful to regard all these conditions as degenerative, with some having an unknown cause and others due to a deficiency of certain enzymes. Among the degenerative diseases of unknown cause are senile atrophy, presenile atrophy (Alzheimer's disease), parkinsonism, and multiple sclerosis.

The most common of these, although not a primary disorder of cerebral tissue, is the atrophy that takes place in old age. It is associated with advancing atherosclerosis in the cerebral vessels. The cerebral tissue gradually shrinks and the ventricular chambers slowly enlarge. The spaces thus created become filled with cerebrospinal fluid, and the compensatory alteration is known as hydrocephalus ex vacuo. When pronounced, dementia may be the clinical manifestation (senile dementia).

Atrophy of the brain also occurs as a primary cerebral disorder before the age of 60 years. It is accompanied by a psychosis, it may begin in early adulthood, and the cause is unknown. It is a presenile dementia termed Alzheimer's disease. In addition to the uniform atrophy, senile plaques occur irregularly in all portions of the cerebral cortex. The plaques are composed of eosinophilic fibrils arranged spherically and surrounded by reactive astrocytes. Neurofibrillary tangles consisting of twisted neurotubules within neurons also occur although they are visible only with special stains. The lesions of Alzheimer's disease are thus atrophy, senile plaques, and neurofibrillary tangles, all occurring within the cerebrum. Progressive personality deterioration accompanies these changes. The course lasts one to 10 years, with final development of incontinence and infection.

Pick's disease is less common and clinically similar, although the cortical atrophy tends to be localized to the frontal and temporal lobes. It is twice as frequent in women as in men.[14] The course is progressive and usually fatal within five to 10 years. The cause is unknown. Spinocerebellar degeneration, primary spinal atrophy, and peroneal muscular atrophy are rarer degenerative disturbances of unknown cause.

Parkinsonism (paralysis agitans) affects the sexes equally, begins in older age, and is gradually progressive. It is characterized by "pill-rolling" tremors, emotionless expression, stooped posture, and a cogwheel rigidity of skeletal muscles. In addition, the gait is mincing and rapid, suggesting that the patient hastens on his way in order to avoid falling forward. The cause is depletion of dopamine (3,4-dihydroxyphenethylamine) from the cells of the basal ganglia. Dopamine is a neurotransmitter produced largely in the pigmented cells of the substantia nigra. The main morphologic changes are focal softening and depigmentation of the substantia nigra with round eosinophilic masses (Lewy bodies) in the dopamine-producing cells. The cause is unknown, although some cases are postencephalitic and others follow the prolonged use of phenothiazine tranquilizers. Dopamine cannot be restored by parenteral use because it does not pass the blood-brain barrier. L-Dopa (levodopa), the immediate precursor of dopamine, does, however. About 75 per cent of patients respond favorably to this agent.[15]

Multiple sclerosis is also a primary, common, important degenerative disease of the central nervous system. It occurs in the population at the rate of 50 to 60/100,000. It begins in young adults, usually between the ages of 15 and 35 years, and is characterized by recurrent unpredictable attacks that include some combination of paresthesias, sensory loss, spells of ataxia, thick speech, tremor, nystagmus, diplopia, oculomotor palsy, and transient blindness. Pain and dementia are uncommon. Patients characteristically maintain a light spirit throughout this devastating, progressive illness. The attacks are intermittent so that the course is relapsing and prolonged. Some residual impairment persists after each attack, and spastic paraplegia gradually develops. There is no specific test for the diagnosis of multiple sclerosis although the spinal fluid protein is increased and the cell count may be slightly raised, to between 10 and 50 cells/cu mm. Bladder dysfunction is a late sign, and infection of the urinary tract is a common terminus. The mean duration of life is 20 years from the clinical onset.

Myelin is produced by oligodendrocytes, and myelin sheaths insulate axon cylinders

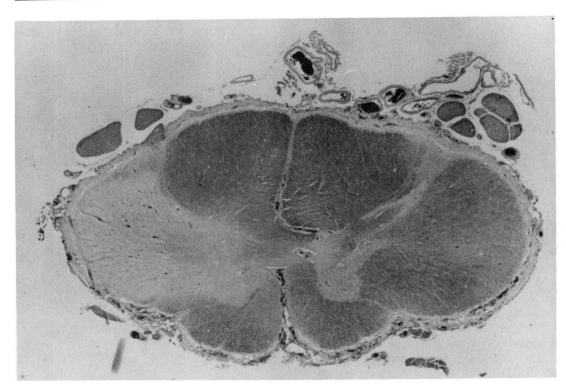

**Figure 22-5.** Focal pallor from demyelination of the spinal cord in multiple sclerosis

and increase the velocity of nerve impulses. Multiple sclerosis is a patchy disintegration of myelin with preservation of the axon cylinders.[16] It is therefore a demyelinating disease. The foci of demyelination are scattered throughout the brain and spinal cord, with special frequency in the paraventricular regions of the cerebrum, the optic tracts and chiasm, the brainstem, and the white matter of the cerebellum. The foci of demyelination, which are often referred to as "plaques," measure up to 2.0 cm in greatest dimension and present translucent, pale gray, irregularly shaped areas that are sharply demarcated from the adjacent white matter. Extension to gray matter also occurs. The microscopic feature is pallor at the site of the demyelination (Figure 22-5). Oligodendrocytes are absent, and localized perivascular cuffing with microglial cells is present in the early lesions. Later the cuffing disappears and marginal gliosis around the sites of demyelination becomes pronounced. It is from the multiplicity of sites and the conspicuous gliosis around them that the term multiple sclerosis comes. Although the cause is not known, attention is currently focused on the possibilities of an immunologic disturbance, a slow viral infection, or perhaps a combination of these. A rare condition of similar pathologic change is Schilder's disease, which affects children, involves the cerebral tissue only, and follows an unremitting, rapidly fatal course.

The disorders of enzyme deficiency are better understood. Without certain enzymes, complex lipids, mainly gangliosides and cerebrosides, accumulate in the cerebral tissue. Accumulation of gangliosides causes Tay-Sachs disease, also known as familial amaurotic (blind) idiocy. The disturbance is an intrinsic disorder of neural tissue. The accumulated lipid causes the brain to swell, and by the age of 6 months the infant, who appeared normal at birth, develops the characteristic clinical triad of a cherry-red macula, exaggerated response to sound, and psychomotor arrest. Blindness gradually follows. The course is progressive, no treatment is known, and death occurs at the age of 3 to 5 years. The condition affects mainly Ashkenazic (Eastern European) Jews. Prenatal diagnosis is possible through amniocentesis, and prevention may be achieved by abortion.[17]

Other enzyme deficiencies affect mainly the liver, spleen, and bone marrow with only incidental involvement of the brain. These include Niemann-Pick disease, in which sphingomyelin accumulates, Gaucher's disease, in which the substance is a glucocerebroside, and gargoylism, in which a mucopolysaccharide accumulates.

In contrast to demyelination, accumulation of cerebrosides causes dysmyelination—the abnormal formation of myelin. This occurs mainly in the white matter of the cerebrum, with loss of axons and widespread gliosis as secondary changes. The accumulation of cerebroside sulfate is known as metachromatic leukodystrophy, and that of galactocerebroside, as globoid cell leukodystrophy.[18] The latter, which is also referred to as Krabbe's disease, is less common than metachromatic leukodystrophy and affects only children.

Huntington's chorea is also a genetic metabolic fault in which γ-aminobutyric acid is depleted from the brain.[19] This substance is an inhibitory synaptic neurotransmitter without which chorea and dementia develop. The onset occurs in middle life, and the course is progressive. The patient develops writhing, purposeless (athetoid) movements of the hands and a characteristic sidewise movement of the head.[14] Later rigidity develops and dementia follows.

Death from inanition and infection occurs 12 to 15 years after the clinical onset. The pathologic change is depletion of neurons, especially from the basal ganglia. The lesion is thus a localized atrophy. The faulty gene is transmitted as an autosomal dominant, and it may be passed to offspring before signs of the disorder develop.

## VASCULAR DISEASE

Circulatory disorders, or "strokes," are the commonest form of neurologic disease. Because the cerebral tissue has a high metabolic rate without any reserve of oxygen or glucose, it depends on a continuous flow of oxygenated blood, and interruption for only a few minutes causes irreversible damage. The main circulatory disturbances of the brain are anoxic encephalopathy, localized infarction, intracerebral hemorrhage, and subarachnoid bleeding from rupture of an aneurysm of the circle of Willis. Anoxic encephalopathy is a secondary disturbance, and aneurysmal ruptures are relatively uncommon. Of the common primary vascular lesions, therefore, 60 per cent are due to atherosclerotic thrombosis, 30 per cent to embolic thrombosis, and 10 per cent to intracerebral hemorrhage.

Anoxic encephalopathy occurs with underoxygenation of cerebral tissue from pronounced anemia, respiratory failure, or shock with low perfusion pressure. In a normotensive person histologic changes develop when the systolic pressure falls below 60 to 70 mm Hg.[20] The neurons swell, degenerate, and drop out; gliosis follows and cortical atrophy results. The clinical manifestations vary from slight confusion to marked dementia. An especially serious hypoxic situation exists when a patient on a respirator develops congestive heart failure. In this event underperfusion becomes pronounced, stasis thrombi form in veins, and the entire brain may undergo infarction with liquefaction necrosis (global ischemia). The patient displays mental deterio-

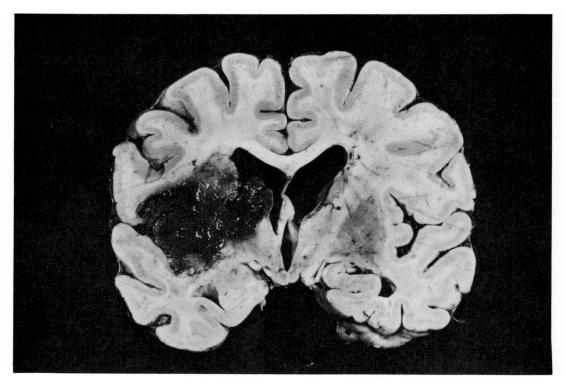

**Figure 22-6.** Recent hemorrhagic infarct of brain. Also shown in color section, p C-11.

ration, deepening coma, and slowing of electroencephalographic activity. The pituitary may also become necrotic. The condition is known as the respirator brain death syndrome.[21]

The brain is supplied by two internal carotid and two vertebral arteries that anastomose around the circle of Willis. Infarction is due to obstruction of these vessels or their branches. The consequence is a focus of coagulation necrosis. Such infarcts are the most frequent lesions of the brain. They occur commonly in normotensive elderly adults and are due to thrombi that form as a result of atherosclerosis, or to emboli that arise elsewhere. The common sites of embolus formation are the left atrial appendage in atrial fibrillation, a mural thrombus overlying a recent infarct of the left ventricle, or a valvular vegetation from

bacterial or nonbacterial endocarditis. From whichever cause, most infarcts of the brain occur in the distribution of the middle cerebral artery or in the basilar-vertebral vessels.

Infarcts are regarded as recent within three weeks of onset, as organizing between three and six weeks, and as old after six weeks. In recent infarcts no changes are visible for six to eight hours. After that, nuclear pyknosis and cytoplasmic eosinophilia affect neurons and there is light infiltration with neutrophilic leukocytes. The brain swells, the necrotic tissue softens, and asymmetry of the hemispheres becomes evident with herniation around the falx or tentorium. The necrotic tissue is pallid ("anemic") and poorly demarcated from the adjacent viable cortex or white matter. When small vessels are damaged

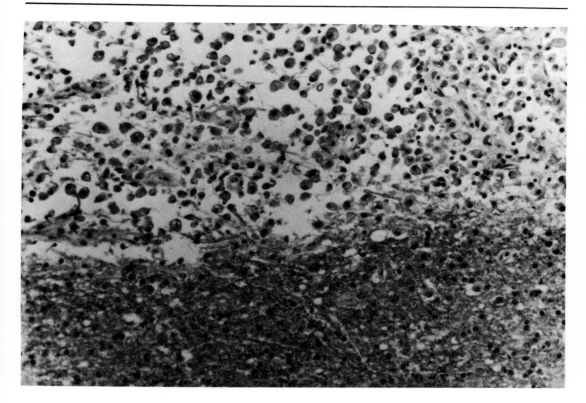

**Figure 22-7.** Macrophages ("gitter cells") phagocytizing the necrotic debris of a recent infarct

by hypoxia, hemorrhage may be extensive. In such hemorrhagic infarcts the cerebral tissue is still intact so that it is distinguishable from primary intracerebral bleeding (Figure 22-6; see color section, p C-11). In the organizing period the tissue dissolves and masses of macrophages ("gitter cells") take up the task of removing the necrotic debris (Figure 22-7). At the same time astrocytes proliferate to form a marginal scar. After six weeks a cavity is left in which the margins are dull yellowish-orange, the surface is covered by a thin curtain of transparent meninges, and the chamber is traversed by a lacework of vessels supported by connective-tissue septa.

With a small infarct of a few millimeters, the patient may experience a transient ischemic attack with only temporary neurologic dysfunction. When the infarct is large, however, the onset is sudden with headache followed by confusion and unsteadiness. Within minutes permanent deficits such as aphasia, dysarthria, diplopia, visual field defects, or hemiparesis become evident. The spinal fluid reveals a slight rise in protein and a small increase in lymphocytes. The patient often survives although the neurologic dysfunction persists.

Primary intracerebral hemorrhage is a catastrophic event. It is the most common cause of death among the circulatory disorders of the brain. The vessels are sclerotic and the patient is hypertensive. The clinical onset is sudden: The patient collapses and becomes unconscious, and the spinal fluid reveals increased pressure and gross blood. Four-fifths of hemorrhages occur in the cerebral hemispheres, and about 80 per cent of these are located in the region of the

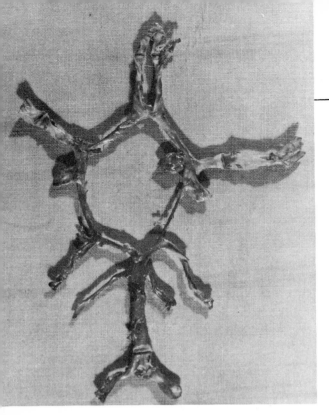

**Figure 22-8.** Saccular (berry) aneurysm of circle of Willis. Also shown in color section, p C-11.

basal ganglia. The bleeding arises from small arteries, but it is not clear whether the cause is necrotizing arteriolitis, rupture of a microaneurysm (Charcot-Bouchard), or hemorrhage into an earlier infarct.[22] Whatever the cause, the hemorrhage splits the tissue apart, forming a solid hematoma that often displaces over half the cerebral hemisphere. As a consequence the lateral ventricle is compressed and the midline structures are displaced toward the opposite side. Edema of the white matter adjacent to the hemorrhage becomes pronounced. The hematoma tends to break outward through the cortex into the subarachnoid space, or inward into the lateral ventricle on the affected side. The increased cerebral volume forces the brainstem downward so that the cerebellar tonsils herniate into the foramen magnum and pressure is exerted on the medulla. Over 90 per cent of patients die, mostly within 96 hours.[22] When the hemorrhage is small, however, the blood is resorbed, a cavity forms, and the yellowish-orange surface covers an immediately underlying glial scar. Neurologic deficits depend on the size and place of the cavity.

Berry aneurysms of the circle of Willis are saccular dilations that measure 0.5 to 1.0 cm in diameter. They are due to a focal absence of muscle cells and elastic fibers so that a portion of the wall consists only of intima overlying adventitia. These musculoelastic gaps are located mainly at the crotch of arterial bifurcations. Although they are presumed to be congenital, they are not seen in infancy but arise in adulthood and are found (unruptured) in 2 to 5 per cent of autopsy examinations.[23] They are located in the anterior part of the circle of Willis six times more often than in the posterior part. The common sites are therefore the internal carotid, middle cerebral, anterior communicating, and anterior cerebral arteries. An example is shown in Figure 22-8 (see color section, p C-11).

The aneurysms tend to rupture at a mean age of 50 to 55 years. Rupture is often the first indication of the lesion, and it frequently takes place during mild exertion. The clinical manifestation is sudden, excruciating headache that mimics a heavy blow to the head. Collapse and unconsciousness follow. Papilledema and retinal hemorrhages signify increased intracranial pressure. The blood flows directly into the subarachnoid space and spreads over the base of the brain. The hemorrhage may rupture through the arachnoid to enter the subdural space, and in 60 to 70 per cent of cases it also lacerates the overlying cortex, extends into the cerebral tissue, and forms a large hematoma that may reach the ventricular system.[14] The event is fatal in about 30 per cent of patients, and death occurs within a few hours. For those who survive, the greatest risk of recurrence is 10 to 15 days later. Diagnosis is established by arteriography, and surgical treatment isolates the supplying artery, which is clipped to prevent further hemorrhage.

## TUMORS

Intracranial neoplasms may be regarded as "inside" when they arise from the brain, and as "outside" when they arise from the coverings of the brain or adjacent structures. Inside tumors are chiefly gliomas, and outside tumors include meningiomas, eighth-nerve tumors, and craniopharyngiomas. Inside tumors are two to three times more common than outside tumors.[24]

The brain is composed of two kinds of cells: neurons and neuroglia. Neuroglia are stromal cells of a supportive nature. They consist of astrocytes, oligodendrocytes, ependymal cells, and microglial cells. There are thus only five different cell types from which inside tumors might arise. However, intracerebral tumors never arise from either neurons or microglial cells and develop only occasionally from oligodendrocytes and ependymal cells. Most inside tumors are therefore composed of astrocytes. The relative frequency of these tumors is shown in Table 22-2.[24]

Astrocytomas are separated into four grades according to the degree of malignancy, with grade IV the most malignant. Glioblastoma multiforme is another name for grade IV astrocytomas. This cancer, the most common and most malignant of the inside tumors, occurs in adults and arises exclusively from the cerebral hemi-

Table 22-2. _____

### Incidence of inside tumors of the brain

| Type of tumor | Incidence |
| --- | --- |
| Astrocytoma | 75% |
| Ependymoma | 6% |
| Medulloblastoma | 6% |
| Oligodendroglioma | 5% |

spheres. The tumor is large, soft, and well demarcated with a cut surface that reveals hemorrhage, cyst formation, and focal necrosis (Figure 22-9; see color section, p C-12). Edema of the adjacent white matter becomes pronounced so that the midline structures are dislocated toward the opposite side. Microsections reveal marked anaplasia with hyperchromatism, abnormal mitotic figures, and multinucleated giant cells. The astrocytic cell type is identified by means of the gold sublimate stain of Cajal. Growth is rapid. Surgical removal is occasionally possible, but the outlook is unfavorable. Astrocytomas of lower grades are white on the cut surfaces with poor demarcation from the adjacent normal tissue. They arise in the cerebellar lobes of children as well as in adult cerebrum. In children the tumors are cystic, often small, and frequently amenable to cure by surgery. None of the astrocytomas is radiosensitive, and none spreads outside the skull.

Oligodendrogliomas also occur in adults, grow slowly, and produce foci of calcification (calcospherites) that are useful in diagnosis because they are visible on X-ray examination of the head. The duration of the illness often exceeds a decade. Ependymomas arise from the ventricles of the brain, occur in children and adults, and grow slowly, often with the production of hydrocephalus (Figure 22-10). These uncommon tumors may arise in the cerebrum, cerebellum, or spinal cord. The characteristic microscopic feature is rosette formation with cells that reveal cilia or their vestiges, termed blepharoplasts. Therapy consists of surgical removal when the location of the lesion permits.

The common brain tumor of children is the medulloblastoma. These occur before the end of adolescence, and half arise during the first decade of life. The tumor develops only in the cerebellum, usually from the midline vermis, and it consists of undifferentiated cells of uncertain origin. The cut surface is soft, pink, and sharply de-

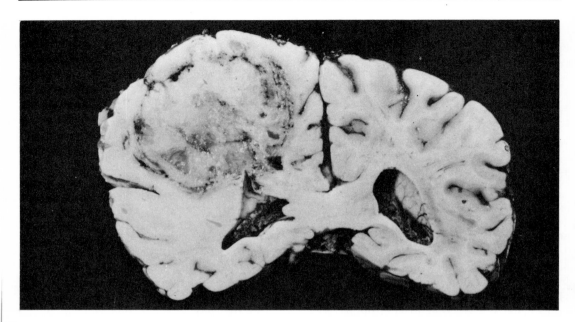

**Figure 22-9.** Cut surface of brain with glioblastoma multiforme. Also shown in color section, p C-12.

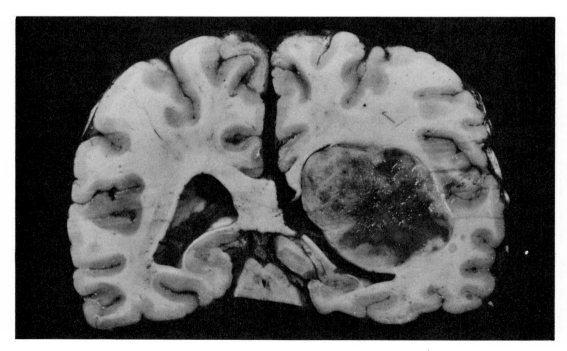

**Figure 22-10.** Cut surface of brain with ependymoma arising from surface of lateral ventricle

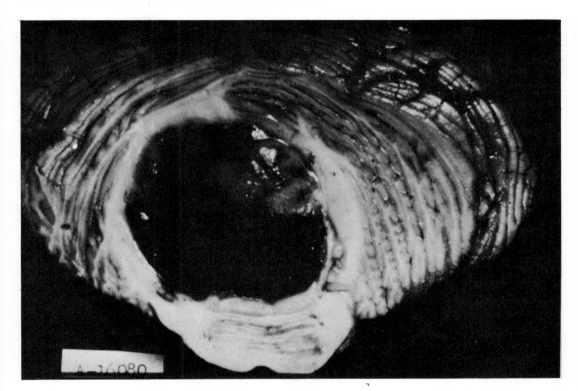

**Figure 22-11.** Medulloblastoma of cerebellum

marcated (Figure 22-11). The fourth ventricle is often obstructed so that internal hydrocephalus develops. The tumor cells are small, round, and occasionally arranged in a rosette-like pattern. They float away in the subarachnoid fluid and seed the meninges of all surfaces, including the spinal cord. The tumor is highly radiosensitive, but this treatment provides only symptomatic relief and recurrence is common within two to three years.

The most common of the outside tumors is the meningioma, which arises from the mesothelial cells of the arachnoidal villi. It therefore occurs especially along the sagittal venous sinus of the dura and the interhemispheric falx of the cerebrum, and over the base of the skull in the anterior and middle cranial fossae. The tumor is benign, grows with extreme slowness, and presents a firm, coarsely trabeculated cut surface that indents the cerebral tissue and is sharply demarcated from it. The tumor occasionally grows to enormous size (Figure 22-12; see color section, p C-12). It is always attached to the dura, and it usually can be shelled out easily from the adjacent tissue. The histologic characteristic is trabeculae of dense connective tissue with interspersed masses of calcium known as psammomas (sandy bodies) (Figure 22-13). Clinical manifestations develop gradually and depend on the site and size of the lesion. Cure is achieved by surgical excision, although this is sometimes difficult because of pronounced bleeding.

Uncommonly the perineural fibroblasts (Schwann cells) of the eighth cranial nerve undergo neoplastic transformation. From this a benign tumor develops at the junction of the cerebellum with the pons. The lesion is therefore often known as a cerebel-

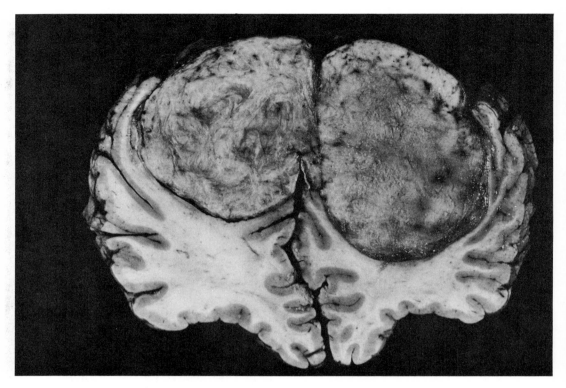

**Figure 22-12.** Large meningioma of dura markedly indenting the subjacent brain. Also shown in color section, p C-12.

lopontine angle tumor. Nerve deafness on one side is an early sign. The tumor is spherical, solid, and firm with indentation of the adjacent structures (Figure 22-14), including other cranial nerves. Involvement of the seventh nerve causes facial palsy; numbness of the face indicates involvement of the fifth cranial nerve. In addition, compression of the fourth ventricle causes internal hydrocephalus. The histologic feature is a solid mass of fibrillary cells in which palisading of nuclei is characteristic. Cure is possible through surgical excision although care is necessary because of the proximity of the medulla to the cerebellum and pons.

The least frequent of the outside tumors is the craniopharyngioma, which arises in the region of the pituitary from remnants of Rathke's pouch. It is a tumor of children,

usually occurring before the age of 15 years. The size ranges from 1 to 6 cm. The lesion is cystic, and the lining surfaces are a mixture of squamous and glandular elements with interspersed foci of calcification. The cysts contain a somewhat viscous black fluid in which cholesterol crystals abound. The tumor remains localized and is not malignant. However, it exerts pressure on the optic chiasm, causing visual field defects; on the hypothalamus, causing obesity; and on the pituitary, causing hypopituitarism manifested by retarded growth, amenorrhea in girls, polyuria, and a low metabolic rate. A useful diagnostic sign of craniopharyngioma is suprasellar calcification seen on lateral X-rays of the head. Enlargement of the tumor occurs extremely gradually, and cure is achievable by surgical removal.

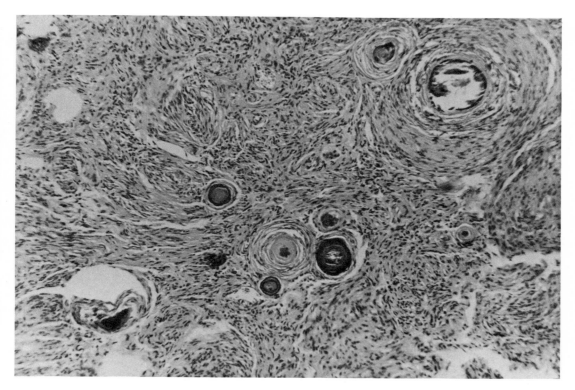

**Figure 22-13.** The fibroblastic nature of the meningioma with characteristic psammoma (sandy bodies)

A review of intracranial neoplasms, however brief, must include a note on metastatic tumors of extracranial origins. They are extremely common and arise especially from carcinomas of the lung, colon, and breast. The outstanding gross feature is the multiplicity of tumor deposits. Cerebral signs may antedate the clinical manifestations of the primary cancer. Rarely, intracranial metastasis occurs in the form of a fine dispersion of loose tumor cells in the subarachnoid space. They are not visible grossly, gastric cancer is the most frequent primary site, and clinical signs are extremely variable.[25]

**Figure 22-14.** Cerebellopontine angle tumor arising from the Schwann cells of the eighth cranial nerve

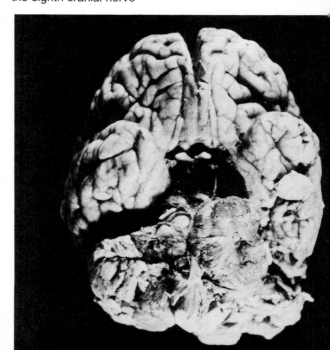

# REFERENCES

1. Ellsworth J, Marks MI, Vose A: Meningococcal meningitis in children. *Can Med Assoc J* 120:155, 1979

2. Kennedy DH, Fallon RT: Tuberculous meningitis. *JAMA* 241:264, 1979

3. Mintz AA: Tuberculous meningitis in children before and since isoniazid. *South Med J* 69:1061, 1976

4. Ellner JJ, Bennett JE: Chronic meningitis. *Medicine* 55:341, 1976

5. Blackwood W, Corsellis JAN: *Greenfield's Neuropathology*, 3rd ed. Chicago: Year Book Medical Publishers, 1976

6. Powell KE, Blakey DL: St. Louis encephalitis: Clinical and epidemiological aspects, Mississippi, 1974. *South Med J* 69:1121, 1976

7. Escourolle R, Poirier J: *Manual of Basic Neuropathology*, 2nd ed. Philadelphia: Saunders, 1978

8. Gajdusek DC: Slow virus diseases of the central nervous system. *Am J Clin Pathol* 56:320, 1971

9. Plotkin SA, Koprowski H: Phobia of hydrophobia justified. *N Engl J Med* 300:620, 1979

10. Gajdusek DC, Zigas V: Degenerative disease of the central nervous system in New Guinea. The endemic occurrence of "Kuru" in the native population. *N Engl J Med* 257:974, 1957

11. Jenis EH, Knieser MR, Rothouse PA, et al: Subacute sclerosing panencephalitis. Immunoultrastructural localization of measles-virus antigen. *Arch Pathol* 95:81, 1973

12. Narayan O, Penney JB Jr, Johnson RT, et al: Etiology of progressive multifocal leukoencephalopathy. Identification of papovavirus. *N Engl J Med* 289:1278, 1973

13. Lampert PW, Gajdusek DC, Gibbs CJ Jr: Subacute spongiform virus encephalopathies. Scrapie, Kuru, and Creutzfeldt-Jakob disease: A review. *Am J Pathol* 68:626, 1972

14. Robertson DM, Dinsdale HB: *The Nervous System. Structure and Function in Disease Monograph Series*, vol 5. Baltimore: Williams & Wilkins, 1972

15. Bianchine JR: Drug therapy of parkinsonism. *N Engl J Med* 295:814, 1976

16. Prineas J: Pathology of the early lesion in multiple sclerosis. *Hum Pathol* 6:531, 1975

17. Volk BW, Adachi M, Schneck L: The gangliosidoses. *Hum Pathol* 6:555, 1975

18. Suzuki K: Genetic leukodystrophies. *Trans Am Neurol Assoc* 101:116, 1976

19. Perry TL, Hansen S, Kloster M: Huntington's chorea. Deficiency of gamma-aminobutyric acid in brain. *N Engl J Med* 288:337, 1973

20. Garcia JH: The neuropathology of stroke. *Hum Pathol* 6:583, 1975

21. Towbin A: The respirator brain death syndrome. *Hum Pathol* 4:583, 1973

22. Chason JL, Mahoney WF, Landers JW: Massive intracerebral hemorrhage. *Minn Med* 49:27, 1966

23. Chason JL, Hindman WH: Berry aneurysms of the circle of Willis. Results of a planned autopsy study. *Neurology* 8:41, 1958

24. Rubinstein LJ: *Tumors of the Central Nervous System. Atlas of Tumor Pathology*, fasc 6. Washington, DC: Armed Forces Institute of Pathology, 1972

25. Smith JC, Kish GF, Jannotta FS: Metastatic meningeal carcinomatosis. *Med Ann DC* 41:736, 1972

# Index

Hepatic (hepatocellular) jaundice, 98, 99
Hepatic porphyrias, 96-*98*
Hepatitis, 246, 251, 252
  carriers, 252
  cirrhosis and, 252, 256
  immune complexes and, 73
  immunity, 251, 252
  infectious, 251, 252
  serum, 252
Hepatolenticular degeneration, 101, 102
Heredity; *see* Genetics *and specific topic, e.g.,* Chromosomes
Herniated intervertebral disc, 393
Herpes simplex
  cold sores, 62, 64
  encephalitis, 407
Herpesvirus
  carcinogenesis, *131*, 132, 311
  classification, *46*
Herpes zoster (shingles), 62, 64
Heterotrophic viruses, 61, 62
Heterozygous, 81
High-density lipoproteins (HDL), functions, 175
Hirschsprung's disease, 232, 233
Histamine, inflammation and, 16, 18
Histiocyte, 19
Histoplasmosis, 188, 189
Hodgkin's disease, 356-*359*
  classification, 349, 356, 357, *359*
  histology, 356-*358*, *359*
  incidence, 357, *359*
  metastases, 357, *358*, 359
  staging, 357, 359
  Sternberg-Reed cell, 356, *358*
  treatment and prognosis, 359
Holocrine gland, 323
Homans' sign, 30, 192
Homozygous, 81
Honeycomb lung, *203*, 204
Hormones; *see also specific hormones, e.g.,* Estrogens
  in cancer chemotherapy, *126*
  transport and function, 363
Horseshoe kidney, 274, *275*
Host responses to viral infections, 61, 62
Humoral immunity, 61, 62
Huntington's chorea, 155, 411
Hutchinson's triad, 60
Hyalinization, 3-5
  blood vessels, 4, 172
  brain, in aging, 4, 5
Hydrocarbons in carcinogenesis, 127, 128
Hydrocele, 292
Hydrocephalus, 402, 409
  brain tumors and, 415, 418
  maternal toxoplasmosis and, 402

meningitis and, 402, 404
Hydrocephalus ex vacuo, 409
Hydronephrosis, 280, *282*
Hydropericardium, 163, 164
Hydrophobia, 407
Hydropic degeneration
  gallbladder, 259
  mechanism of, 3, 4
Hydrosalpinx, 316
Hydrostatic pressure, blood vessel edema formation and, 16, 17, 26
  fluid balance and, 26
Hydrothorax, 27
5-Hydroxytryptamine; *see* Serotonin
Hyperchromic macrocytic anemia, 339-342, *341*; *see also* Pernicious anemia
Hyperemia, 27-28
  exercise and blushing and, 27
  heart failure and, 27, 28
  inflammation and, 15-27
  liver, *27*, 28, 248
  lung, 31, 186, 191, 192
Hyperparathyroidism, 383
  bone deficiency in, 384, 385
  metastatic lung calcification in, 385, *386*
  primary, 377, 378, 385
  secondary, 375, 384
Hyperpituitarism, 365-367
Hyperplasia, 118
  atypical epithelial, 119
  endometrium, 311
  parathyroids, 377, 378
  prostate, 119, 293, *294*, *295*
  uterus, carcinoma and, 315
Hypersensitivity, 69, 71-*74*
Hypersensitivity vasculitis, 162
Hypersplenism
  anemia and, 348
  cirrhosis and, 254, 348
Hypertension
  atherosclerosis risk and, 174, 175
  cirrhosis and, 254
  essential, 9
  obesity and, 114
  portal, 249
  pulmonary, 142, 192, 193
  renal failure and, 9, 282
Hyperthyroidism, 333, 372, *373*, *374*
Hypertrophic cardiomyopathy, 168, 169
Hypertrophic gastritis, 221, *222*
Hypertrophic pulmonary osteoarthropathy, 386, 387
Hypertrophy, 118, 119
Hypoadrenalism, 367, 368
  acute (Waterhouse-Friderichsen syndrome), 48, 367

chronic (Addison's disease), 54, 101, 367, 368
Hypochromic microcytic anemia, 339, *340*
Hypoparathyroidism, 378
Hypophysis; *see* Pituitary
Hypopituitarism, 364, 365
Hypoplasia, 117
Hypospadias, 290
Hypotension, renal effects, 275
Hypothalamus
  anatomic relations with pituitary, 363
  Fröhlich's syndrome and, 364
  pituitary hormone release and, 364, 366, 372, 374
Hypothyroidism, 88, 89, 372, 373

**I**
Idiopathic atrophy of adrenal cortex, 368
Idiopathic cardiomyopathy, 168, 169
Idiopathic interstitial pulmonary fibrosis, 197
Idiopathic pulmonary hemosiderosis, 196, *198*, 199
Idiopathic thrombocythemia, *349*, 352, 353
Ileitis, malabsorption and, 230
Ileoabdominal ulcer, 20
Ileocolic ulcer, 20
Ileovesical ulcer, 20
Immune complex reactions
  classification, *74*
  glomerulonephritis and, 277
  hepatitis and, 73
  hypersensitivity and, 73
  lupus and, 75
Immune mechanism
  amyloidosis and, 10, 11
  antibodies in, 70, 71
  antibody-antigen reactions, 69-71
  capillary permeability and, 27
  classification, *74*
  complement system and, 71
  humoral, viral infections and, 61, 62
  inflammation and, 19
  inhaled particles and, 199, 204
  lymphocytes and, 19, 73, 74, 353
  macrophages and, 71, 73, 74
  myasthenia gravis and, 397, 398
  transformation in carcinogenesis and, 136
  Weil-Felix reaction, 67
Immunization. *See* Vaccines/vaccination
Immunodeficiency disease, 69, 71, *72*

pneumonia in, 54
reinfection, 53
retina, 55
scrotum, 292
spinal column, *C-9*, 54, 383, *384*
treatment, 51, 52, 55
Tuberculous arthritis, 391
Tuberculous endometritis, 311
Tuberculous meningitis, 404, *405*
Tuberculous pneumonia, 54
Tuberculous retinitis, 55
Tubo-ovarian abscess, 312
Tularemia, 51
Tumor, 120, 121; *see also specific topic, e.g.,* Adenocarcinoma
Turner's syndrome, 92, 93
Typhoid fever, 23, 50, 395
Typhus, 67
Tyrosine metabolism, 101, *102*

**U**
Ulcerative colitis
chronic, *C-3*, *234*, 235
colonic cancer and, 241
regional enteritis and, 235
superficial inflammation in, 20
Ulcers/ulceration
blood vessels, 175
as inflammation complication, 20
lower esophagus, 221
peptic, 19, 20, 219, 222, *223*, 224; *see also* Peptic ulcer
scars and healing, 20, 222
sites, 20, *21*
stasis, 20, 181
stress, 221
Ultraviolet rays, 133
Undernutrition, 107-114
famine and adult, 107, 109
kwashiorkor, 26, *108*, 109
malabsorption and, 107, 113
marasmus, 108
regional enteritis and, 229
starvation, 107, 108
Urban yellow fever, 65
Uremic syndrome, 275, 276
Ureter, tumors, *286*, 287
Urethra; *see also* Urethritis
caruncle, 305, 306
congenital anomalies, 281, 290, 291
prostate cancer and, 295
Urethritis, 65
coliform, 50
nongonococcal, 305
postgonococcal, 305
Uric acid metabolism in gout, 393, 394
Uric acid stones, 281
Urinary bladder; *see* Bladder
Urinary tract obstruction; *see*

Obstructive uropathy
Uterine tubes, 316, 317
endometriosis, 313
pyosalpinx, 303, *304*
salpingitis, 316, 317
Uterus; *see also* Cervix, Endometrium
anatomic relations, *307*
hyperplasia, 315
polyps, 311, *312*, 315
tumors, *314*, *315*

**V**
Vaccines/vaccination
Rocky Mountain spotted fever, 67
smallpox, 62, 63
typhus, 67
yellow fever, 65
Vagina, *306*, *307*
Vaginitis, 306
Van den Bergh test for bilirubin, 99
Varicella (chickenpox), 63, 64, 406
Varicella-zoster virus, 64
Varices, esophageal
cirrhosis and, 254-256
described, 216, 219
Varicocele, 292
Variola (smallpox), 62, 63
encephalitis after, 406
Vasculitis, hypersensitivity, 162
Vasopressin (antidiuretic hormone), secretion and functions, 26, 366, 367
Vasospasm, intestinal necrosis and, 228, 229
Vegetation of acute bacterial endocarditis, *C-1*, 159, *160*, *161*
Veins
cancer spread by, 124
dilation and stasis ulcers, 181
intestinal, obstruction, 228
legs, 29, 30
periprostatic, 293
phlebitis, 181
thrombi, 29, 181, 191, 192
Venereal infection, 289; *see also specific topic, e.g.,* Gonorrhea, Syphilis
Venezuelan encephalitis, 407
Ventricle
aneurysm in myocardial infarction, 153, *154*
papillary muscle rupture, 153-*155*
septal defect, 141, 143, 144
septum rupture, 153, 154
Venules
flow rate in, in inflammation, 17, 18

normal, *268*
Verrucous endocarditis, in rheumatic heart disease, 156, 157
Villous adenoma, colorectum
described, 235, 237, *238*, 239
malignant changes, 237, 241
Viral carcinogenesis, 127, 131-133, 328
DNA viruses, *131*, 132
genome somatic mutation and, 135, 136
history of study, 131
RNA viruses, *131*, 132
Viral hepatitis, 246, 251, 252
carriers, 252
cirrhosis and, 252, 256
immune complex and, 73
immunity, 251, 252
infectious, 251, 252
serum, 252
Viral meningitis, 407
Virchow's node, 225
Viremia, 61
Viridans streptococci, 47
Virilism in adrenogenital syndrome, 368
Virion, 61
Virus(es). *See also specific topic, e.g.,* Variola (smallpox), Viral carcinogenesis, Viral hepatitis
characteristics and structure, 61
classification by tissue affinity, 61
heterotrophic, 61, 62
host responses to, 61, 62
infections, 45, 61, 62
nucleic acids, 61
slow virus infections, 406, 408
Vitamin(s); *see also specific vitamin*
common properties of, 109, 110
deficiency diseases, 110-114; *see also specific topic, e.g.,* Beriberi
discovery and naming, 109
essential, *110*
tryptophan as provitamin, 113
water- and fat-soluble, 109, 110
Vitamin A
deficiency, 110, 111, 119
discovery, 109
functions, 110
overdosage, 110
Vitamin $B_2$ (riboflavin), 109
Vitamin $B_6$ (pyridoxine), 109
Vitamin $B_{12}$ (cyanocobalamin), 110
absorption, 230
discovery, 109
gastric acid and, 339, 340
nerve function and, 341

pernicious anemia and, 339, 340, 342
Vitamin C, 110
    functions in metabolism, 112
    scurvy and, 112
    wound healing and, 24
Vitamin D
    deficiency, 111, 378, 384
    excess, 110
    osteomalacia and, 384
    rickets and, 111, 384
    secondary hyperparathyroidism and, 378
    sources and functions, 111
Vitamin E (tocopherol), 109
Vitamin K
    coagulopathies and deficiency, 110, 113, 114
    sources and functions, 113
Vocal cord papilloma, *204*, 205
Volkmann's contracture, 36
Volvulus, 226, *227*
Von Recklinghausen's disease of bone, 377, 385

Vulva, 305, 306
Vulvovaginitis, 48, 49, 304

**W**
Warm autoimmune hemolysis, 348
Warthin-Finkeldey cells, 63
Water
    aspiration, 38
    balance, 26
Water-hammer pulse, 179, 180
Waterhouse-Friderichsen syndrome, 48, 367
Weil-Felix reaction, 67
Wernicke's syndrome, 112
Whiplash injury, 37
Whipple's disease, 107, 230, 231
Whole-body freezing, 39
Whooping cough; *see* Pertussis
Wilms's tumor (nephroblastoma), 287
Wilson's disease (hepatolenticular degeneration), 101, 102
Wiskott-Aldrich syndrome, 71
Wound(s)

    healing, 24
    infections, 47, 50

**X**
Xeroderma pigmentosum, 134
Xerophthalmia, 110, 111
X-rays, 40, 41, 133
XXX females, 93
XXY males, 298
XYY males, 93

**Y**
Yellow fever, 61, 62, 64, 65
    hepatic necrosis and, 250
*Yersinia (Pasteurella) pestis*, 46, 51

**Z**
Zenker's hyaline degeneration of muscle, 395
Zollinger-Ellison syndrome, 225, 270
*Zuckerguss* (spleen sugar coating), 5